APPLETON & LANGE'S REVIEW OF

PSYCHIATRY

FOURTH EDITION

APPLETON & LANGE'S REVIEW OF

PSYCHIATRY

FOURTH EDITION

William M. Easson, M.D.
Professor, Department of Psychiatry
Louisiana State University School of Medicine
New Orleans

APPLETON & LANGE
Norwalk, Connecticut/San Mateo, California

Copyright © 1989 by Appleton & Lange
A Publishing Division of Prentice Hall

Copyright © 1974, 1978, 1983 by Arco Publishing, Inc.

89 90 91 92 93 / 10 9 8 7 6 5 4 3 2

Prentice-Hall International (UK) Limited, *London*
Prentice-Hall of Australia Pty. Limited, *Sydney*
Prentice-Hall Canada, Inc., *Toronto*
Prentice-Hall Hispanoamericana, S.A., *Mexico*
Prentice-Hall of India Private Limited, *New Delhi*
Prentice-Hall of Japan, Inc., *Tokyo*
Simon & Schuster Asia Pte. Ltd., *Singapore*
Editora Prentice-Hall do Brasil Ltda., *Rio de Janeiro*
Prentice-Hall, *Englewood Cliffs, New Jersey*

Library of Congress Cataloging-in-Publication Data

Easson, William M., 1931–
    Appleton & Lange's review of psychiatry.—4th ed. / William M. Easson.
        p.   cm.
    Rev. ed. of: Psychiatry examination review. 3rd ed. 1983.
    ISBN 0-8385-0111-7
    1. Psychiatry—Examinations, questions, etc. I. Easson, William M., 1931–   Psychiatry examination review. II. Title. III. Title: Review of psychiatry. IV. Title: Appleton and Lange's review of psychiatry.
    [DNLM: 1. Psychiatry—examination questions. WM 18 E13pa]
RC457.E18   1989
616.89′0076—dc19
DNLM/DLC
for Library of Congress   88-37935
CIP

Production Editor: Charles F. Evans

Acquisitions Editor: R. Craig Percy

PRINTED IN THE UNITED STATES OF AMERICA

Contents

Preface

The candidate in a national examination needs to recognize certain facts about these examinations and to prepare accordingly.

Since these examinations are given nationally (and often internationally), the subject matter of each question and each answer must be agreed on and accepted nationally. The examinee will not be asked questions that are based on regional interests or reflect merely individual clinical opinions. Since new medical information and treatments take several years to become nationally accepted, it is unlikely that new clinical or research knowledge or recently developed treatments will appear as the subject for a question for at least 1 to 2 years after general acceptance. The questions in the examinations thus tend to be conservative in outlook and approach.

It may seem unnecessary to emphasize, but the candidate should recognize that questions can only be asked where there is solid data about a subject. Some very important clinical topics appear in the examinations rarely or not at all because there is no definite data. Questions about the cause of many psychiatric syndromes are missing, usually because the cause is not known or is debatable. Death and dying is a most important clinical problem but is rarely the focus of questions because there is so little definite data on this topic. If a subject is controversial or sensitive in some way, it is unlikely to be an examination question. Abortion is a very important clinical problem but the candidate will hardly ever see a question in psychiatry about this controversial clinical situation.

The candidate should recognize that there are only a finite number of topics that can be asked about in each clinical examination. In psychiatry, there are probably not many more than 200 separate possible examination subjects. The examination candidate will recognize that, in this book and in the examinations, questions are frequently repeated, but from a different viewpoint each time.

In any board examination, there are only a limited number of questions, new and old, that can be asked. In the psychiatry examinations, 75–85% of the questions posed in any examination are old questions and only 15–25% are new questions. The candidate who knows the old examination questions thoroughly should have no trouble passing the examination—but, in the process of learning and understanding the old questions, will have thoroughly learned psychiatry.

As always, the author has learned a great deal in preparing this latest edition. It is gratifying to note that examination questions, and thus the teaching of psychiatry, deal increasingly with solid data and much less with vague theories. Questions and answers are becoming more precise. Psychiatry once again is becoming a medical science.

In the preparation of this manuscript, I am most grateful to Miss Dee Anderson for her unfailing assistance.

William M. Easson, M.D.
October, 1988

Introduction

This book has been designed to help you review psychiatry for your clerkship course, National Medical Boards Parts II and III, the Foreign Medical Graduate Examination in the Medical Sciences, FLEX, and residency intraining examinations. Here, in one package, is a comprehensive review resource with over 900 Board-type multiple-choice questions with referenced, paragraph-length discussions of each answer. In addition, the last 151 questions have been set aside as a Practice Test for self-assessment purposes. The entire book has been designed to help you assess your areas of relative strength and weakness.

ORGANIZATION OF THIS BOOK

This book is divided into 11 chapters. Eight chapters provide a review of the major areas of psychiatry. There is a chapter of matching-type questions, and one of case history questions. The last chapter is a Practice Test, which integrates all of these areas into one simulated examination.

This introduction provides information on question types, question-taking strategies, various ways you can use this book, and specific information on the Part II NBME examination.

Questions

The NBME Part II contains four different types of questions (or "items," in testing parlance). In general, about 50% of these are "one best answer—single item" questions, 30% are "multiple true—false items, 10% are "one best answer—matching sets," and 10% are "comparison—matching set" questions. In some cases, a group of two or three questions may be related to a situational theme. In addition, some questions have illustrative material (graphs, x-rays, tables) that require understanding and interpretation on your part. More-

over, questions may be of three levels of difficulty: (1) rote memory question, (2) memory question that requires more understanding of the problem, and (3) a question that requires understanding *and* judgment. In view of the fact that the NBME is moving toward the judgment question and away from the rote memory question, it is the judgment question that we have tried to emphasize throughout this text. Finally, some of the items are stated in the negative. In such instances, we have printed the negative word in italic letters (e.g., "All of the following are correct *except;*" "Which of the following choices is *not* correct;" and "Which of the following is *least* correct").

One best answer—single item question. This type of question presents a problem or asks a question and is followed by five choices, only **one** of which is entirely correct. The directions preceding this type of question will generally appear as below:

DIRECTIONS: Each of the numbered items or incomplete statements in this section is followed by answers or by completions of the statement. Select the ONE lettered answer or completion that is BEST in each case.

An example for this item type follows:

1. An obese 21-year-old woman complains of increased growth of coarse hair on her lip, chin, chest, and abdomen. She also notes menstrual irregularity with periods of amenorrhea. The most likely cause is

   (A) polycystic ovary disease
   (B) an ovarian tumor
   (C) an adrenal tumor
   (D) Cushing's disease
   (E) familial hirsutism

In this type of question, choices other than the correct answer may be partially correct, but there can only be one *best* answer. In the question above (taken from *Appleton's Review for National Boards Part II*), the key word is "most." Although ovarian tumors, adrenal tumors, and Cushing's disease are causes of hirsutism (described in the stem of the question), polycystic ovary disease is a much more common cause. Familial hirsutism is not associated with the menstrual irregularities mentioned. Thus, the *most* likely cause of the manifestations described can only be "(A)-polycystic ovary disease."

TABLE 1. STRATEGIES FOR ANSWERING ONE BEST ANSWER—SINGLE ITEM QUESTIONS*

1. Remember that only one choice can be the correct answer.
2. Read the question carefully to be sure that you understand what is being asked.
3. Quickly read each choice for familiarity. (This important step is often not done by test takers.)
4. Go back and consider each choice individually.
5. If a choice is partially correct, tentatively consider it to be incorrect. (This step will help you lessen your choices and increase your odds of choosing the correct answer.)
6. Consider the remaining choices and select the one you think is the answer. At this point, you may want to quickly scan the stem to be sure you understand the question and your answer.
7. Fill in the appropriate circle on the answer sheet. (Even if you do not know the answer, you should at least guess. Your score is based on the number of correct answers, so **do not leave any blanks.**)

*Note that steps 2 through 7 should take an average of 50 seconds total. The actual examination is timed for an average of 50 seconds per question.

One best answer—matching sets. These questions are essentially matching questions that are usually accompanied by the following general directions:

DIRECTIONS (Questions 2 through 4): Each group of items in this section consists of lettered headings followed by a set of numbered words or phrases. For each numbered word or phrase, select the ONE lettered heading that is most closely associated with it. Each lettered heading may be selected once, more than once or not at all.

Any number of questions (usually two to six) may follow the five headings:

Questions 2 through 4

For each adverse drug reaction listed below, select the antibiotic with which it is most closely associated.

(A) Tetracycline
(B) Chloramphenicol
(C) Clindamycin
(D) Cefotaxime
(E) Gentamicin

2. Bone marrow suppression
3. Pseudomembranous enterocolitis
4. Acute fatty necrosis of liver

Note that, unlike the single item questions, the choices in the matching sets questions *precede* the actual questions. As with the single item questions, however, only **one** choice can be correct for a given question.

TABLE 2. STRATEGIES FOR ANSWERING ONE BEST ANSWER—MATCHING SETS QUESTION*

1. Remember that the *lettered choices* are **followed** by the *numbered* questions.
2. As with the single item questions, these questions have only **one** best answer. Therefore apply steps 2 through 7 of the single item strategies.

*Remember, you only have an average of 50 seconds per question.

Comparison—matching set questions. Like the one best answer—matching set questions, comparison—matching set questions are essentially just matching questions. They are usually accompanied by the following general directions and code:

DIRECTIONS (Questions 5 and 6): Each group of items in this section consists of lettered headings followed by a set of numbered words or phrases. For each numbered word or phrase, select

A if the item is associated with (A) only,
B if the item is associated with (B) only,
C if the item is associated with both (A) and (B),
D if the item is associated with neither (A) nor (B).

Any number of questions (usually two to six) may follow the four headings:

Questions 5 and 6

(A) polymyositis
(B) polymyalgia rheumatica
(C) both
(D) neither

5. Pain is a prominent syndrome
6. Associated with internal malignancy in adults

Note that as with the other matching set questions, the choices precede the actual questions. Once again, only **one** choice can be correct for a given question.

TABLE 3. STRATEGIES FOR ANSWERING COMPARISON—MATCHING SET QUESTIONS*

1. Remember that the *lettered choices* are **followed** by the *numbered questions.*
2. As with the one best answer questions, these questions have **only one** best answer.
3. Quickly note what the lettered choices are.
4. Carefully read the question to be sure you understand what is being asked or what its relationship to the lettered choices is.
5. Focus on choices (A) and (B), and use the following sequence logically to determine the correct answer:
   a. If you can determine that (A) is incorrect, your answer must be either (B) or (D).
   b. If you can determine that (B) is incorrect, your answer must be either (A) or (D).
   c. If you can determine that both (A) and (B) are incorrect, your answer must be (D).
   d. If you can determine that both (A) and (B) are correct, your answer must be (C).

*Remember, you only have an average of 50 seconds per question.

Multiple true—false items. These questions are considered the most difficult (or tricky), and you should be certain that you understand and follow the directions that always accompany these questions:

DIRECTIONS: For each of the items in this section, ONE or MORE of the numbered options is correct. Choose the answer

A if only 1, 2, and 3 are correct.
B if only 1 and 3 are correct.
C if only 2 and 4 are correct.
D if only 4 is correct.
E if all are correct.

This code is always the same (i.e., "D" would never say "if 3 is correct"), and it is repeated throughout this book in a summary box (see below) at the top of any page on which multiple true—false item questions appear.

SUMMARY OF DIRECTIONS				
A	**B**	**C**	**D**	**E**
1, 2, 3 only	1, 3 only	2, 4 only	4 only	All are correct

A sample question follows:

7. The superficial perineal space contains which of the following?

   (1) crura of the clitoris
   (2) the deep transverse perineal muscle
   (3) the ischiocavernosus muscle
   (4) the anal sphincter

You first need to determine which choices are right and wrong, and then which code corresponds to the correct numbers. In the example above, 1 and 3 are both structures contained in this space, and therefore (B) is the correct answer to this question.

TABLE 4. STRATEGIES FOR ANSWERING MULTIPLE TRUE—FALSE ITEM QUESTIONS*

1. Carefully read and become familiar with the accompanying directions to this tricky question type.
2. Carefully read the stem to be certain that you know what is being asked.
3. Carefully read each of the numbered choices. If you can determine whether any of the choices are true or false, you may find it helpful to place a "+" (true) or a "−" (false) next to the number.
4. Focus on the numbered choices and your true/false notations, and use the following sequence to logically determine the correct answer:
   a. Note that in the answer code choices 1 *and* 3 are *always* both either true or false together. If you are sure that either one is incorrect, your answer must be (C) or (D).
   b. If you are sure that choice 2 *and either* choice 1 *or* 3 are incorrect, you answer must be (D).
   c. If you are sure that choices 2 and 4 are incorrect, your answer must be (B).

*Remember, you only have an average of 50 seconds per question. Note that the following two combinations cannot occur: choices 1 and 4 both incorrect; choices 3 and 4 both incorrect.

Answers, Explanations, and References

In each of the sections of this book, the question sections are followed by a section containing the answers, explanations, and references for the questions. This section (1) tells you the answer to each question; (2) gives you an explanation and review of why the answer is correct, background information on the subject matter, and/or why the other answers are incorrect; and (3) tells you where you can find more in-depth information on the subject matter in other books and journals. We encourage you to use this section as a basis for further study and understanding.

If you choose the correct answer to a question, you can then read the explanation (1) for reinforcement and (2) to add to your knowledge about the subject matter (remember that the explanations usually tell not only why the answer is correct, but often also why the other choices are incorrect). **If you choose the wrong answer** to a question, you can read the explanation for an instructional review of the material in the question. Furthermore, you can look up the references at the end of each answer and refer to the specific pages cited for a more in-depth discussion.

Practice Test

The 151-question Practice Test at the end of the book covers and reviews all the topics covered in Chapters 1 through 10. The questions are grouped according to question type (one best answer—single item, one best answer—matching sets, comparison—matching sets, then multiple true-false items), with the subject areas integrated. Specific instructions for how to take the Practice Test are given on page 141.

The Practice Test is followed by a subspecialty list, which will enable you to analyze your areas of strength and weakness to help you focus your review. For example, by checking off your incorrect answers, you may find that a pattern develops in that you are incorrect on most or all of the psychological testing questions. In this case, you could note the references (in the Answers and Explanations section) for your incorrect answers and read those sources. You might also want to purchase a psychological testing text or review book to do a much more thorough review. We think you will find this subspecialty list very helpful and we urge you to use it.

HOW TO USE THIS BOOK

There are two logical ways to get the most value from this book. We will call them Plan A and Plan B.

In **Plan A,** you go straight to the Practice Test and complete it according to the instructions given on page 141. Using the subspecialty list, analyze your areas of strength and weakness. This will be a good indicator of your initial knowledge of the subject and will help to identify specific areas for preparation and review. You can now use the first 10 chapters of the book to help you improve your relative weak points.

In **Plan B,** you go through Chapters 1 through 10 checking off your answers, and then comparing your choices with the answers and discussions in the book. Once you have completed this process, you can take the Practice Test and see how well prepared you are. If you still have a major weakness, it should be apparent in time for you to take remedial action.

In Plan A, by taking the Practice Test first, you get quick feedback regarding your initial areas of strength and weakness. You may find that you have a good command of the material, indicating that perhaps only a

cursory review of the first 10 chapters is necessary. This, of course, would be good to know early in your exam preparation. On the other hand, you may find that you have many areas of weakness. In this case, you could then focus on these areas in your review—not just with this book, but also with textbooks.

It is, however, unlikely that you will not do some studying prior to taking the National Boards (especially since you have this book). Therefore, it may be more realistic to take the Practice Test after you have reviewed the first 10 chapters (as in Plan B). This will probably give you a more realistic type of testing situation since very few of us just sit down to a test without studying. In this case, you will have done some reviewing (from superficial to in-depth), and your Practice Test will reflect this studying time. If, after reviewing the first 10 chapters and taking the Practice Test, you still have some weaknesses, you can then go back to the first 10 chapters and supplement your review with your texts.

SPECIFIC INFORMATION ON THE PART II EXAMINATION

The official source of all information with respect to National Board Examination Part II is the National Board of Medical Examiners (NBME), 3930 Chestnut Street, Philadelphia, PA 19104. Established in 1915, the NBME is a voluntary, nonprofit, independent organization whose sole function is the design, implementation, distribution, and processing of a vast bank of question items, certifying examinations, and evaluative series in the professional medical field.

In order to sit for the Part II examination, a person must be either an officially enrolled medical student or a graduate of an accredited United States or Canadian medical school. It is not necessary to complete any particular year of medical school in order to be a candidate for Part II. Neither is it required to take Part I before Part II.

In applying for Part II, you must use forms supplied by NBME. Remember that registration closes *ten weeks* before the scheduled examination date. Some United States and Canadian medical schools require their students to take Part II even if they are noncandidates. Such students can register as noncandidates at the request of their school. A person who takes Part II as a noncandidate can later change to candidate status and, after payment of a fee, receive certification credit.

Scoring

Because there is no deduction for wrong answers, you

should **answer every question**. Your test is scored in the following way:

1. The number of questions answered correctly is totaled. This is called the raw score.

2. The raw score is converted statistically to a "standard" score on a scale of 200 to 800, with the mean set at 500. Each 100 points away from 500 is one standard deviation.

3. Your score is compared statistically with the criteria set by the scores of all of the examinees who (a) took Part II during the four years before the current exam, (b) took Part II as candidates for Board certification, and (c) were in their final year of medical school at the time they took Part II. This is what is meant by the term, "criterion referenced test."

4. A score of 500 places you around the 50th percentile. A score of 290 is the minimum passing score for Part II; this probably represents about the 2nd to 5th percentile. If you answer 50% or so of the questions correctly, you will almost certainly receive a passing score.

Remember: You do not have to pass all six clinical science components, although you will receive a standard score in each of them. A score of less than 400 (about the 15th percentile) on any particular area is a real cause for concern as it will certainly drag down your overall score. Likewise, a 600 or better (85th percentile) is an area of great relative strength. (You can use the practice test included in *Appleton's Review* to help determine your areas of strength and weakness well in advance of the actual examination.)

Physical Conditions

The NBME is very concerned that all their exams be administered under uniform conditions in the numerous centers that are used. Except for several No. 2 pencils and an eraser, you are not permitted to bring anything (books, notes, calculators, etc.) into the test room. All examinees receive the same questions at the same session. The questions, however, are printed in different sequences in several different booklets, and the booklets are randomly distributed. In addition, examinees are removed to different seats at least once during the test. And, of course, each test is monitored by at least one proctor. The object of these maneuvers is to discourage cheating or even the temptation to cheat.

The number of candidates who fail Part II is quite small; however, individual students as well as entire medical school programs benefit when scores on National Boards are high. No one wants to squeak by with a 350 when a little effort might raise that score to 450. That is why you have made a wise decision to use the self-assessment and review materials available in this, the 4th edition of *Appleton & Lange's Review of Psychiatry*.

References

Throughout this book, each question and chapter is referenced to three one-volume general psychiatry textbooks. Rather than list each textbook and its authors repetitiously with each reference, I have cited them as 1, 2, or 3, at the end of each answer explanation.

Reference 1:
Kaplan HI, Sadock BJ: Modern Synopsis of Psychiatry IV, 4th ed. Baltimore, Williams and Wilkins, 1985

Reference 2:
Kolb LC, Brodie HKH: Modern Clinical Psychiatry, 10th ed. Philadelphia, W.B. Saunders, 1982

Reference 3:
Gregory I, Smeltzer DJ: Psychiatry: Essentials of Clinical Practice, 2nd ed. Boston, Little, Brown, 1983

Also, the three-volume textbook:
Kaplan HI, Freedman AM, Sadock BJ: Comprehensive Textbook of Psychiatry III, 3rd ed. Baltimore, Williams and Wilkins, 1980, is recommended to the student with a special interest in clinical psychiatry and to the psychiatry resident.

APPLETON & LANGE'S REVIEW OF

PSYCHIATRY

FOURTH EDITION

CHAPTER 1

Definitions
Questions

INTRODUCTION

Students may believe that definitions of psychological and psychiatric terms form a large part of any examination because such questions are easier to formulate and score, and undoubtedly this is true in part. There is another more important aspect. If students really understand these terms they are asked to define, they have a very good comprehension of the way people develop, relate, and cope with life stresses, in health and in sickness.

To help their understanding and remembering, trainees should look for examples of these behaviors they will be asked to define in their own day-to-day living and in the interactions of people with whom they come in contact.

REFERENCES

1. Chapter 8   Clinical Manifestations, pp 146–180
2. Chapter 4,   Personality Development, pp 58–79
   Chapter 5,   Adaptive Processes and Mental Mechanisms, pp 80–111
   Chapter 6,   Psychopathology, pp 112–148

DIRECTIONS (Questions 1 through 31): Each of the numbered items or incomplete statements in this section is followed by answers or by completions of the statement. Select the ONE lettered answer or completion that is BEST in each case.

1. In a déjà vu situation the

   (A) subject feels a limb long since amputated
   (B) person, just falling asleep, has false sensory perceptions
   (C) subject incorrectly feels a new experience to be the repetition of a previous experience
   (D) patient uses intellectual reasoning to avoid dealing with an unacceptable feeling or idea
   (E) subject shows sleepwalking and stage 4 sleep

2. Blocking is the

   (A) deliberate resistance to sharing uncomfortable feelings
   (B) arrest of psychological development before full maturation
   (C) stoppage of the flow of thoughts or speech due to unconscious feelings
   (D) slowing down of physical and emotional activity due to depression
   (E) state of unusual calmness in response to adversity, seen in hysteria

3. Akathisia is the

   (A) type of psychotherapy that allows regression to infantile behavior
   (B) unconscious falsification of memory where there are memory gaps
   (C) process of emotional defense where the opposite is stressed
   (D) inability to sit still or keep legs motionless
   (E) type of analytic psychotherapy where the patient is heavily sedated

4. When a person stresses the opposite of his or her true feelings, he or she is showing the defense of

   (A) rationalization
   (B) undoing
   (B) displacement
   (D) reaction formation
   (E) denial

5. Repression is the

   (A) return to earlier patterns of behavior
   (B) unconscious blocking out of disturbing feelings
   (C) stressing of opposite feelings
   (D) deliberate forgetting of distressing emotions
   (E) arrest of emotional development before full maturity

6. Paranoia involves the process of

   (A) introjection
   (B) regression
   (C) conversion
   (D) projection
   (E) isolation

7. A person who experiences night terrors (pavor nocturnus)

   (A) is most commonly aged 6 to 12
   (B) wakens later with total amnesia for the episode
   (C) experiences them during REM sleep
   (D) is able to recall the content of the frightening dream
   (E) experiences them during the latter part of sleep

8. Sensory experiences in the absence of external stimuli are called

   (A) projections
   (B) hallucinations
   (C) illusions
   (D) delusions
   (E) introjections

9. Regression

   (A) occurs commonly and normally with serious physical illness
   (B) always indicates severe emotional disorder
   (C) is the unconscious blocking out of awareness of disturbing emotions
   (D) is mediated mainly through the autonomic nerves
   (E) occurs where there is underlying sexual conflict

10. Bulimia is

   (A) uncontrolled aggressive outbursts
   (B) hypersexuality in the female
   (C) chronic psychogenic constipation
   (D) recurrent compulsive intellectual rumination
   (E) a huge appetite with excessive gorging

11. The Halstead Reitan battery is used to

   (A) measure galvanic skin resistance
   (B) assess impairment due to brain damage
   (C) differentiate infantile autism and childhood deafness
   (D) induce unilateral electroconvulsive therapy
   (E) provide negative reinforcement in operant conditioning

12. In conversion

   (A) feelings that are unacceptable when focused on one object are redirected to a more tolerable focus
   (B) the subject has almost total memory loss for a significant period of his or her past

(C) emotional conflict is expressed in a single organ system controlled by the autonomic nerves

(D) the conflictual anxiety is symbolically manifested in a somatic symptom involving the special senses or voluntary nervous system

(E) an unacceptable drive is rechanneled into socially acceptable behavior

13. A delusion is

(A) a sensory experience in the absence of external stimuli

(B) a misinterpretation of actual perceptions

(C) a false belief not in accord with a person's intelligence or culture

(D) a manifestation of unacceptable feelings projected outward

(E) unconscious blocking of instinctual feelings

14. Delusions occur in all of the following *except*

(A) bipolar disorder, manic type

(B) amphetamine psychosis

(C) senile dementia

(D) paranoia

(E) schizoid personality disorder

15. Paranoid delusions are produced by the mechanism of

(A) displacement

(B) projection

(C) rationalization

(D) sublimation

(E) identification

16. The fetal alcohol syndrome includes all of the following *except*

(A) high birth weight

(B) mental retardation

(C) maternal alcoholism

(D) craniofacial abnormalities

(E) cardiac defects

17. In psychoanalysis, catharsis is the

(A) release of unconscious feelings with appropriate outward emotional expression

(B) investment of emotional energy in a specific purpose or object

(C) conscious or unconscious response of the psychotherapist to the patient

(D) process of knowing and learning

(E) defense whereby an unacceptable feeling is externalized

18. The collective unconscious was a concept introduced by

(A) E. Bleuler

(B) J. Breuer

(C) S. Freud

(D) H. S. Sullivan

(E) C. Jung

19. Transference is

(A) the transfer of feelings from an unacceptable object to a more acceptable focus

(B) a process whereby unacceptable thoughts and ideas are excluded from awareness

(C) a form of identification with a loved and feared parental figure

(D) a manifestation of early psychosis, especially in the adolescent or young adult

(E) the projection of feelings originally linked to nuclear early-life figures onto current objects

20. Somatization disorder is

(A) the misinterpretation of physical signs or sensations

(B) the voluntary, deliberate fabrication of symptoms

(C) the loss or alteration in physical function produced by emotional conflict or need

(D) the expression of emotions through physical symptoms

(E) none of the above

21. Psychosomatic reactions

(A) may be fatal

(B) are mediated through the voluntary motor system

(C) are produced solely by emotional problems

(D) should be treated only by psychotherapy

(E) do not occur in young children

Questions 22 and 23

A religiously devout woman learns of her husband's infidelity with initial anger. Her rage soon passes but somehow she develops weakness of her right arm. No physical cause can be found for her illness and she remains remarkably complacent about her paralysis.

22. The arm weakness is a manifestation of

(A) isolation

(B) undoing

(C) delusion

(D) conversion

(E) projection

23. Her seeming lack of concern can be considered as

(A) autism

(B) la belle indifference

(C) malingering

(D) rationalization

(E) reaction formation

24. In spite of excellent emergency care, a middle-aged man dies suddenly of a myocardial infarction. The emergency room physician is quite upset when the shocked and grieving family become personally abusive to him. The doctor may take these comments less personally if he recognizes that he is the focus of the family's mourning anger, which is being

    (A) suppressed
    (B) sublimated
    (C) displaced
    (D) dissociated
    (E) denied

25. After he has been subjected to a long series of painful injections, a 7-year-old boy keeps telling everyone he actually enjoys needles. The nurses may be able to help him better when he starts parading around the ward with needles stuck under his skin if they realize that much of his behavior is

    (A) compulsive
    (B) repressive
    (C) dissociative
    (D) counterphobic
    (E) negativistic

Questions 26 through 28

26. As she walks home at night, an elderly woman becomes convinced that those shadows moving under her neighbor's trees are really a watching man. Her belief is based on a(n)

    (A) hallucination
    (B) projection
    (C) illusion
    (D) reaction formation
    (E) rationalization

27. When she gets into her house, she prepares a meal but later phones the police to complain that the neighbors are poisoning her food. Her behavior now is a manifestation of

    (A) autism
    (B) dissociation
    (C) isolation
    (D) delusion
    (E) obsession

28. Several hours later she starts shooting wildly toward the neighboring house. She is sure that they are "coming to get her." Her belief that she was going to be attacked is an example of

    (A) dementia
    (B) denial
    (C) regression
    (D) displacement
    (E) projection

29. After he is severely reprimanded by his employer, a man goes home and is extremely nasty to his wife all evening. His behavior at home is an example of

    (A) sublimation
    (B) dissociation
    (C) displacement
    (D) rationalization
    (E) conversion

30. A middle-aged, experienced nurse notes a rapidly growing lump in her breast but does not seek medical treatment. When eventually the mass is noted at her annual physical examination, she says she thought the lump was quite normal near the menopause. Her response is an example of

    (A) dissociation
    (B) repression
    (C) sublimation
    (D) rationalization
    (E) projection

31. A previously shy 16-year-old teenager has his leg amputated following a car accident and is fitted with an artificial limb. Within a week of returning home, his physician learns that the boy has been out dancing every evening. This unusual social interest can be considered evidence of

    (A) dissociation
    (B) conversion
    (C) somatization
    (D) reaction formation
    (E) compulsion

DIRECTIONS (Questions 32 through 116): Each group of items in this section consists of lettered headings followed by a set of numbered words or phrases. For each numbered word or phrase, select the ONE lettered heading that is most closely associated with it. Each lettered heading may be selected once, more than once, or not at all.

Questions 32 through 36

    (A) socialization outside the family
    (B) identity resolution
    (C) stable, satisfying infancy
    (D) instinctual drives
    (E) training and control

32. Basic trust

33. Latency

34. Anal stage

35. Adolescence

36. Id

Questions 37 through 41

    (A) self-centered, demanding, dependent
    (B) conscience
    (C) reality testing
    (D) highest personal goal
    (E) identification with same-sex parent

37. Phallic stage

38. Ego

39. Ego-Ideal

40. Superego

41. Oral personality

Questions 42 through 46

    (A) muscular rigidity and immobility
    (B) markedly egocentric, subjectively based feelings and behavior
    (C) presence of contrasting feelings toward same object
    (D) maintains body position in which he or she has been placed
    (E) temporary loss of muscle tone

42. Ambivalence

43. Autism

44. Waxy flexibility

45. Catatonia

46. Cataplexy

Questions 47 through 51

    (A) emotional response of the psychotherapist to the patient
    (B) return to earlier pattern of behavior
    (C) opposition to developing awareness
    (D) unconscious identification with another person
    (E) warm fellow-feeling

47. Transference

48. Resistance

49. Empathy

50. Countertransference

51. Regression

Questions 52 through 56

    (A) sexual energy and drive
    (B) narcissistic, egocentric, subjective
    (C) investment of emotional energy
    (D) pleasure principle
    (E) reality principle

52. Id

53. Ego

54. Libido

55. Autistic

56. Cathexis

Questions 57 through 61

    (A) primitive egocentric, pre-logical emotions and ideas
    (B) feelings that are unacceptable to the individual
    (C) instincts, drives, emotions
    (D) feelings not usually in awareness but can be easily recalled
    (E) perception, learning, thinking

57. The preconscious

58. Primary process thinking

59. Ego dystonic

60. Cognition

61. Conation

Questions 62 through 66

    (A) organized, logical, related to external reality
    (B) feelings of personal unreality, change, and strangeness
    (C) feelings and drives that ordinarily do not enter awareness
    (D) false perceptions when falling asleep
    (E) coexistence of contradictory feelings toward same object

62. The unconscious

63. Secondary process thinking

64. Ambivalence

65. Depersonalization

66. Hypnagogic state

Questions 67 through 71

    (A) emphasis of opposite feelings and qualities
    (B) primitive total identification
    (C) externalization of personal feelings
    (D) unacceptable feelings and drives productively redirected
    (E) symbolic expression through physical symptoms

67. Projection

68. Reaction formation

69. Introjection

70. Sublimation

71. Conversion

Questions 72 through 76

    (A) sexual gratification from an inanimate object
    (B) repetition of another's words
    (C) arrest of emotional development
    (D) behavior and feelings separated from basic central personality
    (E) newly coined word or several words run together

72. Echolalia

73. Dissociation

74. Neologism

75. Fixation

76. Fetishism

Questions 77 through 81

    (A) deliberate forgetting of disturbing feelings or ideas
    (B) unconscious blocking out of unacceptable feelings
    (C) intellectualized justification
    (D) substitute focus for feelings
    (E) intolerable external reality is removed from awareness

77. Repression

78. Rationalization

79. Suppression

80. Displacement

81. Denial

Questions 82 through 86

    (A) exaggerated, inappropriate feeling of pleasure
    (B) falsification of memory to fill gaps
    (C) memory loss
    (D) abnormally repetitive response to different questions
    (E) sudden stopping of thought or feeling

82. Amnesia

83. Euphoria

84. Perseveration

85. Confabulation

86. Blocking

Questions 87 through 91

    (A) thought disorder
    (B) senile dementia
    (C) affective disorder
    (D) infantile autism
    (E) toxic psychosis

87. Psychomotor retardation

88. Visual hallucinations

89. Blocking

90. Amnesia for recent events

91. Obsessive need for sameness

Questions 92 through 96

    (A) misinterpretation of perceptual stimulus
    (B) false, fixed belief
    (C) irrational fear
    (D) recurrent intrusive disturbing thought
    (E) false perception without reality stimulus

92. Delusion

93. Obsession

94. Illusion

95. Hallucination

96. Phobia

Questions 97 through 101

    (A) human cross-cultural studies
    (B) human relationships, individual and group

(C) species-specific behavior
(D) social and vocational training
(E) clinical work involving individual, family, and society

97. Anthropology

98. Ethology

99. Social work

100. Sociology

101. Occupational therapy

Questions 102 through 106

(A) achievement of sexual pleasure by inflicting pain
(B) achievement of sexual gratification with a child partner
(C) reaching sexual pleasure by watching sexual organs or the sexual activities of others
(D) attainment of sexual gratification by enduring inflicted pain
(E) sexual relations between members of the same family

102. Sadism

103. Masochism

104 . Pedophilia

105. Scopophilia

106. Incest

Questions 107 through 111

(A) psychological dependence
(B) withdrawal symptoms that occur with physical dependence
(C) habitual and compulsive need for drugs (with or without physical dependence)
(D) declining effect of same dose of a drug with prolonged use
(E) excessive drug intake unrelated to medical use

107. Abstinence syndrome

108. Habituation

109. Drug abuse

110. Drug dependence

111. Tolerance

Questions 112 through 116

(A) very rapid process of thinking, at times without obvious connections
(B) urgent and compelling need to move: "restless" feet
(C) sudden interruption in flow of thinking
(D) acute anxiety in organic brain syndrome when patient becomes aware of handicaps
(E) alternating periods of elation and depression

112. Thought blocking

113. Flight of ideas

114. Cyclothymia

115. Akathisia

116. Catastrophic reaction

Answers and Explanations

1. **(C)** In a *déjà vu* situation, the subject feels incorrectly that he or she has lived through the present experience at some time before. This feeling can occur in many emotional states and may be also part of the epileptic aura. *(1:161;2:146;3:16)*
A. When a subject senses or feels a body part that has been amputated or removed, this sensation is called a *phantom phenomenon. (1:537;2:574–576)*
B. *Hypnagogic hallucinations* may occur when a normal person is in the "in-between" stage of just falling asleep. Similar hallucinatory states can occur normally in the awakening *hypnopompic state. (1:163–164;2:124–125;3:16)*
D. When intellectual reasoning is used to avoid dealing with unacceptable feelings, this would be considered *rationalization. (1:80;2:100–101;3:8)*
E. Sleepwalking *(somnambulism)* occurs usually during stages 3 and 4 nondreaming sleep. Sleep talking takes place during all stages of sleep. *(1:570–573;2:706;3:352–353)*

2. **(C)** *Blocking, thought deprivation,* occurs in many situations but, when marked, is usually due to schizophrenia. *(1:148;2:129;3:17)*
A. Deliberate resistance to sharing uncomfortable feelings is usually called *negativism.* In psychotherapy, *resistance* is the term given to unconscious attempts to avoid awareness. *(1:177;2:116;3:5)*
B. *Fixation* is the arrest of psychological development before full maturation. *(1:70;2:104–105;3:10)*
D. *Psychomotor retardation* is the physical and emotional slowing seen in depression. *(1:174;2:115;3:20)*
E. The pathological lack of concern about seeming misfortune, seen sometimes in hysterics, was termed *la belle indifference* by Janet. This symptom is nonspecific and can occur in people who are emotionally healthy *or* ill. *(1:162;2:505;3:290)*

3. **(D)** *Akathisia,* the "restless leg" sydrome, occurs with many psychotropic drugs and is likely to develop, especially at the drug levels necessary to treat the psychotic. *(1:644;2:823;3:118)*
A. *Anaclitic psychotherapy* allows regression to infantile or childlike functioning and is most often used with patients with psychophysiological disorders. *(2:542–545)*
B. In Korsakoff's syndrome, *confabulation,* the unconscious falsification of memory, occurs to fill the gaps produced by the illness. *(1:161;2:145;3:16)*
C. *Reaction formation* is the defense mechanism when the opposite emotion is stressed. *(1:329;2:98–99;3:8)*
E. *Narcoanalysis* and *narcosynthesis* are the terms used for the procedure where narcotic drugs (most often barbiturates) are used to facilitate psychotherapeutic work. *(1:678;2:763–764;3:39)*

4. **(D)** In *reaction formation,* the opposite feeling is stressed—and the important word here is "stressed"—the opposite feeling is emphasized. *(1:329;2:98–99;3:8)*
A. *Rationalization* is the unconsciously motivated use of logical explanations for behavior or feelings prompted by unrecognized reasons. *(1:80;2:100–101;3:8)*
B. *Undoing* is typically seen in obsessive compulsive neurosis where the subject repetitiously and compulsively acts to prevent the feared and fantasized consequences of his or her recurrent obsession. *(1:80;2:94,477–478;3:10)*
C. In *displacement* the emotion is unchanged but is directed to a more tolerable focus. When a child cannot comfortably be angry at a parent, he or she may displace the anger and kick the cat or a younger sibling. *(1:80;2:101–102;3:9)*
E. In the process of *denial,* intolerable reality is blocked out of awareness by this unconscious mechanism. Approaching death may be denied because the whole reality produces unbearable anxiety. In *suppression,* on the other hand, the subject consciously shuts painful facts out of direct awareness. *(1:80;2:107;3:8)*

5. **(B)** Regression is very different from *repression,* which is present in many emotional defense mechanisms where unacceptable or anxiety-arousing feelings are unconsciously blocked out of awareness. *(1:80;2:93–96;3:7)*

A. *Regression* is the return to earlier patterns of behavior—the ill child may go back to thumb sucking or carrying an old worn doll. *(1:80;2:105;3:10)*

C. In *reaction formation,* the intolerable feeling is kept out of awareness by the overemphasis of the opposite emotion or drive. The person who finds his or her angry or aggressive feelings intolerably frightening becomes overly sweet, friendly, and accepting. *(1:329;2:98–99;3:8)*

D. In *suppression,* the individual consciously and deliberately shuts out disturbing feelings from awareness. The conscious decision is "I am not going to think about it." *(1:80;2:95–96;3:7)*

E. *Fixation* is the arrest of emotional development before full maturity and may occur at any stage of personality growth. *(1:70;2:104–105;3:10)*

6. **(D)** In *paranoia,* intolerable feelings are *projected* outward and ascribed to an external person or force. Rather than admit the reality of being upset, the subject may defend against anxiety by projection, by explaining away his or her inadequacies as being due to his or her employer's favoritism to others. *(1:80;2:102–103;3:9)*

A. In *introjection,* the subject takes into his or her own personality make-up the totality of the perceived object. This is a primitive form of identification. *(1:80;2:98;3:9)*

B. *Regression* is a return to earlier patterns of behavior and occurs in normal people under stress, especially physical illness. Severe and sustained regression is a manifestation of emotional illness. *(1:80;2:105;3:10)*

C. In *conversion,* the emotional conflict is kept out of awareness but is expressed ("converted") in a physical symptom. The wife who is angry enough to hit her husband develops an arm weakness. *(1:343–345;2:110;3:10)*

E. In the defense mechanism of *isolation,* the subject can recall or consider a disturbing idea or fact but the distressing feelings that usually accompany such recollections are blocked out of awareness, are isolated away.

Following a tragic car accident, a man may recall the events vividly, including the deaths of his loved family, but talk dispassionately. The emotion is isolated away in an emotional defense reaction to allow him to cope with the tragedy. *(1:80;2:94;3:10)*

7. **(B)** The subject with night terrors usually wakens later with total amnesia for the episode. Night terrors are most frequent in the 3- to 5-year-old age group, occur during non-REM sleep, and are present shortly after falling asleep. *(1:572–573;2:705–706;3:199)*

8. **(B)** *Hallucinations* are sensory experiences in the absence of external stimuli. The schizophrenic hallu-

cinates the voice of Christ; the delirium tremens patient hallucinates seeing animals moving. *(1:163–165;2:122–127;3:16)*

A. In *projection,* unacceptable personal feelings or qualities are externalized—projected outward—onto other persons. *(1:80;2:102–103;3:9)*

C. In an *illusion* the subject perceptually misinterprets a real external sensory stimulus. The fearful woman may see men standing in the shadows under a tree, when, in reality, she is misinterpreting empty shadows because of her fearfulness. *(1:163;2:122;3:16)*

D. A *delusion* is a relatively stable false belief that is incompatible with the subject's intelligence, education, and culture.

The minority-group child may grow up believing that he or she is victimized by the majority culture. The personal belief, valid or otherwise, would not be considered a delusion because it is compatible with his or her upbringing and cultural environment. *(1:152–153;2:129–133;3:18)*

E. *Introjection* is the opposite process of projection. In introjection, the subject takes into his or her own personality external qualities or identities of the people around him or her. This is a more primitive, less selective form of personality development than *identification.* *(1:80;2:98;3:9)*

9. **(A)** The unconscious blocking out of awareness of disturbing emotions is *repression.* *(1:80, 2:93–96;3:7)*

A similar word, but with a very different meaning, *regression* may occur in the face of any stress, including sexual conflict. But sexual conflict in itself does not necessarily lead to regression. Regression is a behavioral reaction and is not mediated through any specific nerve pathway.

Regression does not always indicate severe emotional disorder. Where regression is marked and long lasting, there is a greater likelihood of greater causative stress or more profound preexisting emotional weakness.

Regression, however, does occur normally in the face of severe physical illness. The physically ill person takes to bed and allows himself or herself to be cared for and nursed and may become childishly demanding. *(1:80;2:105;3:10)*

10. **(E)** *Bulimia* is the term for excessive gorging that goes with a huge appetite. The voracious eaters may self-induce vomiting after an eating binge.

Bulimia may precede or coexist with anorexia nervosa. *(1:779–780;2:555;3:195)*

The other terms listed are self- explanatory.

11. **(B)** The Halstead Reitan battery is a series of neuro-psychological tests used to identify and localize brain damage. *(1:133;3:48)*

12. **(D)** In hysterical neuroses, *conversion* is the term used when the underlying emotional conflict is symbolically manifested outwardly in a symptom involving the special senses or the voluntary nervous system. The writer may be unable to face a lack of creativity but can blandly tolerate the physical incapacity of writer's cramp. *(1:343–345;2:110;3:10)*
A. *Displacement* is the term to describe the mechanism whereby feelings that are intolerable when directed at one object or person are made more tolerable by redirecting these feelings toward another focus. In everyday experience, the father who "takes it out on" his family when he is frustrated by his work is displacing. *(1:80;2:101–102;3:9)*
B. When a subject has almost total memory loss for a significant part of his or her life, this would be considered *amnesia*. When this is part of a hysterical neurosis, this amnesia would be considered an example of *dissociation*. Amnesia may be produced by many organic syndromes. *(1:80;2:144–145;3:16)*
C. In a *psychophysiologic* (psychosomatic) *reaction* typically an emotional conflict is expressed in a single organ system controlled by the autonomic nerves. *(1:488;2:535–546;3:321)*
E. When an otherwise unacceptable drive is rechanneled into socially acceptable behavior, *sublimation* has occurred.
    It may not be acceptable to an angry father to beat his children brutally but he can sublimate his rage by chopping wood or painting a wall. *(1:80;2:108;3:9–10)*

13. **(C)** A false belief, not in accord with the individual's intelligence, age level, and culture, is a *delusion*. *(1:152–153;2:129–133;3:18)*
A. A *hallucination* is a sensory experience in the absence of external stimuli—where the perception arises within the individual. *(1:163–165;2:122–127;3:16)*
B. An *illusion* is a misinterpretation of actual perceptions where the quality of the misinterpretation is dictated by the subject's feelings. Because of his or her suspiciousness and feelings of inadequacy, the individual has the illusion that waving branches are pointing fingers. *(1:163;2:122;3:16)*
D. When acceptable inner feelings are projected outward and ascribed to another person, this mechanism is called *projection*. *(1:80;2:102–103;3:9)*
E. Unconscious blocking of any feelings, including instinctually based emotions, is labeled *repression*. *(1:80;2:93–96;3:7)*.

14. **(E)** Delusions do not occur in a subject who has a *schizoid personality*. These people are shy, oversensitive, vague, and often "different," but they are still in reasonable contact with reality. The schizoid personality is one example of a *personality disorder*. *(1:367–369;2:596–598;3:330)*
    The other syndromes listed are psychotic states where delusions can and do occur. The presence of

delusions would not be compatible with the diagnosis of personality disorder.

15. **(B)** Paranoid delusions are produced by the mechanisms of *projection*, where unacceptable inner feelings are externalized outward and projected onto another person. *(1:80;2:102–103;3:9)*
A. In *displacement*, the disturbing feelings are already being directed to an external object but the emotions are redirected, displaced, to a more acceptable object. *(1:80;2:101–102;3:9)*
C. When disturbing feelings or behavior are *rationalized* away, the subject comes up with a personally acceptable or tolerable intellectual reason for these distressing emotions. *(1:80;2:100–101;3:8)*
D. In *sublimation*, an emotion or urge that is personally or socially unacceptable becomes acceptable and often growth productive when it is rechanneled into socially approved behavior.
    Where a youngster is intensely competitive with an older sibling, it is not acceptable to eliminate the elder child with an axe. It is very acceptable for the younger child to strive to beat the other academically and athletically, often with the added reward of personal growth and enrichment. *(1:80;2:108;3:9–10)*
E. In the process of *identification*, the individual integrates into his or her own personality selected qualities of significant people in his or her life. Identification has this quality of selection, integration, and ego work in the process. The more primitive forms of identification, incorporation, and introjection are much less integrative or selective. *(1:80;2:96–98;3:9)*

16. **(A)** Alcoholic women are more likely to have children born with the fetal alcohol syndrome, manifesting low birth weight, small size, craniofacial, limb, and cardiac abnormalities, and mental retardation.
    It has been suggested that the relationship between childhood minimal brain damage and later antisocial behavior may be due primarily to the fetal alcohol syndrome. *(1:421;3:163)*

17. **(A)** *Catharsis* is the psychoanalytic term for the release of previously unconscious feelings, with outward expressions of feelings, that comes usually with an appropriate interpretation in the course of treatment. *(1:615;3:66)*
B. *Cathexis* is the analytic word for the investment of emotional energy in a specific purpose or object. Withdrawal of emotional investment is called *decathexis*.
C. The conscious or unconscious response of the psychotherapist to the patient is designated as *countertransference*. This concept emphasizes the two-way process in any psychotherapeutic interaction where the therapist must be aware of both the patient's transference feelings and also of his or her own logical and illogical feelings toward the patient. *(1:598;2:752–753;3:4)*

D. In psychoanalytic practice, the process of knowing and learning can be designated as *insight. (1:125–126;2:201,753;3:66)*
E. When an unacceptable feeling is externalized and ascribed to an external person, the process is called *projection. (1:80;2:102–103;3:9)*

18. **(E)** *Collective unconscious* was a concept introduced by *Carl Jung* early in his career. It implied the common unconscious that is inherent in humanity, a species-specific unconscious that is then integrated with other aspects of the unconscious that are individual and social. *(1:101–103;2:13;3:11)*

19. **(E)** When feelings originally linked to significant or nuclear early-life figures are projected onto, or transferred to, a current-life person, *transference* has occurred—and occurs in everyday relationships as well as in psychotherapeutic relationships. *(2:751–752;3:4)*
A. *Displacement* is the mechanism whereby feelings are transferred from an unacceptable to a more acceptable object. *(1:80;2:101–102;3:9)*
B. When unacceptable thoughts and ideas are unconsciously excluded from awareness, they are said to have been *repressed. (1:80;2:93–96;3:7)*
C. Identification implies internalization, the taking into the personality of significant aspects of a parent-child relationship. In transference, externally directed feelings are transferred to a new external object. *(1:80;2:96–98;3:9)*
D. Transference is in no way indicative of early psychosis, though an illogical transference or a transference unduly acted out may indicate a psychotic process.

A woman may naturally feel initial dislike for bald, middle-aged men because her brutal father was bald—as part of an understandable transference reaction that is not psychotic. However, if she assaulted these bald men, her behavior would indicate a psychotic break with accepted reality. *(1:597;2:751–752;3:4)*

20. **(D)** In a *somatization disorder,* the patient expresses feelings by having physical symptoms or complaints. This is an automatic or unconscious process. *(1:340–342;2:497–501;3:289–290)*

In *hypochondriasis,* the patient misinterprets real physical signs or sensations. *(1:349–352;2:512;3:291)*

When the individual has a loss or change in physical function produced by an emotional conflict or need, this is designated a *conversion disorder. (1:342–348;2:501–505;3:290)*

The malingering patient deliberately and consciously fabricates symptoms for some recognizable personal gain. *(1:551–555;2:515)*

21. **(A)** Psychosomatic reactions, such as peptic ulcers or ulcerative colitis, may indeed be fatal.
B. They are predominantly mediated through the autonomic nervous system. Hysterical conversion reactions affect the voluntary motor system and the special senses.
C. Psychosomatic reactions are not produced solely by emotional problems. Usually there is a strong physical, constitutional predisposition.
D. Psychosomatic reactions should be treated by all means necessary, usually by more than psychotherapy alone. A child in status asthmaticus requires prompt effective medical and psychiatric treatment. Psychotherapy has little effect on a dead child.
E. Psychosomatic illness occurs in young children, even in the neonate. *(1:488–492;2:535–592;3:321–326)*

22. **(D)** This history outline points out how a good, caring woman finds herself angry at the husband she loves. She deals with the emotional conflict of love-rage by repressing (and undoubtedly also suppressing) the anger. This unacceptable feeling of anger, however, is converted into a physical symptom, the right-arm paralysis. The symptom has a symbolic meaning—if her right arm is paralyzed, she cannot use it to hit out at her unfaithful spouse. The symptom is a manifestation of *conversion.*

23. **(B)** Since this physical symptom does relieve her conflict, she can indeed be relatively unconcerned, manifesting the classical *belle indifference* of the hysteric.

This syndrome is referred to as hysterical neurosis, conversion type. *(1:343–345;2:501–505;3:290)*

24. **(C)** In normal mourning, the grieving relatives must face their sadness and anger at the loss, and they must reinvest emotionally. Often in Western society, mourners find it difficult to deal with the normally felt anger at this pain and separation. It is difficult to be angry at the deceased and it is not acceptable to be angry at God. This mourning anger may be *displaced* onto the nurse or physician—the emotion retains the same quality but is focused on a more acceptable target. *(1:80;2:101–102;3:9)*

25. **(D)** Whistling through the graveyard and singing cheerily while walking down dark deserted alleys are the kind of *counterphobic* reactions seen in normal people. The adolescent and childhood games of "daring" and playing "chicken" have a strong counterphobic quality. In order to avoid admitting or facing fears about a situation, the subject actively seeks out or repetitiously engages in the experience.

With the natural pride of a 7-year-old, this young man finds it difficult to admit just how scared he is of painful needles—and rightfully scared. He copes with his fear by the *counterphobic* measure of seeking out and actively engaging in the feared behavior. Many counterphobic behaviors raise tension in observers who can sense the subject's overreaction and underlying anxiety. *(1:324;2:472;3:8)*

26. **(C)** Due to her fearfulness, the subject misinterprets actual perceptual stimuli. The shadows are actually there, but she interprets her perceptions to see, in these shadows, a watching man. This form of misperception is termed an *illusion*. *(1:163;2:121–122;3:16)*

27. **(D)** When she phones the police to complain that the neighbors are poisoning her food, she is manifesting a false belief that probably is inconsistent with her intelligence and cultural background—she is manifesting a *delusion*. She is now externalizing her inner insecurities and directing these feelings toward her neighbors. *Projection* is occurring. *(1:152–153;2:129–133;3:18)*

28. **(E)** The *projection* becomes more fixed and stronger. She can now justify taking action against these neighbors, in a way that endangers them, under the paranoid justification of her delusion. *(1:80;2:102–103;3:9)*

Answers 26 through 28 describe the development of a paranoid delusion to the point of illogical action. Frequently, however, a paranoid delusion forms around a core of reality. In this instance, the lady's paranoid delusion may be based not only in her own inner conflicts and insecurity but also on the fact that the neighbors were uncooperative, unfriendly, or distressing. (1:226–237;2:444–456;3:18)

If this elderly woman then claimed that her food—for instance the milk—had a bitter taste of poison and no one else could detect this taste, she would be showing a *gustatory hallucination*. Much more frequent are taste illusions where a taste is misinterpreted—everyone can taste a chalky flavor in the milk but the subject interprets this as due to strychnine. *(1:179;2:126;3:16)*

29. **(C)** The man is naturally angry, anxious, and sensitive at being reprimanded by his employer. He has found it difficult to express his feelings toward the disturbing person, the employer, possibly because he could be dismissed or because the employer was fully justified in the reprimand. The man continues feeling upset. He cannot or does not suppress or repress the anger. He does not sublimate his tension in more forceful work. He displaces his anger onto a safer target, his wife. This is an example of *displacement*, an everyday, normal (though unproductive) reaction. *(1:80;2:101–102;3:9)*

30. **(D)** This middle-aged nurse very readily would have diagnosed the possible seriousness of this breast lump in anyone else. In reality, she did realize the potential threat of this growing mass to her physical integrity and continued existence, but the thought was so disturbing that she blocked it out of awareness. She *denied* the reality. *(1:80;2:107;3:8)*
    When she could not avoid facing this reality, she explained away her seemingly illogical behavior with intellectual reasons; she *rationalized*. *(1:80;2:100–101;3:8)*

31. **(D)** When Hamlet's mother pointed out to him "The lady doth protest too much, methinks," (*Hamlet,* Act 3, Sc. 2.242) she was highlighting an example of *reaction formation*.
    For a young man who had been socially backward to become suddenly prominent would necessitate quite a reversal of behavior. A leg amputee would not usually consider dancing the easiest activity. Reasonably he might want to work up gradually to this form of social interaction. The patient described here is handling his understandable anxiety about his amputation by emphasizing the opposite behavior to his fears.
    All normal people show reaction formation in some of their activities. This defense is reality distorting—this boy naturally as an amputee would find it more difficult to dance well—and this form of emotional reaction takes a great deal of psychologic energy to maintain and tends to make other people uneasy or anxious. *(1:329;2:98–99;3:8)*

32. **(C)** *Erik Erikson* theorized that the young infant develops *basic trust* in response to a stable, satisfying mothering experience. *(1:89–92;2:61;3:177)*

33. **(A)** In Freudian theory, *latency* follows the resolution of the *phallic phase* of development and is the time when the youngster first moves outside the family and should become adapted to wider society. This approximates the grade school or elementary school period. *(1:71;2:72–73;3:6)*

34. **(E)** The *anal stage* follows the *oral stage* and is the time of initial training and control within the family according to psychoanalytic theory. *(1:71;2:65–66;3:5)*

35. **(B)** Erikson characterized adolescence as the period when the growing child establishes his or her unique individual *identity*. *(1:89–92;2:61;3:177)*

36. **(D)** In psychoanalytic theory, the *id* is the instinctual gratification-seeking part of the psychic structure. *(1:76;2:60;3:7)*

Answers 37 through 41 refer to psychoanalytic concepts. The ego, ego-ideal, and the superego are components of the psychic structure.

37. **(E)** The *phallic stage,* in the age period 3–4 to 6–7 years, is the time the developing child stabilizes gender, identity, and role. This is the developmental phase when the Oedipus complex is faced and, hope-

fully, resolved; whether this complex is culture specific is under debate. *(1:71;2:72–73;3:6)*

38. **(C)** The *ego* is the coordinating, organizing part of the personality, the part that perceives and evaluates reality. *(1:78–79;2:60–62;3:7)*

39. **(D)** The *ego-ideal,* a less frequently used concept, is the idealized self-image, the private, personal optimal goal. *(2:62;3:7)*

40. **(B)** The *superego,* the conscience part of the personality, is derived largely from significant relationships where standards and models, good and bad, have been set. *(1:79–80;2:62–63;3:7)*

41. **(A)** If a person remains relatively *fixated* at the *oral phase* of emotional development, he or she will show the characteristics of the *oral personality*—a demanding self-centeredness. *(1:71–72;2:65;3:5)*

Answers 42 through 46 deal with symptoms typical of schizophrenia.

42. **(C)** *Ambivalence* is the existence of conflicting emotions or impulses toward the same person or object. In lay terms, this is the quality of having mixed feelings about someone. Ambivalence is a major cause of internal emotional conflict. While normal people constantly have ambivalent feelings, in schizophrenia strong and opposing feelings can coexist side by side and can be acted on by the schizophrenic. Ambivalence is one of Bleuler's cardinal symptoms of schizophrenia. *(1:177;2:138–139;3:20)*

43. **(B)** *Autism* is the quality of thinking that is markedly subjective, egocentric, and idiosyncratic. Autistic thinking is characteristic of the schizophrenic. In *infantile autism* this pattern of thinking and reacting is most severe and pervasive. *(1:178;2:127;3:246)*

44. **(D)** *Waxy flexibility, cerea flexibilitas,* is the syndrome where the subject maintains, often for long periods, the position in which he has been placed. This symptom is usually indicative of catatonic schizophrenia. *(1:177;2:370;3:20)*

45. **(A)** *Catatonia* is the clinical syndrome where the individual is rigid and immobile.

     Sometimes this symptom is designated more specifically *catatonic withdrawal,* immobility, or stupor, depending on the quality of the withdrawal, while *catatonic excitement* describes the disorganized, aggressive, frenzied state that may occur in the same patients. *(1:177;2:373–376;3:248)*

46. **(E)** *Cataplexy* is not a symptom of schizophrenia but must be differentiated from catatonia. Cataplexy is the syndrome where the individual suddenly loses power and muscle tone and falls. *(1:567;2:285–286;3:20)*

Answers 47 through 51 focus on the psychotherapy process.

47. **(D)** *Transference* is the process whereby feelings initially directed to an earlier significant person are *transferred* onto a person in an immediate present relationship. In psychoanalytic psychotherapy, transference toward the therapist or analyst is allowed and then becomes a major focus of the psychotherapy. *(1:597;2:751–752;3:67)*

48. **(C)** *Resistance* in psychotherapy is the conscious and unconscious opposition to bringing to awareness previously unconscious feelings. *(1:597;2:751;3:66)*

49. **(E)** *Empathy* is a warm but objective feeling for another human being; this is contrasted with *sympathy,* where the feeling is subjective. *(1:99;2:98)*

50. **(A)** *Counter-transference* is the conscious and unconscious emotional response of the psychotherapist to the patient in treatment. Many psychotherapists use these reactions elicited by the patient as further diagnostic and therapeutic tools. *(1:598;2:752–753;3:67)*

51. **(B)** *Regression* implies a return to earlier patterns of behavior; this may be a normal reaction to severe stress, as in serious physical illness, or may be a manifestation of emotional disorder. *(1:80;2:105;3:10)*

This set of answers (52 through 56) deals primarily with the quality of relationship and emotional drives as outlined in psychoanalytic theory. This question group also illustrates an examination situation where one answer could be appropriate for two questions but one response is more specifically associated to the question than the other and is thus the required answer. When the examinee deals with a group of questions, he or she must also evaluate the style, pattern, or direction of the question series.

52. **(D)** The *id* is the part of the personality that is bound by the *pleasure principle,* tension buildup and release, and instinctual gratification. The id is also the part of the psyche that is constituted by the instinctual drives—so, in some situations, 52A might have been considered a correct answer—"sexual energy and drive."

     Id energy comes from all psychic drives, sexual and nonsexual. *(1:76;2:60;3:7)*

53. **(E)** The *ego* is that part of the personality that is bound by the *reality principle*—perceiving, evaluating, and directing. *(1:76–79;2:60–62;3:7)*

54. **(A)** *Libido* specifically is the sexual instinctual forces and drives:"sexual" is used in the widest sense of life-directed and living. *(1:70;2:72–73;3:5–7)*

55. **(B)** *Autistic* thinking is markedly subjective, dictated by egocentric standards and perceptions, and profoundly narcissistic. *(1:178;2:127;3:246)*

56. **(C)** *Cathexis* is the psychoanalytic term for the investment of emotional energy in an object, goal, or drive.

57. **(D)** In his theory of psychic structure, the *preconscious* was one of the earlier divisions postulated by Freud. The preconscious is the part of the mind just out of awareness, a part that can be brought to awareness with effort.

   This segment of the personality has the quality, "It is just on the tip of my tongue" or "I have it in the back of my mind"—where all that is needed is a connecting link to bring it to awareness. *(1:74;2:25;3:6)*

58. **(A)** *Primary process thinking* is prelogical, not bound by external reality, and gratification oriented. *(1:146;2:90;3:6)*

59. **(B)** Feelings or ideas that are *ego dystonic* or *ego alien* are unacceptable to the goals and standards of the ego. This is in contrast with *ego syntonic* emotions or concepts that are acceptable and do not provoke anxiety, anger, or rejection. *(3:285)*

60. **(E)** *Cognition* is the psychological term for thinking, sensing, perceiving, and learning. *(1:32;2:83–86;3:15)*

61. **(C)** *Conation* is the feeling, instinctual, driving part of the personality. *(1:172;2:114;3:15)*

62. **(C)** According to Freudian theory, feelings and drives that do not originally enter awareness are located in the *unconscious* part of the personality, where they still have a most important effect on the subject's total personality and behavior. *(1:73–74;2:12;3:6)*

63. **(A)** The *ego* part of the personality structure is motivated primarily by *secondary process thinking,* which is logical, related to external reality, and able to delay gratification. *(1:78;2:90;3:6)*

64. **(E)** *Ambivalence* is the emotional state where the individual feels contradictory and conflicting feelings toward the same object. Ambivalence is part of every normal mature relationship, but the healthy person usually prefers to respond to one side of the ambivalence. In schizophrenia, ambivalence may be marked, and the schizophrenic may act or express both aspects of the ambivalence. *(1:177;2:138–139;3:20)*

65. **(B)** A feeling of personal unreality and strangeness occurs periodically in all humans and is probably most common in adolescence. When this sensation, *depersonalization,* is prolonged or pervasive it may be a manifestation of schizophrenia or of a neurotic disorder. *Derealization* is the sense of environmental unreality, a change in one's environment. *(1:357–360; 2:139)*

66. **(D)** A *hypnagogic state* or *hypnagogic phenomenon* is the experience of illusions and hallucinations that may occur to the normal person during the period of falling asleep. The comparable awakening state is the *hypnopompic phenomenon.* *(1:179;2:124–125;3:16)*

Answers 67 through 71 deal with mental mechanisms and emotional defenses.

67. **(C)** In *projection,* personally unacceptable inner feelings and impulses are externalized and ascribed to another person. The defense in this process is the externalizing or pushing away from one's own self of intolerable emotions and drives and then blaming another person for the exact same feelings and intentions. *(1:80;2:102–103;3:9)*

68. **(A)** In *reaction formation,* the subject defends unconsciously against an anxiety-arousing feeling by outwardly stressing the opposite emotion. This defense is not merely repression of one feeling; it involves the emphasis of just the opposite. *(1:79;2:98–99;3:8)*

69. **(B)** *Introjection* is an early primitive form of identification where the subject takes into his or her personality the whole image of the significant person or relationship. This is an all-or-none process: the more mature process of identification involves greater selectivity of personal qualities that are then integrated. *(1:80;2:98;3:9)*

70. **(D)** In *sublimation,* unacceptable drives and feelings are repressed, but the energy of these emotions is rechanneled in socially acceptable and sometimes growth-productive ways.

   The naturally competitive young boy cannot destroy his father physically but he can learn to beat him in chess or in football, both good sublimations. *(1:80; 2:108;3:9–10)*

71. **(E)** When a disturbing emotional conflict is repressed and manifested through a physical symptom, usually involving the special senses or the voluntary muscles, this mechanism is termed *conversion.* *(1:342;2:110; 3:10)*

72. **(B)** When a subject repetitiously and word for word repeats the words and phrases that are said to him, this symptom is called *echolalia* and is usually a manifestation of schizophrenia.

Question: "What is your name, Sir?"
Response: "Name Sir. Name Sir."
Question: "Where are you now?"
Response: "You now, you now."
Echopraxia is the comparable symptom where the other person's movements are automatically imitated. *(1:177;2:116;3:21)*

73. **(D)** *Dissociation* is used to describe the splitting off of a significant part of the personality from normal, conscious control—the fugue state, multiple personality, sleep walking. *(1:80;2:105–106;3:10)*

Sometimes a thought may be described as being dissociated from the feeling that would normally accompany it, the process of isolation. *(1:329;2:94;3:10)*

74. **(E)** A *neologism* is a newly coined word or a series of words run together to form a seemingly nonsensical word. Typically neologisms occur in schizophrenia or acute manic states. *(1:178;2:364;3:17)*

75. **(C)** When there is arrest of emotional development at a particular developmental phase, the subject is said to be *fixated* at that level or to have a *fixation.* *(1:70;2:104–105;3:10)*

76. **(A)** When an individual gains significant sexual gratification from an inanimate object—often a shoe or piece of clothing—that person is manifesting *fetishism.* The object is the *fetish* and the person is a *fetishist.* *(1:447;2:529;3:303)*

Answers 77 through 81 also deal with mental mechanisms and defenses.

77. **(B)** *Repression* is the unconsciously motivated blocking out of unacceptable feelings from conscious awareness and is a factor in most, if not all, emotional defense mechanisms. *(1:80;2:93–96;3:7)*

78. **(C)** *Rationalization* is the defense where intellectual, seemingly logical reasons are presented to justify feelings or behaviors. This defense is motivated by unconscious factors.

A father rationalizes his sudden eruption of rage at his son because he was overtired—a lame excuse that everyone uses. In reality, the father's anxiety and anger arose when he sensed his son was superior to him intellectually and physically—and recognized momentarily his declining capability. *(1:80;2:100–101;3:8)*

79. **A)** The deliberate conscious forgetting or blocking out from immediate awareness of disturbing feelings or ideas is called *suppression.* This blocking out is conscious ("I will not think about it") as opposed to the unconscious motivated repression. *(1:80;2:95–96;3:7)*

80. **(D)** In *displacement,* the feelings remain the same but they are redirected, displaced, to a more tolerable or acceptable object. *(1:80;2:101–102;3:9)*

81. **(E)** When external reality is too disturbing, the individual may continue to cope by blocking out this reality from awareness—by *denial.* In a fatal illness, the patient may continue to function productively only by denying, by blocking this awareness from reality. Denial is a reality-distorting defense and such denial may be more difficult to maintain as the reality of approaching death becomes more obvious. The denial may suddenly give way, leaving the dying patient to face his or her loneliness, anxiety, and anger. *(1:80;2:107;3:8)*

82. **(C)** *Amnesia* is loss of memory and may be total or partial, reversible or otherwise. Usually, total amnesia is due to organic causes, but partial amnesia is a frequent symptom of emotional illness. *(1:179–180;2: 144–145;3:16)*

83. **(A)** *Euphoria* is an exaggerated, somewhat inappropriate feeling of pleasure. In states of unusual happiness and excitement, normal people experience euphoria, which also is seen frequently in hypomanic and manic states. *(1:165;2:135;3:19)*

84. **(D)** *Perseveration* is an abnormally repetitive response to different questions and is seen most often in senile dementia, after injury to brain speech centers, or in catatonia. *(1:178;2:128;3:17)*

85. **(B)** Classically, *confabulation* occurs in *Korsakoff's syndrome* and is the falsification of memory to fill memory gaps. Confabulation is a type of *paramnesia.* *(1:161;2:145;3:16)*

86. **(E)** *Thought deprivation* or *blocking* is the sudden stoppage of the flow of thought or feeling.

Normal people occasionally have thought blocking—"My mind just went blank"—but severe blocking is usually symptomatic of schizophrenia. *(1:148; 2:129;3:17)*

Answers 87 through 96 focus on symptoms of emotional illness.

87. **(C)** *Affective disorder.* Psychomotor retardation is a common symptom of depression. In affective or mood disorders, the symptoms are caused by the disabling intensity of mood (affect). *(1:238–239;2:404;3:263)*

88. **(E)** *Toxic psychosis.* Visual hallucinations occur early in a toxic psychosis. In a schizophrenic psychosis, visual hallucinations occur late when many other psychotic and regressed symptoms are present. *(1:273–276;2:311–334;3:219)*

89. **(A)** *Thought disorder.* Marked thought blocking is a symptom of a thought disorder and is thus a most important manifestation of schizophrenia. Normal people occasionally have thought blocking, though rarely —"It just slipped my mind." *(1:147–154;2:129;3:16–19)*

90. **(B)** *Senile dementia.* In senile dementia, the patient characteristically has great difficulty recalling recent events but often can remember childhood happenings in great detail (anterograde amnesia). *(1:286–290; 2:232–246;3:215)*

91. **(D)** *Infantile autism.* Many children with severe infantile autism have an obsessive need for sameness. They become upset, even panicky, if they note changes in their accustomed environment. *(1:732–737;2:693–694;3:201)*

92. **(B)** A false belief that is inconsistent with a subject's intelligence, level of maturity, and social background is called a *delusion. (1:152–153;2:129–133;3:18)*

93. **(D)** An *obsession* is a recurrent, intrusive, disturbing thought. The subject may have a repetitive intrusive thought that he or she is going to die or may attack someone.

    The sufferer is quite aware that the thought is illogical and finds the obsession distressing.

    A *compulsion* is an illogical act that the subject feels forced to carry out repetitiously. In *obsessive-compulsive neurosis,* recurrent thoughts are obsessions, recurrent acts are compulsions—both are illogical, repetitive, and intrusive. *(1:327–335;2:133;3:17)*

94. **(A)** An *illusion* is a misinterpretation of an actual perceptual stimulus. The quality of the misinterpretation is a reflection of the subject's emotional state.

    The confused, frightened senile patient may misinterpret the chatter of the nursing staff in the distance as a plan to kill her. *(1:163;2:122;3:16)*

95. **(E)** A false perception without an actual reality stimulus is termed a *hallucination.* The schizophrenic may hear voices where there are no external auditory stimuli. This is different from the illusion described in 94, where an external auditory stimulus is present but is misinterpreted. *(1:163–165;2:122–127;3:16)*

96. **(C)** A *phobia* is a persistent irrational fear. The subject knows that this fear is illogical but cannot prevent the recurrent intrusion of the phobia into his or her thinking. In phobias, the fear is focused on a defined target: fear of germs—mysophobia; fear of open spaces —agoraphobia; fear of heights—acrophobia. *(1:321; 2:133–134;3:20)*

Several of the behavioral science professions are defined in the following answer group (97 through 101).

97. **(A)** *Anthropology* deals with human societies from a cross-cultural viewpoint. *(1:865–867)*

98. **(C)** *Ethology* is the science that focuses on animal behavior, including species-specific behaviors. This is a research field that will have increasing impact on the understanding of human personality and development. *(1:45–53;2:31;3:58–60)*

99. **(E)** *Social work* is a clinical profession dealing with the individual as part of his or her family and community. Social workers carry out individual case work, group psychotherapy, and community and agency coordination. *(1:871)*

100. **(B)** *Sociology* is the study of human relationships from the standpoint of the individual and the group. The sociologist evaluates patterns in populations including sick populations such as those in mental hospitals. *(1:865–867;2:801–803)*

101. **(D)** In *occupational therapy,* patients are provided with social, vocational, and recreational experiences that should enhance their total treatment and prepare them better for a healthier way of coping and growing. *(1:604)*

Answers 102 through 106 define various sexual deviations. (1:433–475;2:520–534)

102. **(A)** *Sadism* is the achievement of sexual pleasure by inflicting pain on the sexual object. Sadism is named after the author de Sade. *(1:448–450;2:530–531; 3:306)*

103. **(D)** *Masochism* is the achievement of sexual pleasure by enduring inflicted pain. Masochism is named after Sacher-Masoch, an Austrian writer. *(1:448–450;2: 531;3:305–306)*

104. **(B)** In *pedophilia,* the sexual deviant achieves sexual gratification through some form of contact with a child. Pedophilia is usually applied to the relationship of an adult with a child and does not refer to activities between children. *(1:450–451;2:529;3:304)*

105. **(C)** *Scopophilia* or *voyeurism* is the pattern of achieving sexual pleasure by watching sexual organs or the sexual activities of others. A "Peeping Tom" is a *voyeur. (1:449–450;2:530;3:305)*

106. **(E)** In *incest* there is sexual activity between close family members. Usually, for the activity to be labeled incest, sexual intercourse or intromission must have occurred. Sex play may be designated as incestuous without coitus occurring. *(1:471–473;2:163)*

Various terms dealing with drug dependence are considered in answers 107 through 111. (1:385–432;2:643–671;3:233–234)

107. **(B)** An *abstinence syndrome* is a term for the physical and emotional symptoms that occur on the withdrawal of a drug to which the subject has been addicted. *Addiction* implies dependence on the drug with the presence of physical withdrawal symptoms. *(1:394;2:644–645;3:233–234)*

108. **(A)** *Habituation* is the psychological dependence on a drug because of its pleasurable or tension-relieving effect. Habituation or *habit formation* implies only emotional dependence; where there is also physical dependence, *addiction* exists. *(1:385;2:644;3:233–234)*

109. **(E)** The term *drug abuse*, as defined by the World Health Organization, is the use of drugs, persistently or sporadically, for other than acceptable medical purposes. *(1:400;2:644;3:233)*

110. **(C)** *Drug dependence*, with the qualifying phrase specifying the drug or type of drugs involved, implies a state of psychological dependence, with or without physical dependence, on that drug or drug type. *(1:385;2:644;3:233)*

111. **(D)** Where there is *tolerance* to a drug, the individual finds a decreasing effect from the same dose of the drug and has to increase the drug dosage to produce the same desired effect. *(1:400;2:644–645;3:233)*

112. **(C)** Where there is *thought blocking,* there is a sudden interruption in the flow of thinking. This *thought deprivation* or blocking can occur in normal people or in milder emotional disorders. Where blocking is marked, the symptom usually indicates a schizophrenic illness. *(1:148;2;129;3:17)*

113. **(A)** Where an individual manifests a very rapid process of thinking, at times without obvious connection between thoughts, he or she is said to be showing a *flight of ideas.* This symptom is most characteristic of the manic state. *(1:178;2:127–128;3:17)*

114. **(E)** *Cyclothymia,* mood swings, is a state of alternating periods of depression and elation. *Kretschmer* suggested that cyclothymia typically occurs in people with *pyknic* constitutional build. *(1:259;2:595–596; 3:268)*

115. **(B)** *Akathisia,* the "restless leg" syndrome, is a side effect of many neuroleptic drugs, especially of the piperazine and butyrophenone group. The patient may feel restless, unable to keep still, and may complain that his or her feet are restless. *(1:644;2:823; 3:118)*

116. **(D)** A *catastrophic reaction* is the acute eruption of anxiety that occurs in patients with organic brain syndromes when the subject becomes unavoidably aware of his or her mental handicaps. The patient may present with a wide range of disruptive symptoms. *(1:149–150;2:304–305)*

Psychological Testing
Questions

INTRODUCTION

For many examinations and certainly for general clinical practice, the professional trainee will need more information about psychological testing than is given in standard psychiatry textbooks. It is difficult, if not impossible, to learn the purpose and the usefulness of psychological testing from books, lectures, or seminars. The student should take every opportunity to see the actual test materials, to watch testing in different settings, and to discuss the validity of testing with the professionals who administer, interpret, and use the tests.

REFERENCES

1. Chapter 7,   Diagnosis and Psychiatry
       7.4,   Psychological Testing of Intelligence and Personality, pp 126–132
       7.5,   Psychological Tests For Brain Damage, pp 132–136
2. Chapter 8,   Examination of the Patient. Psychological Testing, pp 202–217
3. Chapter 3,   Psychological Tests, pp 45–52

DIRECTIONS (Questions 1 through 17): Each of the numbered items or incomplete statements in this section is followed by answers or by completions of the statement. Select the ONE lettered answer or completion that is BEST in each case.

1. Which test would be most helpful in evaluating the emotional boundaries and appreciation of reality in an adult patient?

   (A) Stanford–Binet
   (B) Vineland
   (C) Bender–Gestalt
   (D) Rorschach
   (E) Apgar

2. The scoring of the Rorschach test takes into account all of the following *except*

   (A) use of color and shading
   (B) response to whole blot
   (C) ability to copy the designs
   (D) popular and unusual responses
   (E) use of the white areas

3. All of the following statements are valid about intelligence testing *except*

   (A) affected by subject's motivation
   (B) culturally biased
   (C) tend to emphasize verbal ability
   (D) high scores are incompatible with psychotic illness
   (E) measures skills enhanced by traditional education

4. The galvanic skin resistance (GSR) is a measure often used in psychophysiological studies. It reflects

   (A) skin warmth
   (B) blood flow through superficial tissues
   (C) heart rate and output
   (D) sweat gland activity
   (E) muscle tension

5. All of the following statements apply to the Minnesota Multiphasic Personality Inventory (MMPI) *except*

   (A) subject may be able to predict acceptable answers from the nature of the questions
   (B) may be given to a group at one time
   (C) requires a high level of professional skill in administering and scoring
   (D) questions may arouse or increase subject's anxiety
   (E) places high emphasis on verbal comprehension

6. Some indications of the inner fantasy of a 9-year-old child may be given by all of the following *except*

   (A) modeling clay
   (B) Children's Apperception Test
   (C) Bender–Gestalt Test
   (D) finger painting
   (E) toy soldier play

7. All of the following statements apply to the Thematic Apperception Test *except*

   (A) blank card included in test series
   (B) includes three colored cards toward end of set
   (C) made up of ambiguous pictures
   (D) usually reflects the subject's mood and quality of emotions
   (E) prompts sharing of feeling about intrafamilial relationships

8. The Draw-a-Person Test, the Sentence Completion Test, and the Thematic Apperception Test are similar in that they

   (A) all require the subject to draw
   (B) are all projective tests
   (C) measure intelligence
   (D) diagnose sensory-motor incoordination
   (E) can be machine scored

9. The Word Association Test was first used extensively by

   (A) S. Freud
   (B) A. Adler
   (C) K. Horney
   (D) C. Jung
   (E) H. Rorschach

10. Psychological testing can be reasonably requested for all of the following *except*

    (A) localizing a lesion in the brain
    (B) comparing present intelligence capabilities with previous functioning
    (C) differentiating psychotic and organic states
    (D) measuring vocational aptitude
    (E) testing suitability for psychotherapy

11. The validity of a psychological test refers to

    (A) the ability of the test to measure what it is supposed to measure
    (B) the consistency the test shows in test–retest results
    (C) the absence of cultural bias
    (D) the test usefulness in predicting outcomes
    (E) the lack of examiner bias

Questions 12 and 13

You are evaluating an 8-year-old black girl from a city ghetto-area school. Her school report gives her an intelligence quotient of 80.

12. When you are asked the significance of this intelligence rating, you should state

(A) the child is in the borderline retarded range

(B) the youngster is probably above average in basic intelligence

(C) until you know the type and circumstance of the testing, you do not know

(D) ghetto girls are normally more advanced than boys

(E) all testing at this age level has poor predictive value

13. You learn that this intelligence quotient is based on one group test. You can state that all of the following are true *except*

(A) this would have most likely been a paper-and-pencil test

(B) strongly influenced by verbal and reading skills

(C) biased by sociocultural factors

(D) affected by individual motivation

(E) cannot exclude severe retardation

14. All of the following statements apply to the Bender–Gestalt Test *except*

(A) test cards have geometric designs

(B) subject is asked to copy designs

(C) used in eliciting psychotic responses

(D) useful in diagnosing brain damage

(E) evaluates perceptual-motor coordination

15. The ratio of the Mental Age over the Chronological Age multiplied by 100 is the

(A) rating of mental retardation

(B) Intelligence Quotient

(C) Apgar score

(D) Rorschach F score

(E) performance rating on the Weschler Intelligence Scale

16. The Cattell Infant Intelligence Scale

(A) can be used up to grade school age

(B) predicts intelligence level in childhood and adult life

(C) measures neuromuscular development

(D) cannot detect mental retardation

(E) is based largely on parental reporting

17. Group psychological tests are less reliable than individual tests due to all of the following *except*

(A) dependent on reading ability

(B) they test speed more than other factors

(C) anxiety interferes with reading speed

(D) they are valid only with adults

(E) individual motivation is less easily measured

DIRECTIONS (Questions 18 through 22): Each group of items in this section consists of lettered headings followed by a set of numbered words or phrases. For each numbered word or phrase, select the ONE lettered heading that is most closely associated with it. Each lettered heading may be selected once, more than once, or not at all.

(A) ambiguous pictures

(B) geometric designs

(C) inkblots

(D) reports of social functioning

(E) positive and negative responses

18. Rorschach

19. Thematic Apperception

20. Bender–Gestalt

21. Minnesota Multiphasic Personality Inventory (MMPI)

22. Vineland Scale

Answers and Explanations

1. **(D)** In the *Rorschach test,* the subject is presented with ambiguous stimuli (inkblots) for which he or she must supply the structure. Where the subject being examined lacks a definite sense of individual reality and firm personal boundaries, it is impossible for him or her to give clearly defined, reality-based responses to these unstructured stimuli. *(1:128–129;2:206–209;3: 48–49)*
   A. The *Stanford-Binet test,* developed from the first intelligence tests published by Binet, was used extensively for intelligence testing of children and adults. Child psychologists still find it especially useful in evaluating mental retardation and for testing preschool children. *(1:704;2:675–676;3:184)*
   B. *The Vineland Social Maturity Scale* determines the patient's *Developmental Quotient* based on social function as noted by observers, usually parents. This rating is not based on direct clinical observation. *(2:720)*
   C. The *Bender–Gestalt Test* is used in testing perceptual-visual-motor coordination and immediate visual recall. Though it has been used by some psychologists as a form of projective test, this use needs much more extensive validation. *(1:131;2:210–213; 3:47)*
   E. The *Apgar score* is based on physical evaluation of the newborn in the first 5 minutes of life.

2. **(C)** In the *Rorschach test,* the patient does not copy the designs (as is done with the Bender–Gestalt geometric designs). Several of the cards present color stimuli and all show shadowing tones. The subject's ability to respond to the whole card is significant, as are responses to the white or unshaded areas of the card. Each inkblot has responses that are usual, common, or popular, but the range of unusual responses is limitless and all reflect the personality of the subject. *(1:128–129;2:206–209;3:48–49)*

3. **(D)** Many psychotic patients can score well on intelligence tests. Paranoid patients are especially good on these tests: high scores in intelligence tests are in no way incompatible with psychotic illness.

   Testing results are highly affected by the patient's motivation and level of energy at the time of testing. If the patient does not try or does not wish to cooperate, the scores will be lowered.

   Most intelligence tests tend to emphasize verbal ability and often reading ability also—especially group paper-and-pencil tests, on which many school intelligence ratings are based.

   Intelligence tests tend to be biased against minority groups or lower socioeconomic populations. They emphasize skills learned in traditional education rather than survival ability, the capacity for productive action, or nonverbal skills. Intelligence testing may set up a self-fulfilling prophecy. A minority group child can test at a low score level because the test is culturally biased. Nevertheless the child's educational program is often geared to the level of his or her test score, to meet the needs only of a retarded child. Intellectually, the youngster may then be stunted by an insufficiently stimulating or an unrewarding academic program, thus leading to equally low or lower intelligence test scores later. *(1:128;2:202–205;3:46–47)*

4. **(D)** The *galvanic skin resistance* (GSR) is a manifestation of changes in skin resistance to the passage of a weak electric current and is largely responsive to sweat gland activity. This measure has often been used in the evaluation of the physical aspects of emotion. *(1:629;2:137)*

5. **(C)** One of the most useful attributes of the *Minnesota Multiphasic Personality Inventory (MMPI)* is that it can be administered and scored by a relatively untrained person. The final evaluation of the score should be done by a professional clinician. Response C is thus incorrect.

   A reasonably alert subject can guess from many of the questions what is likely to be the expected and acceptable answer. The MMPI is frequently given as a group paper-and-pencil test. Both the group test and the individual test require that the subject read and understand the long series of questions. Because of the nature of the questions and the directness of each question, the individual may be made quite anxious. *(1:130–131;2:214–215;3:49–51)*

6. **(C)** When children are *modeling clay* or *finger painting* on blank paper, they are forced to express themselves to give form, integration, and quality to their activities. With *toy soldiers,* the stimulus is more specific but still allows for freedom of self-expression and the use of inner fantasy. The *Children's Apperception Test (CAT)* is merely a more formal way of presenting ambiguous stimuli on which children must express (project) themselves and show their own personalities and inner fantasies. *(1:707–708;3:49)*

   The *Bender–Gestalt Test* measures visual motor coordination and immediate visual recall and is not usually used to elicit a child's fantasy. *(1:131;2:210–213;3:47)*

7. **(B)** The *Thematic Apperception Test* does not have any colored cards. Answer B is wrong.

   The test is a series of ambiguous picture scenes that are planned to bring out the subject's mood and feelings. Many of the pictures show situations that are easily perceived as a family interaction and thus prompt the expression of feelings about family relationships. The card series has one blank card that may be given to the subject, who is asked to make up a story completely without external stimuli. *(1:129–130;2:210;3:49)*

8. **(B)** The *Draw-a-Person Test,* the *Sentence Completion Test,* and the *Thematic Apperception Test* all are similar in that they require subjects to give of themselves, to project, to do or to complete the test. Thus they are all projective tests.

   Only the Draw-a-Person Test requires the subject to draw. None of them specifically measure intelligence though they are all strongly affected by the subject's motivation, intelligence, and academic and cultural background.

   On the Draw-a-Person Test, sensory-motor incoordination may be apparent but this is better measured by other tests.

   None of the three tests can be machine scored. *(1:129–132;2:210–214;3:48–49)*

9. **(D)** *Carl Jung* (1875–1961), the Swiss analyst, developed the use of the *Word Association Test* to show emotional drives and conflicts. *(1:101–103;2:214;3:11)*

10. **(A)** Psychological testing results are too nonspecific to give more than a very gross localization of a *brain lesion.* In the hands of a few specialized testers, localization may be fairly good, but in general clinical practice other localizing techniques are much more efficient.

    Otherwise, psychological testing is useful clinically in comparing past and present intellectual functioning, to differentiate psychotic and organic states, to measure vocational aptitude, and to evaluate suitability for psychotherapy. *(1:132–136;2:203–205;3:47–48)*

11. **(A)** The validity of a psychological test refers to the level of accuracy with which it measures what it is supposed to measure. The validity of intelligence testing has been shown by the way these scales accurately assess mental retardation levels. The reliability of a test refers to its ability to show consistent test–retest results. *(1:126–127;2:202–203;3:45)*

12. **(C)** The clinician does not know the significance of any *intelligence quotient score* of any person until he or she knows the circumstances of the testing, the tests given, and the subject's social and academic background. In the situation described there is not sufficient information.

    Unfortunately many children are labeled "borderline retarded" solely on the basis of an Intelligence Quotient rating. *(1:127–128;2:715–722;3:46)*

13. **(E)** Because a *group test* is most often a paper-and-pencil test, strongly influenced by verbal and reading skills, biased by sociocultural factors, and markedly affected by individual motivation, you can indeed state that a youngster who scores even moderately well is unlikely to be severely retarded.

    With all these factors against a high score, you can accept the fact that the child's intelligence level is not below IQ 80—that is, the test result does indeed exclude severe retardation. *(1:704–705;2:737–738;3:45)*

14. **(C)** Although the subject may show psychotic responses to the *Bender–Gestalt Test,* this test is not used specifically to elicit psychotic responses.

    The subject is usually asked to copy geometric designs from test cards and then sometimes by memory. The test measures perceptual motor coordination and visual recall and is thus useful in diagnosing brain damage. *(1:131;2:210–213;3:47)*

15. **(B)** $$\frac{\text{Mental age}}{\text{Chronological age}} \times 100 = \begin{array}{c}\text{Intelligence}\\\text{Quotient}\end{array}$$

    Mental retardation can then be rated as an intelligence quotient level, but the IQ in itself is not a specific rating of retardation.

    The *Apgar score* is a measure of the physical condition of the newborn within 5 minutes of birth.

    The *F score* on the *Rorschach test* is the measure of good or poor form responses to the inkblots.

    The *Performance Scale* on the Weschler Intelligence Scale is a summation of the five nonverbal tests. The *Verbal Scale* measures the verbal subtests. *(1:128;2:203–204;3:46–47)*

16. **(C)** The *Cattell Infant Intelligence Scale* primarily measures *neuromuscular ability,* the ability to grasp, sit, stand, walk, talk, self-feed, and self-care in children from 3 to 36 months. The test can detect moderate degrees of mental retardation that are usually evident in the child's slower neuromuscular develop-

ment. The test does not go beyond 3 years of age, after which the Stanford–Binet is used. This test, while it can detect moderate to severe retardation, has no predictive ability to indicate the level of intelligence the child may attain in later life. Infant tests are notoriously poor at predicting.

The Cattell Scale is based on direct child testing; the Vineland Scale uses parental observations. *(1: 705;2:206)*

17. **(D)** *Group psychological tests* are used extensively with *children* as well as with *adults.* Most routine school psychological tests are given in group situations.

The other statements are reasons why group tests are less reliable. They are dependent on verbal and reading ability. They do place high emphasis on speed. Anxiety can markedly interfere with reading and writing speed. In individual testing, motivation is much more easily evaluated. *(1:704;2:202–203;3:45)*

18. **(C)** The *Rorschach test* uses *inkblots* as the unstructured stimuli to produce personality projection. The *Holtzman Test* also uses inkblots. *(1:128–129;2:206–209;3:48–49)*

19. **(A)** In the *Thematic Apperception Test,* the subject is asked to respond to a set of cards showing *ambiguous pictures. (1:129–130;2:210;3:49)*

20. **(B)** The subject is asked to copy a series of *geometric designs* in the *Bender–Gestalt Test* with the original in front of him or her and sometimes also from memory. *(1:131;2:210–213;3:47)*

21. **(E)** In the *Minnesota Multiphasic Personality Inventory (MMPI)* the subject is asked to respond "true," "false," or "cannot say" to a long series of questions. From the *positive, negative,* and uncertain *responses* the inventory is scored. *(1:130–131;2:214–215;3:49–51)*

22. **(D)** The *Vineland Social Maturity Scale* is most often used with children. From reports of the child's functioning, usually from parents and teachers, the youngster's social development is evaluated and his or her *Developmental Quotient* measured. *(2:720)*

Child and Adolescent Psychiatry
Questions

INTRODUCTION

Most examinations have questions on how to manage the child as a member of the family. Often the questions are awkwardly stated but they are trying to elicit some principle. The answers required are often seemingly rigid or dogmatic because only one response is sought when usually there are various reactions that are correct to different degrees.

REFERENCES

1. Chapters 28–37,   Child and Adolescent Psychiatry, pp 691–854
2. Chapter 28,   Disorders Usually First Evident in Infancy, Childhood, and Adolescence, pp 672–714
    Chapter 29,   Mental Retardation, pp 715–744
3. Chapter 11,   Mental Retardation, pp 159–174
    Chapter 12,   Other Disorders of Infancy, Childhood, and Adolescence, pp 175–212

DIRECTIONS (Questions 1 through 38): Each of the numbered items or incomplete statements in this section is followed by answers or by completions of the statement. Select the ONE lettered answer or completion that is BEST in each case.

1. You get a phone call from a mother whose 4-year-old son has just asked, "Mommy, where do I come from?" You should advise her to

   (A) pretend she did not hear the question
   (B) find out what the child wants to know
   (C) demonstrate on herself and the child's father the differences between the sexes
   (D) punish him for asking such a nasty question
   (E) bring the child in for the next available appointment when you will teach him the facts of life

2. A worried mother asks you how to manage her 4-year-old son, who she says is stealing. Apparently he keeps bringing home toys that belong to other children. You should advise her to

   (A) take the toys back herself, without any fuss, and buy him similar toys
   (B) tell him that if he stops stealing, he will have a reward every weekend
   (C) point out that this is stealing and spank him
   (D) make sure he has enough toys and see that he returns the toys to the owners
   (E) ignore the whole affair; this is a developmental phase that will soon pass.

3. The hospital attendants find a 16-year-old girl wandering confused in the hospital parking lot where apparently her friends have left her.
   She seems physically normal and allows you to do a thorough physical. Periodically she asks you to be quiet as she listens to sounds that no one else can hear and to look at the little animals "like rabbits or small dogs" that she sees running around the emergency room. All of the following are applicable *except* that

   (A) she is likely to be suffering from an acute toxic psychosis due to drug abuse
   (B) you reassure, reorient, and support
   (C) reduced sensory stimulation may be helpful
   (D) even after these present symptoms clear, she may have recurrent hallucinatory episodes ("flashbacks") even without further drug use
   (E) you can be sure that she will recover fully from the episode

4. A 16-year-old diabetic teenager insists on a weekly physical check up but nevertheless does not cooperate in his necessary medical treatment. He is probably showing manifestations of

   (A) schizophrenia, disorganized (hebephrenic) type
   (B) organic brain syndrome
   (C) malingering

   (D) obsessive–compulsive neurosis
   (E) oppositional disorder

5. A teenage boy in psychotherapy says to his psychotherapist, "Nobody cares for me." The therapist knows the adolescent is receiving at least the usual family love and attention. The doctor should respond

   (A) "Of course your family cares for you."
   (B) "I wonder why that should be so."
   (C) "I care for you."
   (D) "How much caring do you need?"
   (E) "Maybe you are not worth caring for."

Questions 6 through 9

6. In classical school phobia, the problem typically arises because the

   (A) child has been a scapegoat in school
   (B) teacher is rigid, punitive, and overly demanding
   (C) parents have unreasonably high academic standards
   (D) child is mentally retarded
   (E) child has difficulty separating from the parents

7. Separation anxiety disorder is seen

   (A) only in boys
   (B) only in kindergarten or first-grade children
   (C) where the Oedipus complex is not resolved
   (D) at every age level in childhood and adolescence
   (E) mainly in unusually intelligent, sensitive children

8. To prevent school refusal, parents should

   (A) make sure children know the sexual facts of life
   (B) encourage the gradual development of independence from early childhood
   (C) convince children that they will always have their parents to care for them
   (D) point out how stupid they are to be afraid of school
   (E) make sure they are protected from frustrations and anxiety as they grow

9. The optimum treatment for school refusal is

   (A) immediate assignment of a homebound teacher
   (B) family therapy for the parents and child
   (C) return the child to school and then work on the underlying problem
   (D) arrange for a change of teacher or school, with family therapy
   (E) hospitalize the child to evaluate his or her functioning when separated from the family

10. A previously normal 4-year-old boy is hospitalized for an emergency appendectomy. When he returns from the hospital, he is irritable and demanding. He starts to such his thumb and, after he has wet his bed several nights in succession, his mother brings him for pediatric examination. The pediatrician will tell the mother that

    (A) these symptoms may be the early signs of severe personality pathology and should be further evaluated
    (B) his behavior is an outward manifestation that the boy is working through his Oedipal conflict
    (C) these regressive symptoms indicate undue psychological dependency and suggest the need for greater independence training
    (D) this is a normal transient reaction to a stressful situation, and with care and support the child should soon revert to his preoperative behavior
    (E) this infantile behavior suggests the possibility of operative anoxia and the child should have further neurological and psychological examination

11. In Tourette's Disorder all of the following are applicable *except*

    (A) multiple tics
    (B) compulsive swearing
    (C) childhood onset
    (D) haloperidol therapeutic
    (E) grandiose delusions

12. The syndrome of infantile autism

    (A) occurs more frequently in urban ghetto residents
    (B) may show symptoms similar to those seen with congenital deafness
    (C) commonly occurs in other siblings
    (D) does not occur in black children
    (E) was first described by Bleuler

13. All of the following symptoms tend to occur in infantile autism *except*

    (A) insistence on sameness
    (B) hallucinations
    (C) twirling
    (D) fascination with moving objects
    (E) walking on toes

14. After a visit to the physician, two 5-year-olds play "hospital" all afternoon. Their behavior is a manifestation of

    (A) projection
    (B) identification
    (C) rationalization
    (D) displacement
    (E) dissociation

15. As part of an adjustment disorder in adolescence, all of the following symptoms may be present *except*

    (A) school failure
    (B) delinquency
    (C) paranoid delusions
    (D) depression
    (E) stomach and head pains

Questions 16 and 17

When the supermarket checker does not charge for a can of peas, the parents are delighted. Later that evening at the drive-in movie they claim their 13-year-old daughter is only 11 so that they can avoid paying. Yet they are most upset when their 8-year-old son is caught stealing from lockers in school.

16. The parents' attitude at the supermarket and drive-in is evidence of their

    (A) reaction formation
    (B) intellectualization
    (C) superego lacunae
    (D) undoing
    (E) repression

17. They should remember that their 8-year-old develops his conscience by all of the following mechanisms *except*

    (A) introjection
    (B) projection
    (C) imitation
    (D) internalization
    (E) identification

Questions 18 and 19

In the course of a routine physical examination, a mother mentions that her 4½-year-old son has been sleeping with her and her husband for the past two weeks. The little boy had been having scary dreams of ghosts and witches and felt much safer with his parents.

18. The pediatrician should

    (A) inquire gently about the mother's sexual feeling toward her son
    (B) anticipate that time and family sensitivity will take care of the problem
    (C) assume that the parental marital relationship is unstable
    (D) recommend firmly that the little boy be required to sleep in his own bed
    (E) all of the above

19. The doctor appreciates that

(A) the little boy is showing early homosexual tendencies
(B) scary dreams are an early sign of childhood psychosis
(C) the father must be evaluated also
(D) scary dreams are often part of the normal 4-to 5-year-old's maturation experience
(E) none of the above

20. Adjustment reaction in childhood may include all of the following symptoms *except*

(A) autism
(B) phobias
(C) nail biting
(D) bed wetting
(E) nightmares

21. On Intelligence Quotient scales, average intelligence is taken as

(A) 50
(B) 60–80
(C) 80–100
(D) 90–110
(E) 100–120

22. In which age group is the highest incidence of mental retardation?

(A) infant
(B) preschool
(C) kindergarten
(D) adolescent
(E) adult

23. The social group with the highest reported incidence of mental retardation is

(A) urban ghetto residents
(B) second-generation immigrants
(C) Jews of Eastern European origin
(D) blond haired, blue-eyed Scandinavians
(E) drug addicts

Questions 24 through 27

24. When you are asked to see an 8-year-old patient with enuresis, you anticipate that the child is likely to be

(A) a girl
(B) a boy
(C) mentally retarded
(D) autistic
(E) obsessive–compulsive

25. As you take the history, you recognize that

(A) enuresis usually has encopresis as an accompanying symptom

(B) both parents have usually been toilet trained early
(C) a family history of enuresis is more common
(D) diurnal enuresis is more common than nocturnal
(E) usually an organic defect of the urinary tract is the main cause

26. Enuresis usually occurs

(A) during REM sleep
(B) during non-REM sleep
(C) when the child has wakened
(D) when the child is hungry
(E) during weekends and vacation periods

27. In the treatment of enuresis, you may wish to use all of the following *except*

(A) psychotherapy for the child
(B) imipramine
(C) conditioning device
(D) parental counseling
(E) barbiturates

28. The following statements are applicable to petit mal *except*

(A) onset usually in childhood
(B) disappear before adulthood
(C) often replaced by grand mal seizures
(D) usually associated with borderline retardation
(E) treated with trimethadione

29. X-rays of long bones of children suffering from chronic lead poisoning show

(A) increased thickness and density at zones of provisional calcification
(B) multiple poorly healed fractures
(C) calcified periosteal hemorrhages
(D) cupping and fraying of the distal ends with generalized reduction in shaft density
(E) premature closure of epiphyses

30. The child with attention deficit disorder

(A) always grows out of the symptoms by the end of adolescence
(B) may benefit from treatment with stimulants
(C) is most likely to be a grade-school girl
(D) frequently develops a convulsive disorder
(E) commonly becomes an adolescent schizophrenic

31. At 4:00 AM you are called by the mother of an 11-year-old asthmatic boy who has had recurrent severe asthma for three years. She is really convinced about the emotional etiology of asthma—described as "cry for mother"—she has read. The boy is in the midst of an acute asthmatic attack. The mother thinks you should see him now so you can begin to deal with the basic emotional problems. Considering the above course of events, you should

(A) make an appointment to see the mother and the boy in your office that morning at 9:00 AM
(B) tell the mother that this is a case for a pediatrician
(C) tell the mother you will be willing to help the boy but only in conjuction with close pediatric care
(D) see the boy an hour later in your office for his first psychotherapy session
(E) realize that this early morning call must be prompted by the mother's psychopathology so you arrange to see her alone in your office the next morning

32. The normal child can appreciate that death is irreversible when he or she is

(A) 2 years old
(B) 3 years old
(C) 5 years old
(D) 7 years old
(E) 12 years old

33. Sleepwalking

(A) occurs during REM sleep
(B) is most common in preschool children
(C) is caused by emotional tension
(D) episodes are remembered later
(E) occurs during the latter part of night sleep

34. In withdrawing barbiturates from a chronically addicted patient, the physician should plan

(A) sudden, complete withdrawal
(B) abrupt withdrawal with covering paraldehyde
(C) immediate barbiturate withdrawal with intramuscular chlorpromazine
(D) slow graduated withdrawal of barbiturates
(E) abrupt withdrawal and substitution of methadone

35. About 50% of children will have physical and/or mental defects if the mother has rubella

(A) during her adolescence
(B) in the first month of pregnancy
(C) in the fourth month of pregnancy
(D) in the sixth month of pregnancy
(E) just before delivery

36. In diagnosing phenylketonuria, you might find all of the following *except*

(A) musty odor to urine
(B) hydrocephalus
(C) retardation in siblings
(D) dermatitis
(E) blond hair, blue eyes

37. School refusal is usually a manifestation of

(A) mental retardation

(B) infantile autism
(C) separation anxiety
(D) malingering
(E) attention deficit disorder

38. The childhood syndromes of fire-setting, enuresis, and infantile autism are similar in that they

(A) are much more common in boys
(B) should be treated in a hospital setting
(C) respond to imipramine
(D) were first described by Leo Kanner
(E) lead to childhood schizophrenia

DIRECTIONS (Questions 39 through 81): Each group of items in this section consists of lettered headings followed by a set of numbered words or phrases. For each numbered word or phrase, select the ONE lettered heading that is most closely associated with it. Each lettered heading may be selected once, more than once, or not at all.

Questions 39 through 43

(A) urine with musty odor
(B) reversal of letters and words
(C) twirling
(D) elderly mother
(E) separation from mother in the second six months of life

39. Infantile autism

40. Phenylketonuria

41. Anaclitic depression

42. Down's syndrome

43. Strephosymbolia

Questions 44 through 47

(A) autosomal recessive inheritance
(B) butyrophenones therapeutically effective
(C) barbiturates contraindicated
(D) imipramine most effective drug

44. Acute porphyria

45. Childhood enuresis

46. Phenylketonuria

47. Tourette's Disorder

Questions 48 through 52

    (A) coprolalia
    (B) fecal soiling
    (C) 45 chromosomes
    (D) lead poisoning
    (E) hairpulling and baldness

48. Encopresis

49. Tourette's Disorder

50. Trichotillomania

51. Turner's syndrome

52. Pica

Questions 52 through 57

    (A) 46 chromosomes
    (B) xxy–47 chromosomes
    (C) 45 chromosomes
    (D) trisomy 21

53. Klinefelter's

54. Turner's

55. Down's

56. Tourette's

57. Korsakoff's

Questions 58 through 60

    (A) 2 months
    (B) 6 months
    (C) 10 months
    (D) 2 years
    (E) 3 years

When does the normal child begin to

58. Reach for and grasp a toy?

59. Ride a tricycle?

60. Pick up a small object using thumb and index finger?

Questions 61 through 63

    (A) 2 months
    (B) 5 months
    (C) 6 months
    (D) 12 months
    (E) 18 months

At what age level does the growing infant normally show the following social activities?

61. Smiles

62. Holds out arms to be held

63. Says two or three words

Questions 64 through 66

    (A) 1 month
    (B) 2 months
    (C) 4 months
    (D) 6 months
    (E) 10 months

Match each level of development with the appropriate age level.

64. Begins to hold up head

65. Sits for brief periods

66. Stands without support

Questions 67 through 71

    (A) neurofibroma, optic glioma
    (B) cerebral angioma, convulsions, retardation
    (C) ovarian dysgenesis, sexual infantilism, xo–45 chromosomes
    (D) retardation, brain glioma, pulmonary and renal cysts
    (E) progressive intellectual and motor deterioration, hepatic cirrhosis

Match the physical findings with the appropriate syndrome.

67. Facial "port wine stain"

68. Adenoma sebaceum of the face

69. Café au lait spots and skin polyps

70. Greenish-brown ring in the iris

71. Short stature, webbed neck

Questions 72 through 76

    (A) 47 chromosomes, xxy pattern
    (B) lack of phenylalanine hydroxylase
    (C) Jewish infants of Eastern European extraction
    (D) Rh incompatibility between mother and fetus
    (E) chromosome 5, short arm deletion

Match the syndrome with the predisposing or etiologic factor.

72. Progressive weakness, cherry-red spot on macula, early death

73. Severe retardation, dermatitis, convulsions, blonde hair, blue eyes

74. Marked retardation, microcephaly, catlike cry in childhood

75. Mild retardation, asthenic build, testicular atrophy, gynecomastia

76. Retardation, choreo-athetosis, deafness, yellow-pigmented basal ganglia

Questions 77 through 81

(A) trimethadione
(B) haloperidol
(C) calcium disodium versenate
(D) methylphenidate
(E) imipramine

Match the illness with the appropriate treatment.

77. Attention deficit disorder

78. Tourette's Disorder

79. Petit mal

80. Enuresis

81. Lead poisoning

Answers and Explanations

1. **(B)** This question highlights the fact that the supportive parent should answer the child's curiosity in a fashion the youngster can use productively.

   To answer a question, the parents need to know what the child really wants to know. The 4-year-old in this example may just want to know whether he comes from Detroit or Philadelphia. By the nature of his question the inquiring youngster indicates what he is seeking and also what information he can usefully integrate. There is no point in overwhelming (or in this case overstimulating) the youngster with information he is not seeking. *(1:694–696;2:71–73;3:175–181)*

2. **(D)** This question deals with the level of comprehension that usually can be expected from a 4-year-old child. This is the age period when the child's conscience (superego) is being established and the parental model is especially important.

   A 4-year-old finds it difficult to grasp the abstract concept of stealing. His sense of time is still limited so he cannot usefully integrate the idea of a reward after a week.

   The parents need to know why the child is taking others' toys. The child should understand that taking other people's possessions is not acceptable. The youngster can be starting to be responsible for his behavior and this can be emphasized by his returning the toys himself. *(1:694–696;2:71–73;3:190–191)*

3. **(E)** The 16-year-old girl presents the symptoms of an *acute psychosis,* most likely due to one of the hallucinogens. It is not uncommon for such patients to be brought in by the police who have found them wandering or to be dropped off near a treatment center by friends or relatives who hesitate to be more closely involved for fear of legal difficulties.

   If the patient is in contact with her surroundings, her anxiety may be relieved by constant reassurance, reorienting, and support. If the girl is out of contact, her symptoms are more likely to improve in an environment of reduced sensory stimulation.

   The patient may indeed have recurrent *flashbacks* after the acute episode is over.

   One of the major hazards of hallucinogen use is the fact that the outcome of the reaction is never total-

ly predictable. A good or a bad "trip" cannot totally be forseen. The disturbing effects of a drug trip may hang on unexpectedly, and the user has no guarantee that the next trip may not result in a more prolonged disturbed or psychotic state. *(1:410–414;2:663–667; 3:219–224)*

4. **(E)** This teenage diabetic is showing both an insistent dependency and a constant resistance, symptom patterns that together are typical of the *oppositional disorder.*

   In reality, most adolescents are scared, angry, and bitter when they suffer from a chronic illness such as diabetes or epilepsy. They have no prospect of getting well. They are different, handicapped. Often they manifest both their anger and their anxiety in passive-aggressive behavior—behavior that is sometimes self-destructive.

   This patient shows no manifestations of delusional or hallucinatory behavior usually seen in the disorganized hebephrenic schizophrenic teenager. He is not deliberately feigning illness, as would be seen in *malingering.* He is not manifesting the memory loss or emotional liability of the organic brain syndrome, which would be a very late development due to diabetic arteriosclerosis.

   Though his behavior has some of the repetitiveness of the compulsive *neurotic,* this teenager is not compelled to carry out these acts nor does he feel personal anxiety at his recurrent behaviors; others feel the pain. *(1:786–789;2:692;3:192)*

5. **(B)** Many examinations have questions about the process needed to facilitate psychotherapy. The task in psychotherapy is to help the patient understand why he feels the way he does. This means that concrete answers, even socially appropriate answers, may have to be delayed.

   In the psychotherapy relationship, especially with an adolescent, the reponse of the psychotherapist is often factual and direct.

   To facilitate the teenager's introspection and self-awareness, the appropriate response is "I wonder why that should be so." *(1:813–820;2:708–711;3:181–183)*

   School phobia, or *school refusal,* as it is sometimes called, is often a manifestation of *separation anxiety* in children. This is a favorite examination topic. The answers sought by the examination are often much more specific than is possible in clinical practice.

6. **(E)** Classically, *school phobia* arises because the child has difficulty separating from the parents—and the parents from the child.

All the other reasons listed in this question will indeed make the school experience more anxiety-arousing to the child and, in some situations, become major etiological factors in maintaining school refusal. *(1:791–795;2:687–689;3:193)*

7. **(D)** *Separation anxiety disorder* can occur whenever there is a significant emotional separation from previously gratifying and supportive relationships. The school phobia, or the equivalent form of separation, can occur throughout life. "Homesickness" is one form of separation anxiety with which most people cope reasonably well.

Separation anxiety is more liable to occur where the youngster is less mature and more dependent at the time of first leaving home and going to school. When school phobia, *separation anxiety,* manifests in older children or adults, it suggests a level of emotional weakness more indicative of severe psychopathology at that age. The correct response is that school phobia can occur at every age level in childhood and adolescence (and in adult life). *(1:791;2:687–689;3:193)*

8. **(B)** The optimum way to minimize or prevent *separation anxiety* and *school refusal* is to encourage the gradual development of the child's independence over the years, from early childhood onward. Overprotection may lead to the stunting of growth; overloading with responsibility or with "facts" may overwhelm the youngster. *(1:794–795;2:687–689; 3:193)*

9. **(C)** Once the child has left or been removed from school, it is usually more difficult to get him or her back into school. With a clear separation, the child's fears become less reversible and school peers and teachers tend to grow away from him or her.

If at all possible the child should be returned to school and maintained there, even in a tenuous fashion—visiting the counselor's office—while the underlying factors producing the school refusal are defined and handled. In clinical practice it may not be possible to keep the child in school due to factors in the school, the family, and the child—in which case the other measures may be indicated. *(1:794–795;2:687–689;3:193)*

10. **(D)** *Adjustment disorder in childhood.* Regression is a return to earlier patterns of behavior. At times of illness we all normally tend to regress. We allow ourselves to be cared for, and we act in a more self-centered, childlike fashion.

Regression is a normal response in childhood to the stress of separation, hospitalization, and the trauma of operation. With a little extra caring and support, the child should soon return to his more mature preoperative behavior. *(1:841–843;2:694–695;3:204–205)*

11. **(E)** *Tourette's Disorder* has been the subject of wider interest recently due to the apparent therapeutic effectiveness of *haloperidol.* The etiology of this syndrome is not fully understood.

Usually the onset is in early childhood, with *multiple tics,* compulsive swearing (*coprolalia*), and often *echolalia.*

Patients do not manifest delusional thinking. *(1:763–765;2:700–701;3:196–197)*

12. **(B)** *Infantile autism* is very rare, occurring in probably less than 2 in every 10,000 preadolescent children. The syndrome is important to diagnose early and is extremely significant in research into early personality development and the etiology of emotional illness.

Typically, infantile autism occurs in intellectual middle- and upper-class families, though it may appear in other socioeconomic groups.

Autism was described as one of the cardinal symptoms of schizophrenia by Bleuler, but it was *Leo Kanner* who first defined the syndrome of infantile autism.

Autism is uncommon in other siblings and family members, whereas there is a higher incidence of schizophrenia in the relatives of the schizophrenic.

Children who are born with or develop early or severe hearing loss are likely to develop symptoms very similar to infantile autism. *(1:732–737;2:693–694;3:201)*

13. **(B)** *Hallucinations* do not occur in infantile autism. If hallucinations are present in a child younger than age 7 or 8, a toxic or organic disorder is likely to be present. *(1:732–737;2:693–694;3:201)*

14. **(B)** *Identification* in these 5-year-old children could be an attempt to imitate someone they admire or an effort to cope with their anxiety about someone they fear. *(1:77,694–696;2:71–73;3:9)*

Projection has the quality of externalizing the anxiety and projecting the blame. *Rationalization* is a means of intellectually explaining away the illogical. In *displacement* the feeling is directed at a more acceptable object or target, and in *dissociation* disturbing feelings are split off from the rest of the personality. *(1:80;2:100–103;3:8–9)*

15. **(C)** An *adjustment disorder* at any age is a temporary, transitional period of maladaptation in response to unusual stresses.

    Paranoid delusions, or delusions of any kind, would be such a major disruption of reality contact as to indicate a deeper level of psychopathology than implied in the diagnosis of adjustment disorder.

    The other symptoms—school or job failure, delinquency or antisocial behavior, depression or emotional discomfort, and somatic symptoms—all indicate a personality under stress, but stress from which recovery can reasonably be expected with appropriate management, support, and understanding. *(1:808–809;2:694–696;3:204–205)*

Answers to 16 and 17 are concerned with conscience development.

16. **(C)** Question 16 portrays the kind of *conscience defects (superego lacunae)* that are present in normal parents and families—the conscience lapse that is almost socially acceptable—in avoiding payment at the drive-in movie or cheating the income tax authorities but is not socially tolerable when acted out in other settings—like stealing from other children in school. In reality, stealing and dishonesty are the same wherever the behavior or the victim. Children learn from parental examples. *(1:79–80;2:117;3:5–7)*

17. **(B)** The growing child develops a conscience by taking into his or her personality the qualities and the models he or she sees in the significant people in his or her life.

    Introjection, imitation, internalization, and *identification* are all ways the child has of taking in and of establishing his or her conscience.

    Projection, on the other hand, is a pushing out or extruding and attributing to someone else feelings that are otherwise unacceptable. *(1:80;2:60–63;3:7)*

18. **(D)** The pediatrician should recommend that boy sleep in his own bed. Gently but firmly, the youngster must be taught to tolerate reasonable separation. The parents should support and reward healthy age-appropriate independence. If the parents find it difficult to allow the boy to grow up, time may not take care of the situation.

    When a child routinely sleeps in the parental bed, the parents' sexual activities are likely to be curtailed. In some situations then, a child may be encouraged to stay in the parental bed to help perpetuate sexual distance. However, this would not be the first assumption of the physician.

    In any clinical situation, it is best to look for the common patterns of behavior adaptation and maladaptation. It is premature to ask about the mother's sexual feelings toward her son.

19. **(D)** Scary dreams and even nightmares are often part of normal 4-and 5-year-olds' growing up. At this age, the maturing child understands that he(she) is a separate, unique individual and also is a very small being in a very big world. At night, this awareness of vulnerability may lead to frightening dreams that the youngster gradually outgrows.

    As in any family evaluation, the father should be interviewed. But it is even more important to recognize that the child's behavior is not pathologic, homosexual, or prepsychotic. *(1:694–696;2:71–73;3:176–180)*

20. **(A)** *Phobias, nail biting, bed wetting,* and *nightmares* can all be transitional reactions to stress in a child who basically is emotionally healthy—part of an *adjustment disorder.*

    Autism and autistic behaviors indicate a much more serious and pervasive emotional disorder. *(1:839–840;2:694–695;3:204–205)*

21. **(D)** Average intelligence is usually taken as the Intelligence Quotient levels 90–110—100 mean, plus or minus 10.

    None of the other ranges overlap the mean. *(1:128;2:716–717;3:46)*

22. **(D)** The *highest incidence* of diagnosed or recognized *mental retardation* is the adolescent age group when the growing youngster is faced with the responsibility of complicated social and academic tasks.

    The *borderline retarded,* who may not be diagnosed until the teenage years, often adapt productively to society and, in later years, are no longer recognized as being retarded. *(1:860–862;2:717;3:161–162)*

23. **(A)** The highest incidence of reported mental retardation is among urban ghetto residents.

    Complex cultural factors play a profound role in producing intellectual stunting in children who may already be at risk intellectually and medically.

    In culturally biased tests, these children will tend to test at a lower score level. *(1:860–862;2:717;3:169)*

The diagnosis and treatment of enuresis is referred to in answers 24 through 27.

24. **(B)** An enuretic child is more apt to be a boy with a *family history* of enuresis. Autistic children are often relatively easy to toilet train, while obsessive-compulsive children are typically overtrained. Mentally retarded children may be slower at being trained. The enuretic child is much more likely to be intellectually normal than retarded.

25. **(C)** *Encopresis, psychogenic soiling,* is relatively uncommon but, when present, often coexists with enuresis. Enuresis, a common symptom, only rarely has coexistent encopresis.

There is frequently a parental history of enuresis rather than early toilet training.

Nocturnal enuresis is more common than *diurnal*. Organic defects of the urinary tract are demonstrated in only a small percentage of enuretics.

26. **(B)** Enuresis usually occurs in stage 4 periods of deep sleep, not associated with REM.

27. **(E)** A wide range of treatments has been used in enuretics with varying success. It does appear that many enuretic children are damaged more by being shamed, abused, and overtreated than by the symptom itself. In the total treatment of the child in the family, *psychotherapy* for the child and *counseling* for the parents are often beneficial. With the cooperation of the child, a *conditioning device* or *imipramine* may be effective.

Since enuresis occurs during non-REM deep sleep, *barbiturates* would not be indicated. *(1:843-846;2:697-699;3:197-198)*

28. **(D)** *Petit mal* is not associated with borderline mental retardation. The symptom usually does begin in *childhood*, is treated by *trimethadione*, nearly always disappears before *adulthood*, and often is replaced by *grand mal* attacks. *(1:299-305;2:279-280;3:226)*

29. **(A)** X-rays in cases of *lead poisoning in children* may show increased thickness and density at the zones of provisional calcification of the long bones. However, lead poisoning may be present even in the absence of radiologic signs.

Other diagnostic features would be basophilic stippling of the red cells with hypochromic anemia, coproporphyrinuria, and excessive concentrations of lead in the urine and the blood.

Multiple poorly healed fractures might indicate a *battered child,* a severe nutritional deficiency, or a hypoparathyroid syndrome.

Calcified periosteal hemorrhages would suggest healing lesions of *scurvy.*

Severe vitamin D deficiency, *rickets,* would lead to cupping and fraying of the epiphyseal ends with generalized reduction in shaft density.

Premature closure of the epiphyses may be due to one of the endocrine syndromes producing *premature sexual development. (1:298;2:329-331;3:163)*

30. **(B)** Paradoxically, the child with *attention deficit disorder* may benefit from treatment with stimulants, amphetamines, or, more commonly, methylphenidate.

The youngster with this diagnosis is much more likely to be a boy. The symptoms tend to start in the preschool years but the syndrome is often not diagnosed until grade school.

Increasingly it is being recognized that many of these children do not grow out of their symptoms.

However, in adolescence and adulthood they may be better controlled or expressed in socially less disruptive fashions. *(2:681-683;3:187-190)*

31. **(C)** The youngster (and his family) need immediate treatment. Unless you are competent to handle all pediatric medical treatment, you should plan any treatment program in the closest association with a pediatrician who can treat the boy intensively from a medical aspect.

It is relatively useless to begin psychotherapy in the midst of a life-threatening asthmatic attack. The immediate reality must be handled therapeutically and efficiently before the underlying factors can be elucidated and managed.

Since the mother called you for help, you have the responsibility to see that she and her son have all the assistance they need—and they need it at once, not at an appointment the next day. You must join with her in getting the necessary total treatment and evaluation, medical and psychiatric.

Asthma was at one time considered to be a "cry for mother" or "cry for help." It is now agreed that this is much too simplistic an explanation of an illness with multiple etiological factors. *(1:512-514;2:586-587;3:325)*

32. **(D)** To understand the irreversibility of death, the child must be aware of the continuity of time, be able to fantasize, and have a solid sense of his or her own individuality. This level of maturity usually comes between the ages of 6 and 10 years. The child is typically 7 or 8 years old when he or she begins to understand the basic irreversibility of death. *(2:76;3:179-180)*

33. **(C)** Emotional tensions do not appear to cause sleepwalking. In children who sleepwalk there is usually no evidence of increased psychopathology. Sleepwalking tends to occur during the first half of the night, during non-REM stage 3-4 sleep, and the subject is amnestic for the episode later. Sleepwalking is most common in the 6-12 year age group. *(1:570-572;2:706;3:352-353)*

34. **(D)** If a *barbiturate addict* is abruptly withdrawn from barbiturates, a potentially fatal *abstinence syndrome* may occur. To minimize this abstinence syndrome and to reduce the possibility of withdrawal convulsions, the patient should be taken off barbiturates gradually, in graduated reduced dose levels.

Methadone, paraldehyde, and *chlorpromazine* are inadequate to prevent a disabling abstinence syndrome. *(1:408-409;2:658-661;3:219-220)*

35. **(B)** When the mother has *rubella* in the first month of pregnancy, the risk of *congenital defects* in the child is 50%. The frequency of congenital malformations due to rubella decreases inversely with the duration of pregnancy at the time of the disease.

As a prophylactic measure, before rubella immunization teenage girls were encouraged to contract rubella before marriage. *(1:723;2:723;3:162-163)*

36. **(B)** Children with *phenylketonuria* tend to have head measurements smaller than normal. Hydrocephalus is not a typical finding.

These patients quite often have *blond hair* and *blue eyes*. They frequently have *dermatitis* or *eczema*. *Convulsions* are common. Other siblings may be affected by this disorder, which is transmitted as a simple recessive trait.

The musty odor of the urine was the initial finding that led to the demonstration of this syndrome. *(1: 711–714;2:729–731;3:166)*

37. **(C)** *School refusal* is usually a manifestation of *separation anxiety*. This separation anxiety often affects both the child and the caring person.

The *mentally retarded* child who is more dependent on the parent may have greater difficulty in becoming separate and independent, but school phobia is not specifically associated with retardation.

The *autistic child* who is markedly egocentric often separates easily. He or she may, however, become upset because his or her routine has been disturbed.

Malingering is relatively rare in childhood. *Attention deficit disorder* and school refusal are not directly interrelated. *(1:791–795;2:687–689;3:193)*

38. **(A)** *Fire-setting, enuresis,* and *infantile autism* are all more common in boys.

Enuresis certainly does not need to be treated in hospital. Inpatient care may be needed for the other two syndromes.

Enuresis may respond to *imipramine* but the syndromes of fire-setting or infantile autism are not affected by this drug.

Leo Kanner first described infantile autism.

Fire-setting and enuresis are usually not precursors to childhood schizophrenia. Though infantile autism is included in the childhood psychoses, it is often differentiated from childhood schizophrenia. *(1:592,843–846;2:684–686;3:174–211)*

39. **(C)** *Twirling* is not a major symptom of *infantile autism* but it was described early in the literature. It is still a common question subject and so needs to be remembered. The autistic child is more readily diagnosed by an extreme aloofness, a lack of communicative skills and interpersonal sensitivities, an obsessive need for sameness, and an unusual body posturing. *(1:734–735;2:693–694;3:201)*

40. **(A)** *Phenylketonuria* was first recognized by the musty smell of the urine of these children—due to phenylalanine and its derivatives. *(1:711–714;2:729–731;3:166)*

41. **(E)** *Anaclitic depression, reactive attachment disorder of infancy,* is the withdrawn, overwhelmed "depressed" condition that can develop in infants who are separated from the mothering person in the second 6 months of life—that is, after the infant has developed an emotional bond to another. *(1:771–779;2:691–692; 3:205)*

42. **(D)** *Down's syndrome, mongolism,* is more common in children born to older mothers; these retarded children are more typically the 47-chromosome nondisjunction type of the syndrome. *(1:718–719;2:734–736;3:168)*

43. **(B)** *Strephosymbolia* means, specifically, reversal of letters and words and is one manifestation of dyslexia. Characteristically the child sees *b's* for *d's, p's* for *g's, was* for *saw.* *(1:748–751;2:702–704;3:203)*

44. **(C)** In *acute porphyria,* barbiturates may precipitate or worsen symptoms and are absolutely contraindicated. Acute intermittent porphyria is an autosomal dominant trait. *(1:309–310;2:319–323;3:228)*

45. **(D)** In *childhood enuresis,* imipramine is still often used. Benefit tends to be time limited. The clinician should be alert to the potential toxic effects of this not innocuous drug on children. *(1:843–846;2:697–699; 3:197–198)*

46. **(A)** *Phenylketonuria* is an automosomal recessive metabolic deficiency syndrome that, untreated, can lead to severe mental retardation and convulsions. *(1:711–714;2:729–731;3:166)*

47. **(B)** Butyrophenones are the drugs of choice in treating *Tourette's Disorder* (multiple tics, explosive grunting noises, and coprolalia). *(1:763–765;2:700–701;3:196–197)*

48. **(B)** *Encopresis* is the syndrome of psychogenic *fecal soiling.* The symptom may be due to fecal leakage in a state of chronic constipation or it can be a manifestation of total lack of bowel control. *(1:846–847;2:699–700;3:198)*

49. **(A)** In *Tourette's Disorder,* the patient—usually a child—shows multiple tics, recurrent compulsive swearing (*coprolalia*), and sometimes *echolalia.* The disease may respond to haloperidol. *(1:763–765;2:700–701;3:196–197)*

50. **(E)** *Trichotillomania* is the syndrome, usually seen in children, where the patient compulsively pulls out her (or his) hair, sometimes leading to patchy baldness. These bald areas are in scalp regions accessible to the favored hand. *(1:526;2:695)*

51. **(C)** *Turner's syndrome, gonadal dysgenesis,* occurs in females with 45 xo chromosomes. These patients are typically short-statured, with webbing of the neck and typical facies. Without replacement hormone therapy

they do not develop sexually at puberty. *(1:720;2: 737;3:80)*

52. **(D)** *Lead poisoning* characteristically affects ghetto-area children who have a *pica*—compulsive eating of nonfood substances—for lead-containing plaster or paint from walls. *(1:298;2:329–331;3:163)*

    Chromosome labeling (karyotyping) is becoming increasingly important in psychiatry, especially in understanding the retardation syndromes. The trainee must be acquainted with the more common syndromes.

53. **(B)** *Klinefelter's syndrome* is found in xxy–47 chromosome males. Characteristically, these subjects are tall and thin, with small testes and often moderate gynecomastia. There is a higher incidence of mental retardation in this syndrome. *(1:720;2:736–737;3:168)*

54. **(C)** *Turner's syndrome,* female gonadal dysgenesis, is manifested by females with the 45 chromosome xo pattern.

    These patients are short, somewhat stocky, with webbing of the neck and lack of secondary sexual development at puberty. *(1:720;2:737;3:80)*

55. **(D)** *Trisomy 21* is associated with Down's syndrome. The trisomy may be associated with 46 or 47 chromosomes, depending on the underlying chromosome defect. *(1:718–719;2:734–737;3:168)*

56. **(A)** *Tourette's Disorder*—multiple tics, compulsive swearing, and echolalia in children—is not associated with chromosome defects. These patients have the normal 46-chromosome complement. *(1:763–765;2: 700–701;3:196–197)*

57. **(A)** *Korsakoff's syndrome* is not associated with chromosome defects and these subjects have the normal 46-chromosome count.

    The patients show *confabulation* to cover their severe memory deficit caused by nutritional deficiency, chronic alcoholism, or organic brain damage. *(1:279–281;2:631–633;3:218–219)*

The student must know the basic developmental milestones. A few of these are indicated in the answers to 58 through 66. (1:692–693;2:63–73;3:177)

58. **(B)** The normal child reaches for and can *grasp* a toy at *6 months* of age.

59. **(E)** The growing youngster has adequate muscular coordination and balance to ride a *tricycle* at *3 years. (1:693)*

60. **(C)** The average child can *pick up a small object* with thumb and forefinger by *10 months of age.*
    In the Cattell Infant testing the child is expected

to pick up a pellet with a "scissor" grasp at 9 months and a "pincer" grasp at 11 months. *(1:692;3:177)*

61. **(A)** The growing child *smiles* and cries tears by about *2 months* of age. *(1:692)*

62. **(C)** At *6 months,* the average infant will be *holding out his or her arms* to be taken and held. *(1:692)*

63. **(D)** By *12 months,* the young child should be saying *two or three words* like "Mama" and "Dada" communicatively. *(1:692;3:177)*

64. **(C)** At *4 months,* the child usually starts to *hold up his or her head. (1:692)*

65. **(D)** Normal youngsters can *sit for brief periods* at *6 months* of age. They can sit for longer times when they lean forward, supporting themselves on their hands. *(1:692)*

66. **(E)** At *10 months,* the growing youngster can stand without support. *(1:692;3:177)*

Congenital or hereditary syndromes are discussed in answers 67 through 76. (1:711–722)

67. **(B)** In the *Sturge-Weber-Dimitri syndrome,* classically, the child has a large facial telangiectasis or *port wine stain* involving the trigeminal distribution in the face, most often the ophthalmic division. Associated with this stigma are *intracranial angioma* with resultant focal *seizures* and *paralyses.* Many other symptoms coexist and *mental retardation* is common. *(1:721;2:734;3:166)*

68. **(D)** In *tuberous sclerosis,* the patient may be first recognized by the *adenoma sebaceum* over the nose and cheeks. These patients often have hemangioma, *cysts,* or tumors of the kidney, liver, spleen, and lungs, and *glioma* of the brain (which may become calcified).

    These patients tend to present with *mental retardation* and *seizures. (1:720;2:734;3:166–167)*

69. **(A)** In *neurofibromatosis* (von Recklinghausen's disease), the syndrome tends to be first recognized by the multiple *café au lait spots* and the cutaneous and subcutaneous *neurofibromata* along the nerves. Many of these fibroma become pedunculated.

    Meningiomata and optic and acoustic glioma are not uncommon.

    These patients may present with normal intelligence or with varying degrees of retardation. Epilepsy is a frequent presenting symptom. *(1:720–721;2:734;3:166)*

70. **(E)** The *Kayser–Fleisher ring,* a greenish-yellow ring near the margin of the iris, is characteristic of *Wilson's disease, hepatolenticular degeneration,* where, due to inborn metabolic copper metabolism defect, there is progressive intellectual and motor deterioration with gradually developing hepatic cirrhosis.

    In these patients there is increased urinary excretion of copper. The illness can be treated by penicillamine. *(1:716–717;2:323–324;3:166)*

71. **(C)** In *Turner's syndrome,* the young girl is short-statured with neck webbing or extra neck skin. At puberty there is no development of secondary sex characteristics and the child shows persistent sexual infantilism unless replacement hormonal therapy is given for the ovarian dysgenesis.

    On chromosome testing, the subject shows the 45 chromosome xo pattern. *(1:720;2:737;3:80)*

72. **(C)** The *infantile cerebral lipoidosis, Tay–Sach's disease,* is most common in young children of *Eastern European Jewish* origin. These infants present with progressive hypotonic weakness and lack of development.

    On examination, they show the bilateral *cherry-red spot* on the macula. Death usually occurs in 1 to 3 years.

    Prenatal diagnosis is possible from culture of amniotic cells. *(1:715;2:725–728;3:164)*

73. **(B)** In *phenylketonuria,* the patients are deficient in phenylalanine hydroxylase.

    Frequently these children have blond hair and blue eyes, with dermatitis or eczema. Often they develop convulsions.

    Untreated they become severely retarded. *(1:711–714;2:729–731;3:166)*

74. **(E)** The *cri-du-chat syndrome,* "cat cry" syndrome, occurs in children with a *deletion of the short arm the 5 chromosome.* The subjects are usually markedly retarded and microcephalic with craniofacial anomalies. *(1:720;3:167–168)*

75. **(A)** In *Klinefelter's syndrome,* the subject is an xxy-47-chromosome male, usually of asthenic build. He tends to have small or underdeveloped testes and, commonly, gynecomastia. Mild mental retardation is quite common. *(1:720;2:736–737;3:168)*

76. **(D)** In *bilirubin encephalopathy, kernicterus,* due to Rh incompatibility between mother and fetus, yellow pigmentation of the basal ganglia, cerebellum, and brain stem can be shown on autopsy. These lesions lead to cerebral palsy, deafness, choreoathetosis, and retardation in children who survive.

    This reaction also occurs where there is incompatibility of other blood factors between mother and fetus. *(2:724;3:163)*

The answers to questions 77 through 81 are examples of the use of psychopharmacology in childhood disorders.

77. **(D)** *Attention deficit disorder* is treated with *amphetamines* or methylphenidate. Childhood attention deficit disorder is too often diagnosed on the basis of inadequate and overly vague behavioral and physical criteria. *(1:741–747;2:681–683;3:187–190)*

78. **(B)** *Haloperidol* is presently an effective symptomatic treatment for the *Tourette's Disorder* of multiple tics, coprolalia, and echolalia. *(1:763–765;2:700–701;3:196–197)*

79. **(A)** *Trimethadione* is usually effective in treating children with *petit mal.* *(1:305;3:226)*

80. **(E)** In enuresis, many treatment approaches work when used with enough confidence and consideration for the child patient. *Imipramine* is used in the pharmacological management of this symptom. *(1:843–846;2:697–699;3:197–198)*

81. **(C)** Chronic *lead poisoning* in children is usually treated with calcium disodium versenate. *(1:298;2:329–331;3:163)*

Adult Psychopathology
Questions

INTRODUCTION

Examination questions dealing with adult psychopathology may be focused on a discrete symptom, syndrome, or treatment, but often one question touches on a wide variety of loosely related concepts. The candidate should not assume that topics included in the same questions are necessarily associated.

REFERENCES

For this chapter the reader must be prepared to use the whole range of the standard textbook.

DIRECTIONS (Questions 1 through 64): Each of the numbered items or incomplete statements in this section is followed by answers or by completions of the statement. Select the ONE lettered answer or completion that is BEST in each case.

1. The drift hypothesis is one theory to explain

   (A) the higher incidence of schizophrenia in urban ghetto areas
   (B) the occurrence of Rorschach contamination responses in schizophrenia
   (C) the frequency of illusions in senile dementia
   (D) recurring flashbacks after hallucinogen intake
   (E) the incidence of twin autism

2. Typically, an amphetamine-induced psychosis is preponderantly

   (A) paranoid
   (B) depressive
   (C) grandiose
   (D) confusional
   (E) manic

3. In depression all of the following occur *except*

   (A) early-morning awakening
   (B) chronic tiredness
   (C) loss of appetite
   (D) flattened affect
   (E) low self-esteem

4. The highest suicide rate is likely to occur in

   (A) adolescent black girls
   (B) elderly white males
   (C) middle-class menopausal women
   (D) adolescent white males
   (E) married teenage females

5. The acutely depressed patient may be treated with one or a combination of the following *except*

   (A) monoamine oxidase inhibitors
   (B) electroconvulsive therapy
   (C) imipramine
   (D) leucotomy
   (E) psychotherapy

6. A serious suicide attempt is more likely in patients who

   (A) are quietly depressed
   (B) threaten suicide
   (C) have made previous serious attempts
   (D) have received bad news
   (E) are given inadequate antidepressant medication

7. A suicide attempt may be a manifestation of

   (A) self-punishment
   (B) wish to rejoin loved ones
   (C) angry retaliation
   (D) effort to end a painful situation
   (E) all of the above

8. Bleuler described all the following as fundamental symptoms of schizophrenia *except*

   (A) autism
   (B) affect inappropriate
   (C) aggression uncontrolled
   (D) ambivalence
   (E) associations loosened

9. All of the following are true about obesity *except*

   (A) more common in lower socioeconomic groups
   (B) diagnosed when body weight is above 120% standard weight
   (C) women show higher prevalence of obesity than men
   (D) weight reduction more effective where obesity started in childhood
   (E) group self-help treatment programs are often most helpful

10. Suppression is

   (A) unconscious blocking out of unacceptable emotions
   (B) conscious effort to block out disturbing feelings
   (C) return to earlier patterns of behavior
   (D) redirection of drives in a socially acceptable fashion
   (E) emphasizing the opposite of the true feelings

11. Displacement is

   (A) externalization of inner feelings or conflicts
   (B) separating an idea from the accompanying feelings
   (C) symbolically doing the opposite of the true feelings
   (D) blocking external reality from awareness
   (E) changing focus of emotions to a substitute

12. Barbiturates affect REM sleep by

   (A) increasing REM periods
   (B) reducing REM sleep time
   (C) increasing REM sleep and producing frightening dreams
   (D) increasing REM sleep to as much as 50% of sleep cycle
   (E) no change of REM cycles but rise in arousal threshold

13. When barbiturates are withdrawn from chronic users, there is

   (A) increased REM time, often with nightmares
   (B) temporary abolition of REM sleep
   (C) increased REM sleep without disturbing dreams

(D) unchanged REM cycles but production of nightmares

(E) no change in REM activity but lowering of arousal threshold

14. All of the following traits are characteristic of the anal character *except*

(A) punctuality
(B) dependency
(C) neatness
(D) miserliness
(E) obstinacy

15. Three times in the past month, a 42-year-old married woman has arrived unexpectedly for consultation after the doctor's regular office hours. She has complained of abdominal pain but no specific physical findings can be discovered. The next time she arrives to see the doctor when he is working alone in the evening, he should

(A) tell her firmly that there is nothing wrong with her and she should see a psychiatrist
(B) point out she needs careful, thorough evaluation and give her the next available appointment during scheduled office hours
(C) sit down and have a long heart-to-heart talk with her
(D) show her that she has many things to be thankful for and should pull herself together
(E) refuse to answer the office doorbell

16. An 18-year-old girl comes to see the physician. Soon after she begins talking, she starts to cry. Usually the doctor should

(A) comfort her and put her at ease by gently patting her arm or shoulder
(B) quickly apologize for disturbing her
(C) reassure her that everything will soon be all right
(D) ignore her crying and firmly continue the history taking
(E) acknowledge her crying but gently try to find out what led the girl to cry

17. The chronic emotional handicapping produced by severe maternal deprivation has been shown most clearly by

(A) Harlow's studies of primates
(B) Freud's "Little Hans" study
(C) Piaget's investigation of growing children
(D) Kallmann's twin studies
(E) Hollingshead's and Redlich's social studies

18. The following are examples of dissociation *except*

(A) multiple personality
(B) fugue state
(C) sleep walking
(D) waxy flexibility
(E) automatic writing

19. The following patterns are all common in obsessive-compulsive disorder *except*

(A) intellectualization
(B) magical thinking
(C) recurrent obtrusive thoughts
(D) repetitive rumination
(E) dissociation

20. All of the following are correct about depression *except*

(A) psychomotor retardation common
(B) tends to be more common in men
(C) frequent appetite loss and weight reduction
(D) frequent sleep difficulties
(E) males may become impotent

21. Cross-cultural studies of emotional disorders have shown greatest agreement on prevalence of

(A) psychophysiological disorders
(B) phobias
(C) psychoses
(D) personality disorders
(E) sexual deviations

22. All of the following characteristics are typical of the oral personality *except*

(A) dependency
(B) narcissism
(C) inability to delay gratification
(D) obstinacy
(E) greed

23. All of the following are associated with REM sleep *except*

(A) rapid eye movements
(B) peak plasma testosterone levels
(C) penile erection
(D) enuresis
(E) dreaming

24. All of the following are associated with delirium tremens *except*

(A) visual and tactile hallucinations
(B) irregular flapping tremor of arms
(C) uncommon before age 30
(D) disoriented for time and place
(E) marked motor restlessness

25. In the management of the elderly patient, the following are useful *except*

(A) nighttime barbiturates for insomnia
(B) vitamin supplements
(C) well-lighted, simplified home environment
(D) hospital care if markedly confused or agitated
(E) counseling for the family

26. Electroconvulsive treatment is most specifically therapeutic for

    (A) delirium tremens
    (B) senile dementia
    (C) major depression
    (D) schizophrenia, residual type
    (E) obsessive–compulsive

27. The evidence for genetic factors in the etiology of schizophrenia is most clearly demonstrated by

    (A) adopted away studies
    (B) Sheldon's constitutional studies
    (C) Harlow's infant-rearing primate research
    (D) Spitz's studies on infant deprivation
    (E) Freud's Schreber study

28. The prognosis in schizophrenia is liable to be unfavorable when all of the following factors are present *except*

    (A) insidious onset
    (B) lack of obvious precipitating factors
    (C) previous schizoid personality
    (D) clearly apparent anxiety
    (E) parental and familial psychopathology

29. A depressed patient is most likely to commit suicide when

    (A) the depression is most profound
    (B) he or she is starting to recover from the depression
    (C) he or she receives bad news or a disappointment
    (D) he or she becomes physically ill
    (E) he or she has completed a course of electroconvulsive treatments

30. In bipolar disorder, manic type, all the following symptoms commonly occur *except*

    (A) hyperactivity
    (B) disturbed sleep
    (C) episodes of depression
    (D) auditory and visual hallucinations
    (E) excitement and elation

31. Sensory deprivation is a causative factor in each of the following *except*

    (A) factory assembly-line accidents
    (B) psychosis in coronary care patients
    (C) psychotic states in body cast patients
    (D) petit mal seizures
    (E) highway accidents

32. Freud postulated that paranoia was a manifestation of

    (A) unresolved dependency needs
    (B) identification with the aggressor
    (C) an anaclitic depressive reaction
    (D) repressed homosexual impulses
    (E) introjection and symbolization

33. Weight loss, early-morning wakening, and general tiredness are usually symptomatic of

    (A) paranoia
    (B) schizophrenia
    (C) obsessive–compulsive
    (D) depression
    (E) phobias

34. Folie à deux is

    (A) mercury poisoning
    (B) psychotic reaction seen in Malayans
    (C) form of presenile dementia
    (D) result of infant maternal deprivation
    (E) communicated psychosis

35. The largest single group of hospitalized psychiatric patients in North America have the diagnosis

    (A) bipolar disorder
    (B) schizophrenia
    (C) organic brain syndrome
    (D) alcoholism
    (E) drug abuse

36. In treating posttraumatic stress disorder, acute combat neurosis, which of the following is appropriate?

    (A) remove immediately to base hospital for intensive psychotherapy
    (B) handle in front-line station with brief, firm support and temporary sedation
    (C) return to home country for rehabilitation
    (D) insist that the soldier remain in front-line duty and pull himself together
    (E) none of the above

37. A 37-year-old man complains of chronic lower back pain. Repeated physical, laboratory, and radiological examinations are negative. The doctor should

    (A) tell the patient that he is absolutely healthy and should forget the pain
    (B) tell the patient that the pain is all in his mind
    (C) tell the patient that such pain usually indicates personal or family problems
    (D) ask the patient about his individual, family, and work situations
    (E) prescribe medication to relax his back muscles

38. In using the muscle relaxant succinylcholine during electroconvulsive therapy, the physician must be alert to the rare complication in which the

    (A) relaxant may potentiate the convulsive effect
    (B) patient may constitutionally lack succinylcholinesterase and so stay apneic

(C) succinylcholine may precipitate a toxic psychosis

(D) muscle relaxant may cause acute hemolysis

(E) patient is resistant to the succinylcholine

39. An idiot savant is a(n)

(A) intellectually superior person who has one limited clearly defined area of retardation

(B) basically retarded individual who has a very limited specialized area of superior functioning

(C) mentally defective person with a mental age of 3 to 7 years

(D) adolescent or young adult, diagnosed as retarded in school, but now functioning as an acceptable member of society

(E) socially deprived youngster who scores low on standard intelligence testing

40. In the treatment of acute mania, all of the following may be appropriate *except*

(A) lithium carbonate

(B) chlorpromazine

(C) electroconvulsive therapy

(D) hospitalization

(E) imipramine

41. All of the following statements are true about obesity *except*

(A) more common in lower socioeconomic groups

(B) more common in women, especially after age 50

(C) those affected commonly have oral, demanding personalities

(D) individual psychotherapy usually unsuccessful over the long term

(E) juvenile-onset obesity tends to persist

42. In law, criminal responsibility may be determined on the basis of all the following guidelines *except*

(A) M'Naghten rule

(B) Durham Decision

(C) irresistible impulse test

(D) testamentary capacity

(E) right and wrong test

43. In addicts using morphine, heroin, or methadone, an abstinence syndrome may be precipitated by the injection of

(A) *n*-allyl normorphine

(B) meperidine

(C) codeine

(D) chlorpromazine

(E) methadone

44. With chronic dependency, convulsions may occur on sudden withdrawal from

(A) marijuana

(B) amphetamines

(C) lysergic acid diethylamide

(D) meprobamate

(E) monoamine oxidase inhibitors

45. Chronic amphetamine use may lead to a clinical syndrome similar to

(A) manic–depressive illness, manic type

(B) schizophrenia, paranoid type

(C) schizophrenia, hebephrenic or disorganized type

(D) delirium tremens

(E) catastrophic reaction

46. Tricyclic antidepressants should be avoided where there is (are)

(A) senile dementia

(B) urinary retention

(C) sleep disturbances

(D) weight and appetite loss

(E) myopia

47. Hypnosis would be therapeutically useful in treating

(A) schizophrenia, residual type

(B) dysthymic disorder

(C) conversion disorder

(D) senile dementia

(E) bipolar disorder, manic type

48. Which premorbid personality type has the greatest predisposition to involutional melancholia?

(A) paranoid

(B) schizoid

(C) obsessive–compulsive

(D) histrionic

(E) asthenic

49. Patients taking monoamine oxidase inhibitors should be warned to avoid

(A) cholesterol

(B) butter

(C) polyunsaturated fats

(D) cheese

(E) salt

50. Electroconvulsive therapy is most useful in treating

(A) hypochondriasis

(B) major depression

(C) schizophrenia, residual type

(D) senile dementia

(E) infantile autism

51. A 17-year-old giggling, weeping, schizophrenic girl is brought to your office because "her head is turning to one side." Your best initial procedure would be

    (A) immediate electroconvulsive therapy
    (B) intramuscular benztropine
    (C) intramuscular amobarbital
    (D) oral propanolol
    (E) intramuscular haloperidol

52. Stressful life events have been shown to lead to increased incidence of physical and psychiatric illness. The life event found to be most stressful is

    (A) death of a close family member
    (B) marriage separation
    (C) death of a husband or wife
    (D) retirement
    (E) personal injury

53. Hallucinations may occur in all of the following *except*

    (A) bipolar disorder, manic type
    (B) cyclothymic disorder
    (C) schizophrenia, disorganized type
    (D) major depression
    (E) delirium tremens

54. In psychoanalytic theory, the major factor in producing depression is

    (A) projection
    (B) sublimation
    (C) introjection
    (D) dissocation
    (E) displacement

55. The work of grief or mourning is the

    (A) continued absence of obvious feelings following the death of a loved one
    (B) lengthy prolongation of sadness after a loss
    (C) emotional process of adapting to a loss and reinvesting in others
    (D) denial that is necessary to shield the bereaved from awareness of loss
    (E) accentuated grief reactions due to guilt or ambivalence

56. All of the following are characteristic of delirium *except*

    (A) impulsive behavior
    (B) labile mood changes
    (C) neologisms
    (D) disorientation
    (E) memory loss

57. Peripheral neuropathy is most liable to occur with chronic use of

    (A) reserpine
    (B) chloral hydrate
    (C) disulfiram
    (D) thioridazine
    (E) paraldehyde

58. Systematic desensitization is most often therapeutically beneficial in

    (A) passive–aggressive personality
    (B) conversion disorder
    (C) depression
    (D) phobia
    (E) attention deficit disorder

59. Parental superego lacunae are liable to lead to

    (A) paranoia
    (B) delinquency
    (C) phobia
    (D) schizophrenia
    (E) mental retardation

60. A mother asks her 15-year-old daughter where she is going this evening. The daughter hesitates. When she does tell, her mother is very likely to respond "I don't know why you need to ask my permission all the time. You're a big girl now!" On the other hand, when she does not tell in extensive detail, her mother will complain loudly that she is not being loved, appreciated, and respected. This situation is an exmaple of

    (A) Von Domarus Principle
    (B) double-bind
    (C) superego lacunae
    (D) reaction formation
    (E) folie à deux

61. A black physician has a series of patient deaths in spite of his meticulous treatment. He is depressed by his clinical results but begins to be less guilt ridden; he now feels that his patients were probably poisoned by the hospital pharmacy medication so he would not be so obviously better than his white colleagues. He has now developed a

    (A) dissociative reaction
    (B) paranoia
    (C) sublimation
    (D) reaction formation
    (E) phobia

Questions 62 and 63

A 26-year-old woman is hospitalized at the request of her husband. In recent weeks she has refused to leave home, saying the Communists were trying to kill her. She has twice tried to telephone the president to offer her assistance in the War of Liberation. When her husband tries to reason with her, she tells him that her special "messages" tell her what to do.

62. The probable diagnosis is

    (A) paranoid personality disorder
    (B) schizophrenia, disorganized type
    (C) phobic disorder
    (D) histrionic personality disorder
    (E) schizophrenia, paranoid type

63. The most appropriate treatment is

    (A) amphetamines
    (B) imipramine
    (C) haloperidol
    (D) phenobarbital
    (E) methylphenidate

64. A 24-year-old married man comes for marital counseling. At his request, the counsellor gives fairly specific advice. The patient does not attempt to carry out certain suggestions and even seems to be acting directly counter to other directions of the counsellor. The patient may be showing which of the following personality disorders?

    (A) cyclothymic
    (B) histrionic
    (C) compulsive
    (D) passive–aggressive
    (E) schizoid

DIRECTIONS (Questions 65 through 113): Each group of items in this section consists of lettered headings followed by a set of numbered words or phrases. For each numbered word or phrase, select the ONE lettered heading that is most closely associated with it. Each lettered heading may be selected once, more than once, or not at all.

Questions 65 through 68

    (A) general neurone lipid deposition
    (B) frontoparietal cortical atrophy
    (C) congestion and hemorrhage around third ventricle and aqueduct and in mamillary bodies
    (D) cavity formation in basal ganglia

65. General paresis (paralysis)

66. Wilson's disease

67. Wernicke's encephalopathy

68. Tay-Sach's disease

Questions 69 through 73

    (A) stupor, excitement, negativism, automatisms
    (B) shallow, apathetic, moody, vague, illogical
    (C) aloof, distrustful, suspicious, grandiose, sometimes assaultive

    (D) silly, giggling, hallucinating, regressed
    (E) bizarre ideas with depression and elation, anxious

Schizophrenia

69. Residual

70. Disorganized

71. Paranoid

72. Catatonic

73. Schizoaffective

Questions 74 through 78

    (A) episodes of REM sleep
    (B) three-per-second spike and wave
    (C) diffuse slow activity on electroencephalogram
    (D) temporal lobe EEG foci
    (E) increased REM sleep with nightmares

74. Following alcohol withdrawal

75. Petit mal

76. Psychomotor epilepsy

77. Narcolepsy

78. Delirium

Questions 79 through 83

    (A) up to 50% sleep cycle is REM sleep
    (B) suppression of REM sleep
    (C) rebound increase in REM sleep with nightmares
    (D) non-REM stage 4 sleep
    (E) alpha rhythm declines with increasing slow-wave activity

79. After barbiturate withdrawal in chronic users

80. Newborn

81. During sensory deprivation

82. Amphetamines

83. Sleepwalking

Questions 84 through 88

    (A) basophilic stippling
    (B) neurofibrillary tangles and cortical plaques
    (C) elevated urine porphobilinogen
    (D) lowered srrum ceruloplasmin
    (E) lowered basal ganglia dopamine

84. Acute intermittent pophyria

85. Hepatolenticular degeneration

86. Chronic lead poisoning

87. Parkinsonism

88. Alzheimer's disease

Questions 89 through 93

    (A) more organized delusions of persecution and grandiosity
    (B) loss of interest and drive; aimless, apathetic; illogical; loose
    (C) autism, retardation, toe walking
    (D) grinning, grimacing, and silly; hallucinations
    (E) mutism, posturing, rigidity, stupor

89. Schizophrenia, residual

90. Schizophrenia, disorganized type

91. Schizophrenia, paranoid type

92. Schizophrenia, catatonic type

93. Schizophrenia, childhood type

Questions 94 through 98

    (A) conversion disorder
    (B) Korsakoff's syndrome
    (C) bipolar disorder, manic type
    (D) Ganser syndrome
    (E) transvestism

94. Confabulation

95. Cross dressing

96. La belle indifference

97. Approximate answer

98. Flight of ideas

Questions 99 through 103

    (A) marked impairment of reality contact, often with severe personality disorganization
    (B) stable, maladaptive patterns of interaction during developmental years
    (C) temporary acute reaction to marked stress
    (D) maladaptive reaction to anxiety without severe reality distortion or personality disorganization
    (E) chronic fixed maladaptive behavior patterns

99. Psychosis

100. Neurosis

101. Conduct disorder

102. Adjustment disorder

103. Personality disorder

Questions 104 through 108

    (A) sexual gratification from an inanimate object
    (B) desire to change to the opposite sex
    (C) pathological sexual interest in children
    (D) dressing in clothing of opposite sex
    (E) sexual gratification through self-exposure

104. Pedophilia

105. Transvestism

106. Fetishism

107. Transsexualism

108. Exhibitionism

Questions 109 through 113

    (A) acute agitation in brain-injured person unable to solve problem
    (B) unacceptable feelings repressed but symbolized in physical symptoms
    (C) obsessive overeating
    (D) compulsive chewing and grinding
    (E) illusion of previous experience

109. Conversion

110. Déjà vu

111. Catastrophic reaction

112. Bruxism

113. Bulimia

Answers and Explanations

1. **(A)** The *drift hypothesis* is one theory to explain the higher rates of schizophrenia in populations that are disorganized or highly mobile. The theory needs greater validation. *(1:196;3:144)*

2. **(A)** An *amphetamine-induced psychosis* is typically paranoid in nature and may resemble a paranoid schizophrenic reaction, though the subject usually shows less thought disorder. *(1:403–405;2:663;3:221–222)*

3. **(D)** In *depression* there is an increase in depressive affect. In schizophrenia there may be a flattening of all affect.

   The other symptoms, early-morning awakening, chronic tiredness, loss of appetite, and low self-esteem, are characteristic of depression. *(1:245–284; 2:417–422;3:226–228)*

4. **(B)** The highest *suicide rate* is likely to occur in elderly white males. *(1:575,886;2:118–120;3:270–272)*

5. **(D)** *Leucotomy* is not of therapeutic use with the acutely depressed. Psychosurgery is limited now to chronic intractable and disabling emotional disorders.

   In the treatment of the acutely depressed, *electroconvulsive therapy* has the most prompt therapeutic effect but the *monoamine oxidase inhibitors* or the *imipramine*-related antidepressant drugs are often tried first. *Psychotherapy* is helpful in all phases of the illness. *(1:683–687;2:843–845;3:278–280)*

6. **(C)** When an individual has allowed himself or herself to cross the crucial prohibiting personal and social barrier and makes a serious *suicidal* attempt, that restraining barrier is much weaker on subsequent occasions. The person who has made a previous serious suicide attempt is more liable to make a further serious attempt and to succeed in killing himself or herself.

   Any suicide gesture, comment, or tendency must be taken very seriously in all patients. *(1:575–580;2: 118–122;3:270–272)*

7. **(E)** Suicide and suicidal behaviors are symptomatic manifestations of many feelings, drives, and conflicts.

   Quite commonly a suicide attempt is a form of self-hurting or self-punishment as an expiation for guilt. Following the death of a loved person, suicide may be an attempt to rejoin the dear departed. In the immature and the childish, a suicide attempt may be an angry retaliation akin to "I will eat worms and die—and you will be sorry."

   Suicide is always one way to bring pain to an end or to settle an intolerable problem. *(1:575–580;2: 118–122;3:270–272)*

8. **(C)** In his book *Dementia Praecox or the Group of Schizophrenias,* Eugen Bleuler lists the fundamental symptoms of *schizophrenia* as loosened *associations,* inappropriate *affect,* persistent, pervasive *ambivalence,* and a pathological predominance of the subject's inner life, *autism*—these symptoms are sometimes called the four A's, with a fifth A, the *accessory symptoms,* under which Bleuler included all the symptoms he thought arose from the fundamental symptoms. These accessory symptoms are hallucinations and delusions. *(1:194,203;2:347;3:246)*

9. **(D)** Obesity, diagnosed when the body weight is greater than 120% of the standard body weight listed in height–weight tables, is more common in women and, in both sexes, is more prevalent in lower socioeconomic groups.

   Group self-help programs, such as TOPS (Take Off Pounds Sensibly), provide what is often the most effective therapeutic approach available.

   The prognosis for effective weight reduction is especially poor when obesity has been present from childhood. *(1:495–499;2:550–554;3:324–325)*

10. **(B)** The *unconscious blocking out* of unacceptable feelings or drives is called *repression.* *(1:80;2:93–96; 3:7)*

    Suppression is the *deliberate* or *conscious* effort to block out disturbing feelings. These are emotions that are in conscious awareness but the subject decides not to think about them. *(1:80;2:95–96;3:7)*

Regression is a return to earlier patterns of behavior. This can occur in normal people during times of severe stress and may also be part of socially accepted relaxation—at a party, participants may act in a regressed fashion, acting "childish" or "letting their hair down." *(1:80;2:105;3:10)*

The redirection of otherwise unacceptable drives in a socially acceptable fashion is called *sublimation.*

Many occupations can be said to be examples of sublimation. *(1:80;2:108;3:9–10)*

The emotional defense where the subject unconsciously copes with his or her anxiety by emphasizing the opposite of his true feelings is *reaction formation. (1:79;2:98–99;3:8)*

11. **(E)** In *displacement,* externally directed feelings are displaced away from an unacceptable focus to a more tolerable target. It may not be considered nice to be angry with God when a loved relative dies. The understandable anger at this loss may be displaced onto the physician. *(1:80;2:101–102;3:9)*
A. *Projection* is the mechanism whereby unacceptable inner feelings are externalized and attributed to an external source or person. *(1:80;2:102–103;3:9)*
B. When an idea is separated from the accompanying feelings, the unconscious defense process of *isolation* has occurred. *(1:80;2:94;3:10)*
C. *Undoing* is the symbolic, ritualistic, or magical behavior carried out to undo the fantasied effects of underlying true emotions. *(1:80;2:477–478;3:10)*
D. When external reality has been blocked from awareness, *denial* has occurred. Denial distorts reality and takes a high expenditure of psychic energy to maintain. *(1:80;2:107;3:8)*

12. **(B)** *Barbiturates* reduce *REM sleep* time. *(1:563;2:44;3:345)*

13. **(A)** When *barbiturates* are *withdrawn* from chronic users, the electroencephalogram shows an increase in *REM sleep,* a "rebound" phenomenon. Often this increased REM sleep is accompanied by *frightening nightmares. (1:563;2:44;3:345–346)*

14. **(B)** In psychoanalytic theory, the person with an *anal character* (due to fixation at the anal training stage of psychosexual development) is characteristically punctual, neat, tidy, somewhat miserly, and has a marked tendency to be obstinate or stubborn.
Dependency is more a characteristic of the oral character. *(1:70–71;2:65–66;3:5)*

15. **(B)** This question presents the problem of the seductive patient. While the clinician must be aware of and sensitive to the seductive patient, he must also give her the medical and psychological care she needs. This is the correct approach. The patient is entitled to thorough medical care. To maintain a therapeutic

clinical distance, the doctor should set up an appointment during office hours when he can have his nurse in attendance. If the physical examination is still negative, it would be appropriate to suggest that her symptoms might be a sign of stress, strain, or difficulty. A psychiatrist then might be called in consultation.
A. If there is "nothing wrong with her," she does not need to see a psychiatrist either. This is an example of poorly sublimated anger on the physician's part.
C. To sit down and have a heart-to-heart talk with her, alone after office hours, would mean that the doctor was allowing himself to be seduced. He has become vulnerable and he may or may not then be able to help the patient in this relatively unstructured intimacy.
D. This woman is hurting somewhere, somehow. She feels pain. She is seeking closeness. The "pull yourself together, woman" approach may ask her to use emotional strengths she does not have and leave her feeling more inadequate and guilty when she cannot fulfill the physician's demands.
E. To refuse to answer the door bell is personally rude and unprofessional, the bluntest form of rejection. When a patient is in pain and asking for help, the doctor should not refuse to respond. *(1:112–116;2:195–202;3:31–43)*

16. **(E)** The doctor does not really know why the patient is crying. A pat on the arm or shoulder may appear seductive, threatening, or intrusive to the patient. The physician must learn to cope with pain and not apologize in the presence of pain, physical or emotional—he or she can be empathetic but not apologetic. It is presumptuous to assure a patient that everything will be all right when this may be totally untrue. If the situation is indeed dreadful, by this comment the physician will have made it more difficult for the patient to share the anguish and the cause of the anguish. Too many physicians take this path of steadfastly reassuring because they find it difficult to tolerate anxiety or uncertainty. To ignore the patient's crying would be totally unrealistic and insensitive and probably would reflect the doctor's own discomfort.
The correct approach is quietly to recognize with the patient that she is crying and then try to find out with her why she is so bothered. *(1:112–116;2:195–202;3:31–43)*

17. **(A)** *Harlow's primate studies* at the University of Wisconsin have most clearly shown the chronic emotional handicapping produced by severe *maternal deprivation. (1:45–53;2:69–70;3:59–60)*
B. In his *"Little Hans" study,* using the father as intermediary, *Freud* evaluated and treated the phobia of a 5-year-old boy. *(1:322;2:471)*
C. *Piaget's* investigation of *normal growing children,* starting with his own family, has led to an extensive theory of child development. *(1:34–37;2:85–86; 3:177)*

D. *Kallman's twin studies* suggest a genetic basis for schizophrenia and for homosexuality. Later studies have challenged the significance of Kallmann's findings. *(1:197;2:155;3:249)*

E. *Hollingshead's and Redlich's studies* pointed out the different incidence of emotional illness in different socioeconomic groups and the varying availability of care. *(1:865;2:167;3:145–146)*

18. **(D)** *Waxy flexibility, cerea flexibilitas,* is the motor symptom where the patient maintains a posture in which he or she has been placed. Typically, waxy flexibility occurs in catatonic schizophrenia. *(1:211–212; 2:115;3:248)*

    Multiple personality, fugue states, sleep walking (somnambulism), and *automatic writing* are all examples of *dissociation. (1:353–357;2:105–107;3:291–292)*

19. **(E)** *Dissociation,* as detailed in answer 18, is a manifestation of dissociative disorders.

    Intellectualization, magical thinking, recurrent obtrusive thoughts, and *repetitive rumination* are all typical symptoms of an *obsessive–compulsive* disorder. *(1:353;2:476–482;3:288–289)*

20. **(B)** Depression tends to be more common in women. Psychomotor retardation, loss of appetite and weight, sleep difficulties, and male impotence are common symptoms of depression. *(1:240–241;2:417–422;3:263–268)*

21. **(C)** Across cultures, it is easiest to define what is intolerable, crazy, hospitalized, or, in modern terms, psychotic. *Cross-cultural studies* of emotional disorders have shown greatest agreement on the incidence of psychoses.

    The definition of sexual deviations and personality disorders varies from culture to culture. Phobias are more difficult to measure, as they are not hospital directed. There is still much discussion about the etiology and syndrome definition of the psychophysiological disorders. *(1:54–59;2:151–153;3:139–148)*

22. **(D)** In psychoanalytic theory, an *oral personality* or a person with an *oral character,* fixated at the *oral phase* of psychosexual development, is primarily dependent, narcissistic and self-centered, greedy, demanding, and unable to delay gratification.

    Obstinacy is more characteristic of the *anal* personality, a fixation at the training phase. *(1:70–71; 2:65–66;3:5)*

23. **(B)** Enuresis occurs most often during non-REM sleep.

    Plasma testosterone increases during sleep with maximum levels during REM phases. REM specifically denotes *rapid eye movements* and during these

REM sleep stages dreaming predominantly occurs. Phasic penile erections tend to precede REM sleep phases by several minutes. *(1:558–560;2:41–45;3:197–198)*

24. **(B)** In *delirium tremens,* a coarse tremor of the hands, lips, and face is a common symptom. An *irregular flapping tremor* of the extended arms is an ominous sign of *hepatic failure* and is not part of the delirium tremens syndrome.

    Delirium tremens is relatively uncommon in young adults under age 30. The typical delirium tremens patient shows visual and tactile hallucinations, disorientation for time and place, and often a marked motor restlessness that may exhaust the patient. *(1:419–420;2:628–631;3:217–218)*

25. **(A)** In *elderly* patients, nighttime *barbiturates* are liable to precipitate confusion and disorientation. *(1:882;2:239;3:357)*

    In the general management of the elderly, it is necessary to ensure a *good balanced diet,* with *vitamin supplements* as indicated. The family may be helped by *counseling* in the management of elderly relatives. To prevent the development of confusional states, a *well-lighted, simplified home environment* is often beneficial. If the geriatric patient does become markedly confused and agitated, it will help the patient and the family to suggest *hospital care. (1:881–886;2: 241;3:215–216)*

26. **(C)** *Electroconvulsive therapy* is the most specific therapy for major depression. This treatment is ineffective or contraindicated in delirium tremens, senile dementia, schizophrenia, residual type, or obsessive–compulsive neurosis. *(1:682;2:836–840;3:131)*

27. **(A)** The evidence for *genetic factors* in the etiology of *schizophrenia* is clearly demonstrated by adopted away studies. *(1:197;2:349–353;3:250–251)*

    B. *Sheldon* attempted to correlate body type with personality. His main constitutional types were the *ectomorph, endomorph,* and *mesomorph. (2:156–157)*

    C. *Harlow's* primate studies focus on the effect of mother–child separation and infant deprivation. *(1: 47–53;2:69–70;3:59–60)*

    D. *Spitz* did his research on the effects of human mother–child separation and of institutionalization. *(1:774;2:692;3:186)*

    E. In the study of the *Schreber case, Sigmund Freud* outlined his theoretical concepts for the development of paranoid thinking. *(1:226–227;2:444;3:4–10)*

28. **(D)** The *prognosis* in *schizophrenia* is less favorable when the onset of the illness is *insidious,* with no obvious *precipitating factors,* in a person with a previously *schizoid* personality coming from a family with a high incidence of *psychopathology.*

    Where the schizophrenia patient is clearly anxious and distressed, the prognosis is more optimistic. *(1:220–221;2:285–289;3:252–255)*

29. **(B)** When the depression is most profound, the depressed patient is more likely to be immobilized by the absolute depth of the depression. When beginning to recover from the depressive apathy, he or she is still profoundly depressed but is more mobile and active, and can act out the depression in *suicide.*

Bad news, disappointment, and physical illness can certainly deepen the depression of a patient already depressed.

A course of electroconvulsive treatments should symptomatically have alleviated the depression. *(1: 579;2:118–122;3:270–272)*

30. **(D)** *Hallucinations* in the *manic* type of *manic-depressive illness* are not common and more typically are illusionary distortions. Clearly formed visual and auditory hallucinations are unusual even in *delirious mania.*

Excitement, elation, hyperactivity, disturbed sleep, and periodic brief episodes of *depressive affect* are common symptoms in *bipolar disorder, manic type. (1:249;2:413–417;3:264–266)*

31. **(D)** *Sensory deprivation* is not a specific causative factor in producing *petit mal seizures.* Sensory deprivation does lead to accidents on the highways (highway hypnosis) and on monotonous factory assembly-line work. Sensory deprivation is a major factor leading to psychotic reactions in coronary care patients and in patients immobilized in body casts. *(1:59–64;2:177–178;3:58)*

32. **(D)** Freud postulated that *paranoia* was a manifestation of unresolved *homosexual* conflicts (Schreber case). *(1:226–227;2:450–453;3:4–10)*

33. **(D)** Weight loss, early-morning awakening, and general tiredness are usually symptomatic of *depression.* *(1:246;2:417–421;3:266–268)*

34. **(E)** *Folie à deux* is a form of *communicated psychosis* where a submissive or passive person takes on the psychosis, most often paranoid, of the dominant partner, relative, or friend. *(1:229–230;2:453;3:257)*
A. *Chronic mercury poisoning,* which used to be an occupational disease of hatters and is depicted in the Mad Hatter in *Alice in Wonderland,* may lead to irritability, depression, and sometimes hallucinations. *(1:298–299;2:331)*
B. *Latah* is a profound startle reaction or sudden eruption of bizarre behavior seen in Malaysian women due to acute disruptive anxiety or an exacerbation of more serious underlying psychopathology. *(1:549–550)*
C. *Pick's disease* and *Alzheimer's disease* are the two most common forms of *senile dementia. (1:286–289; 2:242–246;3:215–216)*

D. Children seem to be most vulnerable to *maternal deprivation* between the ages of 6 and 24 months. Separation from the mother leads to a wide range of infant symptoms and may predispose to the development of serious psychopathology in later life. *(1:772–779;2:691–692;3:60–61)*

35. **(B)** The largest group of *hospitalized psychiatric patients* in North America have the diagnosis of schizophrenia. *(1:196;2:348;3:141)*

36. **(B)** In treating the soldier with an *acute combat neurosis* (posttraumatic stress disorder), the patient should be treated promptly and firmly with strong psychological support, temporary sedation as needed, and early return to duty if possible. Withdrawal from duty and hospitalization tend to accentuate or perpetuate emotional disability. *(1:335–339;2:490;3:289)*

37. **(D)** Before making any diagnosis, including a psychiatric diagnosis, the physician must show by examination that the condition does exist. Just because an organic illness cannot be proved at that time does not allow the physician to diagnose a psychiatric illness. Neither medical nor psychiatric illnesses are diagnosed merely by excluding the other. In order to verify whether an emotional illness does exist, the doctor should make the requisite examination, which, in this case, could begin by asking about the patient's life situation.

To prescribe medication for a symptom without a clearly defined etiology is dubious medical care that may lead to concealment of a serious disorder, medical or psychiatric. *(1:136–138;2:184–202;3:31–43)*

38. **(B)** When using the muscle relaxant *succinylcholine* during electroconvulsive therapy, the anesthetist must be cautious lest the patient is one of the rare people who lack active *succinylcholinesterase.* These patients are deficient in their ability to break down the drug so the induced apnea may continue for an extended period. *(1:680;2:838;3:131–134)*

39. **(B)** An *idiot savant* is a *retarded* individual who has a very *limited specialized talent.* Such a person may have an unusual ability to memorize mathematical details, a special artistic talent, or a unique vocational skill. *(1:735;2:721–722)*

40. **(E)** *Imipramine* would have little benefit in the treatment of *acute mania* where the patient (and society) needs rapid relief from his or her symptoms. Antidepressants may worsen mania.

These patients need *hospitalization* where they may be treated with *lithium carbonate, chlorpromazine,* or *electroconvulsive therapy. (1:253–254; 2:432–433;3:280)*

41. **(C)** No one specific personality pattern has been shown to lead to obesity. Obesity is indeed more common in the poor and in women, especially older women. Obese children tend to become obese adults, and early-onset obesity is especially difficult to treat.

    Long-term results with individual psychotherapy of patients for treatment of their obesity have been poor. *(1:495–499;2:550–554;3:324–325)*

42. **(D)** *Testamentary capacity* is the legal capacity to make a will. *(1:893–894;2:859;3:152)*

    The *Durham Decision* states that the patient is not responsible for his or her behavior if this behavior is a product of a mental illness. *(1:896;2:865;3:153)*

    Under the *irresistible impulse test,* the person is not responsible for behavior that is the result of an irresistible impulse. *(1:895–896;2:865;3:153)*

    The *M'Naghten rule* or the *"right and wrong test"* states that persons cannot be held responsible for their behavior if they did not know the nature or quality of their behavior or if they could not appreciate that their actions were wrong. *(1:894–895;2:864–865;3:153)*

43. **(A)** *N-allyl normorphine* may precipitate an *abstinence syndrome* in chronic users of *morphine, heroin,* or *methadone. (1:393;2:665;3:220)*

44. **(D)** Convulsions may occur in *chronic meprobamate users* who are suddenly withdrawn from the drug (and also with chronic users of barbiturates or alcohol). *(1:409;2:660;3:238–239)*

45. **(B)** *Chronic amphetamine use* may lead to a clinical syndrome similar to *paranoid schizophrenia* but usually with less thought disorder. *(1:403–405;2:663;3:221–222)*

46. **(B)** *Tricyclic antidepressants* may produce *urinary retention* so should not be used in patients who already have this tendency. Because of this effect, it has been used in treating childhood *enuresis. (1:654–655;2:826–827;3:197–198)*

47. **(C)** *Hypnosis* is often effective in producing a symptomatic cure of *conversion disorder.* Under hypnosis the hysterical patient may be instructed to regain use of a hysterically paralyzed limb or recover sight or hearing lost as part of a hysterical conversion syndrome. *(1:348;2:764–766;3:72)*

48. **(C)** *Involutional melancholia* is more liable to occur in the lifelong *obsessive-compulsive,* the person who has always been inhibited, inflexible, and overly conscientious. *(1:246–247;2:435–440;3:335)*

49. **(D)** Patients taking *monoamine oxidase inhibitors* should be warned about the hypertensive effects they could suffer due to the dietary tyramine in cheese, beer, wine, chicken liver, and beans. *(1:658–659;2:828–829;3:110–112)*

50. **(B)** Electroconvulsive therapy is most useful in treating *major depression.* This treatment has little beneficial effect in *hypochondriasis, schizophrenia, residual type,* or *infantile autism.* Patients with *senile dementia* may be made more confused. *(1:682;2:836–840;3:131)*

51. **(B)** Intramuscular benztropine. Extrapyramidal drug side effects can be mistaken for the bizarre movements and posturing of the schizophrenic patient and vice versa. Drug-induced dyskinesias will be quickly and dramatically reduced or relieved by intramuscular antiparkinsonian drugs such as benztropine, which, however, will have no effect on psychotic mannerisms. Some patients, however, enjoy the emotional lift they get from benztropine or trihexyphenidyl and may fake extrapyramidal symptoms to get the medication.

    Amobarbital would sedate the patient but possibly make her confused, with no symptomatic relief. Electroconvulsive therapy and oral propanolol are not indicated. *(1:644–645;2:823;3:120)*

52. **(C)** In the social readjustment scale of Holmes and Rahe, the death of a spouse is rated as most stressful and thus most likely to cause disruption of healthy adaptation.

    Divorce, marital separation, and being jailed also rate high as stress factors. *(1:863;2:225;3:269)*

53. **(B)** *Hallucinations* do not occur in personality disorders. The *cyclothymic personality* is subject to wide mood swings but these excessive emotions do not cause a psychotic hallucinatory break with reality.

    Bipolar disorder, manic type, disorganized schizophrenia, major depression, and *delirium tremens* are all psychotic states where hallucinations may occur. In manic states, hallucinations are relatively uncommon and are more illusionary. *(1:163–164;2:122–127;3:16)*

54. **(C)** In psychoanalytic theory, the major factor in producing *depression* is *introjection* of hostile feelings once directed against others but now inwardly directed. *(1:83;2:423;3:272)*

55. **(C)** The *work of grief or mourning* is the emotional process of adapting to a loss and of reinvesting in other people and other goals.

The continued absence of obvious feelings following the death of a loved one would be an example of *denial.* The lengthy prolongation, more than 6 months, of acute sadness following a loss is *pathological mourning.* In all mourning there is some denial to allow gradual adapation to the loss and to permit individual repression of intolerable feelings. Accentuated grief reactions due to guilt or ambivalence are further examples of pathological mourning. *(1:264–270;2:180–182;3:269–270)*

56. **(C)** In *delirium,* disorientation, memory loss, labile mood changes, and impulse behavior are common symptoms. *(1:273–276;2:141–142;3:214)*

Neologisms, the forming of new idiosyncratic words, are most often found in schizophrenia. *(1:208;2:364;3:17)*

57. **(C)** Disulfiram (Anatbuse), used to treat alcoholics, may produce confusion, sleepiness, and worsening of schizophrenic symptoms. With chronic use, it may produce delirium, parkinsonism, and peripheral neuropathy. *(1:426;2:639–640;3:237–238)*

58. **(D)** *Phobias* are most often benefited therapeutically by *systematic desensitization. (1:325–327;2:470–476; 3:296)*

59. **(B)** *Parental superego lacunae, conscience defects,* are liable to lead to *juvenile delinquency* in the children who identify with the messages the parents give, consciously and unconsciously. *(1:858;2:117;3: 338)*

60. **(B)** The classical message of the *double-bind* situation is "Get away closer." The subject is faced with two equally imperative contradictory messages and, in the schizophrenogenic situation, cannot escape. *(2:357; 3:254–255)*
A. The *Von Domarus Principle* points out that the normal person accepts similarity of identity on the basis of identical subjects, but the primitive thinker—in this case the schizophrenic—accepts similar identity on the basis of predicates.

The schizophrenic can think, "Jesus Christ is a man. I am a man. Jesus Christ and I are both men, therefore I am Jesus Christ," or "Grass is green. Money is green. Therefore grass is money." *(1:207; 3:16–17)*
C. *Superego lacunae,* or *conscience defects,* allow the subject to act in an antisocial fashion. Superego lacunae in parents may be one factor leading to delinquency in their children who identify with them: parents consciously and unconsciously convey their own basic conscience standards to their children. *(1:858;2:117;3:338)*

D. *Reaction formation* is an emotional defense whereby the individual stresses the opposite of his or her underlying basic feelings. Unlike this situation presented in the question, both opposing feelings or messages are not outwardly apparent in reaction formation; the feeling intolerable to the subject is unconsciously suppressed as he or she emphasizes the opposite. *(1:79; 2:98–99;3:8)*
E. *Folie à deux* is a form of communicated psychosis where a psychosis, usually paranoid, is communicated or imposed by a dominant individual on a more passive or submissive partner. *(1:229–230;2:453; 3:257)*

61. **(B)** The brief history given outlines the development of a *paranoia.* Because it is intolerable to this perfectionistic physician to feel that he has been therapeutically unsuccessful, he represses this feeling of inadequacy and failure and unconsciously externalizes his blame. Rather than blame himself, he projects the blame outward and blames an external agency for what he feels to be failures.

As in many cases of *paranoia,* there is liable to be a kernel of truth in the subject's suspiciousness. As a minority-group member, this doctor is likely to have been treated differently from his majority peers in the past. *(1:226–229;2:444–457;3:257–258)*

62. **(E)** This lady has a well-integrated delusion of persecution and of grandeur. She feels she is being specially victimized by the Communists and she is important enought to ally herself with the president. Her delusional thinking and her hallucinations reinforce her psychosis.

Socially, her behavior is not markedly bizarre, disorganized, or disruptive.

This is the clinical picture of *schizophrenia, paranoid type. (1:215;2:376–377;3:248)*
A. A patient with a *paranoid personality* state might be suspicious or grandiose but would not be having auditory hallucinations. *(1:365–367;2:596;3:330)*
B. The *disorganized schizophrenic* fits the layman's concept of "craziness." These patients are more openly inappropriate, socially bizarre, uncontrolled, and regressed. *(1:215;2:372;3:248)*
C. An individual with a *phobia* has a fixed fear which he or she realizes is illogical. There is no delusional or hallucinatory thinking. *(1:321;2:470–471;3:286–288)*
D. *Histrionic personalities* are theatrical, self-centered, demanding, and excitable. They seek attention by overreacting, by demanding, and sometimes by lying, but they do not have delusions or auditory hallucinations. *(1:370–371;2:598–602;3:331)*

63. **(C)** The appropriate drug treatment for acute paranoid schizophrenia is *haloperidol. (2:394–396;3:255–256)*

Chronic amphetamine use can lead to a psychosis very similar to a paranoid schizophrenia. *(1:403–405; 2:663;3:241–242)*

64. **(D)** Persons with *passive–aggressive* personalities are characteristically demanding and manipulatively dependent and yet act in such a way as to ensure that the help and support they are given is rendered ineffective.

　　They want, they need, and they should be given but they cannot allow themselves to receive constructively and trustingly.

　　The young man described in this question manifests some of these symptoms and personality characteristics. *(1:381–383;2:612–613;3:335)*

65. **(B)** In *syphilitic meningoencephalitis, general paresis (paralysis),* there is inflammation and degeneration initially involving the frontoparietal cortex but later the other cortical areas. Macroscopically the *frontoparietal cortical areas* show atrophy. *(2:256–264;3:224)*

66. **(D)** *Wilson's disease, hepatolenticular degeneration,* is characterized pathologically by degeneration in the brain lenticular nuclei, especially in the putamen and the caudate nuclei, leading to cavity formation in the *basal ganglia.* *(1:716–717;2:323–324;3:228–229)*

67. **(C)** *Wernicke's encephalopathy or syndrome* occurs most commonly in chronic alcoholism and severe nutritional deficiencies. This rare syndrome is manifested pathologically by congestion, hemorrhages, and necrosis in the areas around the third ventricle and aqueduct and in the mamillary bodies. *(1:420;2:325–326;3:218–219)*

68. **(A)** The most common form of infantile cerebral lipoidosis is *Tay-Sach's disease,* where there is loss of cortical architecture due to general neuron lipoid deposition. *(1:715;2:725–728;3:164)*

Answers 69 through 73 deal with the schizophrenic syndromes.

69. **(B)** *Residual schizophrenia.* After at least one episode of overt psychosis there are still symptoms of continued illness, now no longer florid. *(1:217;2:380; 3:248–249)*

70. **(D)** The *disorganized schizophrenic* appears typically "crazy" in the popular sense of the term. These patients are frequently silly, giggling, grimacing, and inappropriate. They show bizarre delusions and hallucinations and their behavior is often markedly regressed. *(1:215;2:372;3:248)*

71. **(C)** *Paranoid schizophrenia* tends to occur at a later age, often in the 30s, and there is less overt personality disorganization. Characteristically these patients are suspicious, distrustful, and aloof. They have delusions of grandeur and persecution. These persecutory delusions may provoke them into aggressive or assaultive behavior. *(1:215;2:376;3:248)*

72. **(A)** In *catatonic schizophrenia,* there may be episodes of stupor, excitement, or both alternately. Automatisms and negativism may lead to grotesque posturing and bizarre behavior. *(1:214–215;2:376;3:248)*

73. **(E)** *Schizoaffective disorder* presents with schizophrenic personality disorganization plus strong affective symptoms. The affective disorder may be prominent but the personality decompensation denotes a schizophrenia. These patients show depression and elation, often with marked anxiety, together with generally bizarre thought processes. *(1:216;2:460;3:258)*

Answers 74 through 83 deal with electroencephalogram recordings. (2:41–45;3:343–362)

74. **(E)** *Following withdrawal of alcohol* (or barbiturates) in chronic users, there is a *rebound increase in REM sleep,* often with disturbing *nightmares. (1:563;2:44; 3:345–346)*

75. **(B)** *Three-per-second spike and wave* patterns on the electroencephalogram are characteristic of *petit mal. (1:301;2:279;3:226)*

76. **(D)** In *psychomotor epilepsy* usually 4- to 8-per-second *temporal lobe* discharge foci can be noted on the electroencephalogram. *(1:303–304;2:280–281;3: 225)*

77. **(A)** Episodes of *REM sleep activity* on the electroencephalogram are associated with *narcolepsy* attacks. *(1:567–568;2:283–285;3:349–350)*

78. **(C)** In delirium, commonly there is an increase in *diffuse slow-wave* activity on the electroencephalogram as the subject becomes more clouded intellectually. *(2:141;3:214)*

79. **(C)** After *barbiturate withdrawal,* in chronic users, there is a "rebound" increase in total REM sleep, often with frightening nightmares. *(1:563;2:44;3:345–346)*

80. **(A)** In the *newborn,* up to 50% of the sleep cycle is taken up with REM sleep. *(2:43;3:344)*

81. **(E)** During *sensory deprivation,* the alpha rhythm of the electroencephalogram decreases and there is increasing slow-wave activity. *(2:177)*

82. **(B)** *Amphetamines* suppress or block *REM sleep.* Since *narcolepsy* is associated with REM sleep patterns, amphetamines are specifically used in the treatment of this disorder. *(1:403,568;2:44;3:345)*

83. **(D)** Sleepwalking usually occurs in the course of deep sleep, during stage 3 or 4 *non-REM sleep. (1:570–572;2:706;3:352–353)*

84. **(C)** In *acute intermittent porphyria,* there are excreted in the urine large amounts of uroporphyrin and porphobilinogen, which give the classical "port-wine" reddish-brown urine. *(1:309–310;2:319–323;3:228)*

85. **(D)** A *lowered serum ceruloplasmin* level, with increased copper deposition especially in the liver and brain, is found in *Wilson's disease, hepatolenticular degeneration. (1:716–717;2:323–324;3:228–229)*

86. **(A)** *Basophilic stippling* of the red cells on the peripheral blood film is a readily available sign of chronic lead poisoning. Usually there is a co-existent hypochromic anemia. *(1:298;2:329–331;3:163)*

87. **(E)** There is a reduction of *dopamine* levels in the basal ganglia in *parkinsonism.* Levodopa is used specifically to treat the parkinson syndrome. *(1:305–306;2:337–339;3:227)*

88. **(B)** Pathologically, *neurofibrillary tangles* and *senile plaques* are typically found in the frontal cortex and the hippocampal region in *Alzheimer's disease,* a form of senile dementia. *(1:286–288;2:242;3:216)*

Answers 89 through 93 deal with the symptoms typically seen in the schizophrenic syndromes. (1:214–219;2:272–284; 3:248–249)

89. **(B)** The *residual schizophrenic* is left lacking in energy, apathetic and aimless, and withdrawn, with illogical thinking and loose associations. *(1:217;2:380; 3:248–249)*

90. **(D)** The *disorganized schizophrenic* usually is socially *silly.* Frequently the patient shows inappropriate *grinning, grimacing,* and *regressed behavior.* Bizarre *hallucinations* are common. *(1:215;2:372;3:248)*

91. **(A)** The *paranoid schizophrenic* usually shows less grotesque personality disorganization. The psychotic process is often not diagnosed until the third or fourth decade of life. In this illness, the patient presents with *organized delusions of persecution or grandiosity.* *(1:215;2:376–378;3:248)*

92. **(E)** The *catatonic schizophrenic* may show stupor or excitement. In both syndromes negativism is often marked. The stuporous catatonic is mute and frequently posturally rigid. Bizarre posturing is a common symptom. *(1:214–215;2:373–376;3:248)*

93. **(C)** In *childhood schizophrenia, autism* is a common symptom even where infantile autism is not present. Early pervasive psychopathology leads to severe social and intellectual *retardation.* Many of these children end up in hospitals for the retarded. Autistic children show many unusual posturings and body movements, including a tendency to walk on the toes, *toe walking.*
    The diagnosis *schizophrenia, childhood type,* at present covers a wide range of syndromes that may not all be interrelated. *(1:217;2:280–284;3:201–202)*

94. **(B)** *Confabulation,* the falsification of memory to fill remembrance gaps, is most often seen in *Korsakoff's syndrome* and associated organic brain disorders. *(1:180;2:145;3:16)*

95. **(E)** Transvestism is a sexual perversion, starting most frequently in adolescence and occurring usually in males, where the subject obtains sexual pleasure by dressing in clothing of the opposite sex. *(1:447–449; 2:528–529;3:303–304)*

96. **(A)** *La belle indifference,* an unusual equanimity in the face of usually distressing physical or psychological symptoms, is typically manifested by patients showing a *conversion disorder.* However, this symptom occurs in other syndromes and in normal people. *(1:347;2:505;3:290)*

97. **(D)** In the *Ganser syndrome,* sometimes called "prison psychosis," the subject gives an approximate answer to even simple basic questions.
    "What is two plus two?"
    "Five."
    "How old are you?" (correct answer 36)
    "Thirty seven."
    "How many brothers have you?" (correct answer two)
    "One brother." *(1:544–545;2:516–517)*

98. **(C)** When the flow of thought is excessively rapid and there is said to be a *flight of ideas,* the subject is usually manifesting symptoms of a bipolar disorder, manic type. *(1:178;2:127–128;3:17)*

Answers 99 through 103 deal with the definitions of diagnostic terms.

99. **(A)** A *psychosis* is present where the subject shows a *marked impairment of reality contact,* often with *severe personality disorganization. (2:463–464)*

100. **(D)** In *neurosis,* there is a *maladaptive reaction to anxiety* without, however, severe reality distortion or personality disorganization. In the neurotic syndrome, the subject is constantly attempting to cope with inner anxiety. *(1:315;2:463–464;3:285–286)*

101. **(B)** A *conduct disorder* is a *stable maladaptive pattern* of interacting seen in the growth and *developmental years.* This is a relatively fixed but unproductive way of coping where, however, the personality is not yet finalized. There is always the hope with these

children and adolescents that they will grow out of it. Many do not. *(1:800;2:683–687;3:190–192)*

102. **(C)** An *adjustment disorder* at any age is a *temporary acute reaction* to *stress*. When the stress is removed or reduced or the subject learns to cope more effectively, the individual returns to the preexisting level of adaptation. *(1:476;3:289)*

103. **(E)** A *personality disorder* is characterized by chronic fixed maladaptive behavior patterns that are usually recognizable by the teenage years. People with personality disorders typically feel little anxiety themselves about their behavior that, however, makes other people anxious. *(1:361–362;2:593–594;3:329)*

Answers 104 through 108 deal with sexual deviations. (1:432–452;2:520–534;3:301–306)

104. **(C)** The *pedophile* achieves sexual *gratification* through contact with *children*. This diagnosis usually implies adult sexual interest in a child. Sexual play between children would not be included in deviant sexuality. *(1:450–451;2:529;3:304)*

105. **(D)** In *transvestism*, the subject is satisfied with his or her own gender but gains erotic pleasure through dressing in the *clothing of the opposite sex*. *(1:447–449;2:528;3:303–304)*

106. **(A)** In *fetishism*, the *fetishist* gains sexual gratification through contact with an inanimate object, such as a shoe or a piece of clothing (the *fetish*). *(1:447–448;2:529;3:303)*

107. **(B)** The *transsexual* does not accept his or her anatomic sex and has a need to be changed to the opposite sex, usually by surgical means. *(1:434–437;2:525–527;3:302)*

108. **(E)** The *exhibitionist,* usually a male, gains sexual gratification by *genital self-exposure,* usually to members of the opposite sex. *(1:449–450;2:529–530;3:304–305)*

109. **(B)** In a *conversion disorder,* unacceptable feelings are repressed but are manifested outwardly in *symbolic* fashion by a *physical symptom* involving the voluntary musculature or the special senses. *(1:342;2:501;3:290)*

110. **(E)** When the subject has a *déjà vu* reaction, he or she has the *illusion* of having experienced his or her present reality at some time past. This sensation occurs with normal people especially during the teenage years but may also indicate a developing emotional illness. *(1:161;2:146;3:16)*

111. **(A)** A *catastrophic reaction* is manifested by acute disruptive agitation that develops when a brain-injured person cannot solve a problem and is faced suddenly with the reality of his or her intellectual handicap. *(1:150;2:304–305)*

112. **(D)** *Bruxism* is the symptom of *compulsive chewing* and *teeth grinding.* Chronic bruxism can wear down the teeth. *(1:573–574;2:559;3:354)*

113. **(C)** *Bulimia* is obsessive overeating and food gorging that sometimes alternates with bouts of dieting and self-starvation. *(1:779–807;2:555;3:195)*

Somatic Treatments
Questions

INTRODUCTION

For examination purposes and, more important, for general clinical practice, the standard psychiatry textbooks give too generalized a discussion of the somatic therapies. The student and the practitioner should supplement their understanding of these most important procedures from more specialized volumes.

REFERENCES

1. Chapter 27,   The Organic Therapies, pp 632–690
2. Chapter 32,   Pharmacological Therapy, pp 809–834
    Chapter 33,   Shock and Other Physical Therapies, pp 835–846
3. Chapter 8,   Psychotherapeutic Drugs and Electrotherapy, pp 93–138

DIRECTIONS (Questions 1 through 19): Each of the numbered items or incomplete statements in this section is followed by answers or by completions of the statement. Select the ONE lettered answer or completion that is BEST in each case.

1. Before therapeutic response is evident, imipramine may have to be given for a period of

   (A) 3 days
   (B) 10 days
   (C) 3 weeks
   (D) 3 months
   (E) 5 months

2. All of the following statements are true about treatment with lithium carbonate except

   (A) therapeutic serum level 0.8–1.2 mEq/L
   (B) may produce goiter
   (C) slurred speech may indicate toxic levels
   (D) additive therapeutic effect with amphetamines
   (E) convulsions can occur with high blood levels

3. Side effects of chlorpromazine include

   (A) photosensitivity
   (B) gynecomastia
   (C) urinary retention
   (D) none of the above
   (E) all of the above

4. Before giving patients a course of modified electroconvulsive therapy, they should be warned of side effects, which include all of the following except

   (A) amenorrhea in women for 2 to 3 months
   (B) headaches
   (C) loss of memory for recent events
   (D) increase in weight
   (E) sleeplessness for 1 to 2 weeks

5. Convulsions may develop on drug withdrawal after chronic use of

   (A) chlorpromazine
   (B) reserpine
   (C) lithium
   (D) meprobamate
   (E) imipramine

6. For the effective treatment of bipolar disorder, depressive type, the number of shock treatments necessary for full benefit would be

   (A) 1–3
   (B) 5–10
   (C) 15–25
   (D) 25–50
   (E) over 50

7. A 21-year-old student is brought to the student clinic by his roommate. The young man is anxious, restless, and confused. The roommate reports that the patient has been taking large amounts of a popular over-the-counter sleeping preparation. In treating this patient, you may want to use intramuscular injections of

   (A) scopolamine
   (B) amphetamine
   (C) ergotamine
   (D) diphenhydramine
   (E) physostigmine

8. Electroconvulsive therapy is often very effective in

   (A) opioid abuse
   (B) ulcerative colitis
   (C) conversion disorder
   (D) schizophrenia, catatonic type
   (E) phobic disorder

9. Pigmentary retinopathy is seen in patients receiving high doses of which drug?

   (A) phenobarbital
   (B) lithium carbonate
   (C) sodium bromide
   (D) methylphenidate
   (E) thioridazine

10. When insulin coma therapy was used more frequently in the treatment of emotional disorders, the main therapeutic indication was

    (A) major depression
    (B) phobic disorder
    (C) involutional melancholia
    (D) acute early schizophrenia
    (E) chronic paranoid schizophrenia

11. You have maintained a 55-year-old depressed man on tranylcypromine for 8 weeks with only moderate symptomatic relief, so you decide to change his medication to amitriptyline. Accordingly, you plan to

    (A) gradually decrease the tranylcypromine as you give increasing dosages of amitriptyline
    (B) stop the tranylcypromine; after 14 days, start amitriptyline in increasing doses
    (C) stop the tranylcypromine and immediately begin amitriptyline
    (D) continue tranylcypromine at present levels as you give amitriptyline in increasing doses to a therapeutically effective level
    (E) check thyroid and kidney functions

12. A dangerous effect of reserpine is

    (A) bilateral nerve deafness
    (B) acute manic state
    (C) aggressive hypersexuality
    (D) acute schizophrenic reaction
    (E) suicidal depression

13. Electroconvulsive therapy has its therapeutic effect due to

    (A) increase in total REM sleep
    (B) elevation of serum catecholamines
    (C) behavior modification
    (D) all of the above
    (E) none of the above

14. Chlorpromazine is indicated in all of the following except

    (A) senile dementia
    (B) acute schizophrenia
    (C) bipolar disorder, manic type
    (D) major depression
    (E) chronic schizophrenia

15. Hexafluorodiethyl ether (Indoklon) is used in

    (A) narcotherapy
    (B) anaclitic therapy
    (C) desensitization
    (D) convulsive therapy
    (E) testing chronic alcoholics who wish to abstain

16. Electroconvulsive therapy is usually contraindicated by

    (A) pregnancy
    (B) age over 65
    (C) brain tumor
    (D) hypotension
    (E) angina pectoris

17. All the following statements are true about tardive dyskinesia except

    (A) may appear or worsen after phenothiazine is stopped
    (B) lip sucking and smacking, choreiform arm movements
    (C) persists during sleep
    (D) antiparkinsonian drugs do not help and may worsen symptoms
    (E) may be caused by amoxapine

18. Akathisia is

    (A) a form of mutism seen in profound barbiturate overdose
    (B) an extrapyramidal symptom most commonly associated with piperazines
    (C) the type of bluish-gray skin coloration in exposed areas, occurring with prolonged high dosage of chlorpromazine
    (D) form of sudden death, possibly due to ventricular fibrillation, in cases with long-term phenothiazine intake
    (E) cholestatic jaundice possibly due to individual sensitivity to chlorpromazine

19. When imipramine is therapeutically effective in treating the depression of a bipolar disorder, the drug should be maintained

    (A) 3 weeks from starting the drug
    (B) 3 to 6 months after good therapeutic response is noted
    (C) 1 to 2 years after depression is cleared
    (D) until hypomanic state occurs
    (E) 3 weeks from time of beneficial response

DIRECTIONS (Questions 20 through 45): Each group of items in this section consists of lettered headings followed by a set of numbered words or phrases. For each numbered word or phrase, select the ONE lettered heading that is most closely associated with it. Each lettered heading may be selected once, more than once, or not at all.

Questions 20 through 25

    (A) chlorpromazine
    (B) barbiturates
    (C) monoamine oxidase inhibitors
    (D) amphetamines

20. Paranoid psychotic reactions

21. Hypertensive crisis precipitated by cheese

22. Produces acute confusional state in elderly

23. May induce exacerbation of acute intermittent porphyria

24. Purplish-gray suntan reaction

25. Thin, watery breast lactation

Questions 26 through 30

    (A) disulfiram
    (B) lithium carbonate
    (C) chlordiazepoxide
    (D) penicillamine
    (E) ammonium chloride

26. Delirium tremens treatment

27. Chronic alcoholism treatment

28. Chronic bromism treatment

29. Bipolar disorder, manic type treatment

30. Wilson's disease treatment

Questions 31 through 35

    (A) electroconvulsive therapy
    (B) physostigmine salicylate
    (C) chlorpromazine
    (D) levodopa
    (E) ergotamine tartrate

31. Toxic psychosis due to scopolamine-containing sleeping preparations

32. Acute intermittent porphyria

33. Migraine

34. Mania

35. Paralysis agitans (Parkinsonism)

Questions 36 through 40

    (A) chlorpromazine
    (B) amphetamines
    (C) trimethadione
    (D) phenobarbital
    (E) calcium disodium versenate (EDTA)

36. Narcolepsy

37. Grand mal

38. Petit mal

39. Mania

40. Lead Poisoning

Questions 41 through 45

    (A) haloperidol
    (B) methylphenidate
    (C) dimercaprol
    (D) methadone
    (E) imipramine

41. Childhood hyperkinesis

42. Enuresis

43. Tourette's Disorder

44. Chronic mercury poisoning

45. Heroin addiction

Answers and Explanations

1. **(C)** Though *imipramine* may have a mood-elevating effect in 3 to 5 days, in many situations a significant improvement is not noted until the medication has been given for at least *3 weeks*. When effective, the medication should be maintained for 3 to 6 months. *(1:652–653;2:826;3:113–117)*

2. **(D)** *Lithium* has no symptomatic additive effect with amphetamines. The therapeutic blood serum level for lithium is 0.8–1.2 mEq/L, though some clinicians suggest a safer therapeutic level is 0.7–1.0 mEq/L, especially in the elderly.

   Slurred speech and convulsions may occur as toxic symptoms of lithium overdose. Goiter may also be a side effect of lithium treatment. *(1:675–678;2: 829–831;3:125–129)*

3. **(E)** In patients taking *chlorpromazine,* excessive photosensitivity can occur, leading to disabling sunburn. Like many tranquilizers, chlorpromazine may produce constipation and *urinary retention.* The drug should be used with caution where there are preexisting micturition difficulties. Male patients, especially adolescents and young adults, may become very disturbed at the *gynecomastia* that is sometimes produced by the hormonal changes induced by chlorpromazine. *(1:641–650;2:822–826;3:103–110)*

4. **(E)** *Sleeplessness* is not a major side effect of electroconvulsive therapy.

   Amenorrhea is likely to be present in women patients for 2 to 3 months after a course of convulsive therapy. Headache is a frequent complaint after the treatments and usually responds readily to symptomatic treatment.

   After several treatments, the patient usually develops moderate memory loss for more recent events. The amnesia should clear gradually within 2 to 4 weeks of cessation of treatment. *(1:683;2:838–839; 3:133–134)*

5. **(D)** *Convulsions* may occur when *meprobamate* is withdrawn after a period of chronic use. Convulsions can also occur on withdrawal of *barbiturates* or *alcohol* in chronic users. *(1:665;2:832;3:238–239)*

6. **(B)** Usually 5–10, with an average of 9 or 10, *electroconvulsive treatments* are necessary to treat and maintain therapeutic benefits in bipolar disorder, depressive type. Symptomatically the depression is usually relieved by 3 or 4 treatments, but further treatments are necessary to prevent early relapse. *(1: 682;2:839;3:133)*

7. **(E)** A *toxic psychosis* due to the chronic ingestion of over-the-counter sleeping medication is often caused by the scopolamine or belladonna-related compounds in the preparation. Intramuscular injection of physostigmine salicylate 1 mg repeated after 15 to 20 minutes is the treatment of choice. Patients may develop serious hypotension when given phenothiazines. *(1:295,588–589;2:333;3:223)*

8. **(D)** *Catatonic schizophrenia,* especially the excited type, often responds very well to a course of electroconvulsive therapy. Apathetic or stuporous catatonia may show symptomatic improvement, but relapse is common.

   Convulsive therapy would not be indicated for ulcerative colitis, conversion or phobic disorders, or opioid abuse. *(1:682;2:837;3:131)*

9. **(E)** *Pigmentary retinopathy* has been reported in patients receiving 800 mg or more of *thioridazine* over several weeks or months. *(1:649;3:124)*

10. **(D)** Though *insulin coma therapy* is rarely used now, four decades ago it was the preferred treatment of *acute early schizophrenia.* At present, drug treatment or electroconvulsive treatment would be used in this illness.

    Insulin coma therapy requires long-term intensive treatment with specially trained staff. Prolonged or irreversible coma is the main danger. *(1:687–688; 2:840–843;3:93–94)*

11. **(B)** Stop the tranylcypromine and only after 14 days start amitriptyline in increasing doses.

When a monoamine oxidase inhibitor is given in combination with a tricyclic antidepressant, the patient may develop potentially fatal restlessness, twitching, hyperpyrexia, and convulsions.

If the patient has been taking monoamine oxidase inhibitors, a minimum 7 day washout period is recommended before a tricyclic is started. Some clinicians prefer to wait 14 days to insure the patient is free from this cross-reaction. Under very carefully controlled clinical conditions, these drugs may be used in combination and may prove effective in previously refractory depressive states. *(1:659;2:829;3:112)*

12. **(E)** The most dangerous side effect of *reserpine* is the production of depression or the increase of existing *depression* in patients taking the drug. These depressive states may result in *suicide* or may require intensive antidepressant treatment.

Reserpine is rarely used now for its tranquilizing effect. *(1:296;2:822;3:103)*

13. **(E)** *None* of the suggested theories about the effect of *electroconvulsive therapy* has been *validated*—and there are now hundreds of proposed theories. The use of this treatment procedure is solely based on its demonstrated efficacy in certain psychiatric states. *(1:682;2:839–840;3:131)*

14. **(D)** Many tranquilizers, including *chlorpromazine,* tend to maintain or even *accentuate* feelings of *depression.* Chlorpromazine would not be used generally in a patient with *major depression* unless the patient was acutely psychotic or delusional.

The drug is often very effective in reducing anxiety or agitation in *senile dementia, acute schizophrenia, acute mania,* and *chronic schizophrenia.* *(1:633–636;2:820–821;3:103–110)*

15. **(D)** *Convulsive therapy* can be induced by the drug hexafluorodiethyl ether (Indoklon) given by inhalation or intravenously. The therapeutic results are comparable to electroconvulsive treatments. *(1:679;2:840; 3:93–94)*

16. **(C)** With full treatment and support facilities, there are probably very few absolute *contraindications* to the use of *electroconvulsive therapy* in a psychiatric emergency. However, a *brain tumor* is usually considered a specific contraindication. The rise in intracranial pressure during an induced convulsion can prove fatal in patients with brain neoplasm. *(1:682–683;2:837–838;3:131–132)*

17. **(C)** *Tardive dyskinesias* do not persist during sleep.

Tardive dyskinesia may occur at any time during phenothiazine treatment and can appear or worsen when the drug treatment is stopped. Amoxapine may produce tardive dyskinesia.

Symptoms of the syndrome include lip sucking and smacking, tongue protrusion, choreiform arm movements, and tonic spasms of the neck and back muscles.

Antiparkinsonian drugs do not relieve the symptoms and may indeed cause them to worsen. *(1:644–646;2:823–824;3:121–122)*

18. **(B)** *Akathisia* is an *extrapyramidal* symptom, most often associated with the *piperazine* group of tranquilizers. With this side effect, patients feel restless, cannot sit still, pace about, and tend to complain that their feet or legs are "restless." *(1:644;2:823;3:118)*

19. **(B)** *Imipramine,* given in adequate dosage, may take 3 weeks to achieve full therapeutic effect in the treatment of *depression* and should then be continued for 3 to 6 months to maintain the improvement and to prevent relapse. *(1:652–653;2:826–827;3:113–117)*

20. **(D)** *Amphetamines* typically produce *paranoid psychotic reactions,* especially with chronic use. *(1:403–405;2:663;3:221–222)*

21. **(C)** Patients taking *monoamine oxidase inhibitors* must be warned against ingesting aged cheese, beer, wines, chicken liver, pickled herring, and other foods rich in tyramine.

The hypertensive effect of the dietary tyramine is potentiated by the monoamine oxidase inhibitor, and *severe hypertensive crisis* may occur. *(1:657–659;2: 828–829;3:111–112)*

22. **(B)** *Barbiturates* should not be used for sedation in the *elderly* because they are liable to precipitate *acute confusional states.* Chloral hydrate is a much safer drug for nighttime sedation. *(1:276–279;2:239;3:214–215)*

23. **(B)** *Barbiturates* are absolutely contraindicated in patients with *acute intermittent porphyria* because the drug can precipitate an acute attack.

Chlorpromazine is useful in the symptomatic treatment of an acute episode of porphyria. *(1:309–310;2:319–323;3:228)*

24. **(A)** Chronic users of *chlorpromazine* are liable to develop a *purplish-gray suntan* reaction due to the development of skin pigmentation. Penicillamine has been used with benefit to treat the pigmentation. *(1:649;2:825;3:123)*

25. **(A)** *Chlorpromazine* and similar drugs may produce *pseudopregnancy, gynecomastia,* and *thin, watery breast secretion.* *(1:649–650;2:822–826;3:123–124)*

26. **(C)** The acute psychotic confusional state of *delirium tremens* is best treated by *chlordiazepoxide* with high-calorie, high-carbohydrate, and high-vitamin intake. The fluid balance may have to be corrected and maintained. *Morphine* and *barbiturates* must be avoided. *(1:419–420;2:628–631;3:217–218)*

27. **(A)** In treating the *chronic alcoholic* who wishes to give up drinking, *disulfiram* (Antabuse) can be used to help make alcohol intake disagreeable. *(1:426;2:639–640;3:237–238)*

28. **(E)** *Chronic bromide intoxication, chronic bromism,* is treated by discontinuing all bromide ingestion and eliminating bromide from the body.

    Clearing of bromide is accelerated by taking extra salt and fluids to flush out the bromide. Bromide excretion is hastened by the use of *ammonium chloride* rather than *sodium chloride.* The ammonium salt itself has a diuretic action. *(1:292–293;2:667–669)*

29. **(B)** *Lithium carbonate* is used in the treatment of *bipolar disorder, manic type,* especially in the treatment of moderate manic states and in the prevention of manic recurrences. In acute manic states, lithium carbonate is usually too slow-acting to be useful, and one of the stronger tranquilizers is used. *(1:675–678; 2:829–831;3:125–129)*

30. **(D)** *Penicillamine* is used to increase copper excretion and to prevent or minimize symptoms in *hepatolenticular degeneration, Wilson's disease,* where there is increased deposition of copper in the tissues, especially of the basal ganglia and the liver. *(1:716–717;2:323–324;3:228–229)*

31. **(B)** *Toxic psychoses* may occur due to chronic use of nonprescription *scopolamine-containing sleeping preparations.* Intramuscular *physostigmine salicylate* is the specific antidote. *(1:295,588–589;2:333; 3:223)*

32. **(C)** *Chlorpromazine* gives optimum symptomatic relief in acute crises of *intermittent porphyria.* Alcohol and barbiturates must be avoided since they may precipitate acute attacks. *(1:309–310;2:319–323; 3:228)*

33. **(E)** The treatment for *migraine acute attacks* is *ergotamine tartrate* by mouth or subcutaneous injection. Ergotamine may be combined with caffeine, antispasmodics, or sedatives. *(1:531–532;2:579–581; 3:326)*

34. **(A)** Electroconvulsive therapy will quickly bring manic symptoms under control. *(1:682;2:836–840; 3:280)*

35. **(D)** *Levodopa* is now the treatment of choice in most cases of *paralysis agitans (Parkinsonism).* This medication may produce severe depression or toxic psychoses as complications of treatment. *(1:305–306; 2:337–339;3:227)*

36. **(B)** *Amphetamines* are the drugs specifically used for *narcolepsy.* Many narcoleptic patients show REM sleep patterns on their electroencephalograms during attacks; amphetamines inhibit REM sleep. *(1:567–568;2:283–284;3:349–351)*

37. **(D)** *Phenobarbital* is still one of the most effective and least toxic drugs used in the treatment of *grand mal epilepsy.* It has little beneficial effect in *petit mal.* *(1:305;2:291)*

38. **(C)** For *petit mal epilepsy, trimethadione* and associated drugs are the treatment of choice.

    Dilantin is most effective with psychomotor seizures and may be used alone or in combination with phenobarbital in the treatment of grand mal, especially where phenobarbital alone has not controlled the seizures. *(1:305;2:291–293)*

39. **(A)** Chlorpromazine in high dosages is very effective in treating mania. *(1:633;2:431–432;3:106)*

40. **(E)** For *lead poisoning,* a treatment program of *calcium disodium versenate (EDTA)* should be instituted after the source of the lead intake has been blocked. *(1:298;2:329–331;3:163)*

41. **(B)** *Methylphenidate* is the medication presently most used for the syndrome of *childhood hyperkinesis* (attention deficit disorder with hyperactivity). This diagnostic syndrome covers a wide range of symptoms and disorders. This treatment should be prescribed with caution: growth stunting with chronic use is being reported. *(1:744–745;2:681–683;3:187–190)*

42. **(E)** In childhood *enuresis,* many different treatments work with different clinicians and different children. *Imipramine* has shown therapeutic benefit in the treatment of enuresis of all the drugs presently used though improvement is often short-lived. *(1:845;2: 697–699;3:197–198)*

43. **(A)** *Haloperidol,* one of the butyrophenones, is most efficacious in producing symptomatic improvement in patients with *Tourette's Disorder.* The multiple tics, coprolalia, and echolalia shown by these subjects are often totally incapacitating without effective treatment. *(1:547–548;2:700–701;3:196–197)*

44. **(C)** In the treatment of *mercury poisoning*, the patient should be removed from the source of the mercury. Usually this is an occupational hazard. *Dimercaprol (BAL)* is used to increase mercury excretion. *(1:298–299;2:331;3:229)*

45. **(D)** *Methadone* is used to withdraw a patient from heroin or to substitute as a maintenance drug instead of heroin in *heroin addiction. (1:395–397;2:655–656; 3:239–240)*

Psychological Treatment and Management
Questions

INTRODUCTION

Examination candidates will be expected to know in general about different types of psychological treatment but should anticipate more detailed questions on two very different aspects of clinical practice: the management of the difficult patient and the process and planning of psychoanalytic psychotherapy.

The trainee will face questions about difficult patients, such as those who are seductive, manipulative, aggressive, or otherwise disturbing. The questions will be phrased in such a way that the student is expected to recognize the problem posed by these persons, to be aware of the doctor's natural human reaction to such a patient, and yet to be able to plan the necessary examination, management, and treatment that these people, like any other patients, should have.

Frequently in clinical psychiatry examinations, there are questions about the theoretical aspects of psychotherapy, usually from the psychoanalytic standpoint. These questions test the student's understanding of the way the psychotherapy process can be developed and strengthened in a treatment situation where the task is to help patients understand what they are feeling, thinking, saying, and doing. In order to make these questions about psychotherapy sufficiently specific, the questions posed and the answers required may sometimes seem rather unrealistic.

The standard textbooks deal with psychological treatment and management somewhat unevenly. Most students learn this aspect of clinical psychiatry in seminars and direct clinical work rather than in lectures or through reading.

DIRECTIONS (Questions 1 through 16): Each of the numbered items or incomplete statements in this section is followed by answers or by completions of the statement. Select the ONE lettered answer or completion that is BEST in each case.

1. Behavior therapy

   (A) deals with observable behavior
   (B) does not attempt to uncover underlying dynamics
   (C) is based on reinforcement
   (D) all of the above
   (E) none of the above

2. Behavior modification has been used successfully with

   (A) autistic children
   (B) phobic adults
   (C) sexual deviates
   (D) none of the above
   (E) all of the above

3. Behavior modification is based on

   (A) transference
   (B) reinforcement
   (C) counseling
   (D) hypnosis
   (E) group interaction

4. Psychoanalysis is of greatest value in treating

   (A) schizophrenia
   (B) borderline retardation
   (C) adolescent identity crises
   (D) major depression
   (E) neuroses

5. Transference is the

   (A) manifestation of the psychotherapist's feelings toward the patient
   (B) development of warm feelings between patient and psychotherapist
   (C) carryover of feelings from an earlier relationship to the psychotherapist
   (D) ability to feel with the other person and to understand his or her feelings
   (E) splitting of an idea from its accompanying emotion

6. You are seeing a 24-year-old woman in psychotherapy. During the third session she begins to cry loudly as she talks about her marriage. To enhance the treatment process, you should

   (A) encourage her to continue crying, to let out her feelings
   (B) point out that she is trying to share information and crying may be her way of not sharing
   (C) acknowledge her crying and gently continue to discuss this topic with her

   (D) bring the session to an end so that the patient does not become too upset
   (E) change the subject and deal with something less tension provoking

7. A 35-year-old unmarried schoolteacher is too fearful to go to work. She begins psychotherapy. In her third interview, she admits she is afraid she will be attacked by some of her older students and adds, "All the other women teachers are scared too. Several have been assaulted." To facilitate her treatment, you should say

   (A) "Well, it is reassuring to know you have the same anxieties the other teachers have."
   (B) "But they have been able to continue working in school."
   (C) "When you say 'assaulted,' perhaps you are worried about sexual attack."
   (D) "First let us try to understand your feelings and what these feelings do to you."
   (E) "Working in our schools is certainly difficult nowadays."

8. During her fourth psychotherapy session, a 26-year-old married woman asks, "Do you like my new hairstyle?" She really looks dreadful. Your response should be

   (A) "No, you look dreadful."
   (B) "Yes. You look very attractive."
   (C) "Why do you ask?"
   (D) "Are you trying to make a fool of me?"
   (E) "You should not ask questions."

9. You are a male psychotherapist and have just started to see a 44-year-old man in psychotherapy. At the start of the second interview, he gives you a most attractive tie. You should say something like

   (A) "Why do you want to give me this gift?"
   (B) "You are trying to seduce me."
   (C) "Thank you very much."
   (D) "Have you had homosexual relationships?"
   (E) "I never accept personal gifts."

10. For 2 weeks a paranoid schizophrenic man has been under your care in a general hospital psychiatric unit. During an interview, he shows you a switchblade he carries around for protection. You should

   (A) ask the patient for the knife. If he refuses, keep the matter totally confidential.
   (B) ask the patient for the knife. If he refuses, call in the security personnel to take the knife from him.
   (C) ask the patient for the knife. If he refuses, catch hold of him, refusing to let go until he gives you the knife.

(D) tell the patient that knives are totally forbidden on the unit. Insist that he get rid of the switch-blade.

(E) increase the frequency of his appointments so you can work through his need to carry such a weapon.

11. An 18-year-old college student has been hospitalized for recurrent hyperventilation attacks. When you are called in consultation by his physician, you should

(A) reassure the patient that he is really well
(B) explain the purpose and nature of the interview
(C) try to look the patient directly in the eye
(D) first discuss the situation with the dean of students
(E) recommend the patient be discharged from the hospital

12. While the local family doctor is on vacation, you are looking after his practice for him. For the third time this week, you have been interrupted after office hours by a 45-year-old married woman coming to see "her doctor." She has been complaining of recurrent low back pain but you have found nothing wrong. Your office nurse has just left for home when you hear this woman patient rapping impatiently on the office door. You should

(A) ignore her knocking. Leave by the back door.
(B) give her a firm talking to. Point out that her aches are purely functional and she should pull herself together.
(C) tell her that she requires careful, thorough evaluation. Give her the next available appointment during office hours.
(D) bring her in and give her the most intensive physical examination possible. Then point out her seductive behavior.
(E) call her husband and point out that she obviously wants companionship and understanding.

Question 13

You are starting psychotherapeutic treatment with a 23-year-old man. In his second interview he asks, "What should I do to get well?"

13. To facilitate the treatment process you should answer

(A) "Just trust in me and be sure to share your true feelings."
(B) "That is not up to me to tell you."
(C) "How do you feel about that yourself?"
(D) "It is too early in the treatment to tell you yet."
(E) "Try to avoid being bothered by little things."

Question 14

The wife of a 45-year-old man is very concerned about her husband's increasing alcoholism. She wants you to prescribe something for him that "will settle his nerves." He does not have the time to come to see you himself.

14. You should

(A) prescribe a mid-potency tranquilizer such as chlordiazepoxide
(B) insist on seeing the husband before you prescribe any treatment
(C) suggest that he would be better with Antabuse
(D) point out that his inability to come to see you is a sign of his resistance to treatment
(E) give the wife some sedation to help her relax

Question 15

One Sunday afternoon you are asked to see a 19-year-old male college student as an emergency consultation. His parents, who bring him to your office, complain that he is "totally out of control," "weird," and "unable to look after himself." The young man looks unkempt and rather dirty and steadfastly refuses to talk with you; he states he is not sick and "it is none of your business."

15. The only correct statement that follows is

(A) he should be hospitalized for further evaluation
(B) you have insufficient information to take any definite action
(C) he is most likely an early schizophrenic and should repond to chlorpromazine
(D) he is probably emotionally normal. You are being used in a purely family conflict.
(E) the parents may well be sick and themselves need counseling

Question 16

A 43-year-old married woman comes to see you about her 75-year-old mother. The mother lives by herself in a big old house, her home for the past 40 years. Her memory is not as good as it used to be and she leaves lights on, doors unlocked, and water faucets running. The daughter wants her mother to have the protection and care of the local state hospital.

16. You should

(A) prepare a commitment certificate for the mother
(B) point out to the daughter that she is obviously out to get her mother's possessions
(C) agree to interview and examine the elderly woman if she is willing to be examined
(D) refuse to be a part of the whole scheme
(E) suggest that the daughter herself may be undergoing emotional difficulties common at menopause

DIRECTIONS (Questions 17 through 26): Each group of items in this section consists of lettered headings followed by a set of numbered words or phrases. For each numbered word or phrase, select the <u>ONE</u> lettered heading that is most closely associated with it. <u>Each lettered heading may be selected once, more than once, or not at all.</u>

Questions 17 through 21

    (A) patient's emotional reaction to the therapist as if he or she were another significant person

    (B) conscious or unconscious emotional reaction of the psychotherapist to the patient

    (C) the planned giving of insight into the dynamics of feelings and behavior

    (D) uncensored verbalization of thoughts and feelings

    (E) opposition to revealing unconscious material

17. Resistance

18. Counter-transference

19. Free association

20. Transference

21. Interpretation

Questions 22 through 26

    (A) unpleasant stimulus paired with stimulus that causes maladaptive behavior

    (B) rewards for desired behavior

    (C) remove reward for inappropriate behavior so maladaptive response decreases

    (D) produce paired response antagonistic to undesired behavior

    (E) gradually increased exposure to stimulus, so even high intensity no longer produces maladaptive behavior

22. Positive reinforcement

23. Conditioned avoidance

24. Reciprocal inhibition

25. Desensitization

26. Extinction

Answers and Explanations

1. **(D)** *Behavior therapy* deals with *clearly observable behavior* of the subjects. This treatment approach does not attempt to uncover underlying *dynamics* for the maladaptive behavior. When the desired behavior occurs, it is strongly *reinforced positively* while the unwanted or unacceptable behaviors are *negatively reinforced* or the undesired behavior meets with no results, leading to *extinction* of this behavior. *(1:605–608;2: 769–773;3:69–71)*

2. **(E)** *Behavior modification* treatment has successfully treated *autistic children, phobic adults* (and children), and *sexual deviates*. *(1:605–608;2:770–771;3: 69–71)*

3. **(B)** *Behavior modification* is based on *reinforcement* where desired behavior is rewarded and sometimes undesired behavior brings an unpleasant result. *(1:605–608;2:772;3:69–71)*

4. **(E)** Psychoanalysis is of greatest value in treating *neuroses*.

    Psychoanalytic techniques can be used or modified in the treatment of patients with schizophrenia, borderline retardation, adolescent identity crises, and even major depression. In these sydromes, usually the analytic approach must be adapted and combined with other treatment procedures including environmental manipulations, family counseling, and pharmacotherapy. *(1:598;2:748–749;3:66–67)*

5. **(C)** *Transference* is the carryover of feelings from an earlier significant relationship to the psychotherapist. *(1:597–598;2:751–752;3:67)*
   A. *Counter-transference* is the manifestation of the therapist's conscious and unconscious feelings toward the patient. *(1:598;2:752–753;3:67)*
   B,D. The development of warm feelings between patient and psychotherapist would be the development of *empathy* where these feelings were objective, or of *sympathy* where the feelings were subjective. *(1:99;2:98;3:67)*

E. *Isolation* is the defense mechanism whereby an idea is split off or separated from the normal feelings that would accompany the idea but are repressed. *(1:329;2:94;3:10)*

6. **(C)** Whenever the patient manifests a disturbing symptom in the course of psychotherapy, the symptom generally should be openly recognized and the patient gently helped to discover where the symptom arose.
   A. The psychotherapist needs to understand, if possible, why the patient is crying so he can help her. Mere pouring out of feeling without sharing will not necessarily promote therapeutic movement.
   B. Some patients do indeed cry or show emotion not to communicate but to block more meaningful sharing. This interpretation may be correct but the psychotherapist probably needs more information before making such a comment. If the statement is not valid, the patient is liable to feel it to be an attack or a reprimand.
   D. Because the patient is distressed, there is no reason to bring the session to an end. The patient might feel the therapist was also scared of her feelings.
   E. If the psychotherapist changes away from a distressing subject, the patient may believe with good reason that the therapist is also anxious. *(1:595–598; 2:750–755;3:66–67)*

7. **(D)** This would be the most appropriate comment, planned to facilitate further communication. No judgments. No presuppositions.
   A. At the initial stages of psychotherapy, it is more important to gain understanding than it is to reassure the neurotic patient. Reassurance tends to block communication.
   B. This statement may be correct but is directly challenging. At this third session, such a comment may provoke more anger or anxiety than the patient can tolerate and lead her to discontinue therapy. The same interpretation could be made in a more supportive fashion, leading the patient to share and understand her feelings more.

C. This is again a valid comment but a statement that may be out of place. When the psychotherapist raises potentially distressing concepts, he or she should be sure that the psychotherapy bond can tolerate the stress. Also the therapist should beware of raising provoking subjects before having a thorough understanding of the patient, which he or she does not have by the third interview.

E. Reassurance may be comforting to the patient and to the psychotherapist, but reassurance does tend to block rather than facilitate communication. *(1:595–597;2:750–755;3:66–69)*

8. **(C)** While patients need good reality reinforcement, in psychotherapy it is more important for patient and psychotherapist to know why a question was asked than to have an answer.

"Why do you ask?" is the correct answer. The therapist and patient need to know what exactly the patient is asking for and why.

A. Later in the psychotherapy process this might be an appropriate answer when said in a supportive fashion to a patient who needs to know reality. At this stage in treatment, such an answer brings an end to that communication.

B. Not only does this response block communication, it is also untrue and deceitful. The therapist must never base the treatment on deception, however kindly meant. His or her task is to help the patient adapt to generally accepted reality.

D. The psychotherapist should avoid personalizing any issue in psychotherapy. This is a manifestation of counter-transference being acted out.

E. This is a direct block to communication. *(1:595–597;2:750–755;3:66–69)*

9. **(A)** It is more important to gain understanding than to socialize with the patient.

Sometimes patient and psychotherapist will find themselves acting together in a way that delays or minimizes communication.

By bringing a gift the patient is tuning in to the psychotherapist's personality and the therpist must handle the situation with full objectivity.

"Why do you want to give me this gift?" would tend to support increased communication. The psychotherapist is not seduced, threatened, or judgmental. His role is to help the patient and he will not be deflected by a gift.

A. At only the second interview, this is a presumptuous comment by the psychotherapist, who cannot yet know the many reasons for such a gift.

C. To accept any gift without understanding the underlying communication bodes ill for the development of the psychotherapy process. The therapist needs to know much more.

D. This comment has many counter-transference overtones. The psychotherapist is reading into a gesture by the patient much more than the psy-

chotherapist knows. The psychotherapist is reacting to his own counter-transference, to his own projection.

E. The therapist should not make such a comment. He does not know if the tie is a gift, a bribe, a threat—or what.

Again, the therapist and patient must understand what is happening before they feel any need to respond. *(1:595–598;2:750–755;3:66–69)*

10. **(B)** The management of the dangerous patient is a topic that is rarely discussed in standard textbooks. The cardinal rule is that the clinician cannot allow the patient to hurt himself or those around him in any lasting fashion. This responsibility to the individual patient and to society far outweighs any limitations imposed by rules or requirements of confidentiality.

The therapist must attempt to ally himself or herself with that part of the patient's personality that is willing to relinquish this potentially lethal weapon. The physician should emphasize that he or she is not willing to allow the patient, his or her clinical responsibility, to run the risk of hurting himself by using the knife in any fashion. For the patient's sake, he must be relieved of the knife. If the patient refuses to give up the knife, the doctor should call in police or security personnel to relieve the patient of the knife. The patient may need hospitalization.

A. A patient carrying a knife or any other dangerous instrument or weapon is not tolerable in any hospital unit. If the therapist hides behind the barrier of confidentiality, he or she is leaving his or her patient, this paranoid schizophrenic man, and the staff and patients of the unit, liable to be severely hurt.

C. There is no point in appearing to threaten the patient in any way that may provoke a sudden attack. There is no benefit in becoming a dead hero. In society there are people trained to disarm potentially dangerous people. If the paranoid schizophrenic patient seems unlikely to surrender his switchblade to the psychotherapist or to the unit staff, the physician in charge should not hesitate to call on the assistance of the appropriate legal authorities.

D. If the psychotherapist insists that the patient accept the full responsibility of getting rid of the switchblade, the therapist is avoiding his or her clinical responsibility. The physician must make sure that the knife is placed in safe custody or destroyed. If the patient is required only to put it away, he can get it back with equal ease. If he hides it, someone else can find it. The possibilities for acting out are endless.

E. As long as this psychotic patient has possession of a potentially lethal weapon, he is a danger to himself and to society and no number of appointments can get around this reality. Psychotherapy cannot dissolve a weapon. This is one example of a reality where the therapist must act first and then work through the feelings later. *(1:582–583;2:851–852;3:192)*

11. **(B)** As in any consultation, a good introductory move is to introduce yourself and explain the nature and purpose of the visit.

A. Premature reassurance blocks communication that may be vital. Until the consultant has thoroughly evaluated the patient, reassurance is out of place.

C. Too much nonsense is written about looking patients "in the eye." In any evaluation procedure, the consultant notes and considers every communication including the reality of whether there was eye contact or not. Each patient, like each individual, has his or her own way of communicating, and the consultant should not try to impose an unacceptable or uncomfortable communication.

D. The consultant must be careful to maintain routine confidentiality. Unless the patient gives written permission to discuss his situation with the dean of students, even discussing the fact of his hospitalization may be a breach of professional confidentiality. (Even though colleges and universities maintain that a history of emotional illness does not hinder a student's chance of acceptance, it is understandable that admission committees prefer to accept students with no risk of psychiatric difficulty.)

E. Hospitalization can serve many therapeutic functions for the patient, his family, his culture, and his physician. The consultant must thoroughly evaluate all factors before recommending discharge; the consultant should propose alternative treatment or support if such is required. *(1:595-598;2:185-202;3:31-33)*

12. **(C)** The seductive patient is a favorite examination subject. Often these questions seem contrived, but they serve to point out several things: The physician must be able to recognize a seductive patient, male or female; the clinician must be sensitive to his or her own reactions to such a patient; and the doctor must continue to evaluate and treat the patient in the most supportive professional way.

Each patient, even a seemingly neurotic patient, needs to be treated with respect as a first step to maintain or build self-respect. Any patient is entitled to a thorough medical and psychological evaluation. With the office nurse present, the opportunity for seductiveness is minimized and, with support, the patient may communicate in other more direct and appropriate ways.

A. The physician cannot avoid professional responsibilities by rejecting or avoiding the patient. This patient, in her own way, is asking for help.

B. It would be wonderful if we could all "pull ourselves together" on the basis of our own inner strengths, but then we would not really need each other at all. We would cease to be human. Before you, as the physician, make such a demand, you must ask yourself why the patient should be expected to "pull his or herself together." How will this benefit the patient? Or will it? You should know whether the patient has the emotional capacity to pull together and stay together. Most important, you have to recognize that these aches and pains are a communication about something. As the physician, you need to know what this message is before you insist that the communication stop.

D. The doctor should hesitate acting out any patient's wish for private closeness even in order to point out seductiveness. Such an interaction is open to misinterpretation and can easily get out of control.

E. Until the doctor has evaluated the patient thoroughly, medically and psychiatrically, the doctor does not know whether or not the patient does need companionship. If it becomes obvious that this is indeed the situation, it is better to invite the spouse to meet the doctor at the office and discuss the situation. A telephone call can be too abrupt, open to misinterpretation, and too brief for resolution of feelings. *(1:112-114;2:185-187)*

13. **(C)** "What should I do to get well?" is a common question asked by patients and an easy way to pass the responsibility totally over to the psychotherapist. No matter how directly the therapist tries to answer this question, any specific response he or she gives will be wrong in some way. The therapist will help the patient get well by allying himself or herself with the healthy aspects of the patient's personality.

This is an awkward but correct response. The therapist wants to say to the patient that he or she will join with the patient in considering everything together. The psychotherapist's task is to help develop the patient's own individual strengths.

A. By saying, "Trust in me," the therapist has told the patient that the doctor will carry the total burden. If the patient is to grow emotionally, he must learn to carry his own emotional responsibilities more capably. This response is an invitation to regression and dependency.

B. "That is not up to me to tell you" is the opposite quality of response where the psychotherapist refuses to accept any responsibility in what should be a shared therapeutic alliance. Many patients do need guidance, prompting, suggestions, and models.

D. This response blocks communication. The therapist does not know why the patient was asking or what specifically the patient was requesting; so it was bad technique to shut off the communication by this response.

E. Here the therapist is trying to give a specific answer that any patient can quickly make appear ridiculous. *(1:113-114;2:187-189)*

14. **(B)** You must see the husband to evaluate him before deciding on any treatment.

A,C. Never diagnose or treat a patient by proxy or in abstentia. You do not know what this man's alcoholic intake signifies—normality, depression, psychosis, early senility, marital difficulties—the possibilities are endless. You should not treat what you do not understand.

D. You do not know whether his inability to come to see you is a sign of resistance; he may work an inflexible schedule, so you may need to make your schedule more flexible.

E. If the wife is given sedation to block out reality, you are trying to build a barrier of denial. This defense takes a great deal of psychic energy and tends to distort reality. It would be more productive to help the wife cope with the situation with less denial and more productive personal adaptation. *(1:115–116;2:184–185)*

15. **(B)** The doctor who is asked to bring children "under control" is faced with a common problem. It is not the task of clinicians to provide control or to ensure that some individuals, even parents, maintain dominance over other people.

The physician has the responsibility of examining whether the conflict is a manifestation of emotional maladaption or illness. He or she can only evaluate where the patient wishes to be evaluated or where the legally responsible people can insist on maintaining an evaluation.

This 19-year-old man is past the age of full legal responsibility. He states directly that his life is not the physician's concern. Unless the doctor has clear evidence of markedly inappropriate behavior, he or she cannot interfere in this young man's life.

You do not have sufficient information to take any action and you should so inform the parents and the son. However, you can continue to offer to work with them as parents, as a family, or as individuals because their present interaction is mutually unproductive.

A. With no other signs of disturbed behavior, forced hospitalization would grossly infringe on the young man's legal rights and leave everyone involved open to legal suit.

C. The fact that the young man is unkempt, dirty, and refuses to cooperate does not in any way suggest that he is an early schizophrenic. For such a diagnosis, much more information about his personality and relationship ability is needed. The doctor must not confuse a personal dislike for the patient's style of life with evidence of emotional illness.

D. Equally there is insufficient evidence for a diagnosis of normality.

E. The parents may or may not be sick. You have insufficient information.

Here is a family in pain. It is unclear from where the pain is originating. You must not act out family anxieties or psychopathology but you must be supportive to all family members. *(1:112;2:184–187)*

16. **(C)** Unless this elderly woman is grossly incompetent socially or a danger to herself or to society, she cannot be obliged to be examined psychiatrically. At the same time you cannot and must not attempt to diagnose her without seeing her.

A. Commitment necessitates direct examination of the patient.

B. Even if this statement were true, the physician serves little therapeutic purpose by merely antagonizing a patient or a patient's relatives.

D. When a doctor is asked for help, he or she is being requested to respond to some pain, anxiety, or maladjustment in the family. He or she may not like the message or the manner of the request for assistance, but he or she cannot refuse to help or attempt to help this woman and her family.

E. Menopause tensions do indeed lead to many psychological problems, but too often this reason is used to explain away many unrelated physical and emotional difficulties. Before such a diagnostic comment is made, the daughter should be evaluated thoroughly. *(1:112;2:184–187;3:149–152)*

Answers 17 through 21 deal with psychoanalytic technique. (1:595–600;2:748–759;3:66–69)

17. **(E)** *Resistance* is the conscious and unconscious opposition to the revealing of unconscious material, usually by a patient in treatment. *(1:597–2:751; 3:66)*

18. **(B)** *Counter-transference* is the conscious and unconscious emotional reaction of the psychotherapist to the patient.

Many psychotherapists use their counter-transference as a useful diagnostic and therapeutic tool. *(1:598;2:752–753;3:67)*

19. **(D)** *Free association,* a prerequisite for analytic treatment, is the uncensored verbalization of all thoughts and feelings. *(1:596;2:750;3:66)*

20. **(A)** *Transference* is the patient's emotional reaction to the therapist as if the psychotherapist were another significant person. Feelings from an early nuclear relationship are transferred to the therapist in the therapeutic interaction. *(1:597–598;2:751–752;3:67)*

21. **(C)** In psychotherapy, *interpretation* is the psychotherapist's method of giving the patient planned insight into the dynamics of the patient's feelings and

behavior. Sometimes this insight leads to the release of unconscious emotions with the outward release of feelings (catharsis). *(1:598;2:753–754;3:66)*

Answers 22 through 26 deal with behavior therapy. (1:605–608;2:769–773;3:69–71)

22. **(B)** *Positive reinforcement* rewards the subject for producing or manifesting the desired behavior. *(1:607;2:772;3:55–56)*

23. **(A)** When an unpleasant stimulus is paired with the stimulus that usually causes the maladaptive behavior, this is termed *conditioned avoidance.* The alcoholic taking disulfiram (Antabuse) feels physically uncomfortable when he or she tries to enjoy alcohol. *(1:43;2:772;3:69–71)*

24. **(D)** *Reciprocal inhibition* works by pairing a response antagonistic to the undesired behavior with this behavioral response. Wolpe has emphasized the technique of developing progressive relaxation simultaneously with the anxiety-arousing stimulus. *(1:40–41;2:772;3:70)*

25. **(E)** In *desensitization,* the patient is given gradually increased exposure to the anxiety-provoking stimulus, starting from a low intensity, so that eventually even a high-intensity stimulus no longer produces the maladaptive behavior.

The patient who is phobic for white rabbits could be progressively desensitized to white wool, a white rabbit toy, and then a live white rabbit. *(1:41;2:772; 3:70)*

26. **(C)** *Extinction* involves removing the reward for the inappropriate behavior so that the maladaptive behavior gradually decreases and then increases.

Often a child's "bad" behavior is perpetuated by all the attention this behavior brings; when this behavior is ignored, the youngster may gradually cease to act in this fashion and extinction has occurred. *(1:607;2:772;3:69)*

CHAPTER 7

Social Psychiatry and Forensic Psychiatry
Questions

INTRODUCTION

In this era of social awareness, much attention is given to the concept of community psychiatry. Unfortunately, basic principles and goals have yet to be defined and tested. Each standard textbook deals with some aspects of community work, but as yet there is no clear definition of the understanding required from the examination candidate. Most examinations do have specific questions dealing with community psychiatry as one facet of social psychiatry.

Forensic psychiatry is included in this brief chapter as a neglected but essential aspect of the clinician's work. For clinical work and for examinations the student and clinician must know certain basic principles of legal psychiatry, which are asked about in most examinations, often in several different ways.

REFERENCES

Social Psychiatry

1. Chapter 39, Community Psychiatry, pp 869–880
2. Chapter 31, Social and Community Psychiatry, pp 787–808
3. Chapter 9, Community and Social Psychiatry, pp 139–148

Forensic Psychiatry

1. Chapter 41, Forensic Psychiatry, pp 887–898
2. Chapter 34, Psychiatry and the Law, pp 847–867
3. Chapter 10, Psychiatry and the Law, pp 149–158

DIRECTIONS (Questions 1 through 18): Each of the numbered items or incomplete statements in this section is followed by answers or by completions of the statement. Select the ONE lettered answer or completion that is BEST in each case.

1. The fourth pregnancy of a 42-year-old mother has resulted in a child with Down's syndrome. You begin a program of counseling with the parents and encourage them to join the local association of parents of retarded children. Your work with the parents in dealing with their new child could be classified as

    (A) primary prevention
    (B) genetic counseling
    (C) secondary prevention
    (D) tertiary prevention
    (E) suppression

2. Primary prevention programs

    (A) are planned for early identification and treatment of an illness
    (B) minimize the handicapping effect of any illness
    (C) work to lower the incidence of a disease
    (D) deal with the initial symptoms of a disorder
    (E) focus on the outward manifestations of an illness rather than the underlying causes

3. A community is likely to define a substance as a "drug of abuse" when

    (A) the drug is shown to cause liver or brain damage
    (B) the substance is used by a small segment of the population
    (C) the use of the drug conflicts with community standards
    (D) prolonged use leads to physical dependence
    (E) the drug is liable to be impure or diluted with toxic substances

4. In planning a primary prevention program for the management of mental retardation, you would want to establish all of the following *except*

    (A) genetic counseling for parents
    (B) antenatal care programs
    (C) physical rehabilitation services for the retarded
    (D) public education campaigns
    (E) easily accessible pediatric services

5. A 76-year-old woman lives by herself in a small apartment. Her married daughter would like to move her mother to a comfortable rest home. You advise the daughter that

    (A) the move would help encourage her mother to be more socially outgoing
    (B) the move is liable to precipitate physical and psychological deterioration
    (C) the move would lessen her mother's workload and lengthen her life

    (D) the move to a country environment would act as a physical tonic

6. You have just been appointed director of a community health center. Your main professional role should be

    (A) direct care for patients
    (B) clinical supervision of the social workers, psychologists, and paraprofessionals
    (C) consultation with the other agency psychiatrists
    (D) public relations work for the agency
    (E) supervision and coordination of all the agency staff

7. By diagnosis, the largest group of patients in state mental hospitals are

    (A) alcoholic
    (B) senile
    (C) depressed
    (D) schizophrenic
    (E) affected by personality disorders

8. Tertiary prevention

    (A) reduces the residual handicapping of an illness
    (B) provides the earliest possible treatment of a disease
    (C) works for the earliest identification of an illness
    (D) necessitates easily available genetic counseling
    (E) aims to reduce the occurrence of a disorder

9. In a hotly contested political election, you are working actively for one of the candidates. You sincerely believe that the other candidate is unsuited for office. On a radio interview show, you are asked for your clinical opinion of the opposition candidate's mental condition. In response, you should

    (A) give a clear, concise evaluation of the opposition politician but point out that your opinions are not based on direct examination
    (B) give a thoughtful in-depth opinion based on everything you know about the subject
    (C) refuse to give any clinical opinion
    (D) take the opportunity to make known your professional doubts about the opposition candidate's psychological competence
    (E) respond with a joking comment if possible

10. To be competent to stand trial, the accused must be capable of all of the following *except* the ability to

    (A) understand questions
    (B) remember
    (C) distinguish fantasy from reality
    (D) read and write
    (E) cooperate in his or her own defense

11. To make a legally acceptable will, the person making the will must fulfill all of the following criteria *except*

(A) understand that he or she is making a will
(B) be able to read and write
(C) know the nature and extent of his or her property
(D) be aware of the "natural objects of his [or her] bounty"
(E) be able to understand the interrelationship of these factors

12. Once a person has been legally judged incompetent, all of the following usually apply *except* that he or she

(A) is hospitalized
(B) loses his or her voting rights
(C) cannot practice his or her profession
(D) cannot adopt children
(E) loses his or her driver's license

13. The M'Naghten rule

(A) is a test of sanity
(B) provides guidelines for commitment
(C) defines criminal responsibility
(D) indicates criteria for testamentary capacity
(E) outlines the grounds for divorce on the basis of insanity

14. The Durham rule states that the

(A) subject escapes responsibility if his or her criminal behavior was a product of mental illness or defect
(B) accused is not held responsible if he or she does not appreciate the nature and quality of his or her actions
(C) behavior committed as an irresistible impulse cannot be held to the responsibility of the individual
(D) person cannot be held responsible if he or she does not understand the difference between right and wrong
(E) individual cannot be held responsible if he or she lacks the ability to handle himself or herself according to legal requirements

15. Your patient wishes to make a will. To minimize the risk that this will be challenged on grounds of mental incompetency, you should

(A) take a very thorough history from the patient
(B) examine the patient carefully at the time the will is made and record all your findings
(C) make a careful note of your diagnosis at the time the will is being written
(D) discharge the patient temporarily from psychiatric treatment until the will has been written and filed
(E) meet with the family members and do a thorough family evaluation

16. The M'Naghten rule in determining responsibility is concerned with

(A) irresistible impulse
(B) whether the criminal act was a product of mental illness
(C) competence to stand trial
(D) understanding of right and wrong
(E) ability to act as a witness

17. To practice psychiatry in a state requires

(A) specialist board certification
(B) a state medical license
(C) an acceptable residency training
(D) a personal psychoanalysis
(E) none of the above

18. Testamentary capacity is

(A) competency to act as a witness
(B) ability to handle own affairs
(C) competency to make a will
(D) ability to take part in one's own legal defense
(E) the knowledge of right and wrong

Answers and Explanations

1. **(C)** *Secondary prevention* aims to diagnose the illness or malfunctioning early and treat the disease intensively.

   In the case described, you cannot prevent the malfunctioning from occurring (which would have been primary prevention), but you can help the parents deal productively with their anxieties and anger and assist them in working to minimize the immediate consequences of their child's limitations. *(1:877–879; 2:788;3:140)*

2. **(C)** *Primary prevention* programs work to lower the incidence of a disease—to prevent the maladaption or malfunctioning from ever occurring. *(1:876–877;2: 788;3:140)*

   Programs for early identification and treatment that deal with initial symptoms are included in *secondary prevention.*

   Once a disease has occurred and chronic handicapping has developed, programs to limit or reduce the handicapping would be considered *tertiary prevention.*

3. **(C)** A substance is defined as a "drug of abuse" when its use conflicts with community standards. Across the world, alcohol abuse is a major cause of individual, family, and community problems, yet alcohol sale and distribution are socially supported and frequently provide a substantial portion of government revenue. *(1:385;2:644–645;3:233)*

4. **(C)** This is an artificial question since undoubtedly a community planner would not limit a program solely to primary, secondary, or tertiary prevention. This question is designed merely to test the candidates' understanding of primary prevention as a concept. *Primary prevention* prevents the disease from ever occurring. Thus *genetic counseling, antenatal care, public education,* and *accessible pediatric services* all work to prevent mental retardation from occurring. Physical rehabilitation deals with the retarded after they have appeared; that is, after primary prevention has failed or been unavailable. *(1:876–877;2:788;3:140)*

5. **(B)** Most human beings develop a very meaningful sense of belonging—to family and friends, to a place. In the very old and the young, this sense of belonging is a critical and stabilizing part of the individual's adaptation. With the aged, familiar surroundings and faces become even more important and, for many, an integral part of their personality and sense of self. Much more than is often realized, the elderly come to depend on the same accustomed cues and stimuli.

   When an elderly person is removed from his or her own home, emotional disintegration is liable to occur. The healthy elderly man will state that he has lost a part of himself with a move, and psychologically he is correct. The elderly woman may give up physical and intellectual ties to the living world when moved away from her familiar home. A move that lessens an elderly person's workload may also reduce his or her purpose for living. *(1:884–886;2:241)*

6. **(E)** This question attempts to focus on principles of administrative and community psychiatry. The director or focal administration officer must first fulfill the role of decision maker, integrator, and leader for staff. He or she cannot spend time on direct patient care when his or her prime function is to run a mental health center. Clinically-oriented professionals find it difficult not to spend their time in direct front-line patient care when, in reality, they can best use their talents in supervising and teaching others to handle a much wider group of patients than they could have seen in direct patient contact.

   The director of any unit must be director and spokesperson for all the staff, not just any one limited professional group, not even his or her own profession. Similarly the supervisory responsibilities as director take in all the staff, not just the other professions or his or her own profession.

   When a director must do public relations work, he or she cannot work outside the health center at the expense of work with the staff for whom he or she is responsible.

   Thus, the director of a community health center has, as his or her main professional role, the task of supervising and coordinating the work of all the agency staff. *(1:869–872;2:796–798;3:139–140)*

7. **(D)** By diagnosis, the largest group of patients in state mental hospitals are *schizophrenic. (1:196;2:347–349; 3:141)*

8. **(A)** The aim of *tertiary prevention* programs is to *reduce the residual handicapping* of an illness. *(1: 879–880;2:788;3:140)*

　　Primary prevention would include genetic counseling and would aim to reduce the occurrence.

　　Secondary prevention is designed to provide early identification and treatment.

　　Primary, secondary, and tertiary prevention programs are seen in every area of social medicine (and thus in the examination for every specialty).

　　In considering *rheumatic fever, primary prevention* might include prophylactic antibotics to prevent the spread of streptococcal infections.

　　Secondary prevention would offer good pediatric diagnostic and treatment services for children with acute rheumatic fever. The illness cannot now be prevented but heart-valve scarring might be minimized.

　　Tertiary prevention would offer rehabilitation and treatment programs to children with heart-valve scarring: surgery for mitral stenosis and homebound schooling for the incapacitated.

9. **(C)** No clinician gives a clinical opinion without an adequate examination of the patient, and all clinicians are ethically bound to confidentiality about their clinical opinions.

　　A physician, no matter the circumstances, can never avoid his or her professional responsibilities when acting in any fashion in a clinical capacity. *(1:889;2:850)*

10. **(D)** There is no need for the accused to be able to read or write. But to be *legally competent to stand trial* he or she must be able to distinguish fantasy from reality, to answer questions, to cooperate in his or her own defense, and to remember.

　　Competency to stand trial is quite different from criminal responsibility. *(1:879;2:850;3:152)*

11. **(B)** *Testamentary capacity* is a specialized area of competency—the *competency to make a legally acceptable will.*

　　To be considered legally competent, the person making the will must, at the time of making the will, be able to understand that he or she is making a will; know the nature and extent of his or her property; know who are the "natural objects of his [or her] bounty"—wife or husband; children, close relatives; and be able to understand the interrelationship of these factors. He or she does not have to be able to read or write in this situation. *(1:893–894;2:859;3:152)*

12. **(A)** Once a person has been judged legally incompetent, the following usually occur (the word *usually* is included here because the effect of this legal judgment

varies from state to state): he or she loses voting rights, cannot practice his or her profession, cannot adopt children, and loses his or her driver's license.

　　He or she is not necessarily hospitalized. Hospitalization is liable to occur if he or she is judged to be a danger to himself or herself or to society or to require hospital care and supervision.

　　A person judged legally incompetent can be cared for and supervised in his or her own home. *(1:894; 2:859–860;3:151–152)*

13. **(C)** The M'Naghten rule,* established in Victorian Britain, defines *criminal responsibility.*

　　It is not a test of sanity and does not give guidelines for commitment, testamentary capacity, or grounds for divorce. *(1:894–895;2:864–865;3:153)*

14. **(A)** The *Durham rule or decision* states that the subject cannot be held responsible if his or her criminal behavior was a product of mental illness or defect.

　　This rule arose from the legal decision of the District of Columbia Court of Appeals in 1954. In 1972 the same court unanimously discarded this test of insanity. *(1:896;2:865;3:153)*

15. **(B)** To protect your patient or client on any occasion against risk of challenge to his or her *mental competency,* you should examine the patient carefully at the time legal action is taken—in this case making a will—and record all of your findings.

　　A thorough history focuses on the past and may not in any way indicate the patient's mental and emotional state at the time in question.

　　A diagnosis is a subjective opinion, open to later question. You must record observed facts. Even though the patient is not labeled as a psychiatric patient, his or her judgment can always be called in question.

　　A thorough family evaluation may have nothing to do with the patient's mental status. *(1:893–894; 2:859;3:152)*

16. **(D)** The *M'Naghten rule* in defining criminal responsibility is concerned with the accused's understanding of right and wrong—did he or she know the nature and consequences of the act and, if so, did he or she understand that this act was wrong. *(1:894–895;2:864–865;3:153)*

　　The *Irresistible Impulse Rule* states that the accused cannot be held responsible for his or her behavior if he or she could not have resisted the impulse to this behavior, even when understanding the likelihood of being caught or punished. *(1:895–896;2:865;3:153)*

---

*Daniel M'Naghten, after whom the legal rule is named, is listed as McNaugten, M'Naugten, and McNaghten in different textbooks.

17. **(B)** To *practice psychiatry* in a state requires at present only a valid state medical license. *(3:1)*

18. **(C)** *Testamentary capacity* is the *competency to make one's own will. (1:893–894;2:859;3:152)*

Testamentary capacity has nothing to do legally with competency to act as a witness or in one's own defense or with general competency, nor has it any bearing on the capacity to understand the difference between right and wrong.

CHAPTER 8

History of Psychiatry
Questions

INTRODUCTION

Many of the national examinations do not have questions on the historical background of the various branches of medicine. However, even in these examinations, allusions to historical aspects may be part of individual questions. Certainly in other examinations the candidate must be prepared for questions on the historical evolution of the specialty.

In the behavioral sciences, certain key scientists and seminal concepts are important in clinical work and in 20th-century culture. These investigators and their ideas are the focus of this chapter.

REFERENCES

1. Chapters 1–6,   The Life Cycle; Science of Human Behavior; Theories of Personality and Psychopathology, pp 1–111
2. Chapters 1–2,   The Beginnings of Psychiatry: Development of Modern Psychiatry, pp 1–26
3. Chapter 1,   Development and Dynamics, pp 1–14

DIRECTIONS (Questions 1 through 6): Each of the numbered items or incomplete statements in this section is followed by answers or by completions of the statement. Select the **ONE** lettered answer or completion that is **BEST** in each case.

1. In everyday discussion you may hear the phrase "identity crisis." This is a concept of

   (A) S. Freud
   (B) E. Bleuler
   (C) B. F. Skinner
   (D) E. Erikson
   (E) Mesmer

2. "Freudian slip" is a popular term for

   (A) parapraxis
   (B) catharsis
   (C) cathexis
   (D) transference
   (E) counter-transference

3. The "Oedipus complex" is a concept introduced by

   (A) C. Jung
   (B) A. Adler
   (C) P. Janet
   (D) S. Freud
   (E) I. Pavlov

4. The term "inferiority complex" refers to a concept described by

   (A) A. Freud
   (B) J. Piaget
   (C) A. Adler
   (D) J. Sartre
   (E) W. Reich

5. Jung introduced all the following concepts *except*

   (A) inferiority conplex
   (B) collective unconscious
   (C) persona
   (D) introversion and extroversion
   (E) anima

6. In his structuring of the psychic apparatus, Freud included all of the following *except*

   (A) preconscious
   (B) superego
   (C) anima
   (D) id
   (E) ego ideal

DIRECTIONS (Questions 7 through 36): Each group of items in this section consists of lettered headings followed by a set of numbered words or phrases. For each numbered word or phrase, select the **ONE** lettered heading that is most closely associated with it. **Each lettered heading may be selected once, more than once, or not at all.**

Questions 7 through 11

   (A) basic trust
   (B) neurasthenia
   (C) psychobiology
   (D) schizophrenia
   (E) inferiority complex

7. Bleuler
8. Beard
9. Erikson
10. Adler
11. Meyer

Questions 12 through 16

   (A) prefrontal lobotomy
   (B) electroconvulsive therapy
   (C) projective tests
   (D) psychodrama
   (E) therapeutic community

12. Moreno
13. Moniz
14. Maxwell Jones
15. Cerletti
16. Rorschach

Questions 17 through 21

   (A) imprinting
   (B) somatotypes
   (C) schizophrenic twin studies
   (D) primate behavior research
   (E) operant conditioning

17. Sheldon
18. Kallmann
19. Harlow
20. Lorenz
21. Skinner

Questions 22 through 26

    (A) collective unconscious
    (B) infantile autism
    (C) unchaining the mentally ill
    (D) infantile sexuality
    (E) intelligence testing

22. S. Freud

23. Binet

24. Jung

25. Kanner

26. Pinel

Questions 27 through 31

    (A) child development
    (B) phenothiazines
    (C) lysergic acid diethylamide
    (D) electroencephalogram
    (E) insulin coma therapy

27. Hoffman

28. Sakel

29. Piaget

30. Delay

31. Berger

Questions 32 through 36

    (A) *Declaration of Independence* and the first American psychiatry text
    (B) *The Mind That Found Itself*
    (C) *The Anatomy of Melancholy*
    (D) *The Interpretation of Dreams*
    (E) *Confessions of an Opium Eater*

32. Clifford Beers

33. Sigmund Freud

34. Benjamin Rush

35. Thomas DeQuincey

36. Robert Burton

Answers and Explanations

1. **(D)** According to *Erik Erikson, adolescence* is the stage when the growing child establishes his or her individual *identity,* the time of the *identity crisis* of ego identity versus role confusion. *(1:89–92;2:61;3:177)*

   S. Freud was the originator and developer of *psychoanalysis.*

   E. Bleuler introduced the concept of *schizophrenia.*

   B. F. Skinner has developed the concept of operant conditioning.

   Mesmer, an 18th-century German physician, briefly popularized hypnosis—hence our word *mesmerize.*

2. **(A)** A *parapraxis,* or *Freudian slip,* is a slip of the tongue betraying underlying unconscious feelings. *(1:146;2:146;3:6)*

   The other terms also refer to psychoanalytic concepts.

   Catharsis is the release of repressed ideas or feelings with appropriate outward emotional reaction.

   Cathexis is the investment of emotional energy in an object, person, or goal.

   Transference feelings are those emotions, initially linked to a significant life figure, that are transferred onto a person in a present relationship.

   Counter-transference is the feelings, logical and illogical, of the psychotherapist toward the patient.

3. **(D)** The *Oedipus complex* is a psychological concept introduced by S. Freud. *(1:71;2:72–73;3:6)*

   C. Jung, a Swiss analyst, focused more on the heredity aspects of the human personality.

   A. Adler, the founder of Adlerian individual psychology, branched off from traditional psychoanalysis to emphasize more the development of the individual in society.

   P. Janet, a French psychiatrist, wrote extensively on hysteria and obsessive–compulsive neuroses.

   I. Pavlov, a Russian physiologist and Nobel Prize winner, introduced and developed the concept of conditioned reflexes and conditioning.

4. **(C)** *Alfred Adler* emphasized the helplessness of the very young child, a helplessness that leads to a lifelong pervasive feeling of inferiority against which the individual constantly strives.

   The *inferiority complex* was one concept derived from Adlerian principles. *(1:104–105;2:12;3:11)*

   Anna Freud, the daughter of Sigmund Freud, has expanded her father's psychoanalytic theory, especially in the field of child and adolescent psychiatry.

   J. Piaget was an influential Swiss psychologist who developed an extensive theory of child development.

   J. Sartre was a 20th century French writer-philosopher.

   W. Reich, once more the subject of general interest, developed the process of *character analysis.*

5. **(A)** *Carl Jung* introduced the concepts of *collective unconscious, persona, introversion* and *extroversion,* and *anima.*

   Alfred Adler popularized the idea of the *inferiority complex.* *(1:101–103;2:12–13;3:11)*

6. **(C)** *Carl Jung* included the *anima* in his theory of personality structure. The *preconscious,* the *superego,* the *id,* and the *ego ideal* were *Freudian* concepts of psychic apparatus. *(1:101–103;2:11–13;3:11)*

7. **(D)** *Eugen Bleuler* delineated the schizophrenic syndromes and introduced the term *schizophrenia.* *(1:194–195;2:346–347;3:245–246)*

8. **(B)** In the period after the Civil War, *George Beard,* an American physician, introduced the concept of *neurasthenia.*

9. **(A)** *Erik Erikson,* an Austrian psychoanalyst, suggested that infants develop *basic trust* during a stable mother–child interaction. *(1:89–92;2:61;3:177)*

10. **(E)** *Alfred Adler* postulated that all humankind struggles against a basic feeling of inferiority from the time of infant helplessness. He introduced the term *inferiority complex.* *(1:104–105;2:12;3:11)*

11. **(C)** *Adolph Meyer* developed the *psychobiologic* approach, which emphasized the study of the whole person in his or her environment. *(1:110-111;2:13-14)*

12. **(D)** *Jacob Moreno* developed *psychodrama*, a form of group psychotherapy where a person's or a group's relationships are acted out. *(1:619;2:777;3:72)*

13. **(A)** *Egas Moniz* was awarded the Nobel Prize for his pioneering work on *prefrontal lobotomy* in the mid-1930s. Though psychosurgery has been largely superseded by psychopharmacologic treatment, Moniz's work opened up a wide field of research. *(2:843-845;3:94)*

14. **(E)** *Maxwell Jones*, a British psychiatrist, popularized the *therapeutic community* where patients largely govern their own institutional management in alliance with the professional staff. *(2:774)*

15. **(B)** *Ugo Cerletti*, in collaboration with his colleague *L. Bini*, pioneered *electroconvulsive therapy*, following the use of pharmacologic convulsive treatments by *Meduna*. *(1:679;2:836;3:131)*

16. **(C)** *Herman Rorschach* developed the most widely used *projective test*, using a series of ten inkblots as the standard ambiguous stimulus. *(1:128-129;2:206;3:48)*

17. **(B)** *W. H. Sheldon* devised a method of human *somatotyping* and postulated a relationship between personality type and body somatotype. *(2:157-159)*

18. **(C)** *Franz Kallmann*, in the United States, did the first extensive *twin study* on the incidence of *schizophrenia*. *(1:197;2:49;3:249)*

19. **(D)** *Harry Harlow*, at the University of Wisconsin, worked extensively in studies on the effects of *maternal deprivation in primates*. *(1:47-53;2:69-70;3:59-60)*

20. **(A)** *Konrad Lorenz*, in his studies on newly hatched geese, showed the effects of early *imprinting*. *(1:45-46;2:28;3:59)*

21. **(E)** *B. F. Skinner*, a behavioral psychologist, has written extensively about his research in the area of *operant conditioning*. *(1:41-42;2:49;3:55)*

22. **(D)** *Sigmund Freud* first popularized the concept of *infant sexuality* as he was developing his psychoanalytic theory of personality. *(1:70;2:12;3:4-7)*

23. **(E)** *Alfred Binet*, in France, formulated the first widely used form of *intelligence testing*. His test was later modified and is still in use as the Stanford–Binet test. *(1:128;2:203-204;3:46)*

24. **(A)** *Carl Jung*, a Swiss psychoanalyst, developed his own school of analysis and included in his theory of personality growth and structure the concept of the collective unconscious, common to every person. *(1:101-103;2:13;3:11)*

25. **(B)** *Leo Kanner*, in 1943, first delineated the syndrome of *infantile autism*, which has led to extensive research in childhood psychoses and early emotional development. *(1:732;2:384;3:201)*

26. **(C)** Periodically there are waves of treatment reform when the management of the emotionally ill becomes less custodial and repressive. *Philippe Pinel* is famed for *unchaining the mentally ill* in France at the time of the French Revolution. *(2:5)*

27. **(C)** *Albert Hoffman*, a Swiss chemist, accidentally discovered the hallucinogenic effects of lysergic acid diethylamide in 1943. *(3:222)*

28. **(E)** *Manfred Sakel* developed the use of *insulin coma treatment*, which, in the 1940s, was the treatment of choice for acute schizophrenia. *(1:688;2:840;3:93)*

29. **(A)** Based primarily on studies of his own children, *Jean Piaget* developed his theory of cognitive development. *(1:34-37;2:85-86;3:177)*

30. **(B)** *Jean Delay* and *Pierce Deniker* introduced chlorpromazine, the first effective phenothiazine antipsychotic, in 1952. *(2:809;3:103)*

31. **(D)** *Hans Berger* developed the technique of recording changes in brain potential in an *electroencephalogram*. *(2:276;3:343)*

32. **(B)** *Clifford Beers* wrote *The Mind That Found Itself*, the personal story of his recovery from mental illness. *(2:789)*

33. **(D)** *Sigmund Freud* wrote, as one of his earliest and most influential publications, *The Interpretation of Dreams*. *(2:754;3:4)*

34. **(A)** *Benjamin Rush* was one of the signers of the *Declaration of Independence* and wrote the first American psychiatry textbook. *(2:5-6)*

35. **(E)** From his own experiences, *Thomas DeQuincey* wrote *Confessions of an Opium Eater*. *(2:652)*

36. **(C)** *Robert Burton* wrote *The Anatomy of Melancholy*.

CHAPTER 9

Matching-Type Questions
Questions

INTRODUCTION

In most standard examinations there are many matching-type questions where a question is matched to one or several answers. This chapter is devoted to this type of question.

To allow the candidate to test his or her knowledge better, these questions are not subject grouped as they have been in the previous chapters but are in random sequence.

DIRECTIONS (Questions 1 through 129): Each group of items in this section consists of lettered headings followed by a set of numbered words or phrases. For each numbered word or phrase, select the ONE lettered heading that is most closely associated with it. Each lettered heading may be selected once, more than once, or not at all.

Questions 1 through 10

At what age should the normal child be expected to achieve the following developmental milestones? Match the developmental level with appropriate age of first achievement.

   (A) 4 months
   (B) 10 months
   (C) 15 months
   (D) 2 years

1. Aware of strange or different situations

2. Says three to five words with meaningful significance

3. Says "da-da"

4. Speaks of himself or herself by his or her name

5. Spontaneous social smile

6. Sits alone without support

7. Coos, gurgles, and laughs

8. Responds to "peek-a-boo" or smiles

9. Builds tower of six or seven blocks

10. Walks alone

Questions 11 through 15

   (A) lithium
   (B) monoamine oxidase inhibitors
   (C) diphenylhydantoin
   (D) amitriptyline
   (E) glutethimide

11. Toxicity when barbiturates discontinued

12. Restlessness, dizziness, and convulsions when given with tricyclic antidepressants

13. May cause thyroid goiter

14. Withdrawal convulsions

15. Severe urinary retention and paralytic ileus when given with thioridazine and antiparkinsonian drug

Questions 16 through 20

   (A) visual hallucinations
   (B) preoccupation with repetitiously moving objects
   (C) pupils nonreactive to light
   (D) frontal and temporal lobe atrophy
   (E) peripheral neuropathy

16. General paresis

17. Infantile autism

18. Acute intermittent porphyria

19. LSD psychosis

20. Pick's disease

Questions 21 through 25

   (A) opthalmoplegia, memory loss, confusion
   (B) simulated illnesses with multiple hospitalizations
   (C) aggressive, retarded boys with hyperuricemia
   (D) false pregnancy
   (E) rigid, overconscientious, compulsive

21. Pseudocyesis

22. Munchausen syndrome

23. Anankastic Personality

24. Lesch–Nyhan syndrome

25. Wernicke's syndrome

Questions 26 through 30

   (A) an 18-year-old boy with multiple tics, coprolalia, and episodic grunting
   (B) a 24-year-old truck driver, increasingly irritable for the past 3 months; moods have become unpredictable; now is accusing wife of infidelity
   (C) a 32-year-old chronic schizophrenic, maintained as an outpatient with treatment at the local mental health center, develops lip-smacking movements and sideways jaw movements.
   (D) a 54-year-old surgeon recently has forgotten his operative schedules, written incorrect drug prescriptions, and been very abrupt with patients. He walks stiffly and his operative technique seems much slower.
   (E) a 36-year-old man, two weeks after vasectomy, is noted by his wife to be chronically tired, sleeping poorly, and not eating well.

26. Alzheimer's disease

27. Amphetamine psychosis

28. Adjustment reaction

29. Tourette's Disorder

30. Tardive dyskenesia

Questions 31 through 33

Contraindicated:

    (A) tricyclic antidepressants
    (B) barbiturates
    (C) monoamine oxidase inhibitors

31. Cardiac irregularities

32. Senile confusion

33. Wine and cheese

Questions 34 through 38

    (A) subject helped to achieve insight as to dynamic basis for feelings and behavior
    (B) subject helped to develop better coping behaviors by new learning experiences and different rewards
    (C) subject develops a strong emotional reaction to the psychotherapist as if he or she were a significant figure in the patient's earlier life
    (D) subject interprets ambiguous stimuli on basis of feelings and ideas
    (E) subject is helped to strengthen existing defenses and cope with anxiety

34. Projective tests

35. Interpretive psychotherapy

36. Supportive psychotherapy

37. Behavior therapy

38. Transference neurosis

Questions 39 through 44

    (A) Vineland Social Maturity Scale
    (B) Bender–Gestalt Test
    (C) Children's Apperception Test

39. Ambiguous stimuli

40. Tests visual–motor coordination

41. Geometric designs

42. Based on reports rather than direct observation

43. Useful in evaluating brain damage

44. Reveals private fantasies and motives

Questions 45 through 48

    (A) Rorschach Test
    (B) Minnesota Mulitphasic Personality Inventory
    (C) Thematic Apperception Test

45. Ambiguous pictures

46. Color stimuli

47. 550 test questions

48. Can be computer scored

Questions 49 through 51

    (A) autosomal recessive gene; defect in leucine, isoleucine, and valine decarboxylation
    (B) autosomal recessive gene; absence or inactivity of liver phenylalanine hydroxylase
    (C) autosomal recessive gene, deficiency of galactose phosphate uridyl transferase

49. Small size, fair complexion, convulsions, dermatitis, and retardation

50. Urine has characteristic smell and turns blue with ferric chloride; infant convulsions, rigidity, hypoglycemia, and retardation

51. Jaundice, vomiting, diarrhea, and failure to thrive in infancy; mental retardation, cataracts, hepatic insufficiency

Questions 52 through 56

    (A) mercury poisoning
    (B) emotional response to actual external danger
    (C) paranoid reactions
    (D) frontotemporal atrophy
    (E) onset usually in childhood

52. Fear

53. Petit mal

54. Mad Hatter

55. Deafness

56. Pick's disease

Questions 57 through 61

    (A) delusion
    (B) somatization
    (C) denial
    (D) idea of reference
    (E) inappropriate affect

57. "Of course I do not know those people together on the other side of the street, but I know they are talking about me."

58. The nurse has a rapidly enlarging lump in her right breast, but she is not concerned nor does she think she should consult a physician.

59. "The television announcer tells me how to live each day by the way he turns his note pages."

60. The psychotic patient giggles and laughs as she tells how she did her supermarket shopping, deposited money in the bank, and washed the windows of her house.

61. The teenage girl goes upstairs and vomits when she has been refused permission to go out.

Questions 62 through 66

    (A) "Everything seems strange. People are so far away."
    (B) confusion, abdominal pain, limb weakness
    (C) smiling unconcern
    (D) "Two and two is five."
    (E) "My insides are rotting away."

62. Conversion disorder

63. Ganser syndrome

64. Derealization

65. Involutional melancholia

66. Porphyria

Questions 67 through 71

    (A) neologism
    (B) compulsion
    (C) echolalia
    (D) parapraxis
    (E) illusion

67. Slips of the tongue

68. "What time is it?" "What time is it, time is it." "What is your name?" "Name." "What is the date today?" "Date today."

69. The wind is blowing the tree branches. The moving shadow under the tree is interpreted as people pointing.

70. The schizophrenic refers to his wife as "Jinwhanny."

71. On the way home from school, the 8-year-old must walk only on the cracks in the sidewalk. If he steps off a crack he must go back to the beginning and start all over. Sometimes he takes 2 hours to walk a mile.

Questions 72 through 75

    (A) monoamine oxidase inhibitors
    (B) lithium carbonate
    (C) chlordiazepoxide

72. Can be used to prevent recurrent attacks of mania

73. Used in treating delirium tremens

74. Cheeses, wine, and liver may produce paradoxical hypertension

75. May lead to serious hyperpyrexia when given with tricyclic antidepressants

Questions 76 through 79

    (A) REM sleep
    (B) spike and domed waves 3 per second
    (C) lowered EEG frequency and amplitude
    (D) evoked cortical potential

76. Petit mal

77. Hypothyroidism

78. Excludes deafness in autistic child

79. Narcoleptic attack

Questions 80 through 85

    (A) primary prevention of mental retardation
    (B) secondary prevention of mental retardation
    (C) tertiary prevention of mental retardation

80. Reducing the number of adolescent pregnancies

81. Vocational training and sheltered workshops

82. Screening of infants for inborn metabolic disorders

83. Public education about causes of retardation

84. Special education classes for the retarded in public schools

85. Genetic counseling

Questions 86 through 90

    (A) Alzheimer's disease
    (B) Tay-Sach's disease
    (C) Huntington's chorea
    (D) Kanner's infantile autism
    (E) general paresis

86. Loss of nerve cells in putamen and caudate nuclei

87. No demonstrated brain pathology

88. Cortical glial cells markedly reduced, many rod cells, perivascular cuffing

89. Senile plaques and neurofibrillary degeneration

90. Ganglioside accumulation in neurons of brain and retina

Questions 91 through 95

    (A) physical dependence
    (B) marked psychologic dependence
    (C) both
    (D) neither

91. Barbiturates

92. Cocaine

93. Marijuana

94. Caffeine

95. Alcohol

Questions 96 through 105

    (A) interpretive psychotherapy
    (B) supportive psychotherapy
    (C) both
    (D) neither

96. Aims to reduce anxiety to manageable levels

97. Privacy and confidentiality

98. Insight into dynamics of behavior and feelings

99. Empathy with the patient

100. Transference is a focus for discussion and evaluation

101. Attempts to change existing personality structure

102. Counseling, direction, reassurance

103. Used when the personality is disrupting and decompensating

104. More applicable to elderly patients

105. Reassurance about physical complaints immediately, even before examination

Questions 106 through 111

    (A) Minnesota Multiphasic Personality Inventory
    (B) Bender-Gestalt Test
    (C) both
    (D) neither

106. Ambiguous stimuli

107. Geometric designs

108. Tests visual–motor perception

109. Can be machine scored

110. May be used with aphasic patients

111. Results are strongly affected by patient motivation

Questions 112 through 116

    (A) impending hepatic coma
    (B) delirium tremens
    (C) neither
    (D) both

112. May follow bout of heavy drinking

113. Psychomotor retardation

114. Vivid visual hallucinations

115. Flapping tremor of arms

116. Barbiturates for insomnia

Questions 117 through 120

    (A) transsexual
    (B) transvestite
    (C) both
    (D) neither

117. Dresses in clothes of opposite sex

118. Wishes to change anatomic sex

119. Masturbates or self-stimulates during periods of cross-dressing

120. Liable to seek sexual activities with young children

Questions 121 through 125

    (A) mania
    (B) depression
    (C) both
    (D) neither

121. Flight of ideas

122. Disturbed sleep

123. Psychomotor retardation

124. Problems with food intake

125. Grandiosity

Questions 126 through 129

    (A) night terror (pavor nocturnus)
    (B) nightmare
    (C) both
    (D) neither

126. Stage 4 sleep

127. REM sleep

128. Children tend to outgrow

129. Often associated with sleepwalking

DIRECTIONS (Questions 130 through 216): For each of the items in this section, ONE or MORE of the numbered options is correct. Choose the answer

    A if only 1, 2, and 3 are correct,
    B if only 1 and 3 are correct,
    C if only 2 and 3 are correct,
    D if only 4 is correct,
    E if all are correct.

130. Suicide rates

    (1) are lower in American Blacks
    (2) are higher in foreign-born Americans
    (3) are higher in males
    (4) rise with increasing age

131. The incidence of suicide is higher in

    (1) Protestants than in Catholics in America
    (2) the United States than any Western nation
    (3) lower socioeconomic groups
    (4) married adults

132. Male homosexuals

    (1) are incapable of meaningful long-term relationships
    (2) can be recognized by their walk, talk, and dress
    (3) cannot form relationships with women
    (4) may be socially productive citizens

133. Imipramine is used in treating

    (1) hyperkinesis
    (2) enuresis
    (3) amphetamine psychosis
    (4) major depression

134. Usually a teenage girl with anorexia nervosa

    (1) has amenorrhea
    (2) has a male pubic hair configuration
    (3) is active and energetic
    (4) has markedly lowered pituitary hormone levels

135. Females develop anorexia nervosa

    (1) after a difficult labor
    (2) with a craniopharyngioma
    (3) as a manifestation of psychotic depression
    (4) after dieting for previous real or fancied obesity

136. Admissions procedures to a mental hospital include

    (1) voluntary commitment
    (2) civil commitment
    (3) emergency commitment
    (4) commitment by physicians' certificate

137. Which of the following describe lithium blood levels?

    (1) therapeutic level 0.8–1.2 mEq/L serum
    (2) inversely related to phenothiazine levels
    (3) vary with salt intake
    (4) wider therapeutic–toxic margin than most psychotropic drugs

138. Under voluntary commitment, patient

    (1) may request admission
    (2) once admitted, may request discharge
    (3) after discharge is requested, may only be held several days without judicial commitment
    (4) judicial commitment of such a patient can then be only temporary

139. Testamentary capacity is

    (1) ability to act as court witness
    (2) capability of filing suit for damages
    (3) knowledge of right and wrong
    (4) competency to make a will

140. As evidence of legal capacity to make a will, the person making the will must

    (1) know the natural objects of his or her bounty
    (2) leave a reasonable sum to his or her nearest kin
    (3) be substantially aware of what he or she owns
    (4) not be hospitalized in a mental hospital

141. In differentiating a hysterical conversion symptom from an organic paralysis, which of the following are important?

    (1) paralysis does not fit anatomic distribution
    (2) patient seems unduly lacking in concern
    (3) previously immature personality
    (4) absence of all organic factors

142. Histrionic patients are

    (1) usually warm, feminine women
    (2) more often self-centered and childish
    (3) more commonly elderly
    (4) suggestible

143. In severe depression, which of the following are correct?

    (1) depression less in morning but worsens toward evening
    (2) patient wakens early in morning
    (3) delusions and illusions do not occur
    (4) loss of appetite, weight

144. The suicide rate for male American blacks is

    (1) higher than for white males
    (2) lower in urban areas
    (3) falling generally
    (4) lower than for white males

145. Imipramine toxic side effects include

    (1) worsening of narrow angle glaucoma
    (2) cardiac arrhythmias
    (3) twitching, restlessness, convulsions when combined with a monoamine oxidase inhibitor
    (4) hypertensive crisis when alcohol is ingested

146. Involutional melancholia occurs more often when which of the following factors are present?

    (1) male rather than female sex
    (2) prepsychotic, rigid, compulsive personality
    (3) previously socially outgoing and popular
    (4) aged in 40s and 50s

147. With a schizophrenic patient, the lasting benefits of therapy are measured by

    (1) ability to work
    (2) job turnover
    (3) capacity for making and holding friends
    (4) stability of residence

148. The prognosis in schizophrenia is more liable to be favorable if which of the following factors are present?

    (1) obvious external precipitating factors
    (2) prior schizoid personality
    (3) acute onset
    (4) low level of anxiety

149. In childhood autism, the prognosis is more favorable if

    (1) the child is bowel and bladder trained
    (2) there are no autistic siblings
    (3) the youngster is physically healthy
    (4) the child has obvious language ability

150. Reserpine-induced depression

    (1) is dose related
    (2) usually clears when drug is discontinued
    (3) when persistent is relieved by convulsive therapy
    (4) occurs during first week of drug treatment

151. Which statement is usually correct in chronic lead poisoning of childhood?

    (1) seen mainly in urban ghetto families
    (2) mainly due to inhalation of toxic fumes
    (3) produces chronic intellectual retardation
    (4) seen mainly in grade-school children

152. In acute intermittent porphyria, which of the following statements are applicable?

    (1) more common in women
    (2) acute toxic psychosis
    (3) motor paralyses
    (4) barbiturates therapeutic

153. In the management of the chronic alcoholic, which of the following measures may be useful?

    (1) calcium carbamide
    (2) group psychotherapy
    (3) halfway houses
    (4) vocational training

154. Temporary memory defects are likely to result from a course of treatment with

    (1) phenobarbital
    (2) phenothiazines
    (3) tricyclic antidepressants
    (4) electroconvulsive therapy

SUMMARY OF DIRECTIONS

A	B	C	D	E
1, 2, 3 only	1, 3 only	2, 4 only	4 only	All are correct

155. In treating the toxic delirious patient, which of the following may be used?

    (1) diazepam
    (2) haloperidol
    (3) chloral hydrate
    (4) phenobarbital

156. In operant conditioning, which of the following occur?

    (1) the response originates with the subject
    (2) unacceptable thoughts are repressed
    (3) the desired response is reinforced
    (4) the underlying causative factors are revealed

157. Barbiturates affect REM sleep by

    (1) reducing time spent in REM sleep
    (2) increasing REM sleep time
    (3) producing rebound increase REM time after withdrawal
    (4) leaving REM time unchanged but raising arousal threshold

158. Behavior therapy is based on the concepts that behavior

    (1) is learned
    (2) is due to underlying dynamic motivations
    (3) develops in response to rewards
    (4) modification necessitates the understanding of motivational factors

159. A male therapist is treating a 32-year-old married woman in intensive psychotherapy. She sends him a beautiful wristwatch for his birthday. The psychotherapist returns the watch and tries to discuss with her why she sent the gift. She forgets to come to the next session and then has to go to a dentist appointment at the time of the following treatment hour. The psychotherapist is dealing with which of the following reactions with this patient?

    (1) resistance
    (2) secondary gain
    (3) transference
    (4) introjection

160. Which of the following statements are applicable to migraine patients?

    (1) often family history of migraine
    (2) frequently achievement-oriented family background

    (3) hostility tends to be repressed
    (4) usually narcissistic and insensitive

161. In the management of the migrainous patient you may want to use

    (1) psychotherapy
    (2) reserpine
    (3) ergotamine
    (4) electroconvulsive therapy

162. In handling colostomy patients you should

    (1) explain to them preoperatively that they will have a colostomy
    (2) discuss the functioning of the colostomy pre- and postoperatively
    (3) encourage them to join a colostomy club
    (4) continue supportive psychotherapy postoperatively

163. Which of the following statements are correct about mental retardation?

    (1) highest incidence age 10–14
    (2) most are borderline or mildly retarded
    (3) skull x-rays usually normal
    (4) highest incidence in early childhood

164. Which of the following statements are correct about phantom phenomena?

    (1) normally occur after amputation in adults
    (2) are an expression of wish fulfillment
    (3) phantom tends to shrink and disappear with time
    (4) usually are painful

165. Phantom phenomena

    (1) do not occur with congenital absence of a limb
    (2) do not occur after mastectomy
    (3) are accentuated and perpetuated by delayed wound healing
    (4) indicate emotional maladjustment

166. Typically psychosomatic reactions are

    (1) symbolic expressions of emotional conditional conflict
    (2) mediated predominantly through the autonomic nervous system
    (3) reflecting a clearly defined personality pattern (Dunbar)
    (4) due to a combination of psychological stress and constitutional predisposition

167. Which of the following statements commonly apply to ulcerative colitis patients?

    (1) tend to be sensitive and intelligent
    (2) are often basically dependent

(3) never learned to handle rage and frustration productively

(4) tend to manifest hysterical personality traits

168. In managing the renal patient on a long-term hemodialysis program, the psychiatrist may be aware of

(1) high risk of suicide
(2) magical expectations for renal transplant
(3) marked financial and emotional drain on family
(4) potential for violent or aggressive behavior

169. Which of the following predispose to the development of combat neuroses in front-line soldiers?

(1) inadequate group leadership
(2) inactivity under fire
(3) high unit losses
(4) loneliness

170. The combat soldier is liable to decompensate emotionally due to which of the following factors?

(1) conflict over killing
(2) death of close friends
(3) constant threat of being killed
(4) physical exhaustion

171. Even though there is obvious community need, the services of an agency are not being used by the catchment area population. The reasons for the nonuse may include that the

(1) community is not involved in the planning or administration of services
(2) agency goals clash with community standards and needs
(3) agency administration have no direct communication with the established methods of care and treatment in the community
(4) agency funds are inadequate to provide all programs

172. Which of the following side effects have been reported with thioridazine?

(1) inhibition of ejaculation
(2) withdrawal convulsions
(3) pigmentary retinopathy
(4) hypertensive crises with cheese

173. In the treatment of attention deficit disorder with hyperactivity, which of the following drugs may be useful?

(1) amphetamines
(2) pemoline
(3) methylphenidate
(4) phenobarbital

174. Which of the following statements are true in electroconvulsive therapy?

(1) for therapeutic effect it is necessary to produce an obvious muscular convulsion
(2) the patient frequently gains weight
(3) hypertension is an obvious contraindication
(4) amenorrhea for 2 or 3 months may commonly result

175. The risk of suicide is greater where

(1) there has been a previous attempt
(2) there is a family history of suicide
(3) the patient has no close family
(4) the patient is over 60 years old

176. In dealing with former hospital patients, examples of tertiary prevention include

(1) Alcoholics Anonymous
(2) sheltered workshops
(3) halfway houses
(4) vocational placements

177. Programs designed for the primary prevention of emotional disorders in children and adolescents might include

(1) well-baby clinics
(2) readily accessible day-treatment centers
(3) pediatric guidance in normal child development for parents
(4) halfway houses

178. Previously hospitalized chronic psychotic patients are usually readmitted because

(1) their families do not want them
(2) they have no useful job skills
(3) they do not know how to function comfortably in normal social groups
(4) recurrence of their illness is inevitable

179. Dyslexia

(1) is more common in girls
(2) often leads to low self-esteem and depression
(3) is usually associated with a borderline retardation level of intelligence
(4) is found in children with visual–motor perceptual handicaps

180. Behavior therapy would be an appropriate form of treatment for a(n)

(1) mute autistic child
(2) adult woman with fear of enclosed spaces
(3) adult male fetishist
(4) regressed adult chronic schizophrenic

SUMMARY OF DIRECTIONS

A	B	C	D	E
1, 2, 3 only	1, 3 only	2, 4 only	4 only	All are correct

181. A 5-year-old boy is suddenly hospitalized with acute appendicitis. To minimize lasting emotional trauma, the doctor should

    (1) insist that no one discuss the impending operation with the child lest he become frightened
    (2) explain to the child before the operation what will happen and what it will be like postoperatively
    (3) sedate the child heavily immediately on his admission so he does not know what is happening
    (4) encourage the mother to remain with the child during the day and, if possible, overnight

183. In adolescence

    (1) suicide attempts are three times more common in girls than in boys
    (2) suicide is the third most common cause of death in the 15–19 age group
    (3) successful suicide is three times more common in boys than in girls
    (4) suicide is less common in college student population

183. The child's social sexual role depends on

    (1) chromosome patterns
    (2) anatomic sex configuration
    (3) physiologic sex hormones
    (4) what sex the child is reared as

184. To evaluate a child's personality, the examiner may use

    (1) playing with clay
    (2) Rorschach test
    (3) Draw-a-Person Test
    (4) Children's Apperception Test

185. Under temporary stress, a 4-year-old may show

    (1) tantrums
    (2) nightmares
    (3) recurrent tics
    (4) dyslexia

186. Which of the following statements are valid for infant intelligence testing?

    (1) high validity in predicting intelligence level in adolescence and adulthood
    (2) rely mainly on motor–sensory functioning
    (3) measures verbal and abstract ability
    (4) useful in detecting severe retardation

187. Intelligence testing results may be influenced by

    (1) motivation of the child
    (2) previous test experience
    (3) sex and age of the examiner
    (4) purpose of the test

188. Paranoid psychoses occur commonly in

    (1) bromide intoxication
    (2) chronic amphetamine abuse
    (3) myxedema psychosis
    (4) infantile autism

189. In acute intermittent porphyria

    (1) barbiturates are the treatment of choice
    (2) chlorpromazine is contraindicated
    (3) men are affected more often than women
    (4) abdominal pain is a common symptom

190. Racism

    (1) is supported by community attitudes
    (2) is taught by family and culture
    (3) provides a socially acceptable scapegoat
    (4) is not established until the growing child is preadolescent

191. Postpartum depression

    (1) responds well to hormone treatment
    (2) is liable to recur with subsequent pregnancies
    (3) does not respond well to antidepressants
    (4) can be treated with electroconvulsive therapy

192. Feeling that the world is a dream and that one's self is vaguely unreal may be manifestations of

    (1) normal adolescence
    (2) almost falling asleep
    (3) developing psychosis
    (4) hallucinogen effect

193. After a course of electroconvulsive treatments is complete, which of the following commonly occur normally?

    (1) memory impairment for several weeks
    (2) recurrent epileptic convulsions
    (3) amenorrhea for 1 or 2 months
    (4) persistent occipital headaches

194. Exhibitionism is

    (1) equally common in men and women
    (2) normal in young children
    (3) easily treated by psychotherapy
    (4) compulsive genital exposure in public to achieve excitation

195. Binge eaters

    (1) consume large amounts of food in a short time
    (2) tend to be upset and very guilty
    (3) usually eat in response to an obvious frustration
    (4) have morning anorexia and evening overeating

196. Anorexia nervosa

    (1) is often preceded by obesity
    (2) is most common in the second decade of life
    (3) occurs usually in women
    (4) responds well to hormone therapy

197. In treating recurrent manic–depressive depressions, a course of electroconvulsive therapy

    (1) prevents the recurrence of further episodes
    (2) leads to social recovery in the majority of cases
    (3) should not be given during pregnancy
    (4) relieves guilt and suicidal impulses

198. In planning a psychiatric primary prevention program for the elderly, you might

    (1) plan a social club for them
    (2) encourage local businesses to employ social security recipients
    (3) set up a "Welcome Wagon" group to introduce new elderly arrivals into the social community
    (4) contract with the local psychiatric hospital for readily available backup facilities

199. In child abuse, which of the following conditions are commonly found?

    (1) the abuse is often rationalized as necessary discipline
    (2) the male parent is the more frequent abuser
    (3) the abused child is often seen by the parents as being different
    (4) most frequently found in kindergarten-age children

200. Physical dependence on opioids is shown by

    (1) needle marks and signs of phlebitis
    (2) opioids in urine
    (3) drowsiness and pinpoint pupils
    (4) development of abstinence syndrome on withdrawal

201. Delirium may occur due to withdrawal after chronic use of

    (1) chlorpromazine
    (2) barbiturates
    (3) cocaine
    (4) alcohol

202. Regular use of marijuana leads to

    (1) increased aggressive behavior
    (2) increased sexual potency
    (3) addiction to hard drugs
    (4) change in time sense

203. Factors that maintain drug addiction include

    (1) cellular adaptation to the drug
    (2) personal need for immediate gratification
    (3) social acceptance of the successful hustler
    (4) group pressures to experiment with and to use drugs

204. Death may occur from barbiturate overdosage because

    (1) alcohol is taken in addition to barbiturates
    (2) the patient, partially confused by earlier barbiturate dose, automatically takes further doses
    (3) narcotic addict adds barbiturate to narcotic intake
    (4) patient is given N-allyl normorphine (Nalline)

205. In preparation for kindergarten, a 5-year-old boy is brought for examination because he is not yet speaking. You should consider in your diagnosis

    (1) bilateral hearing loss
    (2) infantile autism
    (3) mental retardation
    (4) tongue tie

206. Which of the following statements apply to enuresis?

    (1) may be a manifestation of regressive behavior
    (2) inappropriate management may cause further emotional handicapping
    (3) imipramine may be effective
    (4) found equally in boys and girls

207. In dealing with enuretic children and their families, the physician should be aware that

    (1) enuresis may be the manifestation of emotional difficulties
    (2) chilren always outgrow enuresis
    (3) enuresis often occurs in other family members
    (4) enuresis really requires no treatment if there is no physical cause

208. Which of the following apply to mucopolysaccharidosis?

    (1) abdominal enlargement in childhood
    (2) born with characteristic facial appearance
    (3) lymphocyte metachromatic inclusions
    (4) galactose-free diet prevents clinical manifestations

209. To reduce the incidence of mental retardation, you should

   (1) institute a rubella immunization program
   (2) offer genetic counseling
   (3) develop routine prenatal care programs
   (4) plan postnatal well-baby clinics

210. To treat a 26-year-old woman with a socially incapacitating fear of cats, you may wish to use

   (1) gradual desensitization
   (2) chlorpromazine
   (3) psychotherapy
   (4) methylphenidate

211. Serious adolescent delinquency is much more common in which of the following situations?

   (1) a cultural pattern of delinquency
   (2) mental retardation
   (3) parental conscience defects
   (4) delayed onset of puberty

212. The electroencephalogram

   (1) is always abnormal in hyperkinetic children
   (2) is diagnostically helpful in differentiating most psychiatric disorders
   (3) usually shows abnormalities in children with infantile autism
   (4) may be normal between grand mal seizures

Questions 213 through 216

A 26-year-old married woman brings her third child, a 2-year-old girl, for examination. The mother states that the child slipped and fell downstairs at home.

You note that the youngster is well fed but rather quiet. The child's face is swollen and she has a developing left-sided black eye. The mother explains the bruises on the girl's shoulders and thighs as being due to the fall—"She really came down with a bang, doctor."

X-ray examination of the skull shows a left zygomatic fracture and chest films indicate multiple rib fractures.

213. Your tentative primary diagnosis is

   (1) hyperkinetic child
   (2) cerebral palsy
   (3) mental retardation
   (4) battered child

214. You should now

   (1) report the case to the designated child-protective services
   (2) arrange for more extensive x-ray survey, physical examination, and photography
   (3) admit the child to the hospital
   (4) call in the local police to apprehend the parents

215. Parents of these children

   (1) often have been abused themselves as children
   (2) are most likely to be psychotic
   (3) come from every socioeconomic group
   (4) do not want help

216. These children are more likely

   (1) to have been born prematurely
   (2) to be treated as adults by the parents
   (3) to be preschool age or younger
   (4) to be developmentally retarded

Answers and Explanations

Answers 1 through 10 deal with normal growth and development. (1:692–693;2:63–70;3:175–177)

1. **(A)** At about *4 or 5 months of age,* the infant is aware of *strangeness* or differences in situations and people. The child acts afraid and clings more tightly to the mothering person.

2. **(C)** Usually between *12 and 15 months,* the toddler develops a communication vocabulary of three to five words.

3. **(B)** At *10 months* the average child is *saying "da-da"* and beginning to learn the use of specific verbal sounds to produce environmental effect. The child realizes that the babbling "da-da-da" brings a gratifying response from the significant male in his or her life.

4. **(D)** The *2-year-old* youngster is starting to *refer to himself or herself by name,* a manifestation of his or her increasing self-awareness.

5. **(A)** The newborn infant makes the facial movements of smiling for many reasons but by 2 months the child is smiling *socially and spontaneously* as a sign of pleasure and to produce pleasure.

6. **(B)** The *10-month-old* child can *sit alone* quite well, without having to be propped up and without wobbling unduly.

7. **(A)** The *2-month-old infant* is beginning to be more pleasurable to the family as, by this time, he or she is starting to *coo, gurgle, and laugh.*

8. **(B)** *"Pat-a-cake"* and *"peek-a-boo" games* begin to be exciting and fun for the child about *10 months* of age as he or she experiments with distance, depth, things there, and things not there.

9. **(D)** The *2-year-old* child carefully and methodically can build a *tower of six or seven blocks* and have the greatest glee at knocking it all down—and then building it again.

10. **(C)** As every mother of a *15-month-old* toddler knows, the youngster by this age is *walking alone* and getting into everything. He or she has been standing since 9 to 11 months and walking with a supporting hand since about 1-year-old; at 15 months he or she is moving well on his or her own.

Answers 11 through 15 deal with drug interactions and reactions. (3:108–110)

11. **(C)** Barbiturate enzyme induction speeds up the metabolism of *diphenylhydantoin.* When barbiturates and diphenylhydantoin are given together over any duration and barbiturates are then discontinued, diphenylhydantoin toxicity is likely to occur due to slowed drug breakdown. *(2:291–292;3:108–109)*

12. **(B)** When tricyclic antidepressants and *monoamine oxidase inhibitors* are given concurrently, the patient may develop restlessness, dizziness, convulsions, hyperpyrexia, and intracranial hemorrhage. Fatalities occur. *(1:659;2:829;3:112)*

13. **(A)** In patients taking *lithium,* there is increased incidence of thyroid goiter. *(1:677;2:831;3:128)*

14. **(E)** Users of *glutethimide,* a widely used sedative-hypnotic, are liable to develop withdrawal convulsions after prolonged intake. This drug is also prone to cause drug dependency. *(1:668;3:242–243)*

15. **(D)** When the anticholinergic antidepressant *amitriptyline* is given in combination with the anticholinergic thioridazine or comparable drugs and especially when a further anticholinergic medication, an antiparkinsonian drug is added, severe and potentially fatal urinary retention or paralytic ileus can develop. *(1:654–656;2:827;3:109)*

Answers 16 through 20 deal with diagnostic symptoms.

16. **(C)** In *general paresis,* classically the pupils do not react to light but do react to accommodation—the *Argyll Robertson pupil.*

    Accommodation Reaction Present—Argyll Robertson Pupil. (2:260;3:224)

17. **(B)** Children with *infantile autism* frequently are preoccupied with repetitiously moving objects, mechanical toys, clock mechanisms, and similar objects. *(1:732–737;2:693–741;3:201)*

18. **(E)** *Peripheral neuropathy,* abdominal pain, confusion, and depression may occur together or as discrete symptoms in *acute intermittent porphyria. (1:309–310;2:320–321;3:228)*

19. **(A)** Visual hallucinations occur characteristically in a *toxic* or *organic psychosis.* When visual hallucinations are present in a schizophrenic subject, behavioral regression is usually marked and other psychotic symptoms are apparent. Visual hallucinations are likely to be prominent in an LSD psychosis. *(1:282; 2:126;3:16)*

20. **(D)** In *Pick's disease,* cortical atrophy is most marked in the frontal and temporal lobes, while atrophy is more widespread in Alzheimer's disease. *(2:244–246; 3:216)*

Answers 21 through 30 deal with syndromes.

21. **(D)** In *pseudocyesis* or *false pregnancy,* the woman subject develops the outward signs of pregnancy—absence of menstruation, gradual abdominal distention, breast enlargement, and even labor pains.

    This symptom most often occurs in immature or hysterical females. *(1:66;2:569;3:290)*

22. **(B)** The patient with *Munchausen syndrome, chronic factitious disorder with physical symptoms,* sometimes called a *hospital addict,* simulates a wide range of serious or esoteric illnesses and in this way is admitted to a succession of hospitals where he or she may undergo many procedures, including operative intervention. *(1:522–524;2:516)*

23. **(E)** *Anankastic Personality* is a diagnostic term used more often in European literature and refers to the rigid overconscientious *obsessive-compulsive personality. (3:335)*

24. **(C)** A sex-linked congenital defect that is the focus of increasing research is the *Lesch–Nyhan syndrome.* This occurs in boys who show elevated serum uric acid, mental retardation, and unusual aggressiveness that is self-directed and directed to others. *(1:718;2:731)*

25. **(A)** *Wernicke's syndrome* occurs in chronic alcoholic and severely malnourished or debilitated patients. There is necrosis and hemorrhage in the periaqueductal region and in the mamillary bodies. Symptomatically the patient shows ophthalmoplegia with marked mental confusion or clouding. *(1:420;2:325–326;3:218–219)*

26. **(D)** Dementia developing insidiously in the presenile period should suggest the possibility of *Alzheimer's disease.* Memory loss, especially for recent events, personality change, and neurological deterioration all indicate an organic brain syndrome. *(1:286–289;2:242–244;3:215–216)*

27. **(B)** *Amphetamine psychosis.* Chronic amphetamine use and abuse, as seen in some long-distance truck drivers who use the stimulant drug to stay awake, may cause a psychotic paranoid syndrome that is very similar to paranoid schizophrenia. *(1:403–405;2:663; 3:221–222)*

28. **(E)** *Adjustment disorder* with depressed mood *(reactive depression).* Vasectomy in the male has been a frequent precursor of a postoperative depression, as is hysterectomy in the female. With the increasing social acceptance of vasectomy, it will be interesting to note whether postoperative depressions become less frequent. Sleep and appetite disturbances, lack of energy, and tiredness are common manifestations of depression. *(1:476–479;2:482–483;3:269)*

29. **(A)** *Tourette's Disorder.* Though the syndrome of multiple tics, explosive utterances, and sometimes coprolalia is rare, it must be kept in mind so that treatment for patient and family can be planned appropriately. *(1:763–765;2:700–701;3:196–197)*

30. **(C)** *Tardive dyskinesia.* Lip, tongue, jaw, and face movements, choreiform arm and hand gesturing, and recurrent back and neck contractions may develop in patients taking phenothiazine drugs. Originally the syndrome was described in patients on long-term medications, but increasingly these symptoms are being reported at every stage of phenothiazine treatment and after the cessation of the medication. *(1: 644–646;2:823–824;3:121–122)*

Answers 31 through 33 deal with drug reactions.

31. **(A)** Even within the normal dosage range, *tricyclic antidepressants* cause postural hypotension and tachycardia. Disturbances of cardiac rhythm may develop but these arrhythmias occur most often where there is cardiac pathology or drug overdose. *(1:654; 2:826–827;3:112–117)*

32. **(B)** *Barbiturates* may precipitate or worsen senile confusion. In confusional states in elderly patients, barbiturates or sedatives must always be suspected. Discontinuation of barbiturate use may relieve all confusion symptoms. *(1:274;2:658–661;3:219–220)*

33. **(C)** Hypertensive crisis due to the inhibition of deamination of pressor amines, such as tyramine, is a rare but potentially fatal complication of *monoamine oxidase inhibitor* use. Food rich in tyramine—certain cheeses, beer, some wines, sour cream, chicken liver, avocado, figs—must be avoided with monoamine oxidase inhibitor use. *(1:658–659;2:829;3:111–112)*

34. **(D)** When *projective tests* are used, subjects interpret ambiguous stimuli on the basis of their inner feelings and ideas: they have to project themselves and thus reveal their personality. The best-known projective tests are the Rorschach test and the Thematic Apperception Test. *(1:128–132;2:206;3:48–49)*

35. **(A)** *Interpretive psychotherapy* gives the patient planned insight, through interpretation, into the dynamic basis for his or her feelings and behavior. Optimally this insight should lead to freeing up of emotions and personality restructuring. *(1:598;2:753–754;3:66–68)*

36. **(E)** In *supportive psychotherapy* there is no attempt to change the patient's personality in any profound fashion. Using the strengths and the ways of coping he or she has, the patient is helped to manage his or her life better. Existing defenses are strengthened and the patient is supported in developing more reasonable ways of managing. *(1:600–601;2:769;3:68–69)*

37. **(B)** In *behavior therapy* the subject is taught better coping behavior by allowing him or her to learn new patterns and to experience different rewards. Appropriate behavior is rewarded and *reinforced*. Maladaptive behavior produces a negative reaction or is ignored. *(1:605–608;2:769–773;3:69–71)*

38. **(C)** In *transference neurosis,* which occurs in the course of psychotherapy, the patient develops a strong emotional reaction to the therapist, who is reacted to as if he or she were a nuclear person in the patient's early life. *(1:597;2:752;3:67)*

Answers 39 through 48 deal with psychological testing. *(1:126–136,704–708;2:202–217;3:44)*

39. **(C)** The *Children's Apperception Test,* an adaptation of the *Thematic Apperception Test,* is a set of pictures of animal characters in ambiguous situations. The child is encouraged to project his or her feelings and personality onto these *ambiguous stimuli.* *(1:707; 3:49)*

40. **(B)** The *Bender–Gestalt Test* tests visual–motor coordination and visual recall. *(1:131;2:210–213;3:47)*

41. **(B)** The *Bender–Gestalt Test* is a series of *geometric designs* that the subject is asked to copy and sometimes then to draw from memory. *(1:131;2:210–213; 3:47)*

42. **(A)** The *Vineland Social Maturity Scale* gives a Developmental Quotient based on the child's level of functioning as *reported* by the parents, teachers, or parent surrogates. The test evaluator *does not observe* the child. *(1:705;2:720)*

43. **(B)** The *Bender–Gestalt Test* is one of the more useful procedures to *evaluate brain damage* in patients. *(1:131;2:210–213;3:47)*

44. **(C)** The *Children's Apperception Test* would be one method of revealing a child's private fantasies and motives. *(1:707;3:49)*

45. **(C)** The *Thematic Apperception Test* uses a set of ten *ambiguous pictures* as stimuli to elicit the subject's projection. The Rorschach test also uses ambiguous stimuli but the test cards are inkblots. *(1:129–130; 2:210;3:49)*

46. **(A)** In the *Rorschach test,* several of the inkblot test cards are partially or completely colored to offer *color stimuli* for subjective projection. The Thematic Apperception Test cards are all black and white. *(1:128–129;2:206–209;3:48–49)*

47. **(B)** *The Minnesota Multiphasic Personality Inventory (MMPI)* is a set of 550 test questions to which the subject is expected to answer "True," "False," or "Cannot say." *(1:130–131;2:214–215;3:49–51)*

48. **(B)** Of these three tests, only the *Minnesota Multiphasic Personality Inventory* can be *computer scored* at present. *(1:130–131;2:214–215;3:49–51)*

Answers 49 through 51 deal with mental retardation due to metabolic defects.

49. **(B)** *Phenylketonuria. (1:711–714;2:729–731;3:166)*

50. **(A)** *Maple syrup disease. (1:714;2:731;3:374)*

51. **(C)** *Galactosemia. (1:716;2:732;3:165)*

Metabolic defects are the cause of mental retardation in only a very small percentage of cases, but the clinician must be alert to the more common or easily recognizable syndromes. Early treatment of these disorders may prevent intellectual and physical handicapping. *(1:711–718;2:725–734;3:164–166)*

Sometimes questions are given to test the candidate's awareness of more tenuous associations. In this group of answers, the question phrase has been deliberately kept more brief so that the examinee must be more careful in selecting the appropriate matching answer.

52. **(B)** *Fear* is the *emotional response to an actual specific external danger.* Anxiety is less specifically focused, less directed, and more often aroused by conflictual or illogical factors. *(1:315–316;2:92–93;3:20)*

53. **(E)** Of all the syndromes and symptoms listed, only *petit mal* has *onset usually in childhood.* This form of seizure tends to disappear by late adolescence and may be replaced by other types of convulsive disorders. *(1:301;2:279–280;3:226)*

54. **(A)** *Mercury poisoning* used to be an occupational disease of hatters and furriers. The Mad Hatter in *Alice in Wonderland* is a caricature of the irritability and unpredictability of these patients. *(1:298–299; 2:331)*

55. **(C)** *Paranoid reactions* are more likely to occur in people who suffer from *deafness.* Since they cannot hear clearly, or at all, and are cut off from a great deal of social interaction, the deaf may receive only partial or confusing communications. Because they may not always appreciate environmental reality, difficult situations may occur. Lack of communication, isolation, and social misunderstandings lead to increased suspiciousness and paranoia. *(2:233;3:330)*

56. **(D)** A common macroscopic pathological finding in *Pick's disease,* a form of *presenile* dementia, is *frontotemporal atrophy* of the brain cortex. *(1:287–289;2: 244–246;3:215–216)*

57. **(D)** Although the behavior of the people on the other side of the street does not refer in any way to the speaker, he attributes to this behavior some purpose referring to him. This remark is an illustration of an *idea of reference.* *(1:152;2:103;3:18)*

58. **(C)** Only by massive emotional *denial* could a professional, trained nurse block out of awareness any concern about a rapidly growing breast mass. Denial may have been emotionally necessary as the reality of this lump faced her with intolerable anxiety about her continued existence and femininity. *(1:80;2:107;3:8)*

59. **(A)** The subject who feels that the television personality is communicating to him in a private fashion is manifesting a *delusion,* a fixed false belief, inconsistent with his level of education and cultural background. *(1:152–153;2:129–133;3:18)*

60. **(E)** The psychotic patient who giggles and laughs as she relates her routine activities is showing *inappropriate affect.* *(1:176;2:138;3:20)*

61. **(B)** This adolescent girl is *expressing through a somatic symptom* (vomiting), feelings that she could not express verbally to the controlling parent—she is *somatizing.* *(1:340;2:497;3:289–290)*

62. **(C)** Smiling unconcern, "la belle indifference," is one manifestation of the psychological dissociation that occurs in a *conversion disorder.* Since the subject has dissociated or split off the emotions from the somatic or behavioral manifestation of the illness, he or she may feel no concern about hysterical symptoms that would cause a nonhysteric great concern or anxiety. *(1:342–348;2:505;3:290)*

63. **(D)** "Two and two is five," the approximate answer *(vorbeireden).*

    The *Ganser syndrome,* the syndrome of the approximate answer, is most commonly described in prison populations where the individual, under tension, tries to avoid direct stress by giving an answer that is incorrect but approximates the correct response. This behavior may appear to be deliberately evasive but is not under the patient's conscious control. This maladaptive defense is seen in other stressful situations. *(1:544–545;2:516–517)*

64. **(A)** "Everything seems strange. People are so far away."

    In the state of *derealization,* the subject feels that things around him or her are somehow unreal, almost distant. This feeling occurs occasionally in normal people, especially during childhood and adolescence, but, when the symptom is frequent or incapacitating, it is usually a manifestation of schizophrenia. In depersonalization, the subject feels that his or her body is unreal. *(1:171;2:139)*

65. **(E)** "My insides are rotting away."

    Somatic delusions, especially of a bizarre, malevolent physical process, are characteristic of *involutional melancholia.* These delusions can, of course, occur in other forms of psychotic depression and in other psychotic states. *(1:246–247;2:437–439; 3:267)*

66. **(B)** When the symptoms of confusion, abdominal pain, and limb weakness coexist, especially in young or middle aged women, *acute intermittent porphyria* must be strongly suspected and excluded before any treatment is instituted. Barbiturates are likely to precipitate an acute symptomatic exacerbation. *(1:309–310;2:319–323;3:228)*

67. **(D)** A *slip of the tongue,* a Freudian slip, is a *parapraxis.* These slips give some indication of underlying

unconscious or preconscious feelings. *(1:146;2:146; 3:6)*

68. **(C)** The subject here is echoing the words of the questioner. *Echolalia* most typically occurs in schizophrenia but can occur in other disorders, such as Tourette's Disorder. *(1:210–211;2:116;3:21)*

69. **(E)** When a reality-based external perception, such as blowing tree branches, is misinterpreted due to the subject's emotional maladjustment, this mistaken interpretation is termed an *illusion. (1:163;2:121–122; 3:16)*

70. **(A)** When the schizophrenic patient coins his or her own idiosyncratic words, these words are described as *neologisms. (1:208;2:364;3:17)*

71. **(B)** Children in the grade-school years are normally rather compulsive and rule oriented. The youngster described in this question is pathologically bound by his own rigid regulations. His behavior is markedly *compulsive* and is liable to be increasingly handicapping. *(1:328;2:116;3:17)*

72. **(B)** *Lithium carbonate* is used to treat manic attacks and, in maintenance treatment, to prevent the *recurrence of manic episodes.* Increasingly, lithium is used to prevent the recurrence of *depression* in bipolar *manic depressive illness. (1:575–578;2:829–831; 3:126)*

Chlordiazepoxide would not have a sufficiently strong tranquilizing effect to be used in the treatment of manic states and is less efficient than lithium in preventing recurrence.

73. **(C)** *Chloriazepoxide* is one of the drugs used in treating *delirium tremens.* Diazepam has been commonly used also. *(1:419;2:630–631;3:217–218)*

74. **(A)** *Monoamine oxidase inhibitors* potentiate the dietary tyramine in foods like cheese, wine and beer, pickled herring, and chicken liver, leading to attacks of *paradoxical hypertension. (1:658–659;2:829;3:111– 112)*

75. **(A)** *Serious hyperpyrexia* may occur when patients are given *monoamine oxidase inhibitor drugs in combination with tricyclic antidepressants. (1:659;2: 828;3:112)*

Answers 76 through 79 deal with the electroencephalogram in psychiatry.

76. **(B)** *Petit mal epilepsy* is typically associated with 3-per-second spike and domed waves on the electroencephalogram. *(1:301;2:279;3:226)*

77. **(C)** In *hypothyroidism* there is usually generally *lowered EEG frequency and amplitude. (1:516–517;2: 315–316;3:228)*

78. **(D)** To differentiate *childhood autism* from severe *deafness,* it may be necessary to see whether auditory stimuli *evoke cortical potentials* on the electroencephalogram. The autistic child, who can hear, will show evoked cortical potentials in response to a sound though there may be no outward behavioral response. The deaf youngster will show no sound-evoked cortical potentials. *(1:732–737;2:693–694;3:201)*

79. **(A)** *REM sleep patterns* on the electroencephalogram are associated with *narcoleptic attacks. (1:567–568; 2:283–285;3:349)*

Answers 80 through 85 deal with prevention of mental illness and mental retardation. (1:876–880;2:788;3:140)

80. **(A)** Chromosomal defects and obstetric complications are more common in pregnancies of adolescents (and women over 40). The *reduction in adolescent pregnancies* would be one form of *primary prevention* of mental retardation in children. *(1:876– 877;2:788;3:140)*

81. **(C)** *Vocational training and sheltered workshops* would help the retarded live with their handicaps and find a productive role in society.

Helping the handicapped youngster live productively with his or her handicap is an example of *tertiary prevention. (1:879–880;2:788;3:120)*

82. **(B)** The *screening* of newborn infants for *inborn metabolic disorders* will not prevent the disorder from occurring *(primary prevention)* but will allow for early treatment of the illness *(secondary prevention). (1: 876–879;2:788;3:140)*

83. **(A)** *Public education about the causes* of mental retardation is aimed at preventing the retardation syndromes from occurring *(primary prevention). (1: 876–877;2:788;3:140)*

84. **(C)** *Special education classes* in the public schools help the retarded develop their limited skills and still remain, as far as possible, members of their appropriate age group. These youngsters are helped to cope with their intellectual handicap as efficiently as possible *(tertiary prevention). (1:879–880;2:788;3:170)*

85. **(A)** *Genetic counseling* to parents who potentially carry a gene producing mental retardation informs them of the risk to their future offspring. This counseling is planned to prevent the occurrence of hereditary mental retardation syndromes *(primary prevention). (1:876–877;2:788;3:77–81)*

Answers 86 through 90 deal with neuropathology.

86. **(C)** *Huntington's chorea,* a degenerative nervous system disease, is inherited as an autosomal dominant and is characterized by widespread brain atrophy, especially in the caudate and putamen nuclei. *(1:306; 2:339–341;3:227)*

87. **(D)** *Kanner's infantile autism.* Since 1943, when Kanner first described infantile autism, there has been extensive neuropathological and neurobiochemical research into this syndrome. No pathological brain process has yet been demonstrated in these children. *(1:732–737;2:693–694;3:201)*

88. **(E)** In *general paresis,* there is marked degeneration and disappearance of cortical glial cells, most evident in the frontal cortex. Rod cells are prominent and widely distributed throughout the cortex. Perivascular cuffing with lymphocytes, plasma cells, and mast cells is another manifestation of the chronic syphilitic meningoencephalitis.

    Wagner von Jauregg was awarded the Nobel Prize in medicine for his discovery of malaria-induced fevers as treatment for general paresis. *(2:257–258;3:224)*

89. **(A)** Pathological examination of the brain in *Alzheimer's disease,* one of the senile dementias, shows severe neuron loss, with senile plaques and neurofibrillary tangles. In Alzheimer's disease, the cortical atrophy is widespread but plaques are most often found in the frontal cortex and the hippocampus. *(1:286–289;2:242–244;3:216)*

90. **(B)** *Tay–Sach's disease* is a cerebromacular degeneration, inherited by autosomal recessive dominance. Ganglioside accumulation in the nerve cells of the brain and retina leads to profound mental retardation, convulsions, physical deterioration, and early death. *(1:715;2:725–728;3:164)*

91. **(C)** Subjects can become markedly dependent psychologically on *barbiturates.* Due to the physical dependence that develops, chronic users may manifest a severe and potentially lethal *abstinence syndrome.* *(1:406–409;2:658–661;3:238–239)*

92. **(C)** Users of *cocaine* can become very dependent on the drug psychologically, and, increasingly, cases with physical dependence are being diagnosed. *(1:405–406; 2:661;3:241–242)*

93. **(D)** *Marijuana* use can become a routine way of relaxing and relieving tension, but chronic users can get along without the drug since marked psychological dependence does not occur. Physical dependence does not develop either. *(1:400–403;2:664–665;3:242)*

94. **(D)** Although many coffee or tea users think they could not get through the day without their favorite libation, in reality they could get by. *Caffeine* does not produce either marked psychological or physical dependence. *(1:427–430;3:223)*

95. **(C)** *Alcohol,* still the most common drug of abuse, leads to physical dependence in chronic users, who may suffer a wide range of physical symptoms on withdrawal. Marked psychological dependence is common in chronic alcoholics, who are unable to cope without their alcohol intake. *(1:414–427;2:616–626; 3:236–237)*

Answers 96 through 105 deal with individual psychotherapy. (1:595–605;2:745–786;3:65–76)

96. **(B)** *Supportive psychotherapy* primarily aims to *reduce anxiety* to manageable levels. In interpretive psychotherapy, the psychotherapist uses the patient's anxiety to produce personality changes. *(1:600–601; 2:769;3:68–69)*

97. **(C)** In all forms of psychotherapy, *privacy* and *confidentiality* must be guarded and are an essential part of the treatment contract. *(1:598;2:745–748;3:155)*

98. **(A)** *Interpretive psychotherapy* is planned to give the subject *insight* into his or her behavior and feelings so that behavior change and personality restructuring can occur. *(1:598;2:753–754;3:66–67)*

99. **(C)** In all forms of psychotherapy, the psychotherapist needs *empathy* with the patient—an objective, positive feeling for the person who seeks professional help. *(1:99;2:98;3:66)*

100. **(A)** In *interpretive psychotherapy, transference,* the patient's transferring of feelings about significant earlier people onto the psychotherapist, is supported and becomes a major focus for discussion, evaluation and understanding. *(1:596–598;2:751–752;3:66–67)*

101. **(A)** *Interpretive psychotherapy* aims to remove maladaptive *personality structuring* and inefficient emotional defenses and to produce more effective ways of coping. *(1:598;2:753;3:66–67)*

102. **(B)** *Supportive psychotherapy* involves *counseling, directing,* and *reassuring.* There is only a minimal attempt to restructure the patient's personality. The patient is helped to use his or her existing ways of coping more efficiently. *(1:600–601;2:769;3:68–69)*

103. **(B)** When the patient's *personality* is *disrupting* and *decompensating, supportive psychotherapy* is usually the psychological treatment required. The patient needs help to reorganize and to develop even a limited level of functioning.

Interpretive psychotherapy would tend to increase the patient's anxiety and remove the few emotional defenses left, thus making the patient less able to function. *(1:600–601;2:769;3:68–69)*

104. **(B)** *Supportive psychotherapy* is more appropriate in the *elderly,* where personality patterns are long established and where there is less purpose in producing marked personality changes (even if it were possible). *(1:600–601;2:769;3:68–69)*

105. **(D)** In no form of psychological treatment should the patient be reassured about physical complaints before a thorough medical examination. Such phony reassurance is deceptive and may prevent the development of any trusting patient–therapist relationship. *(1:136–145;3:67–68)*

Anwers 106 through 111 deal with psychological testing.

106. **(D)** Neither the *Minnesota Multiphasic Personality Inventory* nor the *Bender–Gestalt Test* offers the subject *ambiguous stimuli.*

The Minnesota Multiphasic Personality Inventory is a series of 550 specific questions, and the Bender–Gestalt Test offers geometric designs to be copied. *(1:130–131;2:210–215;3:47–51)*

107. **(B)** The *Bender–Gestalt Test* is a set of *geometric designs* that the subject copies directly and sometimes from memory. *(1:131;2:210–213;3:47)*

108. **(B)** The *Bender–Gestalt Test* evaluates *visual–motor coordination* and *perception* and *visual recall.* *(1:131;2:210–213;3:47)*

109. **(A)** The answers to the 550 questions of the *Minnesota Multiphasic Personality Inventory* can be *machine scored.* *(1:130–131;2:214–215;3:49–51)*

110. **(B)** The *Bender–Gestalt Test* can be used with *aphasic* patients and is useful in evaluating brain damage. *(1:131;2:210–213;3:47)*

111. **(C)** The results of both the *Minnesota Multiphasic Personality Inventory* and the *Bender–Gestalt Test* are strongly *affected by patient motivation* and anxiety. *(1:130–131;2:210–215;3:47–51)*

Answers 112 through 116 deal with delirium tremens and liver failure associated with chronic alcoholism.

112. **(D)** Both *delirium tremens* and *impending hepatic coma may follow a bout of heavy drinking.* Delirium tremens can occur after the withdrawal of alcohol in a chronic drinker or may develop in the course of an alcoholic binge.

Hepatic cirrhosis is frequently associated with chronic alcoholism and a heavy drinking bout may finally precipitate liver failure. *(1:308,419–421;2:629–630;3:217–218)*

113. **(A)** The subject who is going into *hepatic coma* is liable to show *psychomotor retardation;* he or she becomes increasingly apathetic, tired, and slow. The delirium tremens patient is more apt to be agitated, restless, and active. *(1:308,421;2:629–630)*

114. **(B)** The patient with *delirium tremens* characteristically has *vivid hallucinations,* while the patient with liver failure becomes disoriented, dull, and unproductive. *(1:419–421;2:628–631;3:217–218)*

115. **(A)** *Flapping tremor of the arms* is an ominous sign of worsening liver failure and indicates *impending hepatic coma.*

The delirium tremens patient usually has the "shakes" but this is a coarse tremor of the hands. "My hand is not as steady as it used to be." *(1:308,419–421)*

116. **(C)** In neither *delirium tremens* nor *impending hepatic coma* should barbiturates be given for insomnia or restlessness. Barbiturates could be fatal in both syndromes. *(1:308,419–421;2:630–631;3:217–218)*

Answers 117 through 120 deal with deviant sexuality.

117. **(C)** Both *transsexuals* and *transvestites* dress in clothes of the opposite sex. *(1:434–437;2:525–529;3:302–304)*

118. **(A)** Only the *transsexual* wishes to be changed anatomically to the opposite sex. *(1:434–437;2:525–527;3:302–303)*

119. **(B)** The *transvestite* achieves sexual gratification by wearing the clothes of the opposite sex and often masturbates to enhance this pleasure during periods of cross-dressing.

The *transsexual* despises and dislikes the sexual anatomy with which he or she was born and tends not to seek masturbatory gratification. *(1:434–437;2:525–529;3:303–304)*

120. **(D)** Neither the *transvestite* nor the *transsexual* seeks children for sexual gratification (pedophilia). *(1:434–437;2:525–529;3:302–304)*

In matching-type questions, not all the answers have to be used. Some answers may be appropriate for several questions and other answers not used at all.

Answers 121 through 125 deal with bipolar disorder. (1:245–249;2:407–434;3:264–268)

121. **(A)** A *flight of ideas,* a markedly pressured flow of thought, is most often symptomatic of *acute mania.* The subject's ideas may be under such pressure that the associations are no longer obvious. *(1:148–149; 2:415;3:17)*

122. **(C)** *Sleep* is *disturbed* both in *mania* and *depression.* The manic patient may be so active that he or she never gets to bed or is no sooner in bed than he or she is up; the depressed patient usually can get to sleep but tends to waken early and stay awake. *(1:245–249;2: 413–423;3:264–268)*

123. **(B)** The *depressed patient* typically shows psychomotor retardation. He or she is slow, tired, or lacks outward initiative. *(1:245–248;2:417–421;3:266–268)*

124. **(C)** Both *manic* and *depressed* patients have problems with food intake. The manic patient may eat voraciously or be too active to eat adequately, while the depressed person may have a poor appetite and low food intake or may eat excessively when he or she feels low. *(1:245–249;2:413–423;3:264–268)*

125. **(A)** The *manic* subject is frequently markedly *grandiose* with expansive ideas of his or her own personal strength, wealth, and potential. *(1:248–249;2:413–416;3:264–265)*

Though grandiosity is correctly attributed only to manic patients, depressed patients state they are the greatest sinner or the main cause of all the world's woes.

Answers 126 through 129 deal with sleep disturbances. (1:558–574;2:704–708;3:343–362)

126. **(A)** *Night terror (pavor nocturnus)* occurs during stage 4 (deep) sleep. The subject appears to be in a confused, panicky state, attempting to flee or defend. Usually the person has no memory of the terror episode the following morning. *(1:572–573;2:705;3:352–353)*

127. **(B)** *Nightmares* occur during REM sleep phases. *(1:573;2:705;3:353)*

128. **(C)** While night terrors and nightmares occur at all ages, they are more common in childhood. Children usually outgrow both nightmares and night terrors. *(1:572–573;2:705;3:352–353)*

129. **(A)** Sleep walking (somnambulism) and night terrors tend to coexist. Sleep walking is common in children and is more often seen in boys; youngsters usually outgrow the disturbance. *(1:570–572;2:705–706;3: 352–353)*

130. **(E)** *Suicide rates* in the United States are lower for *blacks,* though the incidence in urban areas is getting nearer the rates for *Caucasians. Foreign-born Amer-* icans have higher suicide rates. *Males* commit suicide more often than females, who make more frequent suicide attempts. The incidence of suicide tends to increase with increasing *age. (1:575–576;2:118–121;3: 270–272)*

131. **(B)** The *incidence of suicide* in the United States is generally higher in *Protestants* than *Catholics* and is higher in *lower socioeconomic groups.* Several countries, including West Germany, Japan, Denmark, and Sweden, have higher suicide rates than the United States.

Suicide is more common in the single, widowed, and divorced, and is *lower in the married* adult group. *(1:575–576;2:118–121;3:270–272)*

132. **(D)** *Male homosexuals* may be *socially productive* citizens. They are capable of *forming meaningful long-term relationships* with *men* and *women.* They cannot be recognized by a different way of walking, talking, or dressing. *(1:442–445;2:527–528;3:315)*

133. **(C)** *Imipramine* is used in treating *childhood enuresis* and *major depression.* The drug would not be therapeutic with hyperkinetic children or with amphetamine psychosis. *(1:843–846;2:697–699;3:116)*

134. **(B)** Usually a teenage girl with *anorexia nervosa* has *amenorrhea* (the lack of this symptom makes anorexia nervosa more difficult to diagnose in the male). Patients with anorexia nervosa are usually *active* and *energetic. (1:499–504;2:554–558;3:194–195)*

135. **(D)** Females with *anorexia nervosa* often give the history of developing the illness *after dieting for real or fancied obesity.*

After a difficult labor, especially with marked blood loss or infection, pituitary necrosis may occur. A craniopharyngioma may cause pituitary hypofunction by local effects. Hypopituitarism produces a very different symptom pattern. Anorexia nervosa is not associated with psychotic depression. *(1:499–504;2: 554–558;3:194–195)*

136. **(E)** *Admission to a mental hospital* can be *voluntary* or by commitment with a *civil, emergency, or physician's certificate. (1:891;2:852–855;3:150)*

137. **(B)** Lithium blood levels vary with salt intake; toxicity is potentiated by reduced salt use. The therapeutic serum level of lithium is usually stated as 0.8–1.2 mEq/L, though even this range allows toxic reactions in some patients; 0.7–1.0 mEq/L may be safer. As manic symptoms subside, toxic effects may occur at a lower blood level.

Lithium has a narrower therapeutic–toxic margin than most psychotropic drugs, and the blood levels are not related to phenothiazine blood concentration. *(1:676;2:829–831;3:127–128)*

138. **(A)** Under *voluntary commitment procedures,* a patient may *request admission* to a mental hospital. Once admitted, he or she *can request discharge* and *can only be held for several days without judicial commitment* (the specific number of days varies from state to state). However, there is no limitation on the commitment a court may then decide. *(1:891;2:852-855; 3:150*

139. **(D)** *Testamentary capacity* is the *competency to make a will. (1:893-894;2:859;3:152)*

140. **(B)** As evidence of *legal capacity to make a will* (testamentary capacity), the subject should know the *natural objects* of his or her bounty—who are his or her next of kin. He or she should know the *nature and extent* of his or her property—what he or she owns. (He or she should also know he or she is *making a will.*)

    He or she does not have to leave anything to anyone. The subject can be hospitalized in a mental hospital and still have full testamentary capacity. *(1:893-894;2:859;3:152)*

141. **(A)** Many *hysterical conversion reactions* develop in addition to or are superimposed on some organically based symptom.

    In diagnosing a hysterical conversion reaction, it is helpful diagnostically when the hysterical paralysis *does not fit anatomic distribution* and when the patient shows *undue lack of concern—la belle indifference.*

    Hysterical conversion reactions are more likely to occur in *previously immature personalities,* and this supports a diagnosis of hysteria. By itself, however, personality immaturity would not necessarily indicate hysterical conversion. Organic disorders can affect the immature and the mature equally. *(1:342-348;2:501-512;3:290)*

142. **(C)** Histrionic patients are more often *self-centered, childish, and exhibitionistic.* Frequently they are rather suggestible.

    When the histrionic is a woman, usually she is not comfortably warm or feminine. More commonly she is dependent, demanding, and seductive.

    Histrionic personality disorder occurs quite often in the elderly but is not more commonly seen in the elderly. Usually the histrionic has had a life-long neurotic pattern and has been recognized in adolescence or early adulthood. *(1:370-371;2:503-505;3:331)*

143. **(C)** In severe depression the subject is apt to *waken early* in the morning, when he or she *feels worse,* but the *depression may lift* somewhat *during the day.*

    Typically the depressed person has a *poor appetite* and shows *weight loss.*

    Delusions of failure, destructiveness, and evil are common in marked depression, and illusions of a cor-

responding nature are frequent. Somatic delusions are often seen. *(1:245-248;2:417-421;3:266-268)*

144. **(D)** The *suicide rate* for *male American blacks* is *lower* than the rate for *white males* and higher for *urban blacks* than for those in rural areas. The black male suicide rate is *tending to rise* nearer the level of white Americans. *(1:575;2:118-121;3:270)*

145. **(A)** Tricyclic antidepressants, such as *imipramine,* cause a worsening of narrow-angle glaucoma due to their anticholinergic effect. Imipramine may cause T-wave changes in the electrocardiogram of even physically healthy patients; in an overdose, cardiac arrhythmias occur, sometimes with fatal results. Tricyclic and monoamine oxidase antidepressants, when given together, may precipitate twitching, restlessness, convulsions, hyperpyrexia, and even death. As drug abusers have noted, imipramine and the tricyclic antidepressants potentiate the sedative effect of alcohol; in combination these drugs do not produce a hypertensive crisis. *(1:654-656;2:826-829;3:112-125)*

146. **(C)** *Involutional melancholia* is most liable to occur in *women* in their *40s or 50s* who have tended to be *rigid, compulsive,* and overly *conscientious* all their lives. Usually these subjects have not been socially outgoing or popular. Involutional melancholia is now designated *major depression, single episode, with melancholia. (1:246-247;2:436-437;3:267-268)*

147. **(E)** *Therapeutic benefits* in treating a *schizophrenic* patient are measured by *ability to work* and to *hold a job* (job turnover); *capacity for making and keeping friends;* and *stability of residence:* the capability of finding a place to stay and of remaining socially stable. *(1:220-221;2:393-400;3:255-257)*

148. **(B)** Where there are *obvious external precipitating factors* and an *acute onset,* the prognosis for the *schizophrenic* is *more favorable.*

    A prepsychotic *schizoid* personality and a *low level of anxiety* would be indicators of a *poor prognosis. (1:220-221;2:385-389;3:255-257)*

149. **(D)** Most *autistic children* are *physically healthy* and have *no autistic siblings.* Often the autistic child is *easy to toilet train.* However, where the child has no obvious *language ability by the age of 5,* the prognosis is unfavorable. *(1:732-737;2:693-694;3:201)*

150. **(A)** *Reserpine* may induce a depression that is dose-related in severity and usually clears when the drug is discontinued. Sometimes the depression may persist after the reserpine is stopped and antidepressant treatment, including electroconvulsive therapy, may be indicated. Reserpine-induced depression usually does not occur during the first week of reserpine treatment. *(1:242;2:822;3:103)*

151. **(B)** *Chronic lead poisoning* of childhood is usually seen in *young children* living in *urban poverty ghetto areas.* These children *eat lead-containing* paint or plaster from the walls of old or dilapidated houses.

Chronic lead poisoning can lead to *brain damage* and *mental retardation.* *(1:298;2:329–331;3:163)*

152. **(A)** *Acute intermittent porphyria* is more common in *women* and may present with an *acute toxic psychosis, motor paralyses,* or a combination of both.

Barbiturates are absolutely *contraindicated* as the drug may precipitate an acute attack. *(1:309–310;2:319–323;3:228)*

153. **(E)** In managing the *chronic alcoholic, group psychotherapy, halfway houses,* and *vocational training* are useful treatment procedures.

If the alcoholic wishes to stop drinking, *calcium carbamide* (Temposil) can be used to maintain aversion therapy. *(1:424–427;2:637–640;3:236–238)*

154. **(D)** *Electroconvulsive therapy.* Phenobarbital, phenothiazines, and tricyclic antidepressants do not cause memory loss. After several electroconvulsive treatments, the patient is likely to show amnesia, especially for recent events. This memory loss usually clears completely in 1 to 2 months. *(1:683;2:838;3:131–134)*

155. **(A)** In treating the *toxic delirious patient, diazepam, haloperidol,* and *chloral hydrate* are all used effectively.

Barbiturates often produce increased confusion and delirium. *(1:275–276;2:271–272;3:214)*

156. **(B)** In *operant conditioning,* the *response originates with the subject* and, when this response is the *desired behavior,* it is rewarded or *reinforced.*

There is no attempt to elicit underlying causative factors and no effort is made to produce repression. *(1:41–42;2:48–49,771–773;3:69–71)*

157. **(B)** *Barbiturates* reduce the time spent in *REM sleep.* Following the withdrawal of barbiturates, especially after chronic use, there is a "rebound" increase in REM sleep time. This increased REM time may be disturbed by frightening nightmares. *(1:563; 2:44;3:345)*

158. **(B)** *Behavior therapy* is based on the concepts that *behavior* is *learned* and develops in *response* to rewards. There is no attempt to elicit or understand supposed underlying dynamic motivations. *(1:605–608; 2:769–773;3:69–71)*

159. **(B)** By forgetting to come to one appointment and later scheduling a conflicting appointment, the patient is showing her *resistance* to uncovering the reasons for the gift to the psychotherapist. The extent of her resistance confirms that the motives for the gift were not totally logical but were a manifestation of *transference:* she has transferred onto the therapist feelings from an earlier significant relationship. *(1: 597;2:751;3:66)*

160. **(A)** *Migraine* patients more often come from *achievement-oriented families* with a *history of migraine.* Frequently family members show a tendency to *repress or internalize hostility.* These patients are not usually unduly narcissistic and often are very sensitive to others. *(1:531–532;2:579–580;3:326)*

161. **(B)** *Psychotherapy* is often useful in helping *migraine patients* become less tense and less prone to attacks. *Ergotamine* is still the optimum drug to treat migraine.

Reserpine and electroconvulsive therapy would not be beneficial in uncomplicated migraine. *(1:531–532;2:579–581;3:326)*

162. **(E)** In dealing therapeutically with patients about to have a *colostomy,* you should certainly *tell them in advance* and *discuss* with them repetitiously, if required, and in detail *pre-and postoperatively* the functioning of the colostomy. *Postoperative supportive psychotherapy* will help them deal with their anxieties and difficulties adjusting. Membership in a *colostomy club* will give them group acceptance, understanding, and support. *(2:559;3:68–69)*

163. **(A)** The highest reported incidence of mental retardation is in the 10–14 age group, when even borderline retardates are having difficulty with academic work. After they leave school, most borderline or mildly retarded teenagers and adults find socially productive occupations and live healthy normal lives—provided they have not found themselves stigmatized by the label of mental retardation. Skull x-rays are usually normal. *(1:711;2:716–717;3:159–160)*

164. **(B)** *Phantom phenomena* normally occur *after amputation* in *adults;* typically the phantoms tend to *shrink* and *disappear* with time, though they can reappear. Phantom phenomena are not wish fulfillment manifestations nor are they usually painful. *(1:537; 2:574–576)*

165. **(B)** *Phantom phenomena* do *not occur* with *congenital* absence of a limb.

They are *accentuated* and *perpetuated* by *delayed wound healing. Phantom breast phenomena* may occur after breast removal. Normal phantoms do not necessarily indicate emotional maladjustment. *(1:537;2:574–576)*

166. **(C)** *Psychosomatic reactions* occur due to a combination of *psychological* stress and constitutional predis-

position. These reactions mainly affect organs iner-
vated by the *automatic nervous system.*

Dunbar's theory that psychosomatic illnesses reflect clearly defined personality patterns has not been
validated.

Hysterical conversion reactions are more typically symbolically expressive of the underlying emotional
conflict. *(1:488–492;2:535–539;3:321–323)*

167. **(A)** Patients who develop *ulcerative colitis* are usually *sensitive, intelligent,* but basically *dependent* emotionally. Typically they have *never learned how to
handle rage and frustration* productively and tend to
express their feelings in their symptoms.

These subjects are often rather *compulsive.* Many
of their personality traits may have been produced by
the disabling, unpredictable chronic illness. *(1:493–
494;2:549–550;3:324)*

168. **(A)** *Long-term renal hemodialysis patients* have a
high risk of suicide due in part to this continuing
marked financial and emotional drain on them and
their families.

Many of these patients and their families have
magical expectations about receiving a *renal transplant* and about what such a kidney transplant might
do for them.

These patients tend to become depressed and sub-
dued rather than violent or aggressive. *(1:308;2:567–
568)*

169. **(E)** Front-line soldiers are liable to develop disabling
combat neuroses when they are *lonely, under fire but
unable to react actively,* and *lacking competent,
trustworthy group leadership. High unit losses* tend to
undermine morale and accentuate individual and
group anxiety. *(1:476–479;2:485–492;3:289)*

170. **(E)** Other factors leading to disabling *combat neuroses* include personal *conflict over killing, constant
threat of being killed,* and the *death of close friends* or
buddies. *Physical exhaustion* predisposes to emotional decompensation. *(1:476–479;2:485–492;3:289)*

171. **(A)** Even though agency funds are inadequate at any
level, with community cooperation certain useful programs could be established and would be used.

Nonuse of agency services by a community usually indicates lack of community participation in planning and administration, lack of communication with
established community providers of treatment, and
conflict of goals and needs between the agency and the
community. *(1:870–872;2:803–805;3:139–147)*

172. **(B)** *Thioridazine* may cause *inhibition of ejaculation*
and, in high doses, *pigmentary retinopathy.*

Withdrawal convulsions occur more typically
following withdrawal in chronic users of barbiturates,
alcohol, or meprobamate.

Hypertensive crises after eating cheese are liable
to occur in patients taking monoamine oxidase inhibitors. *(1:641–650;2:822–826;3:124)*

173. **(A)** In the treatment of attention deficit disorder with
hyperactivity the stimulants *amphetamines, methylphenidate,* and *pemoline* are effective with individual
patients. Phenobarbital has no therapeutic benefit. In
the United States, this syndrome is grossly over-
diagnosed and overtreated. *(1:741–747;2:681–683;3:
187–190)*

174. **(C)** In using *electroconvulsive therapy,* the patients
should be warned that *moderate weight gain* is common after treatment and women often have *amenorrhea* for a period of *2 or 3 months.*

An obvious muscular convulsion is not necessary:
muscle relaxants are used to minimize this effect of the
treatment.

Hypertension is not a contraindication to electroconvulsive therapy where good anesthetic care is
available. *(1:683;2:837–839;3:131–134)*

175. **(E)** The *risk of suicide* is greater in the elderly subject
over 60 years of age with no close family but with a
family history of suicide, and where there has been a
previous suicide attempt. *(1:886;2:118–121;3:270–
222)*

176. **(E)** *Tertiary prevention* aims to minimize the chronic
handicapping effects of an illness. In dealing with formerly hospitalized psychiatric patients, this could include *sheltered workshops, halfway houses,* and suitable *vocational placement.* For the chronic alcoholic,
contact with *Alcoholics Anonymous* may help maintain productive functioning. *(1:879–880;2:788;3:140)*

177. **(B)** *Primary prevention* is planned to prevent the occurrence of an illness.

To prevent the appearance or production of
emotionally disturbed children, *well-baby clinics* and
parental education in normal child development and
child rearing would be useful.

Day treatment centers and halfway houses deal
with the disturbed youngster when primary prevention has failed. *(1:876–877;2:788;3:140)*

178. **(A)** *Previously hospitalized chronic psychotic* patients usually have to be *readmitted* because the family does not want them (they have nowhere to go), they
have no useful job skills, and they do not know how to
function comfortably in normal social groups.

The reasons for hospital readmission are thus
more *social* than due to any recurrence of the illness.
Recurrence is not necessarily inevitable. *(1:879–880;
2:396–399;3:140–147)*

179. **(C)** *Dyslexia* is more common in *boys*. It is found in children with *visual–motor perceptual handicaps* but is not specifically associated with borderline retardation. After years of failure, these children often feel failures themselves with resultant *low self-esteem* and *depression*. *(1:748–751;2:703;3:203)*

180. **(E)** Behavior therapy has been used effectively with *mute autistic children, phobic* women, male *fetishists,* and regressed *chronic schizophrenics. (1:605–608;2:770–771;3:69–71)*

181. **(C)** To help a *young child* cope with the stress of *emergency surgery,* he or she should have the realistic situation *explained* in terms he or she can understand; it is most helpful if the *mother can stay* with the child, especially over the operative period.

     If the child is not prepared or given added emotional support, an immediate acute emotional reaction and long-term psychological difficulties may result. *(1:839–843;2:694–695;3:204–205)*

182. **(A)** Suicide is more common in *college students* than in their peers in other social settings. *Suicide attempts* are three times more common with teenage girls than with boys but *successfully completed suicide* is three times more common with the male adolescent.

     Suicide is the *third most common cause* of death in the 15–19 age group. *(1:830;2:118–121;3:270–272)*

183. **(E)** The child's *sexual role* in society depends on his or her *chromosome* pattern, *anatomic sex,* level of *sex hormones,* and the *gender role* in which he or she was reared. *(1:433;2:524–525;3:315–317)*

184. **(E)** To evaluate a *child's personality,* the examiner may use *playing* with clay, dolls, or other toys. The *Children's Apperception Test* is a modification of the Thematic Apperception Test for use with children. The *Rorschach test* can be used as a projective test especially with other children and teenagers, while the *Draw-A-Person Test* gives useful information from the preschool years onward. *(1:704–708;2:675–676;3:183–184)*

185. **(A)** *Tantrums, recurrent tics,* and *nightmares* may all be symptoms of an *adjustment reaction of childhood.* The youngster shows signs of emotional maladjustment under stress but returns to normal psychological adaptation and growth when the stress is relieved.

     Dyslexia is not a temporary response to stress. These reading difficulties may be due to neurological immaturity or damage. *(1:839–840;2:694–695;3:204–205)*

186. **(C)** *Infant intelligence testing* has *little predictive* ability in foretelling the later level of intelligence of the subject in adolescence or adulthood. Such testing evaluates mainly *motor–sensory functioning* that is usually adversely affected by *severe retardation.*

     Verbal and abstract ability are only minimally evaluated: these factors are much more important in the intelligence measured in older children. *(1:705; 2:718–719;3:184)*

187. **(E)** The *child's* functioning in *intelligence testing* is strongly influenced by the youngster's *motivation.*

     The *purpose of the test* has a profound effect: if the child knows his or her progress in school will be decided by the test, naturally he or she will be anxious and possibly less productive.

     Previous testing experience allows the youngster to be less anxious and more adept at test taking. Children, and other subjects also, respond differently in the testing situation depending on the *sex and age of the examiner. (1:704–708;2:675–676;3:183–184)*

188. **(A)** *Paranoid psychoses* are commonly seen in *bromide intoxication,* in *chronic amphetamine abuse,* and in *myxedema psychosis.*

     The myxedema patient has blunting of perception, increasing deafness, and slow cerebration due to the metabolic disorder. There may be no obvious outward reason for these changes. The subject feels something is happening to him or her and tends to deal with the anxiety by external projection—by paranoid distortion and delusions.

     Autistic children are usually too self-centered to be concerned about external influences. Paranoid projection implies a high level of awareness of outside forces. *(1:273–276;2:315–316;3:257–258)*

189. **(D)** *Acute intermittent porphyria* occurs more often in *women. Barbiturates* (and alcohol) may precipitate an acute attack and are contraindicated. *Chlorpromazine* is usually the best symptomatic treatment.

     The only correct response—*abdominal pain*—is a very *common symptom* in this disease. *(1:309–310; 2:319–323;3:228)*

190. **(A)** Racism is taught by family and culture and is supported and perpetuated by community attitudes. Racism provides a socially acceptable scapegoat for individuals and social groups. Even in the preschool years, at the age of 2 or 3, children are developing firm racial prejudices. *(1:94;2:160)*

191. **(C)** *Postpartum depression* is liable to recur with subsequent pregnancies. The depression can indeed be treated effectively with *antidepressants* or with *electroconvulsive therapy.*

     The depression does not respond well to hormone treatment. *(1:555–557;2:169;3:229)*

192. **(E)** Feeling that the world is a dream *(derealization)* and that one's self is vaguely unreal *(depersonaliza-*

tion) may be quite normal especially in the *adolescent* years. These sensations commonly occur in the *hypnagogic* state (almost falling asleep) or the *hypnopompic* state (just awakening).

Depersonalization and derealization may also be manifestation of the loosening of reality ties in a *developing psychosis* and are frequent concomitants of a *hallucinogen effect. (1:171;2:139)*

193. **(B)** Following a course of *electroconvulsive therapy,* there is often *memory impairment* for several weeks and, in women, *amenorrhea* of 1 to 2 months.

There should not be recurrent seizures. Persistent occipital headaches are not a normal residual effect. Immediately after a treatment, there may be some muscle aching, but this usually clears in a matter of hours. *(1:683;2:838-839;3:131-134)*

194. **(C)** *Exhibitionism* is still primarily a male syndrome. Even in this era of women's liberation, women are less frequently arrested for exhibitionism, which is the act of public *genital exposure, often compulsive, in order to achieve* some form of *sexual excitement* or gratification.

Exhibitionism is quite normal in young children, who typically may parade around blatantly displaying themselves.

Adult exhibitionists are *not easily treated by psychotherapy.* These patients may have little wish to modify this behavior but are often forced into a form of psychotherapy under legal pressure. *(1:449-450;2: 529-530;3:304-305)*

195. **(A)** *Binge eaters consume large amounts of food in a short time* and tend to be *upset* and *guilty* after their gorging.

They usually eat in response to *frustration* and not to some repetitive daily cyclic pattern. The guilt they feel about eating may make them so upset that they eat again to relieve their tension. *(1:779-780; 2:555;3:195)*

196. **(A)** *Anorexia nervosa* occurs usually in *women,* is most common in the *second decade* of life, and often is preceded (or alternated) by *obesity.*

The syndrome does not respond well to hormone therapy. *(1:499-504;2:554-558;3:194-195)*

197. **(C)** A course of *electroconvulsive therapy* usually *relieves the guilt* and *suicidal* impulses in the depression of manic-depressive illness and leads to *social recovery* in the majority of cases. Electroconvulsive treatment can be given usefully during *pregnancy* when good anesthesia and obstetrical supervision is available.

One course of electroconvulsive therapy will not prevent future episodes of recurrent depression, but this treatment can be used to abort or minimize the severity of later attacks. *(1:682;2:838;3:131-134)*

198. **(A)** *Primary prevention* aims to prevent the development of emotional illness in elderly patients. Prevention should be planned to reduce or eliminate factors that predispose to psychiatric difficulties.

An appropriate *social club, employment opportunities,* and *"Welcome Wagon"* introductions all help prevent isolation, loneliness, and frustration that could lead to emotional illness.

Supporting hospital facilities are not planned to prevent psychiatric decompensation but are needed to treat illness after primary prevention has failed. *(1: 876-877;2:788;3:140)*

199. **(B)** In *child abuse* cases, the abuse is often *rationalized as being merely necessary discipline* and the *abused child is often seen by the parents as being* in some way *different.*

More often the abusing parent is the *mother.* The highest incidence of child abuse is in children *under age 3. (1:834-839;2:680-681)*

200. **(D)** Needle marks, signs of phlebitis, opiates in the urine, drowsiness, and pinpoint pupils may all indicate that the subject is self-administering opioids, but they do not necessarily prove physical dependence.

Physical dependence is proved when the subject develops an *abstinence syndrome* on *withdrawal* of the drug. *(1:385-386;2:645;3:239)*

201. **(C)** *Delirium* may occur in drug withdrawal after chronic use of *alcohol* or *barbiturates:* the symptoms may be very similar with each drug. *(1:273-276; 2:627,660-661;3:217-220)*

202. **(D)** Regular use of *marijuana* has not shown to lead to "hard" drug addiction or to increased sexual potency. Unlike alcohol, marijuana does not increase aggressive behavior but rather tends to soothe and quiet the user.

It has been demonstrated that regular use of marijuana does promote *change or distortion in time sense. (1:400-403;2:664-665;3:223)*

203. **(E)** Factors that *maintain drug addiction* include a body *cellular adaptation* to the drug, the subject's individual *need for the immediate gratification* or relief from tension provided by the narcotic, and *group pressures* to use drugs.

The social acceptance of the *hustler* or drug pusher as the *successful businessperson* continues to promote and allow drug abuse. *(1:388-389;2:646-651; 3:233-236)*

204. **(A)** *Death from barbiturate overdosage* commonly occurs when alcohol is taken in addition to the barbiturate or the *narcotic addict* adds barbiturates to his or her existing narcotic intake.

Fatalities can occur when the barbiturate user, partially confused by earlier barbiturate doses, often prescribed, automatically and repetitiously *takes further doses.*

N-allyl normorphine (Nalline) has no effect on barbiturate users. Nalline is a morphine antagonist and will precipitate an acute withdrawal reaction when injected into morphine addicts. *(1:291–292;2: 658–671;3:219–220)*

205. **(A)** *Tongue tie* does not cause marked delay in talking.

This speech delay, however, could be due to *bilateral severe hearing loss, infantile autism,* or *profound mental retardation.* Often there are multiple factors producing delay or absence of language in children. *(1:752–755;2:81–83;3:203)*

206. **(A)** *Enuresis* is more common in boys.

The symptom may be a manifestation of *regressive behavior.* The *shaming* and *punitive treatment* these enuretic children often face may emotionally *handicap* them much more than the enuresis itself.

Imipramine is presently the drug of choice in the treatment of enuresis. *(1:843–846;2:697–699;3:197–198)*

207. **(B)** *Enuresis* often occurs in other *family* members but may be the outward manifestation of the child's *emotional* difficulties.

Children tend to outgrow this symptom but any army or college physician can testify that children do not always outgrow enuresis. Bedwetting may continue into late adolescent and adult years.

Enuresis should always be evaluated to see what treatment and preventive measures are necessary, even if there is no demonstrable physical cause. Underlying psychological stresses may need treatment. The clinician must help plan the management of the enuresis so children are helped to deal productively with their symptoms and are not burdened by shame, frustration, and resentment. *(1:843–846;2:697–699; 3:197–198)*

208. **(B)** Mucopolysaccharidosis Type I *(Hurler's Syndrome),* transmitted by an autosomal recessive trait, produces accumulation of mucopolysaccharides in the tissues. The leucocytes contain metachromatic inclusions. The child is not born with the characteristic facies and is likely to develop obvious progressive mental deterioration before the gargoyle facial appearance develops. Increasing hepatosplenomegaly eventually leads to abdominal distention in childhood.

Death usually occurs before adolescence. No treatment is effective.

A galactose-free diet prevents the development of clinical manifestations in galactosemia. *(1:717–718; 2:732–733;3:165)*

209. **(E)** To reduce the incidence, the *primary prevention of mental retardation, genetic counseling, prophylactic rubella immunizations,* and *prenatal* and *postnatal clinics* for mother and child would all be helpful. *(1:876–877;2:788;3:140)*

210. **(A)** In treating a 26-year-old woman with a *cat phobia* (ailurophobia), gradual *desensitization, chlorpromazine,* or other *tranquilizers,* and *psychotherapy* can all be helpful as individual treatments or in combination.

Methylphenidate would be of no use in the treatment of a phobia. *(1:326;2:476;3:286–288)*

211. **(B)** Serious *adolescent delinquency* is more common where there is a *cultural* pattern of delinquency.

When the *parents* themselves have *conscience defects (superego lacunae),* their children are more likely to be delinquent.

Mental retardation and delayed onset of puberty make a youngster more vulnerable to emotional problems but they do not specifically predispose him or her to delinquency. *(1:800–801;2:683–687;3:191)*

212. **(D)** The *electroencephalogram* may be normal between *grand mal* seizures.

It is frequently normal in autistic children and may show no abnormalities in *hyperkinetic children.*

The electroencephalogram is usually not helpful in differentiating psychiatric disorders. *(1:299–305; 2:276–277;3:225–226)*

213. **(D)** When a child has bruises and hematomas over several body areas, child abuse should be suspected. It is difficult for anyone to sustain a black eye or a zygomatic fracture from a fall. The history does not match the findings.

Multiple fractures should also suggest the possibility of child abuse.

Some children may give a history of abuse but others may not, out of fear, family loyalty, or ignorance of possible alternative life situations.

Children who are different in some way— premature, hyperkinetic, neurologically handicapped, or retarded—are more liable to be abused: sometimes these syndromes result from the battering or the severe environmental deprivation.

214. **(A)** In a case of suspected child abuse, the clinician should arrange for admission to a hospital and an extensive physical and radiologic examination. Photographs should be taken at the time of admission. The

physician should report the case to the designated child-protective services, which will then take all necessary legal and social steps.

With those measures, it is not necessary or appropriate for the physician to call in the police to apprehend the parents. Too often the community reacts to abusing parents by abusing them. The parents and family situation should be thoroughly evaluated and all appropriate legal measures taken.

215.   (B) Abusing parents, who often have been abused themselves as children, come from every socioeconomic group. Abusing parents are usually not psychotic. Not infrequently, abusing parents seek help with their behavior. Tragically, it is common to note in the history of abused youngsters that parents overtly or covertly acted in some way to bring the child's situation and their abusing behavior to the notice of potentially helping authorities, but they were not heard or understood until the child had been further abused, sometimes irreparably.

Physical abuse is easier to diagnose, treat, and prevent than emotional abuse, but the psychologically battered child may be equally damaged or handicapped.

216.   (E) Abused children more often were premature or of low birth-weight. Frequently their physical and psychological development has been slow.

The abusing parents tend to see the target child as having adult emotions and capabilities and to demand adult functioning or understanding from the child. Most often the physically battered child is of preschool age, typically 3 years old or younger.

It is notable, however, that abused children often have an ability to attract abuse both at home and outside the home. Sometimes these youngsters know only abuse-attracting ways of interacting; at other times these young subjects have physical or emotional qualities that appear to invite abuse. (1:834–839;2:680–681;3:181)

CHAPTER 10

Case Histories
Questions

INTRODUCTION

In many examinations, the student is asked questions based on one- or two-paragraph case histories. Typically there are three to five questions for each case history, though there may be fewer questions or, less commonly, a longer list of questions.

The case history cited may appear unrealistic or forced because the examiner wishes to focus on specific issues. Similarly, the answers offered for selection may sometimes be limited in scope or skewed, as the candidate is expected to respond to one particular cue.

These case history questions are often used to test the trainee's ability to synthesize what he or she has learned. Thus, there are no specific reference chapters for this section as a whole.

DIRECTIONS (Questions 1 through 4): Each group of items in this section consists of lettered headings followed by a set of numbered words or phrases. For each numbered word or phrase, select the ONE lettered heading that is most closely associated with it. Each lettered heading may be selected once, more than once, or not at all.

Questions 1 through 4

You have diagnosed a chromosome translocation in a 15-year-old girl with moderate mental retardation and mild congenital physical anomalies. You undertake certain measures.

(A) primary prevention
(B) secondary prevention
(C) tertiary prevention

1. You advise the teenager and her parents about the likelihood of her passing on these handicaps.

2. You check the child recently born to her sister for similar chromosome anomalies.

3. You arrange for vocational training in a sheltered workshop for the teenage patient.

4. At the parents' request, you arrange for contraceptive instruction for the adolescent patient.

DIRECTIONS (Questions 5 through 118): Each of the numbered items or incomplete statements in this section is followed by answers or by completions of the statement. Select the ONE lettered answer or completion that is BEST in each case.

Questions 5 through 8

A 15-year-old boy is brought to your office by his friends, who say he is "high" on drugs. They are scared of him. As you look at the teenager, you note his sallow complexion and his generally thin appearance. He is constantly restless as he sits in the chair. He grinds his teeth periodically and his eyes shift rapidly as he scans your office. When he talks, his voice sounds thick. You can find no signs of self-injection on physical examination. He admits he is taking "dope."

With some resistance, the adolescent patient responds to your questioning. He reveals a wide range of paranoid thinking and tells how he is planning to "get" those people who are making his life difficult. When you try to sway his ideas by pointing out his lack of logic, he stares suspiciously at you.

5. Your likely diagnosis is

(A) schizophrenia, paranoid type
(B) hallucinogen abuse
(C) amphetamine abuse
(D) heroin abuse
(E) schizophrenia, hebephrenic type

6. Your diagnosis is confirmed best by

(A) urine testing
(B) Rorschach test
(C) serial sevens test
(D) fasting blood sugar
(E) skull x-ray

7. Your treatment may include all the following except

(A) haloperidol
(B) psychotherapy
(C) family counseling
(D) methadone maintenance
(E) hospitalization

8. This illness may be due to the following chronic effect shown on the electroencephalogram

(A) marked increase in REM activity
(B) focal slow waves, especially in temporal lobes
(C) blocking of REM sleep
(D) recurrent 3-per-second spike and wave
(E) triphasic wave pattern

Questions 9 and 10

For almost 2 months after his wife's death, a 49-year-old man was despondent and somewhat instable. During this time, according to his daughters, "he just did not eat" and he did not want to "bother" with his family. After this time, he began to be more outgoing, took more interest in his work, and started to go out with his friends. He still had times when he felt lonely and sad.

9. The man was showing

(A) depression
(B) grief
(C) conversion
(D) reaction formation
(E) helplessness

10. According to statistical data, within 2 years he is most likely to

(A) develop a cardiovascular illness
(B) remarry
(C) kill himself
(D) become an alcoholic
(E) show signs of early dementia

Questions 11 through 15

An intelligent 5-year-old boy had been the only child in a family until a sister was born. Following the birth, he began to wet his bed after being dry for 3 years.

11. You should

(A) avoid doing a physical examination since this is an emotional problem

(B) routinely plan catheterization to test his bladder capacity

(C) take a thorough medical and psychological history and do a careful physical examination

(D) arrange for a battery of intelligence and projective tests including the Rorschach

(E) point out to the mother that this is obviously a minor problem and she should stop worrying

12. Since this is a reaction to the birth of a sister, the parents should

(A) give the patient extra attention and support
(B) hire a babysitter to give him personal care
(C) point out that this bedwetting is very childish
(D) ignore his bedwetting
(E) send him off to the grandparents for a rest

13. Other symptoms that may coexist with the bedwetting include all of the following *except*

(A) nightmares
(B) tantrums
(C) autism
(D) thumb sucking
(E) nail biting

14. All of the following statements are true about enuresis *except*

(A) children tend to grow out of the symptom by adolesence
(B) it is more common in girls than in boys
(C) often there is a history of enuresis in the parents or close relatives
(D) bedwetting occurs most often during deepest sleep
(E) children are often more handicapped by the shame and ridicule than by the symptom itself

15. In the drug treatment of enuresis, the medication presently most effective is

(A) Dilantin
(B) monoamine oxidase
(C) chlordiazepoxide
(D) lithium
(E) imipramine

Questions 16 and 17

You have been treating a severely depressed 52-year-old woman with tranylcypromine. After 3 weeks of treatment, her depression appeared to be clearing. One evening she asks to see you because she is "not feeling herself." She feels sick to her stomach, her neck muscles are stiff, and she has a "dreadful headache."

16. You anticipate that she is suffering from

(A) depressive somatization
(B) cryptococcal meningitis

(C) a hypertensive crisis
(D) early psychotic decompensation
(E) involutional melancholia

17. When you take a history, you will ask especially about

(A) head injury
(B) dietary intake
(C) recent infections
(D) family conflicts
(E) menstrual history

Questions 18 through 22

Father comes home tired from work to find that his two young sons have trampled his rose garden during their ball game. In a fury, he spanks them severely.

18. The younger 5-year-old boy stomps out of the house in a rage. He kicks the sleeping dog as he goes by the front porch. His behavior toward the dog is an example of

(A) projection
(B) isolation
(C) displacement
(D) reaction formation
(E) dissociation

19. His 8-year-old brother, hurt and angry, goes down to the basement and spends the next hour chopping wood. This wood chopping is a manifestation of

(A) identification
(B) intellectualization
(C) introjection
(D) sublimation
(E) suppression

20. Their little sister watched the spankings anxiously and then ran fearfully into the garden. A few minutes later she was heard laughing loudly at a rather dismal television program. Her laughter was an outward sign of

(A) conversion
(B) isolation
(C) repression
(D) reaction formation
(E) rationalization

21. Father is normally a mild-tempered man who does not like to get angry. He is upset that he lost control of his feelings. Later that evening, he develops a pounding headache, an example of

(A) regression
(B) incorporation
(C) conversion
(D) undoing
(E) somatization

22. Mother's parents fought all through her childhood so she does not like any family conflict. Though the noise of the spankings has been clearly audible through the house, somehow mother in the next room has not noticed the tumult. Her reaction is a manifestation of

    (A) negativism
    (B) denial
    (C) autism
    (D) dissociation
    (E) projection

Questions 23 through 27

A 40-year-old farm worker is hospitalized for an infectious pneumonitis. He seems to be responding well to antibiotics but on the third day of his hospital stay he becomes restless, irritable, and wants to leave. He appears to be confused. Restraints are applied and a psychiatrist is called in consultation. The psychiatrist notes from the chart that the patient is a widower, a veteran who lives by himself. The history states that he has been in "good general health," with no accidents, and that he smokes and drinks "moderately." His physical examination is essentially negative apart from the clearing bronchopneumonia. "There is no history of previous emotional illness" according to the hospital record.

The man is lying in bed with arm and leg restraints. He is sweating profusely and the bed is in disarray. He does not acknowledge the doctor's presence but is anxiously watching what he claims to be "big lizards over there in the corner"; he sees these lizards climbing up the wall.

23. The most likely diagnosis here is

    (A) schizophrenia, paranoid type
    (B) hysterical neurosis, conversion type
    (C) delirium tremens
    (D) involutional paranoid state
    (E) pathological intoxication

24. The preferred treatment includes all the following except

    (A) remove restraints
    (B) intramuscular morphine
    (C) parenteral fluids
    (D) chlordiazepoxide
    (E) magnesium sulfate infusion

With treatment, the patient becomes less disturbed but the nursing staff is still concerned. The patient is physically healthy, spends his time walking around the unit, but he does not seem to recognize his surroundings. Even though he is told repeatedly that he is in a hospital, a few minutes later he appears to have forgotten. He states he is in a hotel, on vacation from his work in a local automobile factory. He is just waiting to go home to his wife. His general mood is friendly and cooperative.

25. He is now showing

    (A) la belle indifference
    (B) perseveration
    (C) thought blocking
    (D) confabulation
    (E) flight of ideas

26. This symptom is a manifestation of

    (A) Korsakoff's syndrome
    (B) acute porphyria
    (C) malingering
    (D) Capgras's syndrome
    (E) schizophrenia, simple type

27. Other symptoms that may develop as part of this illness include all of the following except

    (A) acute pancreatitis
    (B) hepatic coma
    (C) pellagra
    (D) Wernicke's encephalopathy
    (E) splenic infarction

Questions 28 through 30

Parents bring their 5-year-old son to you, complaining that he spends all his time winding and rewinding an old beaten clock and becomes most upset if disturbed. Though he does not talk or make communicating sounds yet, he can take apart and put together intricate clock mechanisms; father says he himself could not do so well. The youngster does not play with other children, but may sit for long periods in front of television rocking quietly to the music. The little boy is a healthy looking child. When you lift him up, he hangs heavily in your arms.

28. Your likely diagnosis is

    (A) infantile autism
    (B) mental retardation
    (C) deafness
    (D) adjustment reaction of childhood
    (E) withdrawing reaction of childhood

29. Your most effective treatment is likely to be

    (A) electroconvulsive therapy
    (B) behavior modification
    (C) child psychoanalysis
    (D) long-term institutional care
    (E) methylphenidate

30. This syndrome was first described by

    (A) Anna Freud
    (B) B. F. Skinner
    (C) C. Jung
    (D) E. Bleuler
    (E) L. Kanner

Questions 31 through 33

You are called to the local police station to evaluate a 26-year-old man who has suddenly assaulted a life-long neighbor. He claims that the neighbor has been spying on him and just recently trained his dog to dig up his roses. When you are introduced to the patient, he mutters something like "He sent you."

The man is unwilling to sit down. He paces around restlessly and refuses to be touched. Periodically he stops and seems to talk quietly to himself. At other times he appears to be listening to some private sounds or voices.

31. This disturbed man attacked his neighbor to prevent what he believed to be spying. The emotional mechanism whereby he justified his assault is

    (A) dissociation
    (B) rationalization
    (C) projection
    (D) displacement
    (E) undoing

32. The most likely diagnosis of this patient is

    (A) homosexual panic
    (B) bipolar disorder, manic type, acute
    (C) paranoia
    (D) schizophrenia, paranoid type
    (E) antisocial personality

33. His present symptoms are best treated by

    (A) imipramine
    (B) chlorpromazine
    (C) barbiturates
    (D) amphetamines
    (E) chlordiazepoxide

Questions 34 through 37

A 49-year-old housewife is admitted to hospital because of a "nervous breakdown." She is restless, weepy, and states repeatedly that she is destined for the fires of hell. All her life she has been a hard-working woman, caring for her family, with no physical or emotional illnesses. In recent months she has been increasingly anxious and irritable. She was hospitalized when she refused to go upstairs in her home, claiming that men were waiting up there to kill her.

34. The most likely diagnosis is

    (A) presenile dementia
    (B) involutional melancholia
    (C) adjustment disorder with depressed mood
    (D) schizophrenia, paranoid type
    (E) somatization disorder

35. The preferred treatment is

    (A) chlorpromazine, intramuscularly
    (B) electroconvulsive therapy
    (C) chlordiazepoxide, orally
    (D) intensive psychotherapy
    (E) phenobarbital, orally

36. As longer-term maintenance treatment, the following would be appropriate

    (A) diazepam
    (B) meprobamate
    (C) imipramine
    (D) chlordiazepoxide
    (E) phenobarbital

37. This patient's statement that she should die and go to hell and her fear of going upstairs lest she be killed are examples of

    (A) dissociation
    (B) undoing
    (C) autism
    (D) ambivalence
    (E) isolation

Questions 38 through 41

A previously healthy 8-year-old boy is hospitalized with a malignancy that is diagnosed as inoperable and rapidly progressive. When you go to visit him you find that he is located in a small, isolated room, around a corner from the rest of the unit. The nurses tell you that the patient was moved there to allow him peace and comfort. The nurses are really upset about this boy's illness and find it very difficult to cope with his approaching death.

38. Their reason for his isolation is an example of

    (A) undoing
    (B) sublimation
    (C) dissociation
    (D) rationalization
    (E) compulsion

You find that one nurse has not kept away from the boy. Indeed she is in and out to see him every 15 minutes, to the point of tiring the youngster. You learn that last year the father of this nurse died of a similar malignancy.

39. The nurse's behavior can be considered as

    (A) counterphobic
    (B) schizoid
    (C) cyclothymic
    (D) anancastic
    (E) hysterical

When you visit the 8-year-old patient, he is showing marked weight loss, an intravenous infusion is running, and his mother seems to be wiping away tears. The boy greets you with a feeble smile and within minutes is talking with you about the summer trip he plans to take next year.

40. He is handling the stress of his illness by

    (A) conversion
    (B) denial
    (C) regression
    (D) sublimation
    (E) isolation

These medically knowledgeable parents appreciate that their son is receiving the best possible care. Nevertheless, when you leave the patient, you find the boy's father loudly abusing a nurse about the incompetent treatment his son is getting. You help to calm the father and later you explain to the nurse how the father is handling the normal mourning anger.

41. He is handling the normal mourning anger by

    (A) dissociation
    (B) reaction formation
    (C) suppression
    (D) projection
    (E) displacement

Questions 42 through 48

A 20-year-old male has just been convicted a second time for possession of heroin. He has been addicted for 3 years and on several occasions has unsuccessfully attempted to break the habit. He is put on probation on the condition that he undergoes treatment for his addiction.

42. Withdrawal from heroin is best carried out as an

    (A) outpatient with supportive psychotherapy
    (B) outpatient with methadone cover
    (C) inpatient with heroin antagonist (Naline)
    (D) inpatient with methadone cover
    (E) inpatient with immediate withdrawal and no drug coverage ("cold turkey")

43. A major danger of recurrent self-injections is

    (A) diabetes
    (B) mononucleosis
    (C) hepatitis
    (D) syphilis
    (E) enteritis

44. In spite of the patient's denials, the physician is suspicious of continued heroin self-administration. All of the following signs would indicate self-injection *except*

    (A) recently thrombosed veins
    (B) recurrent skin abscesses
    (C) septicemia
    (D) hepatitis
    (E) syphilis

45. In heroin addiction, withdrawal symptoms include

    (A) runny nose, watery eyes
    (B) vomiting and diarrhea
    (C) muscle and stomach cramps
    (D) all of the above
    (E) A and C only

46. In long-term management of the former addict, what treatment approach would be considered?

    (A) methadone maintenance
    (B) therapeutic community
    (C) psychotherapy
    (D) job training
    (E) all of the above

47. When the addict is withdrawn cold turkey from an addicting opiate, established abstinence symptoms appear in

    (A) 30 to 60 minutes
    (B) 3 to 6 hours
    (C) 12 to 24 hours
    (D) 2 to 3 days
    (E) 1 to 2 weeks

48. Heroin abstinence symptoms clear within

    (A) 12 to 24 hours
    (B) 1 to 3 days
    (C) 4 to 8 days
    (D) 7 to 14 days
    (E) 2 months

Questions 49 and 50

A 35-year-old married woman comes to see you because she is "tired out and draggy." She has no energy. She has put on 30 pounds in weight, her "complexion is a mess" and "life is just not worth living." She received some tranquilizing pills from her local doctor, but this medication only made her feel worse.

As you look at her, she is indeed droopy. She sits hunched in her chair, her round, fat face wet with tears, and she talks in a low monotonous voice.

49. Your most likely diagnosis is

    (A) bipolar disorder, depressive type
    (B) acute intermittent porphyria
    (C) Cushing's syndrome
    (D) involutional melancholia
    (E) psychosomatic gastrointestinal disorder

50. You would confirm your diagnosis by demonstrating

    (A) increased urinary 17-hydroxycorticoids
    (B) abnormal focus on electroencephalogram
    (C) poor form content on Rorschach
    (D) long history of binge eating
    (E) improvement with electroconvulsive therapy

Questions 51 through 53

A 17-year-old boy announces to his parents that, for the past 2 years, he has been actively homosexual. The parents, acutely upset, call to ask you to evaluate the young man, who has agreed to be seen in order to please his father and mother.

51. You agree to see the boy and anticipate that

(A) he will be obviously effeminate
(B) he will want a sex-change operation
(C) he will dislike girls
(D) he will markedly fear his father
(E) none of the above

52. You appreciate that therapeutic attempts to change his sexual orientation from homosexual to heterosexual would depend mostly on

(A) the patient's wish to change
(B) the masculine models he has in his life
(C) the subject's relationship with his mother
(D) the family religious background
(E) the patient's willingness to accept hospital treatment

53. When you discuss the cause of homosexuality with the parents, you point out that homosexuality is caused by

(A) disturbed parent–child interaction
(B) seduction by homosexual adults
(C) hormonal imbalance
(D) xo chromosome type
(E) none of the above

Questions 54 and 55

A 46-year-old woman is hospitalized because she attempted to assault the local mayor, whom, she claimed, was poisoning her water. On examination the woman weeps quietly but profusely. She thinks she may have been mistaken about the mayor, but she is not sure. She has been so confused lately; so tired and so full of aches and pains. She is not good for anything, the children just want to get rid of her, and she cannot even sing in the choir. Her hearing is not what it used to be. She is just old and worn out.

She does indeed look tired and droopy. Her face is sallow, her skin dry, and her hair lifeless. She talks slowly, rather deliberately, and in a dull monotone.

54. Your likely diagnosis will be

(A) chronic bromism
(B) depression
(C) paranoia
(D) schizophrenia, paranoid type
(E) hypothyroidism

55. The specific treatment required would be

(A) chlorpromazine, intramuscularly
(B) electroconvulsive therapy
(C) thyroid extract
(D) chlordiazepoxide
(E) estrogen

Questions 56 and 57

The psychiatrist is called to see a 26-year-old former mental hospital patient. Two days previously the patient was involved in a motorcycle accident. Though he was probably drunk at the time, he was only dazed and shaken up by the crash. His neighbors have now brought him to the emergency room because they found him wandering around his yard, confused and half naked. His previous hospital history is not available. He is disoriented as to time and place. His speech is slow and rather slurred. He is annoyed by all this "fussing" and wants to go home, though he cannot say where his home is. The physical examination is unremarkable apart from superficial skin abrasions from his accident.

56. The most likely diagnosis is

(A) schizophrenia, paranoid type
(B) subdural hematoma
(C) toxic psychosis due to hallucinogens
(D) presenile dementia
(E) schizophrenia, catatonic type

57. The diagnosis is confirmed by

(A) CSF colloidal gold curve
(B) skull burr holes
(C) Rorschach test
(D) urinalysis
(E) serial sevens testing

Questions 58 and 59

A 40-year-old man presents with confusion, agitation, and visual hallucinations. Abdominal x-rays show midline calcification.

58. Your likely diagnosis is

(A) hypersplenism
(B) chronic pancreatitis
(C) hepatic amyloidosis
(D) trichiniasis
(E) acute intermittent porphyria

59. You confirm your diagnosis by measuring

(A) serum amylase
(B) fasting blood sugar
(C) serum bilirubin
(D) blood eosinophils
(E) stool fat

Questions 60 through 65

60. An 8-year-old boy attends a special education class in school. Since he is said to be of borderline intellectual functioning, his intelligence quotient would be in the range

    (A) 30–70
    (B) 71–84
    (C) 72–95
    (D) 61–75
    (E) 80–100

61. Though he is teased mercilessly by other children on the school bus, he does not appear to mind. Indeed he seems to invite their teasing so he can act the fool. His behavior is an indication of

    (A) fixation
    (B) isolation
    (C) undoing
    (D) reaction formation
    (E) displacement

62. Following a minor fight in school, he develops weakness of his right leg. No physical cause can be shown for the leg weakness, which becomes so marked that he cannot go to school. He is now showing a

    (A) depersonalization disorder
    (B) dissociative disorder
    (C) phobia
    (D) anxiety disorder
    (E) conversion disorder

63. His outward lack of concern is categorized as

    (A) autism
    (B) la belle indifference
    (C) illusion
    (D) ambivalence
    (E) displacement

64. This leg weakness has allowed him to avoid the unpleasant school teasing. This result is the

    (A) primary gain
    (B) primary process
    (C) secondary process
    (D) illusion
    (E) rationalization

65. After 2 weeks he is assigned a home bound teacher and his family continues to be very kind and supportive. It will be difficult to remove his emotionally based weakness due to increasing

    (A) negativism
    (B) malingering
    (C) secondary gain
    (D) autistic thinking
    (E) suppression

Questions 66 and 67

In the early evening a 23-year-old man is brought to the hospital emergency room. He is a high school teacher attending a professional convention. He has been working so hard at the convention all day that he has only had time for a coffee break. He had been planning to relax with his colleagues over the evening banquet.

During the afternoon, his fellow teachers found him to be increasingly unstable. His comments seemed at times strange or out of context. Eventually he became quite confused—as another visiting teacher stated, "almost drunk," though he had drunk just one beer.

The young man is restless, sweating, and disoriented to time and place. Physically he is in excellent condition, though there may be needle marks on his thigh.

66. The most likely diagnosis is

    (A) heroin withdrawal
    (B) acute hypoglycemia
    (C) acute anxiety neurosis
    (D) delirium tremens
    (E) methadone intoxication

67. The diagnosis would be confirmed by

    (A) electroencephalogram
    (B) urine testing
    (C) nalorphine, intramuscularly
    (D) blood sugar estimation
    (E) intramuscular chlorpromazine

Questions 68 through 71

In your small town, you are aware that a 37-year-old man has been visiting out-of-town specialized clinics since his accident last year. When you knew him in school, this man was even then a "loner," rather sensitive and irritable. He went on through college and married, but his marriage ended several years ago. He was involved in a minor car accident a year ago, has never been back to work and, you know, has two or three lawsuits pending against the local highway department, the driver of the other car, and the mayor.

He begins his history by telling you how incompetent all his previous doctors have been—but he knows you are most capable. As he gives his history and you do your physical and psychiatric examination, he makes bitter and scathing comments about several of your town acquaintances. You find no evidence of physical disability.

68. In your psychiatric diagnosis, you are most likely dealing with

    (A) bipolar disorder, depressive type
    (B) schizophrenia, paranoid type
    (C) paranoia
    (D) conversion disorder
    (E) malingering

69. The patient asks your opinion of his previous medical examiner and his examination, and you

   (A) agree that the examination was poor and the examiner incompetent
   (B) state you really cannot give an opinion since you did not see the patient yourself at that time and you do not know the findings or recommendations
   (C) tell the patient directly that he is a troublemaker and you are not going to be part of his schemes
   (D) ignore his question
   (E) advise him to contact the local medical society

70. In dealing with this patient, you should

   (A) do a minimal examination and insist on referring him to a psychiatrist
   (B) carry out a thorough examination and note all findings and recommendations clearly on the patient's record
   (C) begin to set up regularly scheduled appointments at least twice a week
   (D) start him on a fairly strong analgesic for the back pain he complains of
   (E) refuse to see him again

71. This man's emotional condition is

   (A) likely to stay the same
   (B) a precursor of senile dementia
   (C) probably going to lead to a florid schizophrenia
   (D) a manifestation of underlying depression
   (E) likely to become completely normal

Questions 72 and 73

"Like a vise crushing my skull" was the symptom a 26-year-old married woman used to describe how "she never slept a wink at night" and never could eat anything. She said she was constantly tired and exhausted by her two children, though she did manage to go out several evenings each week.

Physical examination is negative and indeed the lady seems to be in excellent physical condition, though slightly overweight. She talked freely about herself and her family.

72. Her diagnosis is likely to be

   (A) bipolar disorder, depressive type
   (B) chronic hypotension
   (C) anxiety disorder
   (D) hysterical neurosis, conversion type
   (E) involutional melancholia

73. The appropriate treatment might include all of the following except

   (A) individual psychotherapy
   (B) family therapy
   (C) meprobamate
   (D) diazepam
   (E) electroconvulsive therapy

Questions 74 through 76

Ostensibly, because she has read about community trouble in other cities, a 26-year-old married woman is too scared to travel alone on the local city bus service. She insists that her husband go with her each time.

74. The fact that her husband does accompany her each time and she enjoys this attention may prolong this phobia due to

   (A) reinforcement of the phobia
   (B) secondary gain
   (C) primary gain
   (D) rationalization
   (E) displacement

75. Though they have a car and used to shop near home, she now insists on doing all her shopping downtown and always going by bus. This behavior is an example of

   (A) intellectualization
   (B) sublimation
   (C) fixation
   (D) counterphobic reaction
   (E) suppression

76. A phobia is usually an example of

   (A) conversion
   (B) sublimation
   (C) reaction formation
   (D) displacement
   (E) undoing

Questions 77 through 81

You are asked to see a 14-year-old girl hospitalized because of recurrent nocturnal convulsions. You find her in her hospital room, surrounded by cards, pictures, and flowers, with her boyfriend solicitously holding her hand. Physical examination and laboratory tests have all been normal.

You ask the boyfriend to leave the room. The young girl is friendly, cooperative, and seemingly not too concerned about her illness. She had her first seizure when her boyfriend was walking her home from a movie 3 weeks ago. Since that time the convulsive episodes have tended to recur about the time of day when he is liable to be with her. She tells you that she comes from a devoutly religious family. Her 15-year-old boyfriend is hard-working and good looking. With some more direct questions, she does admit that she and her boyfriend did almost "get carried away" in their embracing a month ago but they both decided "they were too young."

77. The most likely diagnosis is

   (A) malingering
   (B) antisocial personality
   (C) conversion disorder
   (D) schizophrenia, hebephrenic type
   (E) avoidant disorder of adolescence

78. Her symptoms were produced by

   (A) feelings of anger toward her boyfriend
   (B) the wish for closer sexual relationship with her boyfriend conflicting with moral prohibition
   (C) catastrophic reaction
   (D) counterphobic reaction
   (E) identification with mother

79. The defense whereby her conflict is partially repressed and expressed symbolically in a physical symptom is an example of

   (A) displacement
   (B) intellectualization
   (C) conversion
   (D) isolation
   (E) rationalization

80. The fact that she is now the focus of so much care and solicitude by her family and boyfriend may make her illness more difficult to treat. This factor is called

   (A) identification with the aggressor
   (B) fixation
   (C) regression
   (D) secondary gain
   (E) narcissism

81. To produce a rapid symptomatic improvement you may use

   (A) electroconvulsive therapy
   (B) interpretive psychotherapy
   (C) hypnosis
   (D) chlorpromazine
   (E) imipramine

Questions 82 through 84

A 19-year-old, previously healthy female student is referred to you because of "seizures." She is just 2 months into her first year at college. These episodes began 2 weeks after she came to the university. Typically the attacks occur just after she has had breakfast at the dormitory, before she can go to classes. She becomes weak and giddy, her heart beats rapidly, she cannot breathe properly, her hands go numb and tingle, and her legs give way under her. Her friends tell her she is pale and sweating. She wonders if she has heart trouble, a brain tumor, or "something." Physical examination is normal.

82. The likely diagnosis is

   (A) acute schizophrenia
   (B) major depression
   (C) hyperventilation syndrome
   (D) psychomotor epilepsy
   (E) homosexual panic

83. The diagnosis may be confirmed by asking the subject to

   (A) take the Minnesota Multiphasic Personality Inventory
   (B) overbreathe for 2 minutes
   (C) do push-ups for 15 minutes
   (D) breathe in and out of a paper bag
   (E) have a skull x-ray

84. In the management of this patient, you may want to

   (A) explore the stresses she faces on leaving home
   (B) explain the physiological basis for her symptoms
   (C) offer supportive psychotherapy
   (D) all of the above
   (E) none of the above

Questions 85 through 87

A 14-year-old girl is referred for evaluation because of marked weight loss. A year ago she was somewhat overweight, weighing 160 pounds; now she weighs 78 pounds, due to the strict dieting she has been maintaining. Though she claims she is no longer interested in food, she meticulously cuts away fat in her food and always makes sure her brothers have extra food. She started limiting her food when her boyfriend teased her about being "well rounded." Her menses started when she was 11 but stopped 4 months ago. She is active, energetic, and considers herself healthy.

85. The most likely diagnosis is

   (A) hypopituitarism
   (B) anorexia nervosa
   (C) schizophrenia, simple type
   (D) conversion disorder
   (E) depression

86. On physical examination, in addition to her weight loss, it will be noted that she has

   (A) feminine pubic hair distribution
   (B) masculine pubic hair distribution
   (C) no pubic hair
   (D) masculine pubic hair and chest hair
   (E) loss of hair pigmentation

87. This syndrome

   (A) occurs predominantly in women
   (B) occurs equally in men and women

(C) is usually seen in other family members

(D) usually indicates an underlying psychosis

(E) occurs predominantly in young men

Questions 88 and 89

In school the teacher notes that an 8-year-old boy confuses letters and words as he reads. He sees *saw* for *was,* *b*'s for *d*'s, and *p*'s for *g*'s. He really can only read when the book has many pictures. He is an intelligent youngster, but he is becoming frustrated with schools. You examine the youngster physically. He is somewhat awkward, writes with his left hand, and kicks with his right foot but is in good physical condition.

88. Your likely diagnosis is

   (A) brain tumor

   (B) childhood schizophrenia

   (C) school phobia

   (D) strephosymbolia

   (E) obsessive–compulsive disorder

89. Your optimum treatment would then be

   (A) immediate long-term psychotherapy

   (B) methylphenidate

   (C) remedial teacher

   (D) transfer to another school

   (E) phenobarbital

Questions 90 through 92

A 6-year-old boy is brought to you by his mother at the request of his schoolteacher. He is said to be "totally out of control" in school.

   Apparently he spends his time wandering about the classroom, sometimes aimlessly, sometimes talking to other children. He hardly ever sits still, even for their in-school television programs. His mother states he has always been "on the go" but in their farm home he is usually outside with the animals. His parents, however, do worry about his being up at all hours of the night. Group testing in school gives this boy an average intelligence quotient.

90. Your diagnosis is likely to be

   (A) infantile autism

   (B) childhood schizophrenia

   (C) conduct disorder

   (D) attention deficit disorder

   (E) overanxious disorder

91. Factors confirming your diagnosis might include

   (A) amnioaciduria

   (B) "soft" neurological signs

   (C) blonde hair and blue eyes

   (D) café-au-lait spots

   (E) Kayser–Fleischer ring

92. In treating this patient you would likely use

   (A) imipramine

   (B) phenobarbital

   (C) methylphenidate

   (D) thiamine

   (E) haloperidol

Questions 93 and 94

As student mental health consultant you are asked to interview a 21-year-old girl because she is "crazy." Apparently she has been bothering her classmates by her disheveled appearance and her loud laughter during class study periods. When you see her you note that she is indeed a messy dresser. She smiles rather fatuously as she talks, but she is cooperative. As she begins to tell what she is doing, she stops and seems to listen momentarily. She admits readily that she is listening to her voices and she often hears these voices. She continues to talk about her classes, but you find her conversation difficult to follow. Periodically she giggles to herself.

93. Of the following, the most likely diagnosis is

   (A) histrionic personality disorder

   (B) borderline intellectual functioning

   (C) schizophrenia, disorganized (hebephrenic) type

   (D) schizophrenia, catatonic type

   (E) schizoid personality disorder

94. In your treatment you may want to include all of the following *except*

   (A) haloperidol

   (B) electroconvulsive therapy

   (C) hospitalization

   (D) lithium carbonate

   (E) psychotherapy

Questions 95 through 97

A 32-year-old woman is brought to the hospital by her distraught husband. In the past 3 days she has been on a shopping spree and has charged several thousand dollars on various charge accounts. In this time she has bought three fur coats. At home she has cleaned the house daily. Last night at 4:00 AM she decided to retile the kitchen floor so she phoned all her neighbors to ask them to help. She talks and jokes constantly. The husband says she has had three episodes like this before but "this is the worst."

95. It is likely this woman has

   (A) passive–aggressive personality disorder

   (B) pathological intoxication

   (C) schizophrenia, hebephrenic type

   (D) bipolar disorder, manic type

   (E) psychogenic fugue

96. Without treatment, her symptoms would

    (A) clear in 1 week
    (B) evolve into chronic dementia in 6 months
    (C) subside in about 3 months
    (D) continue for 6 to 12 months and then gradually clear
    (E) develop into obvious delirium tremens

97. In managing this patient you should plan

    (A) interpretive psychotherapy
    (B) family therapy
    (C) outpatient electroconvulsive therapy
    (D) supportive psychotherapy
    (E) hospitalization with drug therapy

Questions 98 through 100

You are asked to see a 25-year-old man in the hospital emergency room. Physical examination and laboratory tests have shown nothing abnormal, but he is said to be "acting queer."

When you see him, he is sitting on a bench looking straight ahead. His face is motionless and he does not seem to notice the hustle around him. When you talk to him, he does not answer. You raise his arm, which then remains in an outstretched position.

98. Your most likely diagnosis is

    (A) delirium tremens
    (B) psychogenic amnesia
    (C) conversion disorder
    (D) paranoid personality disorder
    (E) schizophrenia, catatonic type

The patient is hospitalized for further evaluation. Laboratory tests are still normal. Two days later he becomes acutely agitated, shouting and screaming almost incoherently. He seems unable to sit still, has torn his bed sheets and mattress into shreds, and has hit two staff members.

99. He is now showing

    (A) panic disorder
    (B) catatonic excitement
    (C) bipolar disorder, manic type
    (D) catastrophic reaction
    (E) explosive personality

100. Your treatment should be

    (A) inderal orally
    (B) lithium carbonate orally
    (C) barbiturates intramuscularly
    (D) haloperidol intramuscularly
    (E) chlordiazepoxide orally

Questions 101 and 102

You are called to see a previously healthy, stable 63-year-old woman on the opthalmology service. Three days ago she had bilateral cataract operations. Her eyes are healing well, but she became confused, agitated, and assaultive today.

101. She is likely to be suffering from

    (A) schizophrenia, paranoid type
    (B) senile dementia
    (C) psychosis due to sensory deprivation
    (D) involutional paranoid disorder
    (E) major depression

102. The appropriate management includes all the following *except*

    (A) oral barbiturate
    (B) telephone at her bedside
    (C) frequent visitors
    (D) radio or television
    (E) central peephole in eye bandage

Questions 103 through 105

You have been called in consultation to see a 45-year-old widower. He is weepy, depressed, and unable to do his work as company accountant. From the family history, you note that his sister committed suicide. You are concerned that he might be suicidal.

103. You should

    (A) avoid mentioning suicide lest you precipitate the act
    (B) directly raise the question as to whether he has thought of killing himself
    (C) try to talk first with other family members to see if they have seen signs of suicidal intent
    (D) arrange to see him for a series of appointments so you can raise the question at an appropriate time
    (E) avoid distressing him now with pointed questions about suicide, but start him on antidepressant medication

104. The patient admits that he is profoundly depressed and is thinking seriously about killing himself. You should

    (A) point out how stupid and self-defeating such a terrible act would be
    (B) send him home to get his clothes so that he can be admitted to hospital that day or next
    (C) institute or maintain high intake of antidepressants and set up daily outpatient appointments

(D) admit him directly to the hospital from your office. Be sure he is closely accompanied to the hospital unit.

(E) arrange contact for him with one of the suicide prevention groups, like "Rescue." They will care for him.

105. In the hospital your treatment might include all of the following *except*

(A) electroconvulsive therapy
(B) antidepressant medication
(C) psychotherapy
(D) suicidal precautions
(E) lithium carbonate

Questions 106 and 107

A 14-year-old girl has been losing weight in the last 6 months. She has gone down from 110 to 70 pounds. Her menses stopped 3 months ago. She is described as always having been close to her father and somewhat of a tomboy. This weight loss started 1 week after she broke up with her boyfriend.

She is a pert, friendly girl who seems to like her tall, thin appearance. Apart from her thinness, physical examination is normal except for a moderate right-sided papilledema.

106. Your most possible diagnosis is

(A) anorexia nervosa
(B) intracranial tumor
(C) conversion disorder
(D) obsessive–compulsive disorder
(E) histrionic personality disorder

107. Your diagnosis might be confirmed by

(A) fasting blood sugar
(B) skull x-rays
(C) Rorschach test
(D) serial sevens test
(E) serum amylase

Questions 108 through 110

A 12-year-old boy is hospitalized for recurrent "seizures" in school. Otherwise, he is in excellent physical health. A thorough neurological examination including repeat electroencephalograms gives completely normal findings. At the time of your psychiatric consultation, the teenager admits that these spells occur when he is angry at the teasing of his classmates. As you encourage him to talk, he speaks with increasing vehemence about his fury at being "picked on" and then quite suddenly goes into one of his attacks. Physically he becomes motionless, staring downward, his arms fall back to his side. This spell lasts 20 minutes and then he comes around over a period of 2 or 3 minutes.

108. Your likely diagnosis is

(A) schizophrenia, childhood type
(B) schizophrenia, catatonic type
(C) avoidant disorder of adolescence
(D) depersonalization disorder
(E) dissociative disorder

109. Your treatment might include

(A) tranquilizers
(B) psychotherapy
(C) strong symptom-directed suggestion
(D) all of the above
(E) none of the above

110. In such a symptom, conflictual anxiety is

(A) projected outward
(B) redirected onto a more tolerable focus
(C) consciously and deliberately controlled and inhibited
(D) strongly repressed and the opposite impulse emphasized
(E) separated from normal awareness and expressed or acted out

Questions 111 through 113

For the past 5 months a 40-year-old woman has been seeing a succession of physicians about her stomach trouble and eventually she is referred for psychiatric consultation. She knows she has a big deep ulcer—"at least the size of your fist"—that has eaten away her stomach and is now "working on her liver." She can feel the gnawing and biting so she knows. Generally she feels "just no good" and she states she just cannot go on this way. She is no use to anyone. It is just as well her husband died last year and she thinks her children should put her away. She admits she has thought of killing herself and, as God knows, she well deserves to go to hell but she cannot get up the courage. She feel that no one can help her.

Previously she had no history of emotional illness. Extensive physical and laboratory studies are normal.

111. Your diagnosis is likely to be

(A) panic disorder
(B) major depression
(C) schizophrenia, hebephrenic type
(D) bipolar disorder, depressed type
(E) conversion disorder

112. When she talked further about her abdominal discomfort, she described how there was "something like germs in there with teeth, chewing." This symptom is an example of

(A) conversion
(B) phobia
(C) projection
(D) phantom phenomenon
(E) somatic delusion

113. Your treatment might include all of the following *except*

    (A) electroconvulsive therapy
    (B) reserpine
    (C) psychotherapy
    (D) chlorpromazine
    (E) imipramine

Questions 114 through 118

A 30-year-old farmer comes to see you because he is having "another fit of the blues." He just feels tired and miserable. He is waking up early in the morning and lies there in bed thinking and "feeling low." He is not eating well and he is down 15 pounds in weight. As he talks he begins to cry, and he tells you he cries often now but "it does not do any good." He has had these spells before, since he was a teenager, and he had an uncle who "used to get real low." His physical examination is normal.

114. The likely diagnosis is

    (A) adjustment disorder with depressed mood
    (B) bipolar disorder, depressive type
    (C) involutional melancholia
    (D) hypochondriasis
    (E) anaclitic depression

115. With the symptoms he describes and the signs you note, you are worried about possible suicide intent. You should

    (A) avoid raising the subject lest you precipitate suicide

    (B) set up an appointment within the week to ask his wife about suicidal signs
    (C) ask him directly if he ever has thoughts of doing away with himself
    (D) investigate carefully the family history of suicide
    (E) begin treatment to alleviate his symptoms; do not mention suicide

116. If you wish to use medications, your most beneficial treatment would be

    (A) barbiturates
    (B) methylphenidate
    (C) chlorpromazine
    (D) meprobamate
    (E) imipramine

117. According to Kretschmer's studies, subjects with this illness are more likely to be

    (A) asthenic
    (B) athletic
    (C) mesomorphic
    (D) pyknic
    (E) ectomorphic

118. The medication prescribed has only minimally relieved the patient's symptoms. Your most effective treatment now is likely to be

    (A) insulin coma therapy
    (B) leucotomy
    (C) intensive supportive psychotherapy
    (D) electroconvulsive therapy
    (E) hypnosis

Answers and Explanations

Questions 1 through 4 deal with prevention in mental retardation. (1:876–880;2:788;3:140)

1. **(A)** *Genetic couseling* to prevent the birth of further mentally retarded children is a good example of *primary prevention.*

2. **(B)** If the newly born child has chromosome defects, it is now too late to prevent the illness from occurring. *Early treatment* can be instituted to minimize handicapping—*secondary prevention.*

3. **(C)** Specialized training in a sheltered workshop will help the retarded teenager function more productively. She is helped to live with her handicaps—*tertiary prevention.*

4. **(A)** *Contraceptive instruction* may help lower the chances that the retarded adolescent will become pregnant and produce retarded offspring—*primary prevention.*

Questions 5 through 8 deal with amphetamine abuse. (1: 403–405;2:662–663;3:241–242)

5. **(C)** This patient shows the typical symptoms of *amphetamine abuse.* His presenting emotional symptoms are paranoid in nature. While paranoid schizophrenia cannot be totally excluded, this form of schizophrenia usually occurs in the late 20s or the 30s. The teenager does not show the bizarre mannerism, grossly inappropriate affect, and regressed behavior of the hebephrenic schizophrenic.

    LSD intoxication may produce a paranoid syndrome and chronic drug ingestion can produce this debilitated state; however, lysergic acid diethylamide toxicity usually leads to greater disruption of reality contact.

    Heroin abuse is usually manifested by needle marks, phlebitis, and other signs of self-administration. Very often, of course, the amphetamine abuser takes the drug by intravenous injection and may have all the signs seen with heroin abuse.

    When an adolescent presents with a florid paranoid psychosis in this era of more common drug abuse, amphetamine abuse is the most likely diagnosis and must be excluded first.

6. **(A)** The diagnosis is best confirmed by *urine testing* for amphetamines.

    The Rorschach test indicates the patient's emotional state as a paranoid psychosis. The test does not diagnose the etiology.

    The serial sevens test is too nonspecific in an evaluation.

    Fasting blood sugar levels and skull x-rays should be normal.

7. **(D)** Methadone maintenance is not used with amphetamine addiction.

    The teenager with an amphetamine psychosis requires *hospitalization. Haloperidol* or equivalent may be necessary to control anxiety or disruptive behavior. During and following the acute symptoms, *psychotherapy* may help the patient, and *family counseling* may be indicated both for the patient and his family.

8. **(C)** *Amphetamines block REM sleep.* Amphetamine psychosis may be related to this electroencephalogram effect.

    After the withdrawal of barbiturates and other REM-blocking drugs, there is an increase in REM activity, sometimes with nightmares.

    Focal slow waves, especially in the temporal lobes, are characteristic of psychomotor epilepsy.

    Recurrent 3-per-second spike-and-wave EEG readings are diagnostic of petit mal.

    A triphasic wave pattern on the electroencephalogram is seen in about 25% of patients with hepatic failure.

Questions 9 and 10 deal with normal mourning and grief. (1:264–268;2:180–182;3:269–270)

9. **(B)** This middle-aged man is showing a normal grief reaction with sadness, some anger, and eventual emotional reinvestment. The major work of mourning is usually complete within 3 months. Mourning is liable to start when it is recognized that the ill person is dying and does not necessarily wait until death occurs.

10. **(B)** Statistically it has been shown that a middle-aged widower is likely to remarry within 2 years of his spouse's death.

Questions 11 through 15 deal with enuresis. (1:843–846; 2:697–699;3:197–198)

11. **(C)** In any case of *enuresis,* a thorough physical and psychological examination should be carried out by the clinician.

    Where there is a physical symptom, a physical examination is always necessary. Since this boy was previously toilet trained and has an obvious psychological reason for behavioral regression, more traumatic physical examinations can be delayed. Catheterization should be one of the last evaluation procedures and used only when a physical etiology is strongly suspected.

    A child may be traumatized by excessive psychological testing just as much as by overzealous physical examinations. Projective tests and especially the Rorschach test have little value with a 3-year-old patient. Intelligence testing may offer little in the diagnosis of secondary enuresis.

    Until the clinician is sure of the diagnosis and the etiology of any symptom, reassurance is premature and may be counterproductive.

12. **(A)** The child (or patient of any age) showing an *adjustment reaction* benefits best by *increased emotional support.*

    Passing the youngster over to a babysitter or grandparents can be felt as a total rejection by a young child. The youngster may blame himself for being in some way unacceptable to his parents.

    To stigmatize the bedwetting as "childish," without giving extra emotional support and understanding for those reasons he has to be childish, would merely shame the child and burden him further emotionally.

    Bedwetting is a form of communication. While the enuresis need not provoke a punitive rejecting reaction, the message and the behavior should not be ignored.

13. **(C)** Autism is a sign of profound emotional maladjustment; it is *not a temporary adjustment reaction.*

Regressive behavior like nightmares, tantrums, thumb sucking, and nail biting can be temporary. When the stress is relieved, the symptoms clear.

14. **(B)** *Bedwetting* is more common in *boys.*

    Enuresis does tend to *disappear by adolescence.* Children are often more handicapped by the *shame* and *ridicule* they face than by the symptom itself.

    Enuresis frequently occurs in *families* so there is often a history of enuresis in parents or close relatives.

    Bedwetting occurs most often in *stage 3 or 4* deep sleep.

15. **(E)** The present drug of choice in the treatment of enuresis is *imipramine,* which does, however, have significant side effects.

Questions 16 and 17 deal with monoamine oxidase toxicity. (1:657–659;2:828–829;3:110–112)

16. **(C)** This case vignette describes a patient with some of the early symptoms of a *hypertensive crisis.*

17. **(B)** *Dietary intake.* Patients receiving monoamine oxidase inhibitors should be warned that foods containing tyramine—cheeses, wines, chicken liver—may induce a disabling and potentially fatal vasopressor reaction. (The majority of patients on monoamine oxidase inhibitors will not have a hypertensive crisis even when these foods are eaten.)

Questions 18 through 22 deal with mental mechanisms. (1:80;2:80–111;3:7–11)

18. **(C)** The 5-year-old cannot express his anger toward his father but he displaces his rage onto a more acceptable focus—*displacement.* (1:80;2:101–102;3:9)

19. **(D)** The 8-year-old boy partially represses his anger and no longer directs it at his family. Rather he redirects his aggressive tensions into socially more acceptable behavior. He chops wood—an example of *sublimation.* (1:80;2:108;3:9–10)

20. **(D)** Their little sister is scared and upset. Her inappropriate laughter is an overreaction, a manifestation of *reaction formation.* She laughs *too much.* (1:79; 2:98–99;3:8)

21. **(E)** The father does not or cannot totally repress his conflictual anxiety about his temper outburst. He is hurting and his hurt is manifested by direct somatic expression of his feeling state. He has *somatized.* (1:340;2:498–499;3:289)

22. **(B)** The mother's ability to block out disturbing external reality is an example of *denial.* She manages not to hear, though she is not deaf. (1:80;2:107;3:8)

Questions 23 through 27 deal with delirium tremens and Alcohol Withdrawal Delirium (a favorite examination topic). (1:419–420;2:628–631;3:217–218)

23. **(C)** Visual hallucinations are more typically seen in a toxic psychosis like delirium tremens and would be uncommon in paranoid schizophrenia. The paranoid schizophrenic usually has fairly circumscribed paranoid delusions but may function well socially and intellectually. The involutional paranoid would not show these gross visual hallucinations or this confusional state.

In a hysterical conversion, an emotional conflict is symbolically expressed by a physical symptom involving the voluntary musculature or the special senses. Visual hallucinations are not considered visual conversion symptoms.

Some of the hysterical dissociative states, including the latah, amok, and berserk states, may be manifested by agitated frenzy, but marked visual hallucinations would usually not be present.

Pathological intoxication is a term infrequently used now. Often the syndrome is a manifestation of a hysterical dissociative neurosis. Pathological intoxication occurs when the subject is taking or has just taken alcohol and is an excessive intoxication reaction to the alcohol.

24. **(B)** Intramuscular *morphine* can be *fatal* to the patient with delirium tremens.

The *restraints* should be *removed* or the patient may exhaust himself in a struggle to be free. Chlordiazepoxide is often used to produce sedation. *Parenteral fluids* with *vitamin* supplements and *magnesium sulfate* may be necessary to restore body homeostasis.

25. **(D)** *Confabulation* is the falsification of recall to fill gaps in memory—as is described in this question.

La belle indifference, classically seen in hysterical conversion, is an unusual lack of reasonable anxiety in face of disabling or usually distressing symptoms.

Perseveration is present when the subject gives the same response to different and unconnected questions.

Thought blocking or *thought deprivation* is the sudden stopping of the flow of thought due to unconscious processes. "My mind just went blank" can occur normally, but when this symptom is prominent it usually is a sign of schizophrenia.

A *flight of ideas* typically occurs in hypomatic or manic states where the subject shows a very rapid flow of thinking, sometimes so fast that the connections are no longer obvious.

26. **(A)** *Confabulation* is a typical manifestation of *Korsakoff's syndrome. (1:279–281;2:631–633;3:218)*

27. **(E)** Syndromes that can occur as part of *chronic alcoholism* include acute *pancreatitis, hepatic failure, coma, pellagra,* and *Wernicke's encephalopathy.*

Splenic infarction is not typically a manifestation of the alcoholic syndromes.

Questions 28 through 30 deal with infantile autism. (1:732–737;2:693–694;3:201)

28. **(A)** Your likely diagnosis is *infantile autism.* When you lift up the child, he does not respond to you—he just hangs. The autistic child may resist being lifted as this is an intrusion into his private existence, but he will not respond to your lifting by "moulding" his body to your body. Unless the retarded child is autistic, he will show a moulding or resisting reponse. The other youngsters typically would react to you as a person.

The *preoccupation with moving mechanisms,* the *self-rocking,* and the *anxious reaction when disturbed* are characteristics of the autistic child.

The deaf child, who is not autistic, may not communicate in words, but he interacts with sounds and gestures.

The children showing an adjustment reaction or a withdrawing reaction are involved in environmental interaction but their ways of coping are maladaptive.

29. **(B)** In general, no treatment has been very effective with autistic youngsters. *Behavior modification* is the therapeutic approach that has given most predictable improvement by more efficient use of (usually limited) treatment resources.

Electroconvulsive therapy has no long-range beneficial effect. *Methylphenidate* may make the patient more distressed or disturbed.

Long-term institutional care usually leads to profound social and intellectual retardation in autistic children.

Classical *child psychoanalysis* is ineffective with the autistic child. *Modified child psychotherapy* can sometimes successfully intrude into the child's private world and help him or her emerge. However, results of even many years of psychotherapy tend to be rather poor.

30. **(E)** The syndrome of *infantile autism* was first described by *Leo Kanner* in 1943.

Questions 31 through 33 deal with schizophrenia, paranoid type. (1:215;2:376–378;3:248)

31. **(C)** This disturbed patient justified his assaultive behavior on the basis of his paranoid *projections.* He *projected* his own unacceptable and intolerable thoughts onto his neighbor and then attacked the neighbor with the justification of these projections.

32. **(D)** The most likely diagnosis is *schizophrenia, paranoid type* in a man with fairly circumscribed paranoid delusions and auditory hallucinations.

Hallucinations do not occur in personality disorders such as *paranoia* or *antisocial personality*. The gross reality distortion manifested by the hallucinations and the paranoid delusions would not support a diagnosis of *homosexual panic,* an uncertain diagnosis at best.

This patient does not show the incessant driven quality of the *manic.* His affect is inappropriate and contradictory. The emotional state of the manic is excessive rather than grotesque or idiosyncratic. While the most likely diagnosis is that of paranoid schizophrenia, a manic state is not totally excluded.

33. **(B)** This patient is best treated with *chlorpromazine* in *adequate doses.*

Questions 34 through 37 deal with involutional melancholia and major depression with melancholia. (1:246–247;2:417–422;3:267–268)

34. **(B)** This is the typical history of a patient with *involutional melancholia*—a lifelong conscientious, hard-working woman in the involutional period of life, presenting with depression and bizarre self-accusatory delusions.

Presenile dementia would usually manifest with greater confusion and memory loss. A thorough medical evaluation is always indicated when presenile dementia is suspected.

A patient with an *adjustment disorder with depressed mood* would not manifest these bizarre delusions.

A patient with a *somatization disorder* will express emotions through physical symptoms but not to this delusional degree; nor is such a patient profoundly depressed.

Paranoid schizophrenia would not manifest with this exaggerated affect but would present with inappropriate paranoid projection, often with over auditory hallucinations.

35. **(B)** *Electroconvulsive therapy* is most effective in treating first episodes of major depression with melancholia. Recurrent bouts do not respond quite as well.

36. **(C)** *Imipramine* may be used to maintain the patient at a comfortable level of emotional adaptation. Long-term maintenance drug therapy also allows supportive psychotherapy and early detection of symptomatic recrudescence.

37. **(D)** *Ambivalence* is the presence of contrasting and conflicting thoughts or emotions: the wish and need to die coexisting with the fear of death and the wish to live.

Patients with involutional melancholia may act on one side of the ambivalence and commit *suicide.* Suicide is a definite risk in this syndrome.

Questions 38 through 41 deal with the management of the dying child. (1:264–270,593;2:75–76)

38. **(D)** The reality that this boy is dying faces the nurses with intolerable feelings. They deal in part with their problem by isolating the boy and then explain their seemingly illogical behavior by outwardly logical intellectual reasons—by *rationalization. (1:80;2:100–101;3:8)*

39. **(A)** For very understandable causes, this nurse would naturally be made anxious and upset by this patient. She handles her inner conflicts and tension by overdoing the very thing she fears—a specific form of *reaction formation* where the phobic object is sought after rather than avoided—*counterphobic* behavior. (1:324; 2:98–99;3:8)*

40. **(B)** The 8-year-old boy copes with the intolerable life situation by blocking out certain parts of reality—by *denial.* This is a normal way of adapting to dying and should, at least in part, be supported. *(1:80;2:107; 3:8)*

41. **(E)** As part of normal mourning, these parents are angry. They are angry at their little son for leaving them, they are angry at God or Fate for giving them such pain, and they may well be angry with themselves for not in some way preventing this illness. They cannot express this anger at the cause of their rage so they handle it in part by displacing it onto a more acceptable target, in this situation the nurse—*displacement.*

Sometimes the doctors and the nurses become an acceptable focus for displaced anger because they appear so strong and competent and thus able to tolerate the anger. *(1:80;2:101–102;3:9)*

Questions 42 through 48 deal with heroin drug dependence. (1:385–400;2:651–658;3:239–241)

42. **(D)** *Withdrawal from heroin* is best carried out in an *inpatient* setting with *methadone cover.*

No matter how much the patient promises, it is almost impossible to withdraw the chronic addict from this drug on an outpatient basis.

Withdrawal without methadone cover would lead to a marked abstinence syndrome.

Nalline would precipitate an abrupt abstinence syndrome.

43. **(C)** *Hepatitis* is the major danger in the addict's self-injection. Other illnesses carried by dirty syringes include mononucleosis and endocarditis.

44. **(E)** *Syphilis* would not usually be an indication of self-injection. *Phlebitis,* skin *abscesses, septicemia,* and *hepatitis* all may be caused by repeated self-injections.

45. **(D)** The *abstinence syndrome* in *heroin* withdrawal includes runny nose and watery eyes as in an upper respiratory infection, vomiting and diarrhea, and muscle and stomach cramps.

46. **(E)** In the long-term treatment of former heroin addicts, *methadone maintenance* may allow them to stay off heroin. A *therapeutic community* may help them give up drugs and may support them in staying off. *Psychotherapy* can help addicts face and deal with their maladaptive behavior. *Job training* prepares them to function more productively in society.

47. **(C)** When an addict is withdrawn from heroin, *abstinence symptoms* build up gradually but are *established* in *12 to 24 hours.*

48. **(C)** Withdrawal *abstinence symptoms* can be expected to *clear* in *4 to 8 days.* Symptoms persisting longer necessitate further medical or psychiatric evaluation.

Questions 49 and 50 deal with Cushing's Syndrome. (1:517–518;2:312–313;3:227–228)

Occasionally there are examination questions focused on physical illnesses presenting as an emotional problem. Even though the examination subjects may be psychiatry and the behavioral sciences, the candidate should not ignore the significance of physical signs or symptoms detailed in any question.

49. **(C)** This woman presents with the clinical features of *Cushing's syndrome.* She is depressed—"life is not worth living"—but her physical symptoms and hormonal imbalance are reasonable cause for such depression.

    The clinician must always consider the whole range of medical and psychological diagnoses when considering a problem, even though the patient may be suggesting by the presenting complaints that the difficulty is either physical *or* emotional.

50. **(A)** The diagnosis of Cushing's disease is confirmed by demonstrating *increased urinary 17-hydroxycorticoids.*

    The *electroencephalogram* should not show abnormal foci.

    Poor form content on the *Rorschach test* is a nonspecific finding that must be evaluated in the appropriate clinical context.

    Binge eating is symptomatic of a range of disorders, psychological and physical.

If the woman is severely depressed, *electroconvulsive therapy* might give symptomatic relief but this treatment result is not specifically diagnostic of any syndrome.

Questions 51 through 53 deal with homosexuality. (1:442–445;2:527–528;3:315)

51. **(E)** Many male homosexuals are comfortably masculine in attitude and appearance. Usually they do not dislike girls. Homosexuals accept and enjoy their gender anatomy and have no wish for sex change. Transsexuals, not homosexuals, wish operative sex-change procedures. Most homosexuals do not especially fear their fathers and, conversely, many males who hate or fear their fathers do not become homosexual.

52. **(A)** While all procedures designed to change a subject from homosexual to heterosexual orientation have limited or poor results, the major factor in producing or allowing such a sex-orientation change is the motivation of the patient. Other factors have much less change-producing effect.

53. **(E)** At present, no consistent factor has been demonstrated in the etiology of homosexuality, though there are many theories about its causation.

Questions 54 and 55 deal with myxedema (hypothyroidism). (1:516–517;2:315–316;3:228)

54. **(E)** This patient presents with the typical symptoms of myxedema, *hypothyroidism.*

    The cerebration of these patients is slow, their perception is blunted, and they feel different. They see no obvious reason for this change so they tend to blame external factors; *paranoia* is a common symptom in hypothyroidism. Depression also frequently occurs and is precipitated in part by the physical debility and discomfort.

55. **(C)** The specific treatment for hypothyroidism is thyroid replacement—*thyroid extract* or equivalent.

    Myxedema patients who are given thyroid may symptomatically get worse before they get better. The body readjustment precipitated by the thyroid intake may exacerbate emotional and physical difficulties.

Questions 56 and 57 deal with subdural hematoma. (1:276; 2:302–303;3:226)

56. **(B)** This is the typical history of a patient who has developed a *subdural hematoma.* Even patients with previous psychiatric hospitalization can develop the whole range of physical illnesses.

57. **(B)** The diagnosis is confirmed finally by *skull burr holes.*

Questions 58 and 59 deal with chronic pancreatitis. (1: 250;2:319)

Many metabolic, hormonal, or neoplastic disorders may manifest initially or primarily with psychiatric symptoms.

58.   **(B)** The midline abdominal calcification suggests the diagnosis of *chronic pancreatitis,* which can give the symptoms described—*confusion, agitation,* and even *visual hallucinations.*

59.   **(A)** In symptomatic pancreatitis the patient usually has an *elevated* serum amylase.

Questions 61 through 65 deal with the mentally retarded child. (1:709–731;2:715–744;3:159–172)

60.   **(B)** In the *Diagnostic and Statistical Manual* of the American Psychiatric Association, *borderline intellectual functioning* (intelligence quotient in the range 71–84) is included in conditions not attributable to mental disorder.

Level of Retardation	IQ
mild	51–70
moderate	36–50
severe	20–35
profound	under 20

(1:709–711;2:717;3:160–161)

61.   **(D)** The child who acts the class clown is often showing *reaction formation.* Peer teasing can make a child very anxious and upset, especially when the teasing is based on a realistic reason. One way of coping with such teasing or feelings of vulnerability is to emphasize the vulnerability oneself and flaunt it for the amusement of others. By emphasizing the opposite of his true feelings—reaction formation—the youngster can cope with an otherwise intolerable situation. *(1:79;2:98–99;3:8)*

62.   **(E)** He is now showing a *conversion disorder.* His emotional conflict has been repressed but has been expressed symbolically through this symptom affecting his voluntary musculature. *(1:342–348;2:110;3:290)*

63.   **(B)** His outward lack of concern is called *la belle indifference,* a term coined by Janet, a French neuropsychiatrist. The normal person would naturally be most concerned by a physical paralysis. In a hysterical conversion, the subject often shows this seeming total lack of concern. *(1:347;2:505;3:290)*

64.   **(A)** The *primary gain* of a symptom is the relief of the conflictual anxiety. This young man was being mer-

cilessly teased. He could not effectively fight back. He could not escape. His leg weakness has allowed him relief from the anxiety. *(1:82;2:505–506;3:290)*

65.   **(C)** *Secondary gain* is the reward, the attention, and the care the subject begins to receive because of his illness. Secondary gain will tend to perpetuate the emotional illness because the illness becomes rewarding in itself.
       This rather tragic retarded boy is now finding that his hysterical leg paralysis brings him all kinds of support, care, and attention—more than he was able to get before he developed the conversion symptoms. This *secondary gain* from his paralysis will make it more difficult for him to give up his paralysis and go back to being a retarded, inadequate 8-year-old. *(1: 82;2:506;3:290)*

Questions 66 and 67 deal with acute hypoglycemia. (2:316–318;3:228)

66.   **(B)** The most likely diagnosis is *acute hypoglycemia* in a diabetic young man who is taking insulin.
       Hypoglycemia may present with a wide range of emotional symptoms that mimic neurotic, psychotic, or confusional states.

67.   **(D)** The diagnosis is confirmed by *blood sugar estimation* to demonstrate the hypoglycemia.
       In evaluating the patient, the clinician should try to ascertain the previous medical and psychological history. Where the subject has been well adjusted and productive, an acute psychotic reaction, especially with confusion, is likely to be toxic or organic in origin. Thigh needle marks would suggest intramuscular or subcutaneous injections rather than the addict's intravenous "mainlining."
       A simple acute anxiety reaction would not manifest with gross confusion or bizarre actions or comments.

Questions 68 through 71 deal with paranoid disorder. (1: 226–237;2:444–457;3:257–258)

68.   **(C)** This history describes the typical subject with a *paranoid personality*—hypersensitive, suspicious, isolated, often litigious, and usually very insecure beneath his aloofness.
       Though the patient is unusually sensitive, suspicious, and irritable, his behavior and history do not indicate a major break with reality as would be found in paranoid schizophrenia.
       He is angry and aggressive but gives no indication of cyclic depressive swings. This patient is overly involved, anxious, and irritable; the hysteric is liable to appear blandly unconcerned, only superficially involved, and often theatrical.

You have no indication of deliberate falsification of symptoms or history as would be noted in obvious malingering.

69. **(B)** No patient should be able to seduce a clinician into diagnosing or evaluating in retrospect or from hearsay. If you did not evaluate the patient at the time in question or if you do not have all the findings, you *cannot make a competent evaluation.* At the same time, the patient, even a grossly paranoid patient, merits your full attention and a thoughtful response.

70. **(B)** In dealing with the paranoid patient, the clinician is most helpful if he or she deals with immediate reality. The doctor should carry out a thorough examination and keep careful notes of all findings and recommendations, positive and negative. A detailed record of actual history (even quoting the patient's words) and of specific clinical signs allows the doctor to help the patient best and also protects the clinician against later suit.

71. **(A)** This man's *paranoia* is likely to *stay the same.* Treatment should be primarily supportive to help the patient function as productively and tolerably as possible.

Questions 72 and 73 deal with chronic anxiety disorder. (1:315–320;2:473–476;3:288–289)

72. **(C)** The patient with a *chronic anxiety disorder* often expresses emotional tension and pain in a somatic ache—by *somatization*—a headache, stomach ache, backache. This is one way of telling others that she is hurting. These symptoms can occur in depressive states but the depressed patient is more likely to show psychomotor retardation, feelings of worthlessness, and more obvious depressive affect.

This subject does not show the relative unconcern of the hysteric. Anxiety and tension are the main presenting symptoms; in hysterical conversion, anxiety would be repressed and converted into a physical symptom.

Involutional melancholia can present with disabling headaches as a major symptom—but the patient is not yet in the involutional period. The involutional melancholic usually talks with profound affect about her depressive feelings—this patient is describing tension rather than depression.

73. **(E)** Electroconvulsive therapy would not benefit this patient and might even make her symptomatically worse.

Individual psychotherapy, family therapy, and the tranquilizers *meprobamate* and *diazepam* in short-term treatment can all be therapeutically beneficial to the patient with a chronic anxiety neurosis.

Questions 74 through 76 deal with phobia. (1:321–327;2:470–472;3:286–287)

74. **(B)** *Secondary gain* is the emotional reward that comes with being ill—the extra attention, the added support and understanding, and the reduction of responsibility. Secondary gain tends to maintain the illness as the subject becomes reluctant to give up these new gratifications. This woman's phobia is liable to be perpetuated by all the attention her husband now gives her.

75. **(D)** When the phobic individual insists on experiencing the feared situation repeatedly and unnecessarily, this behavior is termed a *counterphobic reaction.*

76. **(D)** Phobic subjects realize that their phobic anxiety is illogical. The phobia arises when conflictual fear and anxiety is dealt with by displacing these feelings onto a specific object or situation—*displacement.*

The young child, who cannot tolerate the anxiety provoked by separation from home and mother, *displaces* this anxiety and focuses it on the school situation in a *school phobia* or *school refusal.*

Questions 77 through 81 deal with conversion disorder. (1:342–348;2:501–507;3:290)

77. **(C)** With the medical, neurological, and laboratory tests all normal, the most likely diagnosis is that of hysterical convulsions, a *conversion disorder.*

A conversion disorder can occur superimposed on an organic illness, so positive physical and laboratory findings would not exclude this diagnosis. Equally, hysterical patients can develop organic illnesses like anyone else. A prolonged period of observation, usually on an outpatient basis, may be necessary to confirm the diagnosis.

In a conversion disorder, the symptom develops due to emotional factors and is not within the patient's conscious control. *Malingering* involves deliberate planning and conscious deciding.

Too often the diagnosis *antisocial personality* merely indicates that the clinician did not like the patient or the patient's life-style. The girl is too young for the diagnosis of a personality disorder. Her behavior is not *antisocial.*

Hebephrenic schizophrenia is manifested by bizarre and regressed behavior, by marked inappropriate affect, and by obvious disruption of reality contact. The patient described in this question does not show this level of psychopathology.

An *avoidant disorder of adolescence* is manifested by shyness, insecurity, and isolation; this 14-year-old girl is able to relate warmly and comfortably. She does not appear to be unduly timid.

78. **(B)** This adolescent is basically a good girl with high moral standards. She is a normal adolescent with rising sexual drives. The closeness with her boyfriend brings these strong sexual and moral feelings into *conflict,* producing anxiety that is difficult to manage.

79. **(C)** Her conflictual feelings are repressed and expressed symbolically in the physical "convulsive" symptoms. This is an example of a *conversion reaction.*

80. **(D)** The extra caring and gratification the patient receives because she is ill is termed *secondary gain.*

81. **(C)** *Hypnosis* would be one way to produce rapid symptomatic improvement. Hysterical neuroses are frequently responsive to hypnotic suggestions.

Questions 82 through 84 deal with hyperventilation syndrome. (1:586;2:584–586;3:288–289)

82. **(C)** The term *seizures* can cover a wide range of physical and emotional disorders. This young woman gives a classical history for a *hyperventilation syndrome.* This is not the complete diagnosis. The clinician needs to find out what is the underlying disorder producing the hyperventilation attacks. Usually these symptoms are a manifestation of an adjustment reaction, but more serious illness such as a *schizophrenia* may first manifest with this nonspecific syndrome.

    A hyperventilation syndrome is typically symptomatic of underlying anxiety rather than depression.

    Psychomotor epilepsy can produce a wide range of episodic physical and emotional symptoms. Usually a temporal lobe focus on the electroencephalogram can be demonstrated in temporal lobe epilepsy.

    Homosexual panic is not a clearly defined or useful diagnosis.

83. **(B)** The symptoms of the hyperventilation syndrome can be reproduced by asking the subject to *overbreathe for 2 minutes.* This is usually the best way of showing the patient the physiological cause and the absence of serious physical pathology.

84. **(D)** In the management of the patient, you would likely wish to *explain* the physiological basis for her symptoms, *explore* the possible factors producing this syndrome, and *offer supportive psychotherapy* if indicated.

Question 85 through 87 deal with anorexia nervosa. (1:499–504;2:554–558;3:194–195)

85. **(B)** The most likely diagnosis is *anorexia nervosa.* There are no indications of the generalized endocrine deficiency seen in hypopituitarism.

Anorexia nervosa is a symptom complex that may be a manifestation of a range of psychiatric disorders.

The patient does not show the vagueness and personal inadequacy of the simple schizophrenic, though a schizophrenic process sometimes underlies the anorexia nervosa syndrome.

86. **(A)** The patient with anorexia nervosa has *sex-appropriate secondary characteristics.* This patient would show feminine pubic hair distribution.

87. **(A)** *Anorexia nervosa* occurs predominantly in *women* and is rare in men. It may be a manifestation of an underlying psychosis. The syndrome can occur in other family members but not frequently.

Questions 88 and 89 deal with strephosymbolia-dyslexia—developmental reading disorder. (1:748–751;2:702–704; 3:203)

88. **(D)** *Strephosymbolia,* reversal of letters, is one manifestation of dyslexia. Right–left incoordination frequently coexists with this reading disability.

    The youngster does not show school phobia or school refusal, but untreated dyslexia may make the school experience anxiety-provoking and unrewarding.

    Medical examination of children with dyslexia is usually noncontributory, but a physical evaluation should be performed to make absolutely certain that this common symptom is not an uncommon manifestation of a serious illness like a brain tumor.

    The symptoms and the behavioral reactions of this patient would not indicate a childhood psychosis or an obsessive–compulsive neurosis.

89. **(C)** The optimum treatment for dyslexia is *remedial teaching.*

    Psychotherapy may help with some patients. Methylphenidate and phenobarbital are not therapeutically beneficial.

    Transfer to another school will not solve the problem without specific remedial education.

Questions 90 through 92 deal with attention deficit disorder. (1:741–747;2:681–683;3:187–190)

90. **(D)** This clinical picture of excessive activity, distractibility, and restlessness is characteristic of the *hyperkinetic reaction of childhood.* These high-energy children are liable to cause anxiety in present-day structured school programs.

    The *infantile autistic child* does not relate meaningfully to other people, is preoccupied with his or her own inner world, and often is fascinated by moving mechanisms.

    The runaway and the overanxious reactions of childhood refer to specific repetitive behavior patterns seen in certain children.

91. **(B)** Children with a *hyperkinetic* reaction often show "soft" neurological signs.

    Aminoaciduria is found in several inborn metabolic disorders.

    Blond hair and blue eyes tend to occur in patients with *phenylketonuria.*

    Café-au-lait spots are found in subjects who have *neurofibromatosis (von Recklinghausen's disease)* or *tuberous sclerosis.*

    A greenish-brown ring in the iris, the Kayser–Fleischer ring, is a pathognomonic sign of *hepatolenticular degeneration* (Wilson's disease).

92. **(C)** *Methylphenidate* or the amphetamines are the drugs usually used in treating hyperkinetic children.

    Imipramine would not be used in childhood hyperkinesis.

    Haloperidol might be helpful because of its tranquilizing action on the hyperactive child, but phenobarbital might make school concentration more difficult due to its sedative effect.

Questions 93 and 94 deal with disorganized (hebephrenic) schizophrenia. (1:215;2:372–373;3:248)

93. **(C)** The layman's concept of being "crazy" is the *disorganized (hebephrenic) schizophrenic,* and this young woman presents with the symptoms of hebephrenic schizophrenia. Her behavior is regressed, bizarre, and poorly controlled; her emotions are inappropriate; and she has obvious distortion of reality contact.

    Patients with personality disorders, hysterical or schizoid, do not show hallucinations or similar signs of loss of reality contact. A patient with uncomplicated borderline mental retardation would not present with psychotic symptoms, but a psychotic subject may test at a borderline retarded level.

94. **(D)** Lithium carbonate is ineffective with the hebephrenic schizophrenic, who may be helped by haloperidol, hospitalization, electroconvulsive therapy, and, in select cases, psychotherapy.

Questions 95 through 97 deal with bipolar disorder, manic type. (1:248–251;2:413–417;3:264–266)

95. **(D)** The pressured activity and speech and the elation of this woman are characteristic of a *manic state.* The history of at least three prior episodes points to the cyclical *bipolar disorder.* Usually, the manic patient is brought for evaluation and treatment because his or her behavior has become intolerable to the people around him or her.

    The behavior of this woman is certainly not passive, not even the intrusive demanding passivity of the passive–aggressive personality. In personality disorders there is not this excessive affect.

The symptoms of pathological intoxication may be largely due to the uncovering of an underlying schizophrenia by the sedating effect of alcohol. The patient described in this question manifests a pathological excess of affect rather than the toxic, sometimes confused state seen in pathological intoxication. This patient does not show the primitive bizarre behavior of the hebephrenic schizophrenic nor the dissociative emotional splitting of psychogenic fugue.

96. **(C)** Without treatment, manic attacks tend to clear in about 3 months.

97. **(E)** The patient with an acute manic state usually has to be hospitalized and treated with drugs or electroconvulsive therapy. In the patient's disturbing, uncontrolled state, outpatient electroconvulsive therapy may not bring the symptoms under control quickly enough. The manic patient may be unwilling or unable to cooperate with outpatient treatment.

    Psychotherapy—interpretive, family, or supportive—has only minimal value until the patient's symptoms are brought under control.

Questions 98 through 100 deal with catatonic schizophrenia. (1:214–215;2:373–376;3:248)

98. **(E)** The mutism, immobility, and waxy flexibility shown by this young man are characteristic of *catatonic schizophrenia.*

    These symptoms do not occur in psychogenic amnesia or in a paranoid personality disorder. The patient does not show the toxic delirium and confusion of delirium tremens.

    A toxic psychosis is also a common cause for this kind of catatonic state.

99. **(B)** The patient is now showing *catatonic excitement*—a state of psychomotor hyperactivity.

100. **(D)** Immediate energetic treatment of catatonic excitement is necessary before the patient injures himself or those around him or before he collapses from exhaustion. *Haloperidol,* parenterally, in high doses, or *electroconvulsive therapy,* or sometimes both together, should be used to produce symptomatic relief.

Questions 101 and 102 deal with psychosis due to sensory deprivation ("Black Patch" syndrome). (1:59–64;2:177–178; 3:214–215)

101. **(C)** Following cataract surgery, elderly patients are liable to develop delirious confusional states due to the enforced sensory deprivation and the postoperative isolation. These disturbed patients may become acutely agitated, assaultive, and uncooperative. This is *psychosis due to sensory deprivation.*

102. **(A)** Barbiturates should never be used with these patients. This sedative drug will further blur their contact with their surroundings and may accentuate their confusion.

This confusional psychosis is best treated by measures that will reestablish the patient's contact with reality—frequent *familiar visitors, radio* or *television* in the room, a *telephone* to talk to people, and, if possible, *uncovering one eye* or a central peep hole in the eye bandage.

Questions 103 through 105 deal with the suicidally depressed patient. (1:575–580;2:118–121;3:270–272)

103. **(B)** If the clinician *suspects* that the patient is *suicidal,* it is usually best diagnostically and therapeutically to *ask the patient directly* in a gentle fashion.

No one else—not even his family—can really say if he is actively suicidal. The prescription of antidepressant medication may merely provide the patient with a drug he can use to kill himself.

If the patient is actively suicidal, he may not be able to delay his suicide until the clinician finds an "appropriate" time to ask the direct question at later appointments. Most patients are relieved when they can talk openly about their suicidal impulses, wishes, and fears. A direct question tends to decrease their inner fears.

104. **(D)** Once the patient admits directly that he is seriously thinking about killing himself, he needs total protection and support at all times. If he is left without support—to get his clothes, to go by himself to the hospital, to contact suicide prevention groups—he may be unable to delay suicidal impulses. When the clinician, family, or society leaves the overtly suicidal patient without support and protection, the subject may feel isolated or impelled to act suicidally. To berate the suicidal patient about his "stupidity" is merely to increase his emotional burden. The patient should be *admitted to hospital, with responsible accompaniment* to get him there.

105. **(E)** Lithium is ineffective with the actively suicidal patient.

The hospitalized suicidal patient initially should have full *suicidal precautions.* For depression, electroconvulsive treatment or antidepressants (under close supervision) can be used. Psychotherapy, in hospital and after discharge, may be beneficial.

Questions 106 and 107 deal with brain tumor. (1:307–308; 2:295–298;3:226)

106. **(B)** The subject may have the most disturbed environment, a history of gross deprivation and emotional trauma and markedly pathological psychological testing—none of these will produce papilledema, a manifestation of increased intracranial pressure.

All causes of *increased intracranial pressure* including an *intracranial mass* must be investigated.

107. **(B)** *Skull x-rays* are most likely to confirm or further the diagnosis.

Questions 108 through 110 deal with dissociative disorder. (1:353–357;2:513–515;3:291–293)

108. **(E)** This is the typical description of a *dissociative reaction*—dissociative trance or twilight state—precipitated by intolerable tension or anxiety. Frequently the subject is partially or totally amnesic for the episode.

109. **(D)** Appropriate treatment might include strong symptom-directed suggestion, tranquilizers to reduce anxiety to a more tolerable level, and psychotherapy to uncover the underlying cause of the dissociative state and to produce a better way of coping.

110. **(E)** In this dissociative symptom, conflictual anxiety is *separated from normal awareness* and is acted out or expressed. Frequently the patient gets much secondary gain from the attention aroused by the dissociative state.

Questions 111 through 113 deal with major depression. (1:245–248;2:417–422;3:266–268)

111. **(B)** A *major depression* is a profoundly depressed state that follows a loss, separation, or disappointment. These patients are markedly depressed, often suicidal, and commonly express this kind of somatic delusion.

There is no previous history of mood swings or cyclic emotional decompensation that would suggest a manic–depressive illness.

The patient shows exaggerated affect, seen in an affective psychosis, rather than the personality fragmentation of the schizophrenic.

Delusions do not occur in depersonalization or conversion disorders.

112. **(E)** This symptom is an example of a *somatic delusion.*

113. **(B)** *Reserpine* would tend to increase this patient's depression and has been known to precipitate suicide.

A psychotic depressive reaction can be treated with *electroconvulsive therapy* or *imipramine* for the depression, *chlorpromazine* for the anxiety or agitation, and psychotherapy for support and *rehabilitation.* The patient should be *hospitalized.*

Questions 114 through 118 deal with bipolar disorder, depressive type. (1:245–251;2:417–422;3:264–268)

114. **(B)** This man describes recurrent episodes of disabling depression. He has a family history of similar affective symptoms. His present symptoms—profound sadness, weepiness, psychomotor retardation, loss of appetite and weight loss, and early-morning awakening—are characteristic of endogenous rather than *reactive depression.*

    As with this case, *bipolar disorder, depressive type* begins in adolescence or early adult life. Manic symptoms tend to occur earlier than depression.

    This 30-year-old man is not showing a *reaction* due to involution or failure of physical or emotional powers.

    His emotional complaint is an expression of an exaggerated painful emotional state rather than a *hypochondriacal* physical disability. *Anaclitic depression* is typically described in infants or young children. A similar syndrome can occur in adults but is usually unrecognized as being anaclitic, that is, due to loss of necessary external support and gratification. This young farmer has been functioning independently and is not responding to the loss of external support.

115. **(C)** If the clinician suspects *suicidal intent,* he or she should *ask the patient directly.*

116. **(E)** In treating the depression of manic–depressive illness, *imipramine* and related drugs are the drugs of choice.

117. **(D)** *Kretschmer* suggested that manic–depressive illness tends to occur in patients with a *pyknic* physical constitution, *Sheldon's* endomorphic type, rather thick-set and stocky.

118. **(D)** If drugs do not bring reasonably prompt symptomatic relief, a course of *electroconvulsive therapy* should be given. Usually five to ten treatments give good therapeutic effect.

CHAPTER 11

Practice Test
Questions

Carefully read the following instructions before taking the Practice Test.

1. This examination consists of 151 questions, covering areas listed in the Table of Contents.
2. The Practice Test simulates an actual examination in question types and integration of subject areas.
3. You should set aside 2 hours of *uninterrupted,* distraction-free time to take the Practice Test. This averages out to 50 seconds per question.
4. Be sure you have a clock (to time and pace yourself) and an adequate number of No. 2 pencils nd erasers.
5. You should tear out and use the answer sheet that is provided on page 165.
6. Be sure to answer all of the questions, and be sure the number on the answer sheet corresponds to the question number in the Practice Test.
7. Use any remaining time to review your answers.
8. After completing the Practice Test, you can check all of your answers on pages 152 through 161. A score of 65% to 70% or higher should be considered as a passing score (99 to 106 correct answers).
9. After checking your answers and your score, you can analyze your strengths and weaknesses on the Practice Test Subspecialty List on page 163. To do this, you should check off your incorrect Practice Test answers on the Subspecialty List. You may find a pattern developing. For example, you may find you do well on the definitions but poorly on adult psychopathology. In such an instance, you can go back and review the adult psychopathology section of this book and supplement your review with your texts and with the references cited in the adult psychopathology section.

DIRECTIONS (Questions 1 through 48): Each of the numbered items or incomplete statements in this section is followed by answers or by completions of the statement. Select the ONE lettered answer or completion that is BEST in each case.

1. Tolerance is the clinical term for

    (A) unconsciously motivated inability to discuss certain topics in psychotherapy
    (B) the psychological splitting off of mental functions from the rest of the personality
    (C) the declining effect of the same dose of a drug on repeated administration
    (D) the physical symptoms that develop on the withdrawal of a drug on which the subject is physically dependent
    (E) the ability to maintain in psychological awareness directly conflicting or opposing emotions about the same object

2. The defense mechanism whereby the subject emphasizes the opposite of his or her true feelings is

    (A) suppression
    (B) denial
    (C) repression
    (D) rationalization
    (E) reaction formation

3. Akathisia is

    (A) reduction in frequency and amplitude of voluntary movements
    (B) continuous involuntary orofacial and lingual movements
    (C) repetitive involuntary muscle spasm, especially involving the neck, face, or tongue
    (D) inner restlessness with the inability to keep still
    (E) isolated tremor of tightly pursed lips

4. The Bender–Gestalt Test is

    (A) a series of nine geometrical designs that the patient copies
    (B) an inventory of 550 statments to which the subject has to respond
    (C) a standard set of ten inkblots to which the patient associates
    (D) a set of ambiguous pictures about which the patient gives a story
    (E) a series of standardized subtests measuring verbal and performance abilities

5. Secondary gain is

    (A) the reduction of emotional conflict and anxiety
    (B) the logical, reality-based thinking that promotes sublimation
    (C) the benefits that come from deliberate malingering

    (D) the sympathy, attention, and rewards that come from being ill
    (E) the process whereby unacceptable emotional drives are converted into socially acceptable behaviors

6. Electroconvulsive therapy is most effective in

    (A) amphetamine psychosis
    (B) major depression
    (C) disorganized schizophrenia
    (D) borderline personality disorder
    (E) conversion disorder

7. To treat the child with attention deficit disorder, you are most likely to use

    (A) lithium
    (B) phenobarbital
    (C) phenelzine
    (D) methlyphenidate
    (E) diphenhydramine

8. When a patient being treated with a tricyclic antidepressant develops confusion, disorientation, and visual hallucinations, you are most likely dealing with

    (A) hypertensive crisis
    (B) paradoxical reaction
    (C) anticholinergic psychosis
    (D) neuroleptic malignant syndrome
    (E) catastrophic reaction

9. An example of primary prevention would be

    (A) the development of halfway houses
    (B) repainting inner-city homes
    (C) early return of a phobic child to school
    (D) use of depot neuroleptics
    (E) initiation of a crisis hotline telephone service

10. You are called to the emergency room to see a 23-year-old schizophrenic male. You find him lying on a bed, mute, with his head arching backward and his eyes turned up. Your best immediate treatment would be

    (A) intramuscular haloperidol
    (B) intravenous barbiturate
    (C) reassurance and "talking down"
    (D) intramuscular benztropine
    (E) hypnosis

11. As they take a shortcut through a graveyard at night, two young men laugh and sing loudly. Their behavior is a manifestation of which defense?

    (A) dissociation
    (B) displacement
    (C) counterphobic
    (D) undoing
    (E) regression

Questions 12 through 14

12. A middle-aged female patient whom you have been treating for some months with depot haloperidol comes to you complaining of "just not feeling well." Her temperature is 38°C and she says her face and leg muscles feel stiff. You should be concerned that she may be developing

    (A) hypertensive crisis
    (B) acute dystonic reaction
    (C) early tardive dyskinesia
    (D) drug-induced catatonia
    (E) neuroleptic malignant syndrome

13. Your diagnosis will be best confirmed by

    (A) increased cerebrospinal fluid protein
    (B) elevated serum creatine phosphokinase
    (C) lowered blood sugar
    (D) high blood eosinophils
    (E) high blood neuroleptic levels

14. In your treatment you would likely use

    (A) physostigmine
    (B) naloxone
    (C) disulfiram
    (D) bromocriptine
    (E) propanolol

15. Electroconvulsive therapy should not be used where there is

    (A) hypertension
    (B) previous myocardial infarction
    (C) increased intracranial pressure
    (D) cervical spondolisthesis
    (E) pregnancy in third trimester

16. Average intelligence is the IQ range

    (A) 80–100
    (B) 100–120
    (C) 70–90
    (D) 90–110
    (E) 90–100

Questions 17 and 18

17. A 62-year-old society matron is involved in a car accident. She is hospitalized for the treatment of her fractured femur. She has no known physical or psychiatric problems. On the day after her hospitalization, she is restless, sweating; her blood pressure is 150/100 and her pulse rate is raised. In a more detailed history-taking, you anticipate

    (A) long-standing bulimia
    (B) chronic alcohol abuse

    (C) spending sprees and hypersexuality
    (D) lifelong compulsive behavior
    (E) recurrent panic attacks

18. Your treatment would include all of the following except

    (A) benzodiazepines
    (B) chlorpromazine
    (C) parenteral vitamin B complex
    (D) high-calorie, high-carbohydrate diet
    (E) supportive psychotherapy

19. Neologisms are most often indicative of

    (A) mental retardation
    (B) dementia
    (C) multiple personality
    (D) malingering
    (E) schizophrenia

20. A young man is referred to you because of recurrent anxiety symptoms. After he has been describing his problems for 15 minutes, suddenly he asks, "Doctor, am I going crazy?" Your best response is

    (A) "Why do you ask?"
    (B) "Certainly not. You will soon be fine."
    (C) "We will have a psychiatrist check you."
    (D) "When did you first think you were going crazy?"
    (E) "Does craziness run in your family?"

21. Penicillamine is an effective treatment for

    (A) Down's syndrome
    (B) Korsakoff's syndrome
    (C) Huntington's chorea
    (D) Klinefelter's syndrome
    (E) Wilson's disease

Questions 22 and 23

22. A 48-year-old man, found wandering in the streets, is brought to the emergency room by the police. He is unkempt and looks much older than his age. Though he is unsteady on his feet, physical examination shows no gross defects. He cannot recall how he came to be in the hospital. You are called away momentarily and on your return you find that he has forgotten your name and cannot remember the questions you asked. Diagnostically you are probably dealing with

    (A) Korsakoff's syndrome
    (B) Ganser syndrome
    (C) Capgras syndrome
    (D) Munchausen syndrome
    (E) Klinefelter's syndrome

23. When another physician comes into the examining room, though the patient has never met him before, the patient talks at length about having been treated by this doctor in a nearby town. The patient is now showing

    (A) rationalization
    (B) confabulation
    (C) la belle indifference
    (D) intellectualization
    (E) catastrophic reaction

24. A conscientious secretary who has been with the company many years is now approaching retirement. Her fellow workers have been noting lately that she is unkempt, almost sloppy, and increasingly forgetful. She surprises her staid employer one day be addressing him as "sweetie." Her recent annual physical examination showed no evidence of drug or medication use. In your evaluation you would anticipate finding evidence of

    (A) developing depression
    (B) incipient dementia
    (C) latent schizophrenia
    (D) histrionic personality
    (E) chronic delirium

25. Paranoia is produced by the emotional mechanism of

    (A) reaction formation
    (B) repression
    (C) projection
    (D) displacement
    (E) undoing

26. Transference is the

    (A) return to an earlier pattern of coping and behavior
    (B) therapist's illogical feelings based on previous experiences
    (C) patient's past relationship feelings transferred onto a new object
    (D) redirection of feeling onto a more acceptable or safer object
    (E) channeling of otherwise unacceptable drives into productive directions

27. The passive–aggressive personality is

    (A) neat, methodical, perfectionistic
    (B) aloof, indifferent to others; has few friends
    (C) lacking self-confidence; lets others make decisions
    (D) stubborn, delaying, forgetful
    (E) unpredictable, intense, impulsive

28. A delusion is

    (A) an irrational fear
    (B) a misinterpretation of a perceptual stimulus
    (C) a recurrent, intrusive distressing thought
    (D) a false perception
    (E) a false, fixed belief

29. Amphetamine psychosis often presents with symptoms similar to

    (A) major depression with psychosis
    (B) disorganized schizophrenia
    (C) paranoid schizophrenia
    (D) presenile dementia
    (E) acute porphyria

30. Mania may be treated on a long-term basis with

    (A) cimetidine
    (B) carbamazepine
    (C) lorazepam
    (D) trazodone
    (E) hydroxyzine

31. Testamentary capacity is the

    (A) measure of ability to stand trial
    (B) measure of criminal responsibility
    (C) measure of competency to make a will
    (D) measure of ability to handle one's own affairs
    (E) measure of ability to act as a witness

32. Electroconvulsive therapy is very effective in treating

    (A) recurrent agoraphobia
    (B) chronic paranoia
    (C) fugue state
    (D) acute mania
    (E) infantile autism

33. The rabbit syndrome

    (A) is improved by antiparkinsonian medication
    (B) is masked by increased dosage of neuroleptics
    (C) is worsened by antiparkinsonian medication
    (D) is the ability to keep still without inner feelings of anxiety
    (E) may worsen after neuroleptics are stopped

34. Pigmentary retinopathy may occur after high doses of

    (A) trifluoperazine
    (B) thioridazine
    (C) nortriptyline
    (D) phenelzine
    (E) alprazolam

35. Attention deficit disorder may be treated with

    (A) diazepam
    (B) benztropine
    (C) disulfiram
    (D) naloxone
    (E) pemoline

36. In sleepwalking, all of the following are true *except*

    (A) occurs during stage 3–4 sleep
    (B) most common at age 6–12
    (C) if wakened, subject is confused and disoriented
    (D) a manifestation of disturbing anxiety
    (E) subject amnestic for sleepwalking behavior when awakens later

37. With Huntington's chorea, all of the following statements are true *except*

    (A) personality changes may precede neurological symptoms
    (B) sexes equally affected
    (C) suicide risk is increased
    (D) autosomal recessive inheritance
    (E) genetic counseling indicated

38. Symptoms of dementia may be produced by all of the following syndromes *except*

    (A) pernicious anemia
    (B) Huntington's chorea
    (C) hypothyroidism
    (D) normal pressure hydrocephalus
    (E) Tourette's Disorder

39. Tactile hallucinations are commonly associated with the following conditions *except*

    (A) cocaine toxicity
    (B) alcohol withdrawal delirium
    (C) opiate withdrawal
    (D) amphetamine psychosis
    (E) lysergic acid diethylamide toxicity

40. Monoamine oxidase inhibitor side effects include the following conditions *except*

    (A) hypertensive crisis with specific foods
    (B) postural hypotension
    (C) insomnia
    (D) neuroleptic malignant syndrome
    (E) seizures, coma with meperidine

41. Hallucinations occur in each of the following syndromes *except*

    (A) delirium
    (B) bipolar disorder, manic
    (C) paranoid personality disorder
    (D) amphetamine psychosis
    (E) chronic disorganized schizophrenia

42. Because his wife is threatening to leave him unless he gives up his chronic heroin use, a 23-year-old man decides to stop completely, "cold turkey." Without treatment for his drug withdrawal, he is liable to experience all of the following symptoms *except*

    (A) vomiting, cramps, diarrhea
    (B) recurrent seizures
    (C) muscle spasms
    (D) insomnia, restlessness
    (E) spontaneous ejaculation

43. All of the following statements are true about bulimia *except*

    (A) episodic binge eating
    (B) high-calorie, sweet, easily eaten foods
    (C) terminated by abdominal pain, sleep, or induced vomiting
    (D) subject recognizes that binge eating is abnormal
    (E) symptoms quickly become life threatening

44. All of the following statements are true about transvestism *except*

    (A) more commonly diagnosed in males
    (B) subject dresses in the clothes of the opposite sex
    (C) subject wishes to change anatomical sex
    (D) behavior used to promote sexual arousal or gratification
    (E) tends to begin in childhood or adolescence

45. In Tourette's Disorder all of the following occur *except*

    (A) coprophagia
    (B) coprolalia
    (C) echolalia
    (D) multiple tics
    (E) childhood onset

46. In enuresis all of the following statements apply *except*

    (A) more common in boys
    (B) treated with conditioning devices
    (C) may benefit from psychotherapy
    (D) occurs during REM sleep
    (E) frequent family history of enuresis

47. All of the following statements apply to lithium treatment *except*

    (A) tremor often helped by propanolol
    (B) therapeutic level in elderly 0.6–1.0 mEq/L
    (C) polyuria and polydipsia may cause noncompliance
    (D) postural hypotension, worse in morning
    (E) often causes diarrhea, may be worse with long-acting compound

48. Delusions occur in all of the following syndromes *except*

    (A) disorganized schizophrenia
    (B) major depression
    (C) primary degenerative dementia
    — (D) psychogenic fugue
    (E) amphetamine toxicity

DIRECTIONS (Questions 49 through 83): Each group of items in this section consists of lettered headings followed by a set of numbered words or phrases. For each numbered word or phrase, select the ONE lettered heading that is most closely associated with it. Each lettered heading may be selected once, more than once, or not at all.

Questions 49 through 52

    (A) L-dopa
    (B) thioridazine
    (C) lithium
    (D) meprobamate

Treatment may lead to

49. Goiter

50. Withdrawal convulsions

51. Pigmentary retinopathy

52. Hypomania

Questions 53 through 55

    (A) akathisia
    (B) rabbit syndrome
    (C) tardive dyskinesia
    (D) acute dystonia

53. Grimacing, sucking, choreiform movements

54. Perioral tremor of pursed lips

55. Restlessness, unable to sit still

Questions 56 through 59

    (A) displacement
    (B) reaction formation
    (C) conversion
    (D) sublimation

56. The man who is angry with his wife kicks the cat.

57. The man who is angry with his wife chops a pile of logs.

58. The man who is angry with his wife unexpectedly buys her a piece of jewelry.

59. The man who is angry with his wife develops a sudden right-arm paralysis.

Questions 60 through 62

    (A) calcium disodium versenate (EDTA)
    (B) meperidine
    (C) disulfiram
    (D) naloxone

60. Chronic alcoholism

61. Opioid overdose

62. Lead intoxication

Questions 63 through 65

    (A) hallucinations
    (B) delirium
    (C) dementia

63. Clouding of consciousness

64. Vitamin B_{12} deficiency

65. Alert and well oriented

Questions 66 through 69

    (A) lithium
    (B) reserpine
    (C) phencyclidine
    (D) amitriptyline

May cause

66. Agitation, depression, suicide

67. Finger tremor, slowing of thought, seizures

68. Nystagmus, hypertension, agitation, violence

69. Postural hypotension, urinary retention, sedation

Questions 70 through 73

    (A) Wilson's disease
    (B) Alzheimer's disease
    (C) Tourette's Disorder
    (D) Wernicke's syndrome

70. Necrosis and hemorrhage in mamillary bodies and adjacent to ventricles

71. Degeneration, cell loss in putamen and caudate

C

72. No gross neuropathology

73. General brain atrophy, most marked in frontal and temporal lobes

Questions 74 through 77

(A) transsexual
(B) transvestite
(C) pedophile
(D) exhibitionist

74. Sexual gratification through self-exposure
D

75. Sexual gratification through dressing in opposite-sex clothing
B

76. Wish for anatomical sex change
A

77. Sexual gratification through actual or fantasied activities with children
C

Questions 78 through 80

(A) amantadine
(B) carbamazepine
(C) pemoline

78. Mania
B

79. Attention deficit disorder
C

80. Akathisia
A

Questions 81 through 83

(A) waxy flexibility, negativism, mutism
(B) silly, giggling, hallucinating
(C) suspicious, litiginous, grandiose

Schizophrenia,
81. Catatonic
A

82. Paranoid
C

83. Disorganized
B

DIRECTIONS (Questions 84 through 103): Each group of items in this section consists of lettered headings followed by a set of numbered words or phrases. For each numbered word or phrase, select

A if the item is associated with (A) **only**,
B if the item is associated with (B) **only**,
C if the item is associated with **both** (A) **and** (B),
D if the item is associated with **neither** (A) **nor** (B).

Questions 84 through 87

(A) bulimia
(B) anorexia nervosa
(C) both
(D) neither

84. Tends to occur mainly in women
C

85. Recognizes eating behavior patterns are harmful
A

86. Liable to be life threatening
B

87. Eating behavior typically followed by depression
A

Questions 88 through 91

(A) neuroleptic malignant syndrome
(B) neuroleptic-induced parkinsonism
(C) both
(D) neither

88. May present with muscle stiffness
C

89. Temperature over 38°C
A

90. Symptoms reversed by benztropine
B

91. Symptoms reversed by physostigmine
D

Questions 92 through 95

(A) tricyclic antidepressants
(B) monoamine oxidase inhibitors
(C) both
(D) neither

92. May cause disturbing hypotension
C

93. Hypertensive crisis with certain foods
B

94. Use may be limited by cardiac toxicity
A

95. Interacts with meperidine to cause fever and blood pressure changes
B

Questions 96 through 99

(A) chronic alcoholism
(B) opiate addiction
(C) both
(D) neither

96. Withdrawal convulsions
A

97. Higher incidence in physicians
C

98. Increased incidence of infective endocarditis
B

99. Usually starts in middle age
D

Questions 100 through 103

(A) nightmares
(B) night terrors
(C) both
(D) neither

100. Peak incidence in 3–6 year age group

101. When wakens later, total amnesia for episode

102. Occurs during REM sleep

103. Indicates emotional problems in child

DIRECTIONS (Questions 104 through 151): For each of the items in this section, ONE or MORE of the numbered options is correct. Choose the answer

A if only 1, 2, and 3 are correct,
B if only 1 and 3 are correct,
C if only 2 and 4 are correct,
D if only 4 is correct,
E if all are correct.

104. Disulfiram therapy

(1) indicated where hepatic cirrhosis present
(2) used where patient will not comply with other treatment regimens
(3) beneficial when patient has Korsakoff's syndrome
(4) may get toxic reaction with use of aftershave

105. Psychogenic amnesia

(1) recovery of memory is usually gradual and partial
(2) amytal interview may recover inaccessible memories
(3) quickly responds to electroconvulsive therapy
(4) recovery of memory is typically abrupt and total

106. In treatment of delirium tremens

(1) chlordiazepoxide 25–50 mg every 2–4 hours as required
(2) chlorpromazine 50–100 mg every 4–6 hours as needed
(3) high-calorie, high-carbohydrate diet
(4) restraints to control confusion and hyperactivity

107. Alcoholic hallucinosis

(1) auditory hallucinations usually present
(2) visual hallucinations usually present
(3) often marked fear and agitation
(4) clouding of consciousness

108. Panic attacks may produce symptoms similar to

(1) pheochromocytoma
(2) hypoglycemia
(3) hyperthyroidism
(4) acute porphyria

109. Paranoid personality disorder

(1) more common in deaf
(2) persistent persecutory delusions
(3) subjects rarely seek treatment
(4) benzodiazepines therapeutic

110. Delirium

(1) clouding of consciousness
(2) hallucinations present
(3) increase or decrease in activity
(4) fluctuates over the course of the day

111. Side effects of lithium

(1) polyuria
(2) difficulty concentrating, memory impairment
(3) acne
(4) fetal cardiovascular abnormalities

112. Diazepam

(1) primary metabolic pathway is conjugation
(2) long half-life in elderly
(3) no long-acting metabolites
(4) may persist longer in obese

113. You are called to the emergency room to see an abused child. You anticipate that

(1) the child is most likely to be under age 3
(2) the parents rationalize the abuse as necessary discipline
(3) the parents state the child is different from the other siblings
(4) one or both of the parents is psychotic

114. Dementia may be caused by

(1) autoimmune deficiency syndrome
(2) multiple schlerosis
(3) pellagra
(4) Huntington's chorea

115. The police bring a 26-year-old man for examination. He has been found wandering through a downtown store. He does not know his name, where he lives, or

where he is going. Physical examination is normal. Your tentative diagnosis is psychogenic amnesia, so you anticipate

(1) his memory return will be gradual and partial
(2) he shows no impairment of consciousness
(3) he has difficulty making and retrieving new memories
(4) hypnosis may show that the inaccessible memories are intact

116. Compliance

(1) increased with good doctor–patient relationship
(2) better in chronic patients
(3) poor compliance may be a direct expression of psychopathology
(4) better when medication is given in multiple doses

Questions 117 and 118

117. Your colleague wishes to refer a child with attention deficit disorder for evaluation. You anticipate that

(1) the patient is most likely to be male
(2) the patient is impulsive
(3) the youngster has difficulty maintaining attention
(4) the symptoms were first noted in the preschool years

118. In treating this patient with methylphenidate, you will advise the parents about

(1) the possibility of height and weight retardation
(2) the major risk of drug abuse in adolescence
(3) the benefits of drug holidays
(4) the absence of benefit from this medication in teenage and adult years

119. Examples of primary prevention programs include

(1) halfway houses for former patients
(2) rubella vaccinations
(3) crisis phone-in services
(4) AIDS education in high school

120. A child with infantile autism has a more favorable prognosis when the following statements are true

(1) no other family members with autism
(2) the child is organized in his or her play
(3) the youngster has an interest in mechanical objects
(4) the child is able to converse meaningfully

121. A 56-year-old woman is brought to the emergency room because she is restless and confused. She appears to be having visual and auditory hallucinations. She complains of a dry mouth. Her pupils are dilated,

reacting only sluggishly, and her skin is warm and dry. She has a tachycardia. This clinical state could be caused by

(1) amitriptyline
(2) thioridazine
(3) scopolamine
(4) benztropine

122. In acute intermittent porphyria, the following statements apply

(1) highest incidence after age 50
(2) may present with acute depression
(3) treated with phenobarbital
(4) can be precipitated by oral contraceptives

123. Neuroleptic malignant syndrome

(1) after stopping the neuroleptic and giving appropriate treatment, restarting the same neuroleptic will always cause recurrence of the neuroleptic malignant syndrome
(2) is precipitated by giving tyramine-containing foods to patients taking monoamine oxidase inhibitors
(3) will be quickly terminated by giving a course of electroconvulsive therapy
(4) may be fatal

124. Lorazepam and oxazepam

(1) acute onset of withdrawal symptoms
(2) may produce sedation 2 or more weeks after stopping
(3) fewer problem side effects in the elderly than diazepam
(4) metabolized by hepatic oxidation

125. In differentiating delirium from dementia you would look for

(1) thought disorder
(2) memory deficits
(3) disturbance of orientation
(4) clouding of consciousness

126. Childhood disturbances that occur during non-REM sleep include

(1) night terrors
(2) enuresis
(3) sleepwalking
(4) nightmares

127. An anticholinergic psychosis may be produced by

(1) imipramine
(2) benztropine
(3) thioridazine
(4) physostigmine

SUMMARY OF DIRECTIONS

A	B	C	D	E
1, 2, 3	1, 3	2, 4	4	All are
only	only	only	only	correct

128. False positive dexamethasone test results may be associated with

   (1) anorexia nervosa
   (2) obesity
   (3) pregnancy
   (4) Addison's disease

129. When a patient presents with mutism, negativism, rigidity, and waxy flexibility, your differential diagnosis should include

   (1) major depression
   (2) encephalitis
   (3) schizophrenia
   (4) neuroleptic toxicity

130. In considering the involuntary psychiatric hospitalization of an adult patient, the following statements apply

   (1) a psychiatrist must evaluate the patient before hospitalization
   (2) hospitalization can be justified on the basis of grave disability
   (3) a responsible relative must consent to the hospitalization
   (4) hospitalization can be required if the patient is dangerous to others

Questions 131 through 133

131. A 56-year-old man is brought for examination because in the past month he has become increasingly socially withdrawn and for the last 2 days has hardly moved. He has been staring blankly, occasionally crying. He has been telling his family that he is too old, that he deserves to die, and that they would be better off without him. He has no history of drug or alcohol abuse. Physical examination is normal. His family fears that he might be suicidal. You recognize that the risk of suicide

   (1) is increased when suicide is discussed with the patient
   (2) is greater when there have been prior suicide attempts
   (3) is lower in older males like this patient
   (4) is higher when the patient is beginning to come out of a depression

132. You decide to treat this patient with tricyclic antidepressants. You advise him and his family that

   (1) mood improvement is likely to take 2–3 weeks of treatment
   (2) dry mouth, constipation, and urinary problems may develop in the first week of treatment
   (3) at therapeutic levels, the medication has a quinidine-like effect on the heart
   (4) potentially fatal hypertensive crisis may occur when certain foods are eaten

133. The family ask whether electroconvulsive therapy would be a suitable treatment. You advise them that

   (1) at his age, electroconvulsive therapy is contraindicated
   (2) electroconvulsive therapy has dangerous hypertensive effects
   (3) his symptoms would not be benefited by electroconvulsive treatment
   (4) electroconvulsive therapy would be a safe and efficient treatment

134. In considering the use of lithium with pregnant women, you recognize that

   (1) lithium passes through the breast milk to the nursing infant
   (2) lithium does not pass the placental barrier and does not affect the fetus
   (3) lithium produces a higher incidence of fetal cardiac deficits
   (4) lithium causes an increased incidence of Turner's syndrome

135. Important factors in determining testamentary capacity include

   (1) the ability to read and write
   (2) the knowledge as to who next of kin are
   (3) the absence of psychotic thinking
   (4) the awareness of what he or she owns

136. Under the M'Naghten rule, a subject will be held criminally responsible if the

   (1) subject knew what he or she was doing
   (2) subject is able to consult rationally with his or her lawyer
   (3) subject knew whether the act was right or wrong
   (4) subject can understand the trial proceedings

137. In considering mental retardation, the following apply

   (1) highest incidence in early childhood
   (2) most are mildly retarded
   (3) the encephalogram typically confirms the diagnosis
   (4) most often diagnosed in teenagers

138. Under the stress of parental separation and divorce, a 4-year-old child may show

(1) thumb sucking
(2) enuresis
(3) tantrums
(4) encopresis

139 . In conversion disorder, which of the following statements apply

(1) not diagnosed with coexistent physical illness
(2) symptoms do not follow anatomical boundaries
(3) la belle indifference is diagnostic
(4) symptoms perpetuated by secondary gain

140. Enuresis

(1) higher incidence in other family members
(2) more common in boys
(3) responds to conditioning devices
(4) occurs during non-REM sleep

141. Somatoform disorders include

(1) hypochondriasis
(2) psychogenic amnesia
(3) conversion disorders
(4) chronic factitious disorder

142. Which of the following statements apply to anorexia nervosa

(1) feels guilty and anxious when does not eat
(2) tends to overestimate body size
(3) usually very active sexually
(4) commoner in people who jog and exercise

143. In the management of anorexia nervosa

(1) early age of onset has better prognosis
(2) patients are often deceitful about food
(3) laxative abuse may precipitate electrolyte imbalance
(4) dexamethasone suppression test is likely to be abnormal

144. The patient with paranoid personality disorder is likely to show

(1) coldness and distance in relating
(2) mistrust of others
(3) hypersensitivity to fancied slights
(4) persecutory delusions

145. Suicidal risk is increased when the following factors are present

(1) history of previous suicide attempts
(2) patient is female
(3) patient is elderly
(4) patient is married

146. There is greater likelihood that a patient will be violent under the following circumstances

(1) patient is paranoid
(2) patient is intoxicated
(3) patient is experiencing command hallucinations
(4) patient is showing signs of dementia

147. The psychological processes whereby a child develops a conscience include

(1) identification
(2) intellectualization
(3) introjection
(4) projection

148. At the request of the school authorities, a 7-year-old boy has been referred to you for evaluation. To an increasing extent he has been missing school because of recurrent abdominal pain. Physical and laboratory examinations have been normal. In your management of this youngster you recommend

(1) that he go to school regularly each day
(2) immediate homebound schooling with a tutor
(3) evaluation of the classroom environment
(4) methylphenidate, in the morning and at lunch time

149. Phencyclidine intoxication commonly causes

(1) tachycardia
(2) nystagmus
(3) anxiety
(4) catatonia

150. Chronic alcoholics treated with disulfiram must be warned to avoid

(1) foods prepared with wine
(2) aftershave
(3) cough syrups
(4) pyridoxine

151. Depression in the elderly

(1) may produce symptoms similar to dementia
(2) has a higher incidence of suicide
(3) may coexist with dementia
(4) does not respond to antidepressants

Answers and Explanations

1. **(C)** *Tolerance* is the declining effect of the same dose of a drug on repeated administration. The subject then has to take larger doses to get the same effect. *(1:400; 2:644–645;3:233)*

   Resistance is the unconsciously motivated inability to discuss certain topics in psychotherapy. *(1:597;2:107;3:5)*

   The psychological splitting off of mental functions from the rest of the personality, as in a fugue state, is the process of *dissociation.* *(1:80;2:105;3:10)*

   Ambivalence is the emotional state when the subject maintains directly conflicting feelings about the same object at the same time, as in a "love-hate" relationship. *(1:170;2:138–139;3:20)*

2. **(E)** *Reaction formation* is a defense mechanism whereby the person emphasizes the opposite of his or her true feelings, as with the individual who deals with disturbing angry feelings by being outwardly very sweet and polite. *(1:79;2:98–99;3:8)*

   Suppression occurs when the subject consciously blots out a problem from awareness: "I do not want to think about it."

   In *repression,* unacceptable thoughts or feelings are automatically or unconsciously kept out of awareness.

   In *denial,* unpleasant realities are emotionally ignored, as is often seen with a life-threatening illness.

   Rationalization is the emotional defense where otherwise awkward or conflicted situations or feelings are given a quasiplausible intellectual explanation that the subject believes.

3. **(D)** Neuroleptic side effects.

   Akathisia is a feeling of inner restlessness with an inability to remain still. When these patients are questioned closely, they will say that they are not anxious, they just have to keep moving.

   Bradykinesia, or *akinesia,* is the reduction in frequency and amplitude of voluntary movements.

   The patient with *tardive dyskinesia* is most readily diagnosed by visual inspection because he or she is liable to show continuous, involuntary, repetitious orofacial and lingual movements, with choreic or athetoid movements of other parts of the body.

   Less commonly, patients will show the *rabbit syndrome:* an isolated tremor of tightly pursed lips, parkinsonian in frequency and responsive to antiparkinsonian medication. *(1:643–646;2:822–824;3: 117–120)*

4. **(A)** In the *Bender–Gestalt Test,* the subject copies a series of nine geometrical designs, initially from cards and then from memory. This test is most often used to evaluate the possibility of organically based psychological problems.

   The *Minnesota Multiphasic Personality Inventory (MMPI)* is a collection of 550 statements to which the subject is required to respond.

   The *Rorschach test,* a set of ten inkblot cards, and the *Thematic Apperception Test,* a set of ambiguous pictures, both evaluate the subject's thinking and associational ability.

   The *Wechsler Intelligence Scale* is a series of six verbal subtests and five performance subtests used to evaluate the subject's intelligence. *(1:128–131;2:205–215;3:46–49)*

5. **(D)** *Secondary gain* is all the sympathy, attention, and rewards that come from being ill; *primary gain* is the emotional relief, the reduction of conflict and anxiety, that is permitted by the neurotic illness.

   Secondary process thinking is logical, reality based, and optimally produces sublimation and development.

   Sublimation is the process whereby unacceptable drives are converted into socially acceptable, growth-oriented behaviors.

   Secondary gain is produced by unconscious factors and maintained by environmental response, while the gain in *malingering* is consciously planned and sought. *(1:82;2:504–505;3:290)*

6. **(B)** *Electroconvulsive therapy* is most effective in *major depression*. This treatment is *not indicated* in *amphetamine psychosis, disorganized schizophrenia, personality disorders,* or *conversion disorders. (1:679–682;2:836–840;3:131–134)*

7. **(D)** *Methylphenidate* is the medication most often used to treat children with the symptoms of an attention deficit disorder. The other medications are not indicated in this disorder. *(1:741–747;2:681–683;3:187–190)*

8. **(C)** The symptoms described are those seen in an *anticholinergic psychosis*. This toxic syndrome may be caused by the tricyclic antidepressants, especially when they are used with other anticholinergic drugs. *(1:588–589;2:826–827;3:223–224)*

9. **(B)** In *primary prevention* the illness is prevented from occurring. Repainting inner-city houses after the removal of lead-containing paint is a major factor in preventing lead intoxication in children. The use of halfway houses is an example of *tertiary prevention*. Depot neuroleptics use, a crisis hotline service, and early return of a phobic child to school are all measures to minimize the effect and severity of an existing emotional illness, all examples of *secondary prevention*. *(1:867–877;2:788;3:180–181)*

10. **(D)** This schizophrenic patient is likely to be suffering from neuroleptic-induced dystonia, which would be relieved by *intramuscular benztropine*. Intramuscular haloperidol would worsen the symptoms, while hypnosis and "talking down" would be ineffective and barbiturates merely sedating. *(1:644;2:822–824;3:119)*

11. **(C)** Whistling through the graveyard is an example of *counterphobic* behavior. These young men are scared but they deal with their fear by overreacting in the opposite emotional direction. *(1:324;2:473;3:8)*

12. **(E)** This is the symptomatic picture seen in evolving *neuroleptic malignant syndrome*. In drug-induced catatonia or dystonia, significant fever would not be present. A hypertensive crisis does not occur with haloperidol use and does not present with these symptoms. Tardive dyskinesia, best diagnosed visually, has different symptoms. *(1:643)*

13. **(B)** Your diagnosis is best confirmed by demonstrating *elevated serum creatine phosphokinase*. When a

neuroleptic malignant syndrome is fully developed, there is likely to be complete breakdown of body homeostasis and most tests will then be abnormal. *(1:643)*

14. **(D)** *Bromocriptine,* a dopamine antagonist, is most commonly used to treat neuroleptic malignant syndrome. Dantrolene, a muscle relaxant, is also used. Neuroleptics must be discontinued and intensive supportive treatment instituted. *(1:643)*

15. **(C)** Increased intracranial pressure is about the only contraindication to the use of electroconvulsive therapy. With careful anesthesia and seizure control, this treatment can be given in the other clinical situations listed. *(1:682–683;2:837–838;3:131–132)*

16. **(D)** *Average intelligence* is the IQ range *90–110*. The Intelligence Quotient (IQ) is the ratio between the Mental Age and Chronological Age, multiplied by 100. *(1:127–128;2:203–204;3:46)*

$$IQ = \frac{\text{Mental Age}}{\text{Chronological Age}} \times 100$$

17. **(B)** This is the classical history of the development of withdrawal symptoms in a *chronic* (unsuspected) *alcoholic. (1:418; 2:626–627;3:217–218)*

18. **(B)** *Chlorpromazine* is not used in treating delirium tremens or alcohol withdrawal symptoms because of the convulsant, hypotensive, and potential hepatotoxic effects of this medication. Benzodiazepines are effective at a lower risk. *(1:418–420;2:626–627;3:217–218)*

19. **(E)** *Neologisms*—idiosyncratic words used by a patient—are almost pathognomonic of schizophrenia. Very rarely a lesion of the superior temporal gyrus of the dominant hemisphere may produce a fluent aphasia with nonsense speech and neologisms (Wernicke's aphasia). *(1:147;2:364;3:17)*

20. **(A)** In evaluating a patient, your task is first to find out *the patient's concerns and feelings*. Before you give answers, you need to find out what the patient is asking and why. *(1:112–116;2:184–189;3:31–33)*

21. **(E)** *Penicillamine,* a copper chelating agent, is used in the treatment of *Wilson's disease*. Early treatment of asymptomatic patients may prevent the development of symptoms. Penicillin-sensitive patients may also show sensitivity reactions to penicillamine. *(1:716–717;2:323–324;3:228–229)*

22. **(A)** This patient is presenting with the type of short-term memory deficit seen in *Korsakoff's syndrome.* Signs of cerebellar dysfunction, peripheral neuropathy, and cirrhosis may be present due to chronic alcohol abuse. *(1:420;2:631–633;3:218–219)*

The *Ganser syndrome,* the syndrome of the approximate answer—"Two and two is five"—was first described as a response of prisoners to interrogation. *(1:544–545;2:516–517)*

The *Capgras syndrome,* the sydrome of twins or imposters, is most often seen in paranoid patients who claim that someone they know well is not really the person they are talking to or seeing but rather someone else, looking exactly like the known person, a twin or someone impersonating that other person. *(1:548; 2:133)*

In the *Munchausen Syndrome,* the patient deliberately feigns symptoms in order to get medical attention or treatment. *(1:522–524;2:516)*

Klinefelter's syndrome, a xyy chromosome disorder, produces a male with testicular atrophy, small penis, and, sometimes, adolescent gynecomastia. *(1:438;2:736–737;3:80–81)*

23. **(B)** This patient is *confabulating.* Automatically he is producing false memories to compensate for his memory deficit. *(1:161;2:145;3:16)*

24. **(B)** When a patient shows increasing forgetfulness, impaired self-care, and a lack of self-control, *early dementia* should be suspected. In early dementia, these symptoms may be apparent only when the patient is tired, stressed, or dealing with new or unexpected situations. *(1:276–279;2:232–246;3:215–216)*

25. **(C)** *Paranoia* is produced by the mechanism of *projection.* The feeling that is unacceptable to the subject is projected outward and ascribed to another person. *(1:226–227;2:444–447;3:257)*

26. **(C)** *Transference* is the situation in psychotherapy (and in all relationships) where the feelings the patient has from past relationships are transferred onto a new relationship object—in psychotherapy, onto the psychotherapist. *(1:597;2:97–98;3:4–5)*

27. **(D)** Patients with a *passive-aggressive* personality classically are stubborn, repeatedly delaying, and forgetful about things they do not wish to do or have to face. *(1:381–383;2:612–613;3:335)*

The *compulsive* personality is neat, methodical, and perfectionistic. *(1:380;2:613;3:335)*

The subject with the *schizoid* personality is aloof, indifferent to others, with few friends, and does not really want friendship. *(1:367–368;2:596–598;3:330)*

The person with a *dependent personality disorder* lacks self-confidence and passively allows others to make major life decisions for him or her. *(1:378–380, 3:35)*

The patient with a *borderline personality disorder* is likely to be unstable, intense, and impulsive: predictably unpredictable. *(1:375–377;2:602–604;3:334–335)*

28. **(E)** A *delusion* is a false, fixed belief, not amenable to logic, and incompatible with the subject's culture and level of maturity. *(1:152–153;2:129–133;3:18)*

29. **(C)** An *amphetamine psychosis* often presents with symptoms similar to paranoid schizophrenia and should be excluded in patients of all ages presenting with these symptoms. *(1:403–405;2:662–663;3:221)*

30. **(B)** On a long-term maintenance basis, *mania* may be treated with *carbamazepine,* especially in patients for whom lithium is contraindicated or ineffective. *(1:297;3:280)*

31. **(C)** *Testamentary capacity* is the measure of a subject's competence to make a legally valid will and should be verified by a detailed mental status examination. *(1:893–894;2:859;3:152)*

32. **(D)** In patients who are *acutely manic, electroconvulsive treatment* given daily or on alternate days, sometimes more frequently, brings symptoms under good control, usually within a few days. Although electroconvulsive therapy was used in the past to treat chronic paranoia, the treatment results were disappointing and frequently short lived. The other syndromes listed are not treated with electroconvulsive therapy. *(1:682;2:837;3:131)*

33. **(A)** The *rabbit syndrome,* a late-onset parkinsonian symptom in which the patient shows a parkinsonian tremor of pursed lips, is improved by *antiparkinsonian medication.* *(1:643–646;2:823;3:119)*

34. **(B)** *Pigmentary retinopathy* occurs after high doses of *thioridazine.* Usually it is stated that this side effect occurs at a dose level above 800 mg daily, but it has been reported at lower dosage levels. *(1:649;3:124)*

35. **(E)** *Attention deficit disorder* may be treated with *pemoline,* a longer-acting amphetamine derivative. Pemoline is usually not recommended for use with preschool children. *(1:745;2:682;3:189–190)*

36. **(D)** *Sleepwalking* is not a manifestation of disturbing anxiety. It is most common in the 6–12 year age group and occurs during stage 3–4 sleep. If the subject is wakened during the sleepwalking, he or she appears to be confused and disoriented: upon awakening later, he or she is amnestic for the sleepwalking behavior. *(1:570–573;2:706;3:352–353)*

37. **(D)** *Huntington's chorea,* an autosomal dominant, affects both sexes equally and may present initially with personality rather than neurologic changes. Suicidal risk is markedly increased in these patients and their relatives. Genetic counseling and investigation is indicated. *(1:306;2:339–341;3:227)*

38. **(E)** *Dementia* is *not* a symptom of *Tourette's Disorder* but can present in the other syndromes listed. The symptoms of *Tourette's Disorder* tend to be less obvious in adult life. *(1:547–548;2:700–701;3:196–197)*

39. **(C)** Definite *tactile hallucinations* do *not* occur in *opiate withdrawal.* The subject undergoing opiate withdrawal will be very uncomfortable with sweating, piloerection, muscle aches and twitching, abdominal cramps, diarrhea, and vomiting but will not become psychotic. *(1:394;2:127;3:16)*

40. **(D)** *Monoamine oxidase inhibitors* do *not* cause the *neuroleptic malignant syndrome.* The dietary-induced side effects are rare and, in clinical practice, monoamine oxidase inhibitors produce fewer distressing side effects than tricyclic antidepressants. *(1:657–659;2:828–829)*

41. **(C)** Hallucinations and other psychotic symptoms do not occur in personality disorders and are not present in a paranoid personality disorder. *Hallucinations* do occur in *mania, schizophrenia, amphetamine psychosis,* and *delirium. (1:163–164;2:445–446;3:330)*

42. **(B)** In the course of *heroin withdrawal "cold turkey," seizures* do *not* occur. If seizures do present during a withdrawal process, it is probably because the subject was also abusing sedatives such as barbiturates or meprobamate in combination with the heroin. *(1:394; 2:653;3:220–221)*

43. **(E)** *Bulimia* does *not* become *life threatening.* The bulimic subject periodically binges on high-calorie, easily eaten food. The binges are frequently terminated by vomiting or sleep, sometimes by abdominal pain, and typically are followed by much guilt and self-blame over this abnormal eating behavior. *(1:779–780;2:551;3:195)*

44. **(C)** The strictly diagnosed *transvestite* does not wish to change anatomical sex: if this wish for sex change is present, the subject would be considered transsexual. Transvestism usually begins in childhood or adolescence. The patient dresses in the clothes of the opposite sex for sexual gratification. In Western societies, women can cross-dress without meeting as much social disapproval and without being labeled as transvestite. *(1:447–449;2:528–529;3:303–304)*

45. **(A)** *Coprophagia,* the eating of feces, does *not* occur in *Tourette's Disorder. Coprolalia,* the compulsive expression of obscenities, was thought to occur in the majority of patients with Tourette's Disorder, but now that less severe cases are being diagnosed the symptoms are found to occur less often. *(1:763–765;2:700–701;3:196–197)*

46. **(D)** *Enuresis* is more common in boys, occurs in families where other family members, especially males, have a history of enuresis, and may be beneficially treated with both conditioning devices and psychotherapy. Enuresis occurs during stage 3–4 non-REM sleep. *(1:843–846;2:697–699;3:197–198)*

47. **(D)** *Postural hypotension,* worse in the morning, is *not* a side effect of *lithium* (but is frequently seen with tricyclic antidepressants). *Polyuria* and *polydipsia,* frequent side effects disturbing to the patient, often lead to noncompliance, as does lithium-produced diarrhea, which may be worse with the slow-release lithium tablets. Lithium-induced tremor is often helped by *propanolol.* While the therapeutic adult serum lithium level is 0.8–1.2 mEq/L, in the elderly 0.6–1.0 mEq/L is an effective and safer therapeutic range. *(1:675–678;2:830–831;3:128–129)*

48. **(D)** *Delusions* do *not* occur in a *psychogenic fugue:* delusions are evidence of psychotic thinking and may be present in the other syndromes listed. *(1:152;2: 514;3:292)*

49. **(C)** *Goiter* is a well-recognized side effect of *lithium* use. In some patients receiving lithium, hypothyroidism may develop, requiring either discontinuation of the lithium or supplemental thyroid intake. *(1:677; 2:830–831;3:128)*

50. **(D)** *Withdrawal convulsions* may occur after chronic *meprobamate* use (and on withdrawal from other sedatives such as alcohol, barbiturates, and benzodiazepines). *(1:409;2:831–832;3:219–220)*

51. **(B)** *Pigmentary retinopathy* is liable to occur in patients given *thioridazine* in doses over 800 mg/day. These eye changes can develop within several weeks. *(1:649–3:124)*

52. **(A)** *Hypomania* and manic states may be precipitated by *L-dopa,* bromocriptine, and amantadine, all dopamine antagonists. Confusion, disorientation, and depression may also be seen in patients receiving L-dopa. *(1:295–296;2:337–339)*

Answers 53 through 55 deal with neuroleptic side effects. (1:643–646;2:822–824;3:117–122)

53. **(A)** *Tardive dyskinesia,* most easily recognized by visual inspection, often presents with orofacial–lingual dyskinesias such as tics and grimaces, lip smacking, chewing movements, and tongue protrusion with choreiform or athetoid movements of the limbs and trunk. *(1:644–646;2:823–824;3:121–122)*

54. **(B)** In the *rabbit syndrome,* the subject shows neuroleptic-induced lip pursing with a slow, steady parkinsonian-rate perioral lip tremor—like the lip movements of a rabbit. This syndrome is responsive to the antiparkinsonian drugs. *(1:644;2:823;3:119)*

55. **(A)** *Akathisia* is manifested by restlessness and the inability to keep still. The subject may feel this constant need to move to be irritating and socially disruptive. These symptoms may be misdiagnosed as manifestations of anxiety. *(1:644;2:823;3:118)*

Answers 56 through 59 deal with defense mechanisms. (1:79–80;2:91–111;3:1–11)

56. **(A)** In *displacement,* feelings are transferred or redirected onto a more acceptable object. In this way, otherwise unacceptable or dangerous feelings are allowed open expression. *(1:80;2:101–102;3:9)*

57. **(D)** In *sublimation,* unacceptable feelings or drives are repressed but the energy behind these emotions is redirected into socially useful and growth-promoting goals. *(1:80;2:108;3:9–10)*

58. **(B)** When a person is struggling emotionally with unacceptable feelings, these emotions may be dealt with by *reaction formation,* whereby the subject responds to the situation outwardly with feelings and behaviors opposite to the underlying emotions, frequently in an exaggerated fashion. *(1:79;2:98–99;3:8)*

59. **(C)** The term *conversion disorder* is one of the few psychiatric diagnoses that suggest a psychological process or mechanism. In conversion, psychological feelings are thought in some way to be converted into a physical symptom, a loss or alteration of function, that relieves the emotional conflict. In this situation described, the man's right-arm paralysis successfully prevents him from acting out his unacceptable urges to hit his wife, for whom he cares—the primary gain of the conversion symptom is the resolution of his emotional conflict. *(1:342–345;2:110;3:10)*

60. **(C)** *Disulfiram* (Antabuse) is used in the treatment of chronic alcoholics who want incentive or assistance to help them stay off alcohol. Disulfiram therapy should only be used as part of a multifaceted treatment program. *(1:426;2:639–640;3:237–238)*

61. **(D)** *Opioid overdose* can be treated with the short-acting opioid antagonist *naloxone.* With opiate abusers naloxone may precipitate a withdrawal abstinence syndrome. *(1:398;2:655;3:220)*

62. **(A)** *Calcium disodium versenate (EDTA),* used in treating lead encephalopathy, is given intravenously over several days. *(1:298;2:330–331;3:163)*

63. **(B)** *Clouding of consciousness* is the primary symptom that distinguishes *delirium* from *dementia* and *hallucinosis.* *(1:273–276;2:140–141;3:214–215)*

64. **(C)** *Vitamin B$_{12}$ deficiency,* pernicious anemia, is one potentially reversible cause of dementia that should be sought in every case of dementia. *(1:312;2:327–328; 3:229)*

65. **(A)** In *hallucinosis,* the subject experiences hallucinations, most often auditory but sometimes involving other perceptual modalities, in a state of wakefulness, alertness, and orientation. *(1:281–283;2:633–635; 3:218)*

66. **(B)** *Reserpine* may produce nightmares, agitation, and depression, symptoms that are dose-related in intensity. Suicide can result from this drug-induced depression. *(1:296;3:278)*

67. **(A)** Even within therapeutic dose range, *lithium* may cause finger tremor and slowing of thought. Many patients find these side effects annoying. At higher toxic lithium levels, seizures may occur. *(1:676–677; 2:830–831;3:128–129)*

68. **(C)** The patient experiencing *phencyclidine* (PCP, "Angel Dust") toxicity is likely to be unpredictable, agitated, violent, and psychotic. Physical examination may show ataxia, muscle rigidity, and tachycardia with blood pressure elevation. *(1:410–412)*

69. **(D)** For the patient taking *amitriptyline,* postural hypotension, most marked on rising in the morning, is likely to be a nuisance and in the elderly quite dangerous. Prostate obstruction, increased by anticholinergic effect, may cause urinary retention. Sedation is present, especially early in treatment. *(1:654–656)*

Answers 70 through 73 deal with neuropathology.

70. **(D)** In *Wernicke's syndrome,* most often due to chronic alcoholism, necrosis and hemorrhage in the mamillary bodies and adjacent to the aqueduct and the ventricular system may be found. *(1:279–281;2:325–326;3:218–219)*

71. **(A)** *Wilson's disease,* hepatolenticular degeneration, is an autosomal recessive disorder of copper metabo-

lism, leading to degeneration and cell loss in the putamen and caudate (the lenticular nuclei of the brain). *(1:716-717;2:323-324;3:228-229)*

72. **(C)** In *Tourette's Disorder* there is no gross neuropathology, though recent studies indicate a possible neurotransmitter defect. *(1:547-548;2:700-701;3:196-197)*

73. **(B)** Autopsy of the patient with *Alzheimer's disease* will show general brain atrophy, which is likely to be most prominent in the frontal and temporal lobes. *(1:287-289;2:242-243;3:216)*

Answers 74 through 77 deal with sexual deviations. (1:445-452;2:528-533;3:303-306)

74. **(D)** The *exhibitionist,* usually a male, gains sexual gratification through genital exposure to strangers, usually of the opposite sex. Typically exhibitionists pose no physical danger to others unless they are prevented from escaping. *(1:449-450;2:529-530;3:304-305)*

75. **(B)** The *transvestite* gains sexual pleasure through dressing in the clothes of the opposite sex. These patients are almost exclusively males. *(1:447-449; 2:528-529;3:303-304)*

76. **(A)** The *transsexual* is dissatisfied with his or her anatomical sex, believes that he or she is really a member of the opposite sex, and seeks surgical and hormonal sex change to make the physical appearance coincide with the sexual self-image. *(1:434-437;2:525-527;3:302-303)*

77. **(C)** The *pedophile* achieves sexual excitement and gratification by engaging in sexual activities, homosexual or heterosexual, with prepubertal children. *(1:450-451;2:529;3:304)*

Answers 78 through 80 deal with less frequently used medications.

78. **(B)** Especially when lithium is ineffective or contraindicated in the treatment of a *manic patient, carbamazepine* may be used. *(1:297;3:280)*

79. **(C)** In *attention deficit disorder,* methylphenidate is the usual initial medication. Where this drug treatment is ineffective or causes unacceptable side effects, *pemoline* is often prescribed. *(1:745;3:189-190)*

80. **(A)** *Akathisia,* neuroleptic-induced motor restlessness, often does not respond to antiparkinsonian medication. *Amantadine* may be more effective in producing symptom relief. *(1:645;2:823;3:120)*

Answers 81 through 83 deal with schizophrenic syndromes. (1:214-218;2:372-384;3:248-249)

81. **(A)** Waxy flexibility, negativism, and mutism are characteristic of *catatonic schizophrenia* (but are now more frequently seen in drug- or neuroleptic-induced catatonic states). *(1:214-215;2:373-376;3:248)*

82. **(C)** The *paranoid schizophrenic* is typically hypersensitive and suspicious, jealous, resentful, and litiginous, sometimes hostile and violent. Frequently the paranoid delusions seen in these patients are grandiose in nature—patients believe they are victimized or persecuted because they are in some way special. *(1:215;2:376-378;3:248)*

83. **(B)** The *disorganized* (hebephrenic) *schizophrenic* displays the layperson's idea of psychosis—silly, giggling, bizarre, hallucinating, and socially markedly disabled. *(1:215;2:378-379;3:248)*

Answers 84 through 87 deal with eating disorders. (1:779-784,499-504;2:554-558;3:194-196)

84. **(C)** Bulimia and anorexia nervosa both occur mainly in women and start most often in adolescence and young adulthood. *(1:499,779;2:554-558;3:194-195)*

85. **(A)** The bulimic patient recognizes that gorging is abnormal and harmful and often feels guilty and anxious about eating. *(1:779-780;2:555-556;3:195)* The anorexia nervosa patient will serenely *insist* that his or her self-starvation is not abnormal in any way. *(1:501; 2:555;3:194-195)*

86. **(B)** Anorexia nervosa is likely to be life threatening but bulimia does not pose a major threat to life. *(1:502,779;2:555-558;3:194-195)*

87. **(A)** Bulimic gorging is typically followed by intense anxiety or guilt, which often lead to further overeating. *(1:779-780;2:555-556;3:195)*

Answers 88 through 91 deal with neuroleptic-induced syndromes. (1:643-646;2:822-826;3:117-125)

88. **(C)** Both neuroleptic malignant syndrome and neuroleptic-induced parkinsonism may present with muscle stiffness. *(1:643-644;2:823;3:119)*

89. **(A)** Neuroleptic-induced parkinsonism does not by itself cause a fever. Pyrexia of 38°C and above should strongly raise suspicion of neuroleptic malignant syndrome in a patient receiving neuroleptics. *(1:643-644;2:825)*

90. **(B)** Neuroleptic-induced parkinsonism is reversed by benztropine, which has no effect or may worsen the symptoms of neuroleptic malignant syndrome. *(1: 643–644;2:823;3:120)*

91. **(D)** In neither neuroleptic malignant syndrome nor neuroleptic-induced parkinsonism are the symptoms reversed by physostigmine. *(1:643–644;3:120)*

Answers 92 through 95 deal with antidepressant side effects. (1:654–659;2:826–829)

92. **(C)** Both tricyclic antidepressants and monoamine oxidase inhibitors produce postural hypotension though this side effect tends to be more disabling with tricyclic antidepressants. *(1:654,658;2:826–829;3:111, 123)*

93. **(B)** Monoamine oxidase inhibitors may cause a hypertensive crisis when certain foods, primarily tyramine-containing, are ingested. This danger has perhaps been over emphasized; in western Europe, monoamine oxidase inhibitors are used widely and safely. *(1:658–659;2:829;3:111–112)*

94. **(A)** The use of tricyclic antidepressants may be limited due to cardiac toxicity. Even at therapeutic levels, these medications have a quinidine-like effect on the heart. *(1:655;2:826–827;3:123)*

95. **(B)** Monoamine oxidase inhibitors may interact with meperidine to produce agitation, hyperpyrexia, convulsions, and even death. *(1:659;2:828–829)*

Answers 96 through 99 deal with drug dependency.

96. **(A)** Convulsions can occur on withdrawal after chronic use of alcohol, barbiturates, and other sedative hypnotics, but they do not occur in opiate withdrawal. *(1:394,406–410;2:626,653–656;3:219–221)*

97. **(C)** Both alcoholism and opiate addiction are more common in physicians than in other groups comparable socially and educationally. *(1:385–386,416;2:617–626,646;3:234–236)*

98. **(B)** The incidence of infective endocarditis is higher in opiate addicts due to the use of contaminated needles. *(1:390–391)*

99. **(D)** Both alcoholism and opiate addiction tend to start in adolescence and young adulthood. Late onset of these addictions is relatively uncommon. *(1:386, 416;2:619–621,646–651)*

Answers 100 through 103 deal with sleep disorders. (1:570–574;2:704–708;3:352–354)

100. **(C)** Both nightmares and night terrors have peak incidence in the 3–6 year age group, with rapidly decreasing incidence thereafter. *(1:572–573;2:705–706; 3:353)*

101. **(B)** The subject with night terrors usually has total amnesia for the terror episodes on later awakening. The child with nightmares will recall the frightening dream. *(1:572–573;2:705–706;3:353)*

102. **(A)** Nightmares occur during REM sleep; night terrors manifest during stage 3–4 non-REM sleep. *(1:572–573;2:705–706;3:353)*

103. **(D)** Neither nightmares nor night terrors indicate emotional problems in a child. Parents can be reassured. When these sleep disturbances occur in adolescents and adults, they are more likely to indicate emotional problems. *(1:572–573;2:705–706; 3:353)*

104. **(D)** The patient using *disulfiram* (Antabuse) may develop toxic symptoms when exposed to any alcohol-containing compound, including aftershave, cough syrup, foods cooked in wine, and other often unsuspected day-to-day commodities. Disulfiram therapy requires unfailing compliance and a good memory. Patients can be given Antabuse under very careful supervision when there is hepatic impairment, but hepatic cirrhosis would certainly not be considered to be an indication for this treatment. *(1:297–298;2:639–640;3:237–238)*

105. **(C)** In patients with *psychogenic amnesia*, recovery of memory is typically abrupt and total. Amytal interview may recover otherwise inaccessible memories. Electroconvulsive therapy is not indicated. The patient with psychogenic amnesia is alert and in full contact with his or her environment. *(1:354;2:513;3:291–293)*

106. **(B)** In the treatment of alcohol withdrawal syndromes and *delirium tremens,* chlordiazepoxide or other benzodiazepines are used with a high-calorie, high-carbohydrate diet. Chlorpromazine lowers the seizure threshold, may be hepatotoxic, and is hypotensive so is contraindicated. Restraints also should not be used as the confused patient may become exhausted by struggling against them. *(1:418–420;2:626–631; 3:217–218)*

107. **(B)** In *alcoholic hallucinosis,* the patient is usually fearful and agitated, especially concerning the audi-

tory hallucinations that are present. Visual hallucinations usually do not occur. The patient is in a clear state of consciousness. *(1:420;2:633–635;3:218)*

108. **(A)** Symptoms similar to *panic attacks* may be caused by pheochromocytoma, hypoglycemia, and hyperthyroidism. Acute porphyria is more likely to produce confused or depressed states. *(1:309–310,319; 2:473–475;3:288)*

109. **(B)** *Paranoid personality disorder* is more common in deaf people. Subjects with this type of personality rarely seek treatment. Delusions that would indicate psychotic thinking do not occur in paranoid personality disorder, though the person is hypersensitive and overly jealous, but not delusional. Benzodiazepines are not indicated. *(1:365–367;2:445–446;3:330)*

110. **(E)** In *delirium* there is clouding of consciousness; perceptual distortions such as hallucinations are present; actively may be increased or decreased; and symptoms may fluctuate over the course of the day. *(1:273–276;2:140–142;3:214–215)*

111. **(E)** *Lithium* often causes annoying polyuria and polydipsia. Even in the therapeutic range, mild memory impairment and difficulty concentrating may be a problem. Acne may develop or worsen if already present. Lithium also causes fetal cardiac abnormalities when taken in the first trimester of pregnancy. *(1:675–678;2:830–831;3:128–129)*

112. **(C)** *Diazepam* is metabolized by hepatic oxidation and has long-acting metabolites. In the elderly, metabolic breakdown tends to be slower, so diazepam has a longer half-life. The medication persists longer in obese subjects. *(1:662–663;2:832;3:129–130)*

113. **(A)** *Abused children* are most often under age 3. Their parents often describe these children as being in some way different from their siblings and rationalize the abuse as being necessary discipline. Usually neither parent is psychotic. *(1:834–839;2:680–681)*

114. **(E)** *Dementia* may be caused by autoimmune deficiency syndrome, multiple sclerosis, pellagra, and Huntington's chorea. *(1:276–279;2:147;3:214–215)*

115. **(C)** In patients with *psychogenic amnesia,* hypnosis may show that the inaccessible memories are intact. The memory return is typically fairly sudden and complete. These patients show no impairment of consciousness and have no difficulty in making and retrieving new memories. *(1:354;2:513;3:291–293)*

116. **(B)** *Compliance* is better where there is a good doctor–patient relationship. Compliance is worse in more chronic illness and where patients are expected to take multiple doses. Poor compliance is very often a direct expression of the patient's psychopathology. *(1:879;2:816)*

117. **E.** Children with *attention deficit disorder* are much more commonly male. Impulsivity is a major symptom in this syndrome, as is difficulty maintaining attention at different tasks. Typically these symptoms are noted in the preschool years, though often these youngsters are not brought for evaluation until their disruptive classroom behavior causes a problem. *(1:741–774;2:681–683;3:187–190).*

118. **(B)** *Methylphenidate* may cause weight retardation and possibly height retardation. With this in mind, drug holidays during vacations and holidays are recommended. There does not appear to be a major risk of methylphenidate drug abuse in the teenage years; increasingly it is noted that a significant number of these patients continue to show symptoms and are benefited by methylphenidate in the adolescent and adult age years. *(1:744–745;2:682;3:189–190)*

119. **(C)** Examples of *primary prevention,* aimed at preventing the illness or disability from occurring, include rubella vaccinations and AIDS education in high school. *(1:876–877;2:788;3:140)*

120. **(D)** The *autistic* child has a more favorable prognosis when the young patient is able to converse meaningfully. These autistic youngsters are prone to be interested in mechanical play and in rigid organization, to the exclusion of interpersonal relationships. It is uncommon for other family members to present with infantile autism. *(1:732–737;2:693–694;3:201)*

121. **(E)** This is the classical picture of an *anticholinergic psychosis,* which can be produced by amitriptyline and the tricyclic antidepressants, thioridiazine and other neuroleptics, scopolamine and atropine derivatives, benztropine and the antiparkinsonian agents, especially when they are used together. *(1:588–589; 2:827;3:223–224)*

122. **(3)** *Acute intermittent porphyria* tends to start in teenagers and young adults and is more common in females. This illness may present as a depression, a confusional state, or with nervousness and irritability. Acute episodes may be precipitated by barbiturates and by oral contraceptives *(1:309–310;2:319–323; 3:228)*

123. **(D)** Neuroleptic malignant syndrome may be fatal. This syndrome is not precipitated by giving tyramine to patients taking monoamine oxidase inhibitors. Electroconvulsive therapy has been tried but found to be ineffective. Restarting the same neuroleptic may cause recurrence of the syndrome but frequently the neuroleptic malignant syndrome does not recur; under these circumstances the neuroleptic can be reintroduced under careful supervision. *(1:643)*

124. **(B)** *Lorazepam* and *oxazepam* are metabolized by glucuronide conjugation to inactive metabolites. Since they are more rapidly broken down and excreted, patients on these medications will show an acute onset of withdrawal symptoms. Hepatic oxidation, the metabolic process for diazepam, takes longer in the elderly, so patients over 60 using diazepam are more likely to experience problem side effects. *(1:662–665;2:832)*

125. **(D)** *Delirium* and *dementia* both produce disturbances of thinking, memory deficits, and disturbances of orientation. In dementia there is no clouding of consciousness, which is the hallmark of delirium. *(1:276; 2:140–142;146–147;3:214–215)*

126. **(A)** In childhood, during non-REM sleep, night terrors, sleepwalking, and enuresis may occur. Nightmares occur during REM-sleep. *(1:570–574;2:705–706;3:353)*

127. **(A)** An *anticholinergic psychosis* may be caused by imipramine, benztropine, and thioridazine. Physostigmine can be used to treat anticholinergic symptoms or, by producing symptomatic improvement, to confirm the diagnosis of an anticholinergic psychosis. *(1:588–589;2:827;3:223–224)*

128. **(B)** Anorexia nervosa and pregnancy may cause false positive results on the *dexamethasone test*. Addison's disease would produce a false negative test. *(1:243; 3:276–277)*

129. **(E)** A *catatonic syndrome* is commonly caused by neuroleptic toxicity but may also be a manifestation of major depression or schizophrenia. Since encephalitis and other neurological disorders may cause this syndrome, careful neurological examination is essential with catatonic patients *(1:214–215,646;2:391;3:248)*

130. **(C)** *Involuntary hospitalization* can be required and justified if the patient is gravely disabled emotionally or dangerous to others or himself or herself. Family consent is not required because this treatment decision is based on the patient's needs. Any licensed physician can initiate the process of involuntary hospitalization; an initial psychiatric evaluation is not required. *(1:891;2:852–855;3:150)*

131. **(C)** *Suicide risk* is greater where there have been prior suicide attempts. When a patient is deeply, overwhelmingly depressed, he or she is likely to be too immobilized by the depression to act suicidally. As the patient begins to improve, he or she may be less overwhelmed, less immobilized, but still deeply suicidal—and now more able to act on the suicidal feelings. Suicidal risk is higher in elderly patients. The risk of suicide is not increased when patients are asked directly about this possibility. *(1:575–580;2:118–121; 3:270–272)*

132. **(A)** *Tricyclic antidepressants* will cause anticholinergic side effects (dry mouth, constipation, and urinary problems) within the first week of treatment and, even at therapeutic levels, have quinidine-like effects on the heart. It is likely to take 2 to 3 weeks before there is significant mood elevation. Food-induced hypertensive crises do not occur with tricyclic antidepressants. *(1:654–656;2:826–828;3:110–124)*

133. **(D)** *Electroconvulsive therapy* would be a safe and efficient treatment. With careful management, age and hypertension do not contraindicate the use of electroconvulsive therapy. *(1:679–683;2:837;3:131)*

134. **(B)** *Lithium* passes through the placenta and produces a higher incidence of fetal cardiac defects. In nursing mothers, lithium passes through the breast milk to the nursing infant. Lithium does not produce a higher incidence of Turner's syndrome. *(1:676–677; 2:829–831;3:127)*

135. **(C)** To be able to make a legally valid will, to have *testamentary capacity,* the subject must know who his or her next of kin are and must know what he or she owns. Psychosis is not in itself a contraindication to testamentary capacity, nor is the inability to read and write, provided the subject fulfills the criteria above. *(1:893–894;2:859;3:152)*

136. **(B)** The *M'Naghten rule* says a subject is criminally responsible if, at the time of the act, he or she knew what he or she was doing and knew whether the act was right or wrong. *(1:894–895;2:864;3:153)*

137. **(C)** The highest incidence of *mental retardation* is in teenagers. Most mentally retarded youngsters are mildly retarded and only have major difficulties in school in the adolescent years. The encephalogram is not diagnostically helpful in most retarded children. *(1:711;2:716–717;3:159–160)*

138. **(E)** Under stress a preschool child may show *regressed behaviors* such as enuresis, encopresis, thumb sucking, and tantrums. *(1:839–840;2:694–695;3:204–205)*

139. **(C)** *Conversion disorder* frequently does coexist with physical illness. Symptoms often do not follow anatomical boundaries and may be perpetuated by secondary gain. La belle indifference is not diagnostic of a conversion disorder and may merely reflect a stoic or phlegmatic way of coping with symptoms. *(1:342–348;2:501–511;3:290)*

140. **(E)** *Enuresis* is more common in boys. There is often a higher incidence of enuresis in family members, especially males. Enuresis responds to conditioning devices and a range of other treatments. The symptom occurs during non-REM stage 3–4 sleep. *(1:843–846; 2:697–699;3:197–198)*

141. **(B)** *Somatoform disorders* include hypochondriasis, conversion disorders, and somatization disorder but not chronic factitious disorder nor psychogenic amnesia. *(1:339–340;2:496;3:289–291)*

142. **(C)** *Anorexia nervosa* is more common in people who jog and exercise. Patients with anorexia nervosa tend to overestimate their body size. They do not feel guilty or anxious when they do not eat and typically have reduced sexual interest. *(1:499–504;2:554–558;3:194–195)*

143. **(E)** Patients with anorexia nervosa are often deceitful about food. Their laxative abuse (and vomiting) may precipitate electrolyte imbalance. As in other starvation syndromes, the dexamethasone test is likely to be abnormal. In anorexia nervosa patients with an early age of onset, the prognosis tends to be better than those who develop the syndrome later in life. *(1:499–504; 2:554–558;3:194–195)*

144. **(A)** A patient with a *paranoid personality disorder* is likely to be emotionally cold and distant, mistrustful of others, and hypersensitive to fancied slights. These subjects do not show psychotic symptoms such as persecutory delusions. *(1:365–367;2:445–446;3:330)*

145. **(B)** *Suicidal risk* is increased when the patient is elderly, male, unmarried, or has a history of prior suicide attempts. Females attempt suicide more frequent, but males are more at risk for successful suicide. *(1:575–580;2:118–121;3:270–272)*

146. **(E)** Patients are more likely to be *violent* when they are demented, paranoid, or intoxicated. Usually patients can resist command hallucinations, but a minority of patients with this kind of perceptual distortion respond to the prompting and the commands of the voices. *(1:582–583;2:117–118)*

147. **(B)** Children develop a *conscience* through *incorporation,* a primitive form of total psychological internalization, and by *identification,* whereby the child selects aspects of another person's personality to internalize. Intellectualization and projection are not involved in basic conscience development. *(1:77;2:62–36;3:7)*

148. **(B)** In the management of *school refusal,* school phobia, early return to school is imperative. Assignment of a homebound teacher tends to perpetuate the school absence and may delay or make more difficult an eventual return to school. There should always be a careful evaluation of the school environment, the family situation, and the child to ascertain factors that might produce or maintain separation anxiety and fear. Methylphenidate is used in treating attention deficit disorder but is not indicated in school refusal. *(1:791–795;2:688;3:193)*

149. **(E)** *Phencyclidine intoxication* can cause extreme anxiety, tachycardia, blood pressure changes, nystagmus, catatonia, violent disruptive behavior, and florid psychosis. *(1:410–412;2:667;3:222)*

150. **(A)** *Chronic alcoholics treated with disulfiram* must be warned to avoid contact with any alcohol-containing substance, including food prepared with wine, aftershave, many cosmetics and cough syrups, and any alcohol-containing medication. Pyridoxine is used to treat the peripheral neuropathy that may develop in disulfiram users. *(1:297–298;2:639–640;3:237–238)*

151. **(A)** In the elderly, *depression* may coexist with dementia. Depression can also cause a "pseudodementia" syndrome. The incidence of suicide is highest in the elderly, especially in males. Depression in the elderly does respond to antidepressants, typically in lower than the usual adult dose. *(1:883;2:254; 3:272–280)*

Practice Test Subspecialty List

DEFINITIONS

2, 5, 9, 11, 25, 26, 28, 56, 57, 58, 59, 119, 147

PSYCHOLOGICAL TESTING

4, 16

CHILD AND ADOLESCENT PSYCHIATRY

7, 35, 36, 45, 46, 72, 79, 100, 101, 102, 103, 113, 117, 118, 120, 126, 137, 138, 140, 148

ADULT PSYCHOPATHOLOGY

1, 10, 17, 18, 19, 22, 23, 24, 27, 37, 38, 39, 41, 42, 43, 44, 48, 63, 64, 65, 68, 70, 71, 73, 74, 75, 76, 77, 81, 82, 83, 84, 85, 86, 87, 96, 97, 98, 99, 105, 106, 107, 108, 109, 110, 114, 115, 122, 125, 128, 129, 131, 139, 141, 142, 143, 144, 145, 146, 149, 150, 151

SOMATIC TREATMENTS

3, 6, 8, 12, 13, 14, 15, 21, 29, 30, 32, 33, 34, 40, 47, 49, 50, 51, 52, 53, 54, 55, 60, 61, 62, 66, 67, 69, 78, 80, 88, 89, 90, 91, 92, 93, 94, 95, 104, 111, 112, 121, 123, 124, 127, 132, 133, 134

PSYCHOLOGICAL TREATMENT AND MANAGEMENT

20, 116

SOCIAL PSYCHIATRY AND FORENSIC PSYCHIATRY

31, 130, 135, 136

NAME _____
         Last   First   Middle

ADDRESS _____
                    Street

_____
City   State   Zip

DIRECTIONS Mark your social security number from top to bottom in the appropriate boxes on the right. Refer to the section "HOW TO TAKE THE PRACTICE TEST" in the introduction to the book for more information. PLEASE USE NO.2 PENCIL ONLY.

MAKE ERASURES COMPLETE

SOC. SEC. NUMBER

	0 1 2 3 4 5 6 7 8 9
	0 1 2 3 4 5 6 7 8 9
	0 1 2 3 4 5 6 7 8 9
	0 1 2 3 4 5 6 7 8 9
	0 1 2 3 4 5 6 7 8 9
	0 1 2 3 4 5 6 7 8 9
	0 1 2 3 4 5 6 7 8 9
	0 1 2 3 4 5 6 7 8 9
	0 1 2 3 4 5 6 7 8 9

PAGE 1 2
TYPE 1 2 3

1 A B C D E   2 A B C D E   3 A B C D E   4 A B C D E   5 A B C D E   6 A B C D E   7 A B C D E   8 A B C D E

9 A B C D E   10 A B C D E   11 A B C D E   12 A B C D E   13 A B C D E   14 A B C D E   15 A B C D E   16 A B C D E

17 A B C D E   18 A B C D E   19 A B C D E   20 A B C D E   21 A B C D E   22 A B C D E   23 A B C D E   24 A B C D E

25 A B C D E   26 A B C D E   27 A B C D E   28 A B C D E   29 A B C D E   30 A B C D E   31 A B C D E   32 A B C D E

33 A B C D E   34 A B C D E   35 A B C D E   36 A B C D E   37 A B C D E   38 A B C D E   39 A B C D E   40 A B C D E

41 A B C D E   42 A B C D E   43 A B C D E   44 A B C D E   45 A B C D E   46 A B C D E   47 A B C D E   48 A B C D E

49 A B C D E   50 A B C D E   51 A B C D E   52 A B C D E   53 A B C D E   54 A B C D E   55 A B C D E   56 A B C D E

57 A B C D E   58 A B C D E   59 A B C D E   60 A B C D E   61 A B C D E   62 A B C D E   63 A B C D E   64 A B C D E

65 A B C D E   66 A B C D E   67 A B C D E   68 A B C D E   69 A B C D E   70 A B C D E   71 A B C D E   72 A B C D E

73 A B C D E   74 A B C D E   75 A B C D E   76 A B C D E   77 A B C D E   78 A B C D E   79 A B C D E   80 A B C D E

81 A B C D E   82 A B C D E   83 A B C D E   84 A B C D E   85 A B C D E   86 A B C D E   87 A B C D E   88 A B C D E

89 A B C D E   90 A B C D E   91 A B C D E   92 A B C D E   93 A B C D E   94 A B C D E   95 A B C D E   96 A B C D E

97 A B C D E   98 A B C D E   99 A B C D E   100 A B C D E   101 A B C D E   102 A B C D E   103 A B C D E   104 A B C D E

105 A B C D E   106 A B C D E   107 A B C D E   108 A B C D E   109 A B C D E   110 A B C D E   111 A B C D E   112 A B C D E

113 A B C D E   114 A B C D E   115 A B C D E   116 A B C D E   117 A B C D E   118 A B C D E   119 A B C D E   120 A B C D E

121 A B C D E   122 A B C D E   123 A B C D E   124 A B C D E   125 A B C D E   126 A B C D E   127 A B C D E   128 A B C D E

129 A B C D E   130 A B C D E   131 A B C D E   132 A B C D E   133 A B C D E   134 A B C D E   135 A B C D E   136 A B C D E

137 A B C D E   138 A B C D E   139 A B C D E   140 A B C D E   141 A B C D E   142 A B C D E   143 A B C D E   144 A B C D E

145 A B C D E   146 A B C D E   147 A B C D E   148 A B C D E   149 A B C D E   150 A B C D E   151 A B C D E   152 A B C D E

153 A B C D E   154 A B C D E   155 A B C D E   156 A B C D E   157 A B C D E   158 A B C D E   159 A B C D E   160 A B C D E

S O C
N U M B E R
S E C

	0	1	2	3	4	5	6	7	8	9
	0	1	2	3	4	5	6	7	8	9
	0	1	2	3	4	5	6	7	8	9
	0	1	2	3	4	5	6	7	8	9
	0	1	2	3	4	5	6	7	8	9
	0	1	2	3	4	5	6	7	8	9
	0	1	2	3	4	5	6	7	8	9
	0	1	2	3	4	5	6	7	8	9
	0	1	2	3	4	5	6	7	8	9
	0	1	2	3	4	5	6	7	8	9

PAGE 1 2
TYPE 1 2 3

161 A B C D E 162 A B C D E 163 A B C D E 164 A B C D E 165 A B C D E 166 A B C D E 167 A B C D E 168 A B C D E

169 A B C D E 170 A B C D E 171 A B C D E 172 A B C D E 173 A B C D E 174 A B C D E 175 A B C D E 176 A B C D E

177 A B C D E 178 A B C D E 179 A B C D E 180 A B C D E 181 A B C D E 182 A B C D E 183 A B C D E 184 A B C D E

185 A B C D E 186 A B C D E 187 A B C D E 188 A B C D E 189 A B C D E 190 A B C D E 191 A B C D E 192 A B C D E

193 A B C D E 194 A B C D E 195 A B C D E 196 A B C D E 197 A B C D E 198 A B C D E 199 A B C D E 200 A B C D E

201 A B C D E 202 A B C D E 203 A B C D E 204 A B C D E 205 A B C D E 206 A B C D E 207 A B C D E 208 A B C D E

209 A B C D E 210 A B C D E 211 A B C D E 212 A B C D E 213 A B C D E 214 A B C D E 215 A B C D E 216 A B C D E

217 A B C D E 218 A B C D E 219 A B C D E 220 A B C D E 221 A B C D E 222 A B C D E 223 A B C D E 224 A B C D E

225 A B C D E 226 A B C D E 227 A B C D E 228 A B C D E 229 A B C D E 230 A B C D E 231 A B C D E 232 A B C D E

233 A B C D E 234 A B C D E 235 A B C D E 236 A B C D E 237 A B C D E 238 A B C D E 239 A B C D E 240 A B C D E

241 A B C D E 242 A B C D E 243 A B C D E 244 A B C D E 245 A B C D E 246 A B C D E 247 A B C D E 248 A B C D E

249 A B C D E 250 A B C D E 251 A B C D E 252 A B C D E 253 A B C D E 254 A B C D E 255 A B C D E 256 A B C D E

257 A B C D E 258 A B C D E 259 A B C D E 260 A B C D E 261 A B C D E 262 A B C D E 263 A B C D E 264 A B C D E

265 A B C D E 266 A B C D E 267 A B C D E 268 A B C D E 269 A B C D E 270 A B C D E 271 A B C D E 272 A B C D E

273 A B C D E 274 A B C D E 275 A B C D E 276 A B C D E 277 A B C D E 278 A B C D E 279 A B C D E 280 A B C D E

281 A B C D E 282 A B C D E 283 A B C D E 284 A B C D E 285 A B C D E 286 A B C D E 287 A B C D E 288 A B C D E

289 A B C D E 290 A B C D E 291 A B C D E 292 A B C D E 293 A B C D E 294 A B C D E 295 A B C D E 296 A B C D E

297 A B C D E 298 A B C D E 299 A B C D E 300 A B C D E 301 A B C D E 302 A B C D E 303 A B C D E 304 A B C D E

305 A B C D E 306 A B C D E 307 A B C D E 308 A B C D E 309 A B C D E 310 A B C D E 311 A B C D E 312 A B C D E

313 A B C D E 314 A B C D E 315 A B C D E 316 A B C D E 317 A B C D E 318 A B C D E 319 A B C D E 320 A B C D E

The History of
The Church

Didache Series

— SEMESTER EDITION —

The Didache

[DID-uh-kay]

The *Didache* is the first known Christian catechesis. Written in the first century, the *Didache* is the earliest known Christian writing outside of Scripture. The name of the work, "*Didache*," is indeed appropriate for such a catechesis because it comes from the Greek word for "teaching," and indicates that this writing contains the teaching of the Apostles.

The *Didache* is a catechetical summary of Christian Sacraments, practices, and morality. Though written in the first century, its teaching is timeless. The *Didache* was probably written by the disciples of the Twelve Apostles, and it presents the Apostolic Faith as taught by those closest to Jesus Christ. This series of books takes the name of this early catechesis because it shares in the Church's mission of passing on that same Faith, in its rich entirety, to new generations.

Below is an excerpt from the *Didache* in which we see a clear example of its lasting message, a message that speaks to Christians of today as much as it did to the first generations of the Church. The world is different, but the struggle for holiness is the same. In the *Didache*, we are instructed to embrace virtue, to avoid sin, and to live the Beatitudes of our Lord.

My child, flee from every evil thing, and from every likeness of it. Be not prone to anger, for anger leads the way to murder; neither jealous, nor quarrelsome, nor of hot temper; for out of all these murders are engendered.

My child, be not a lustful one; for lust leads the way to fornication; neither a filthy talker, nor of lofty eye; for out of all these adulteries are engendered.

My child, be not an observer of omens, since it leads the way to idolatry; neither an enchanter, nor an astrologer, nor a purifier, nor be willing to took at these things; for out of all these idolatry is engendered.

My child, be not a liar, since a lie leads the way to theft; neither money-loving, nor vainglorious, for out of all these thefts are engendered.

My child, be not a murmurer, since it leads the way to blasphemy; neither self-willed nor evil-minded, for out of all these blasphemies are engendered.

But be meek, since the meek shall inherit the earth.

Be long-suffering and pitiful and guileless and gentle and good and always trembling at the words which you have heard.[1]

The *Didache* is the teaching of the Apostles and, as such, it is the teaching of the Church. Accordingly, this book series makes extensive use of the most recent comprehensive catechesis provided to us, the *Catechism of the Catholic Church*. The *Didache* series also relies heavily on Sacred Scripture, the lives of the saints, the Fathers of the Church, and the teaching of Vatican II as witnessed by the pontificates of St. John Paul II, Benedict XVI, and Francis.

1. "The Didache," *Ante-Nicene Fathers*, vol. 7. tr. M.B. Riddle. ed. Alexander Roberts, James Donaldson, and A. Cleveland Coxe (Buffalo, NY: Christian Literature Publishing Co., 1886).

The History of
The Church

SEMESTER EDITION

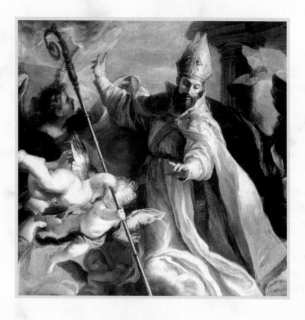

Author: Rev. Peter V. Armenio
Publisher: Rev. James Socias

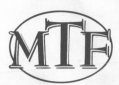

MIDWEST THEOLOGICAL FORUM
Downers Grove, Illinois

Published in the United States of America by

Midwest Theological Forum
4340 Cross Street, Suite 1,
Downers Grove, IL 60515
www.theologicalforum.org

Copyright © 2010–2017 Rev. James Socias
ISBN Hardcover 978-1-936045-15-0
ISBN Paperback 978-1-939231-75-8
First Edition

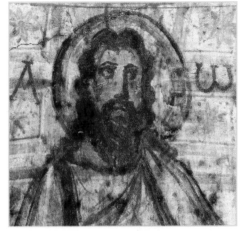

Jesus the Alpha and Omega. Fourth-century wall
painting from the Catacombs of Commodilla, Rome, Italy.

Nihil Obstat
Reverend Martin A. Zielinski, Ph.D.
Censor Deputatus
June 6, 2005

Imprimatur
Reverend George J. Rassas
Vicar General
Archdiocese of Chicago
June 7, 2005

Author: Rev. Peter V. Armenio
Publisher: Rev. James Socias
Editor in Chief: Jeffrey Cole
Editorial Board: Rev. James Socias, Dr. Scott Hahn, Rev. Peter V. Armenio, Mike Aquilina, Jeffrey Cole
Other Contributors: Dan Cheely, Joseph Lechner, Joseph Linn, Russell Shaw, John Shine, Peter Simek
Design and Production: Marlene Burrell, Jane Heineman of April Graphics, Highland Park, Illinois,
Jerzy Miszczyszyn of Lyndon Studio, Downers Grove, Illinois

Acknowledgements

English translation of the *Catechism of the Catholic Church* for the United States of America copyright ©1994, United States Catholic Conference,
Inc.–Libreria Editrice Vaticana. English translation of the *Catechism of the Catholic Church: Modifications from the Editio Typica* copyright ©1997,
United States Catholic Conference, Inc.–Libreria Editrice Vaticana.

Scripture quotations are from the Catholic Edition of the *Revised Standard Version of the Bible*, copyright ©1965, 1966, National Council of the
Churches of Christ in the United States of America. Used by permission. All rights reserved.

Excerpts from the Code of Canon Law, Latin/English Edition, are used with permission, copyright ©1983 Canon Law Society of America, Washington, D.C.

Citations of official Church documents from Neuner, Josef, SJ, and Dupuis, Jacques, SJ, eds., *The Christian Faith: Doctrinal Documents of the
Catholic Church*, 5th ed. (New York: Alba House, 1992). Used with permission.

Excerpts from *Vatican Council II: The Conciliar and Post Conciliar Documents*, New Revised Edition edited by Austin Flannery, O.P., copyright
©1992, Costello Publishing Company, Inc., Northport, NY, are used by permission of the publisher, all rights reserved. No part of these excerpts
may be reproduced, stored in a retrieval system, or transmitted in any form or by any means – electronic, mechanical, photocopying, recording or
otherwise, without express permission of Costello Publishing Company.

*Disclaimer: The editor of this book has attempted to give proper credit to all sources used in the text and illustrations.
Any miscredit or lack of credit is unintended and will be corrected in the next edition.*

Library of Congress Cataloging-in-Publication Data

Armenio, Peter V.
 The history of the church / author, Peter V. Armenio; general editor, James Socías. -- Semester ed.
  p. cm.
 Originally published: 1st ed. c2001, in series: The Didache series.
 Includes index.
 ISBN 978-1-936045-15-0
 1. Catholic Church--History--Textbooks. 2. Christian education--Textbooks for teenagers--Catholic. I. Socías, James. II. Title.
 BX948.A76 2010
 270--dc22   2010018590

Printed in Canada

CONTENTS

CONTENTS

CONTENTS

CONTENTS

CONTENTS

CONTENTS

CONTENTS

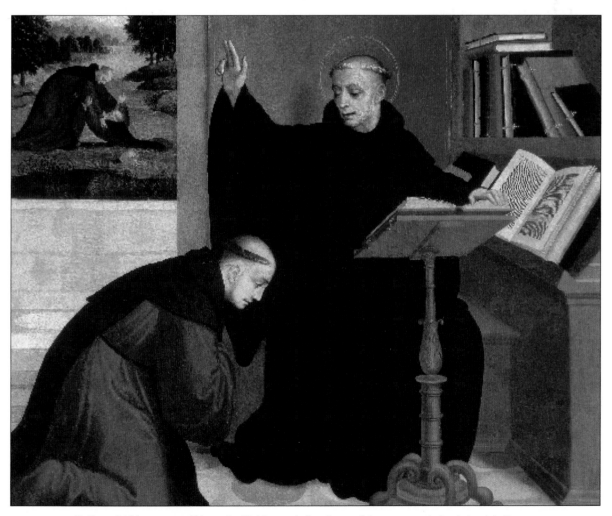

St. Benedict blesses one of his pupils, St. Maurus, before the monk leaves on a mission to teach in France.
In the background is an event from St. Maurus's life when he saved a drowning boy named Placid by walking on the water.

ABBREVIATIONS USED FOR THE BOOKS OF THE BIBLE

OLD TESTAMENT

Genesis	Gen	Tobit	Tb	Hosea	Hos
Exodus	Ex	Judith	Jdt	Joel	Jl
Leviticus	Lv	Esther	Est	Amos	Am
Numbers	Nm	Job	Jb	Obadiah	Ob
Deuteronomy	Dt	Psalms	Ps(s)	Jonah	Jon
Joshua	Jos	Proverbs	Prv	Micah	Mi
Judges	Jgs	Ecclesiastes	Eccl	Nahum	Na
Ruth	Ru	Song of Songs	Sg	Habakkuk	Hab
1 Samuel	1 Sm	Wisdom	Wis	Zephaniah	Zep
2 Samuel	2 Sm	Sirach	Sir	Haggai	Hg
1 Kings	1 Kgs	Isaiah	Is	Zechariah	Zec
2 Kings	2 Kgs	Jeremiah	Jer	Malachi	Mal
1 Chronicles	1 Chr	Lamentations	Lam	1 Maccabees	1 Mc
2 Chronicles	2 Chr	Baruch	Bar	2 Maccabees	2 Mc
Ezra	Ezr	Ezekiel	Ez		
Nehemiah	Neh	Daniel	Dn		

NEW TESTAMENT

Matthew	Mt	Ephesians	Eph	Hebrews	Heb
Mark	Mk	Philippians	Phil	James	Jas
Luke	Lk	Colossians	Col	1 Peter	1 Pt
John	Jn	1 Thessalonians	1 Thes	2 Peter	2 Pt
Acts of the Apostles	Acts	2 Thessalonians	2 Thes	1 John	1 Jn
Romans	Rom	1 Timothy	1 Tm	2 John	2 Jn
1 Corinthians	1 Cor	2 Timothy	2 Tm	3 John	3 Jn
2 Corinthians	2 Cor	Titus	Ti	Jude	Jud
Galatians	Gal	Philemon	Phlm	Revelation	Rv

GENERAL ABBREVIATIONS

AA	Apostolicam actuositatem	GS	Gaudium et spes
AAS	Acta Apostolica Sedis	HV	Humanae vitæ
AG	Ad gentes	IOE	Instruction on Euthanasia
CA	Centesimus annus	LE	Laborem exercens
CCC	The Catechism of the Catholic Church	LG	Lumen gentium
CCEO	Corpus Canonum Ecclesiarum Orientalium	LH	Liturgy of the Hours
CDF	Congregation for the Doctrine of the Faith	MF	Mysterium fidei
CHCW	Charter for Health Care Workers	MM	Mater et magistra
CIC	Codex Iuris Canonici (The Code of Canon Law)	ND	Neuner-Dupuis, The Christian Faith in the Doctrinal Documents of the Catholic Church
CL	Christifidelis laici	OC	Ordo confirmationis
CPG	Solemn Profession of Faith: Credo of the People of God	OCM	Ordo celebrandi Matrimonium
		OP	Ordo paenitentiæ
DD	Dies Domini	PG	J. P. Migne, ed., Patrologia Græca (Paris, 1857-1866)
DRF	Declaration on Religious Freedom		
DH	Dignitatis humanæ	PH	Persona humanæ
DIM	Decree Inter mirifici	PL	J. P. Migne, ed., Patrologia Latina (Paris, 1841-1855)
DoV	Donum vitæ		
DPA	Declaration on Procured Abortion	PP	Populorum progressio
DS	Denzinger-Schönmetzer, Enchiridion Symbolorum, definitionum et declarationum de rebus fidei et morum (1965)	PT	Pacem in terris
		RH	Redemptor Hominis
		RP	Reconciliatio et pænitentia
DV	Dei verbum	SC	Sacrosanctum concilium
EN	Evangeli nuntiadi	SD	Salvifici doloris
EV	Evangelium vitæ	SRS	Solicitudo rei socialis
FC	Familiaris consortio	STh	Summa Theologiæ
GCD	General Catechetical Directory	VS	Veritatis splendor

FOREWORD

"Jesus Christ is the key."

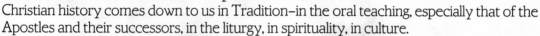
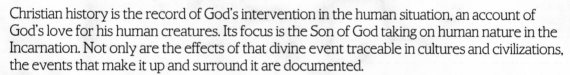

It has been said that to try to do without history is to cease to be Catholic. Faith in Jesus Christ is based on events that have happened and have been witnessed in written records. The truth embodied in the Christian faith came to us from outside ourselves as a revelation. Much more than a reflection or personal experience, the truths of our faith are objective and are reliably handed on.

Much of this Christian story is therefore found in written documents–the Bible, the writings of the Church Fathers, the decisions of early Church councils. Christian history comes down to us in Tradition–in the oral teaching, especially that of the Apostles and their successors, in the liturgy, in spirituality, in culture.

Christian history is the record of God's intervention in the human situation, an account of God's love for his human creatures. Its focus is the Son of God taking on human nature in the Incarnation. Not only are the effects of that divine event traceable in cultures and civilizations, the events that make it up and surround it are documented.

Because Jesus was truly God as well as truly man, human history can take us only so far; faith goes beyond that point to tell us the meaning of the Christ event. The Christ of history is the ground for the Christ of faith; the Christ of faith brings ultimate meaning to the Christ of history. There is only one Christ of God. "Jesus Christ is the key, the center and the purpose of the whole of human history" (Vatican II: *Gaudium et Spes* 10), because in him the boundless mystery of God is manifested in the world.

The Incarnation happened in history as a divine-human event and it continues and is extended in the form of the Church, in her sacraments, in the Eucharist, in her mission. It is a deeply human story of the best and the worst in the human situation; in the end, it is always the story of the victory of grace and of the destiny of humanity.

The Didache Series is remarkably complete and, with this volume, it integrates divine revelation and the story of the Church in light of sound human scholarship. I recommend it warmly for use in the high schools and colleges of the Archdiocese of Chicago.

✠Francis Cardinal George, O.M.I.
Archbishop of Chicago

INTRODUCTION

"Be not afraid!"

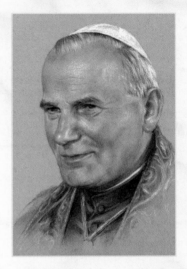

The world is waiting for a new era of holiness among the laity. When St. John Paul II came on to the balcony of St. Peter's Basilica in Rome and spoke about his acceptance of a heavy burden, he declared that no one should be afraid to open the doors of our hearts to the Redeemer. These words became a rallying cry throughout his pontificate. In the midst of an all-pervading moral relativism and dissent within the Church, expressed in a culture of death, the Holy Spirit, through his Pope, has tapped into hidden desires for holiness and spiritual renewal, especially among the laity.

The twenty-first century is calling for a type of Christianity that was practiced during the first few centuries of the Church's history. The signs of the times call for new age of holiness and martyrdom. In a sense the Holy Spirit is moving the laity to put on a repeat performance of what the earliest Christians accomplished almost seventeen centuries ago when they brought the pagan Roman world literally to its knees.

In order to properly understand the fundamental nature of this new evangelization, however, one must be firmly grounded in the history of the Church. For example, if the People of God are being called to a new age of holiness and martyrdom closer to that of the early Church, one must understand what the early Church was. *The History of The Church* is an account of Christian history based solidly on historical fact viewed through the eyes of Faith; students will see both her visible and her spiritual reality as bearer of divine life. The book delves deeply into the heroic lives of the saints and the tremendous achievements of the Church, and will bring those who read it to a deeper understanding of Christ and his calling for a new evangelization.

Two thousand years ago, Christ invited a handful of followers to bring the Gospel message to a world diametrically opposed to everything it stood for. Reading the first chapter of St. Paul's Epistle to the Romans gives an idea of the challenges faced by the early Christians. The task seemed impossible — if not sheer madness! — given the moral corruption, the dislike for matters spiritual, and the deification of the emperor and the state if it were not for Christ's assurance of victory. They indeed believed in Christ's word and accomplished a feat that defies any possible human explanation.

We are now in a new springtime of Christianity, perhaps the same springtime experienced by our first brothers and sisters in the Faith, who generously laid down their lives for Christ. As St. John Paul II habitually recommended, let us resolve to go to the Mother of God so each of us can meet the challenge to extend the Kingdom of God and shoulder the burden of the Church's mission to bring salvation to all.

The Founding Of The Church And The Early Christians

"Christ is the Spouse and Savior of the Church…
The more we come to know and love the Church,
the nearer we shall be to Christ."

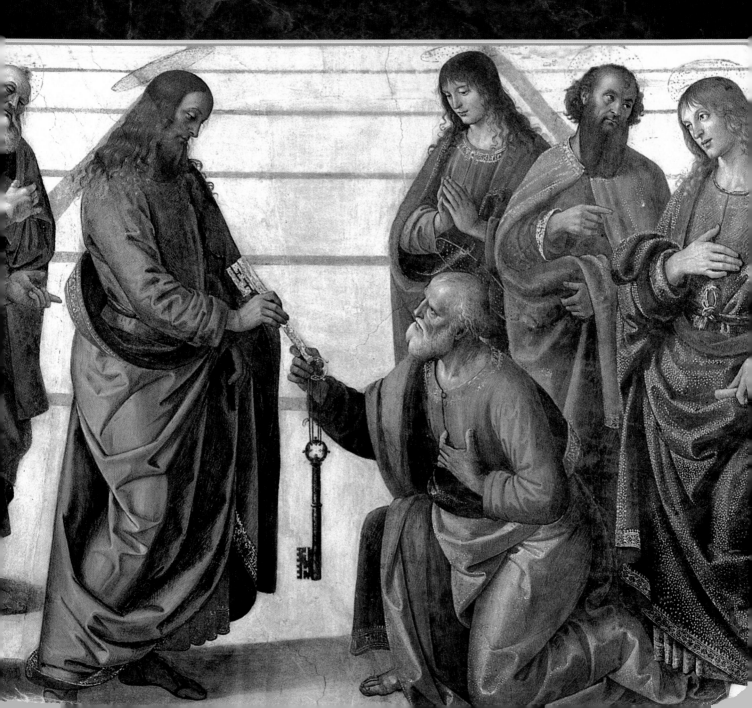

CHAPTER 1

The Founding Of The Church And The Early Christians

In the days directly following the crucifixion of Jesus, his disciples were afraid. The Sanhedrin had condemned their Master to death, and the disciples believed that they would be the next targets of persecution. Since they no longer had Jesus to guide them, they feared for their safety and were uncertain of the future, being for the first time without their leader. At first the Resurrection appearances only increased doubt and fear among the disciples. Though their Master had returned to them, He remained among them for only a short time. After the Ascension into Heaven, the Apostles, Mary, and other followers of Jesus were again suddenly alone.

But God did not leave his infant Church alone and unguided. Before departing, Christ declared to his disciples that they would soon receive the Holy Spirit. Ten days later, on the Jewish feast of Pentecost, the Holy Spirit descended upon the disciples, and subsequently resolved all their doubts, fears, and worries. The Apostles, through the power of the Holy Spirit, were certain that the Church of Christ would stand throughout all time as a living sacrament of his love, truth, and power. Christ is the cornerstone of his Church, and St. Peter is "the rock," Christ's vicar, upon whom the Church would be built. In the years following the Resurrection, the Apostles, filled with the grace of the Holy Spirit, boldly set about the great task of building the Church. They proclaimed the Good News that the long-awaited messiah had come and that he had paid in full the terrible price required for the redemption of all mankind. Christianity began to spread quickly through the ardent and intrepid preaching of the disciples. They carried the message of salvation proclaimed by Jesus all over the known world. Thus began the history of Christianity – a unique history that, simply stated, reflects Christ's constant presence in the world through the Church and how he interfaces with human history. The history of the Church is a record of the life and actions of men and women under the guiding light of the Holy Spirit acting in the Church. This narrative about the development of Christ's kingdom on earth is forged as the Church interacts and responds to every culture and historical situation.

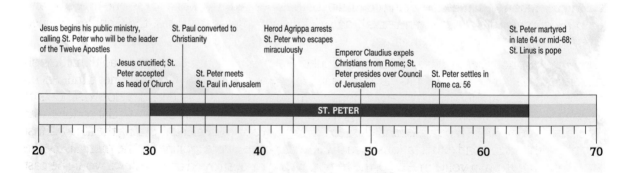

Jesus begins his public ministry, calling St. Peter who will be the leader of the Twelve Apostles

Jesus crucified; St. Peter accepted as head of Church

St. Paul converted to Christianity

St. Peter meets St. Paul in Jerusalem

Herod Agrippa arrests St. Peter who escapes miraculously

Emperor Claudius expels Christians from Rome; St. Peter presides over Council of Jerusalem

St. Peter settles in Rome ca. 56

St. Peter martyred in late 64 or mid-68; St. Linus is pope

ST. PETER

20   30   40   50   60   70

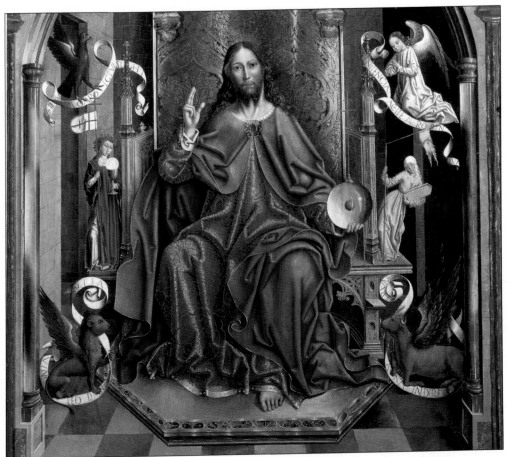

Christ is the cornerstone of his Church, and St. Peter is "the rock," Christ's vicar, upon whom the Church would be built.

PART I

The Jews

The history of the Jewish people is particular to the ancient world. Besides being monotheistic, the Jewish people believed that they had a special role in God's providential plans to serve as his chosen people. One of the unique characteristics of the chosen people was their realization of a personal God. A long history of suffering and oppression molded a people whose faith stimulated their expectation for a messiah. Being cognizant of their obligation to worship the one true God and keep his commandments, they shunned the religions and immoral ways of the Gentiles, typified especially by the Greeks and Romans.

The Jewish world of Jesus was a crossroads of cultures, under Hellenist, Latin, and traditional Jewish influences. This Jewish culture was different than the one depicted in the Old Testament. Influenced by Greek thought and ideas, many new groups of scholars, priests, and ascetics developed schools of Jewish theology. Roman, not Mosaic Law governed society, and despite some special concessions for worship, Jews were held as second class to the Roman citizens. Palestine during the life of Christ was rife with tension and expectations as many Jewish groups were looking for the messiah to free Israel from the Roman yoke. In AD 70, the temple would be destroyed and the Jews would be cast out of Jerusalem.

PART II

The Life of Jesus Christ

Jesus of Nazareth was born in Bethlehem in Judea around the year 4 BC In the humblest of surroundings, the Word of God became Incarnate; love and mercy found perfect expression, and the vessel of God's salvation was born into human history. The foundational principles of Christianity were present there in the quiet little stable in Bethlehem with Jesus, Mary, and Joseph. Peace, simplicity, material poverty, spiritual abundance, God's love, and sacrifice are the chief message of Christ's birth.

The Bible only records a few key events concerning Jesus' childhood. One of them is the Presentation in the Temple. After the birth of Christ, in accordance with the Jewish Law, Joseph and Mary took Jesus to the Temple in Jerusalem to be consecrated to God. Through the power of the Holy Spirit, an old man named Simeon, to whom it had been revealed that he should not die until he had seen the messiah, recognized the Infant, blessed his parents, and spoke of Jesus' destiny. Anna, an elderly prophetess, was also present and, recognizing the messiah, began to speak about the child to all who were waiting for him (Lk 2:22-39).

Shortly after the birth of Jesus, Joseph was warned in a dream by an angel that Herod, the King of Judea, had learned of the birth of the messiah and planned to murder the baby. The angel instructed Joseph to flee to Egypt with Mary and Jesus immediately, so that the Holy Child would escape Herod's wrath. When Herod failed to discover the precise location of Jesus, he sent his soldiers to kill every male child in Bethlehem aged two and under. Known as the "Slaughter of the Innocents," this dreadful massacre was the first shedding of blood among countless unnamed martyrs for the Christian Faith (Mt 2:16-18). After some time in Egypt, an angel appeared to Joseph in a second dream, telling him that it was safe for the Holy Family to return to Israel. Ever obedient, Joseph began the journey back to Israel with Jesus and Mary. Upon hearing that Herod's son Archelaus was now king of Judea, Joseph did not return there, but went to Galilee instead, and settled his family in Nazareth (Mt 2:19-23).

After the Holy Family returned to Nazareth, the Gospels record very little of their lives. One can assume that their lives were very ordinary, consisting of work, observance of the Jewish Law, finding joy in the company of one another and of their friends. Joseph was a carpenter, and Jesus most likely trained in the trade of his father, learning to work with wood and build with his hands. Until the beginning of His public ministry, the only event the Gospels describe is the finding of the twelve-year-old Jesus speaking with the elders in the Temple in Jerusalem. The Holy Family traveled to Jerusalem for the feast of the Passover, and when they set out to return home, Jesus was lost for three days. After frantically looking for their son, his parents finally discovered the child Jesus in the temple, which the boy called his "Father's house." The young Jesus was confidently conversing with the elders, whom he astounded with his wisdom and understanding (Lk 2:41-52).

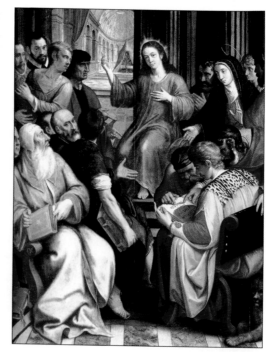

PALESTINE IN THE TIME OF CHRIST

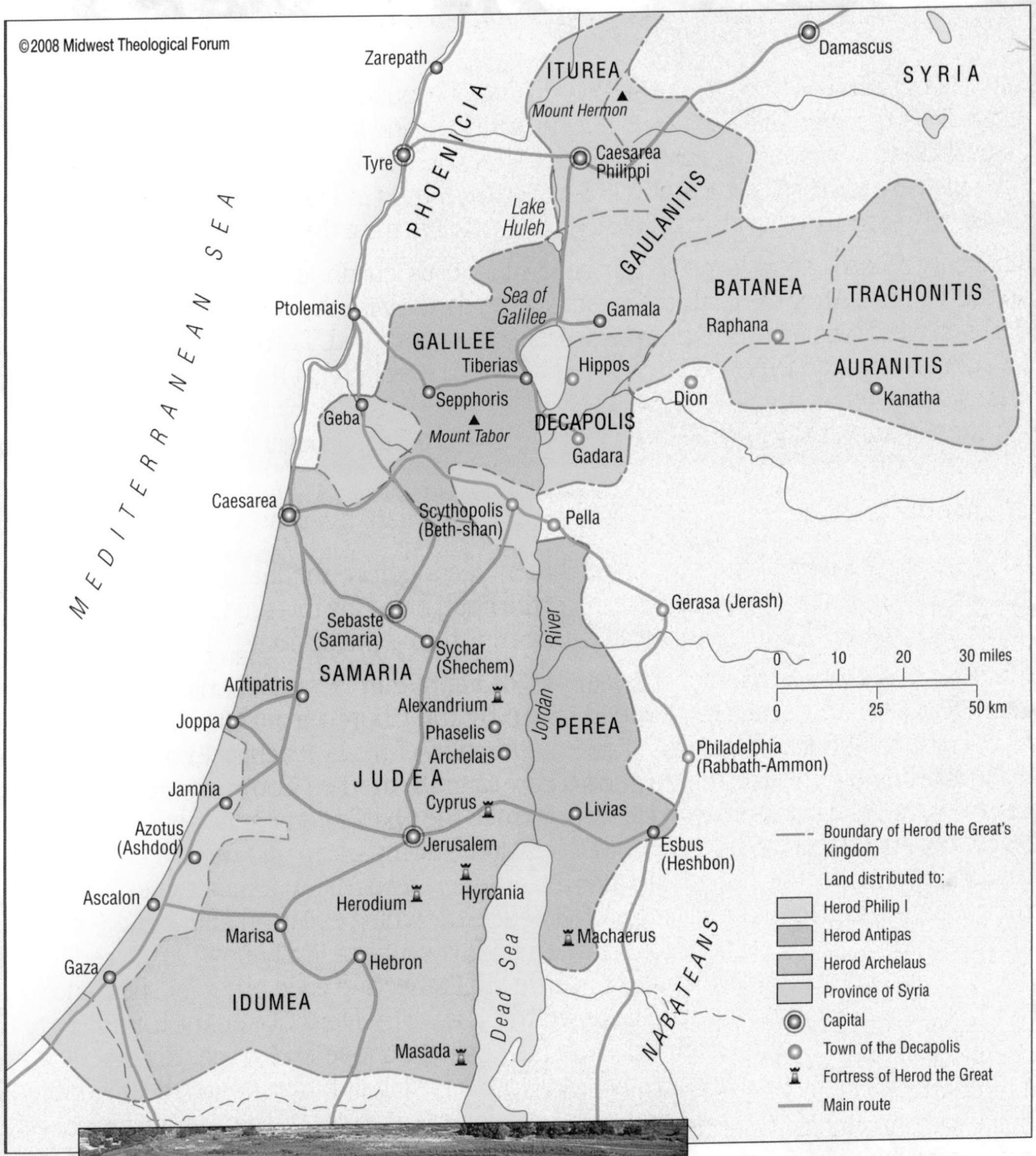

©2008 Midwest Theological Forum

Zarepath

ITUREA
Mount Hermon

Damascus

S Y R I A

Tyre

P H O E N I C I A

Lake
Huleh

Caesarea
Philippi

G A U L A N I T I S

Ptolemais

Sea of
Galilee

Gamala

BATANEA

Raphana

TRACHONITIS

GALILEE

Tiberias

Hippos

AURANITIS

Kanatha

Sepphoris

Dion

Geba

Mount Tabor

DECAPOLIS

Gadara

M E D I T E R R A N E A N   S E A

Caesarea

Scythopolis
(Beth-shan)

Pella

Gerasa (Jerash)

Sebaste
(Samaria)

Sychar
(Shechem)

SAMARIA

Antipatris

Alexandrium

Joppa

Phaselis

Archelais

PEREA

Philadelphia
(Rabbath-Ammon)

Jamnia

J U D E A

Cyprus

Livias

Azotus
(Ashdod)

Jerusalem

Esbus
(Heshbon)

Ascalon

Herodium

Hyrcania

Marisa

Hebron

Machaerus

Gaza

IDUMEA

Masada

Jordan River

Dead Sea

N A B A T E A N S

0   10   20   30 miles
0   25   50 km

---- Boundary of Herod the Great's
Kingdom

Land distributed to:

Herod Philip I

Herod Antipas

Herod Archelaus

Province of Syria

◎ Capital

○ Town of the Decapolis

Fortress of Herod the Great

—— Main route

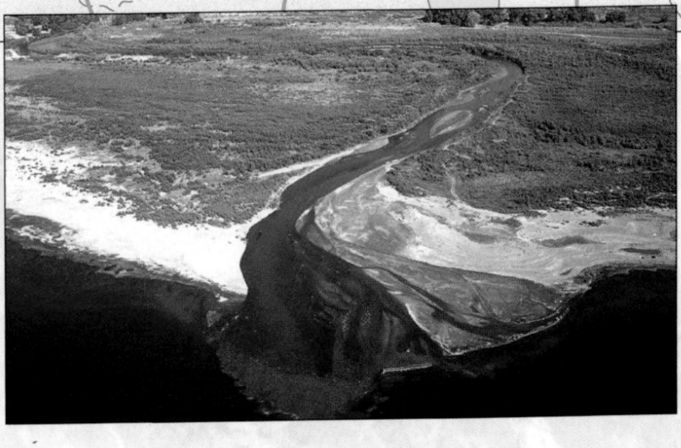

The Jordan River
entering the
Sea of Galilee

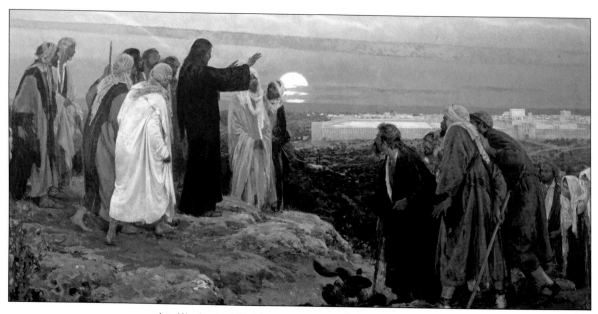

Jesus' New Law taught his followers to love their enemies and to avoid violence.

Following this event, there is a period of eighteen years before the inaugural event of his public ministry: Jesus' Baptism at the hands of St. John the Baptist. During this time it is recorded that Jesus spent time in the desert fasting, praying, and preparing for his public ministry.

Jesus' teaching constitutes part of the Deposit of Faith, that is the heritage of Faith contained in Sacred Scripture and Tradition, handed down by the Church from the time of the Apostles (cf. CCC 84, 1202). The most concise and direct collection of Jesus' teaching is given at the Sermon on the Mount (Mt 5-7). Fulfilling the traditional Law found in the Ten Commandments, Jesus taught the Beatitudes and the Lord's Prayer. He transformed the Old Testament notion of justice, fulfilling and perfecting it with the call to charity, which includes compassion and mercy. In contrast to the Old Law, expressed by the rule of "an eye for an eye," Jesus' New Law taught his followers to love their enemies and to avoid all forms of violence, drowning evil in an abundance of good. The institution of mercy to the point of loving one's enemies was radically new. Jesus redirected the spirit of worship, instructing his followers to serve the Father and each other in "spirit and in truth," thereby rejecting a legalistic interpretation of the Law. The New Covenant founded by Christ would perfect the Old Law through the New Law based on love and grace. His teaching and his many miracles – from the wedding feast at Cana to the raising of Lazarus – laid the groundwork for the contents of the Catholic Faith that would develop in response to the circumstances of every time period.

Jesus' teachings were brought to their fulfillment through the example of Christ's suffering, death, and Resurrection. Around the year AD 33, Jesus and his followers went to Jerusalem to participate in the celebration of the Jewish Passover. Despite his initial warm welcome on Palm Sunday, the Jewish leaders mounted a major opposition against Jesus. They charged him with heresy and blasphemy, but finally they accused Jesus of being insubordinate to Caesar in order to force the civil authorities to execute him. Under tremendous pressure and risk of widespread civil dissent (not to mention his own blindness to the truth of Christ; cf. Jn 18:38), Pontius Pilate condemned Jesus to death by crucifixion. Jesus, according to the plan of the Father, willingly submitted himself to his passion and death on the cross, the perfect sacrifice for the salvation of all mankind. By his Resurrection three days later, he showed his victory over death, thereby calling every person to repentance and the fullness of filiation with the Father.

THE FOUR GOSPELS

Most of what is known about Christ's life comes from the four canonical gospels: Matthew, Mark, Luke, and John. The word "gospel," which means "good news," is applied to these four books that describe the life and teachings of Jesus.

Although all four gospels share the same subject, each has its own point of view and emphasis, depending on the source of the account and the audience for whom it was written. Matthew, Mark and Luke are known as the "synoptic" gospels (from Greek words meaning "seeing together") because their accounts are so similar. The gospel of St. John stands apart because of its more abstract, theological scope.

Both Sts. John and Matthew were themselves Apostles. Both gospels seem to be directed toward a Jewish Christian audience. St. John's was the last gospel to be written. St. Mark's is thought to be the first gospel written. St. Mark, though not an Apostle, traveled with St. Peter, who is very likely the primary source for this gospel intended for the Christians of Rome. St. Luke, who accompanied St. Paul, wrote mainly for gentile Christians and his main source is thought to be Mary the mother of Christ because this gospel includes stories about Christ's origins and early life.

The four authors, known as the Evangelists, are often identified with four symbols. St. Matthew's symbol is a man because his gospel emphasizes Christ's humanity and opens with his genealogy. St. Mark's symbol is a lion because it opens with the command "Prepare the way of the Lord." St. Luke's symbol is a bull because early on it speaks of priestly duties and temple sacrifices. St. John's gospel is symbolized by an eagle because of the lofty language of its opening verses.

These four gospels have always been held as authentic and canonical (officially declared as such at a synod in Rome in AD 382) by the Sacred Tradition of the Church, though there exist several "unofficial" gospels, known as the apocryphal gospels, which appeared in the first centuries of the Church. These gospels were discredited early in the Church's history because of their dubious origins and because many are tainted by errant beliefs.

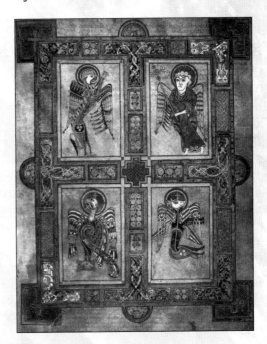

The Book of Kells
"The work not of men but of angels…"
(Giraldus Cambrensis, ca. AD1150)

One of the most famous books in the history of the world completed in AD 800 contains the Four Gospels. It was created by Columban monks who lived on the remote island of Iona, off the west coast of Scotland. The Book is on display at the Trinity College Library in Dublin.

PART III

Pentecost, the Birth of the Church

> When the day of Pentecost had come, they [the Apostles and Mary] were all together in one place. And suddenly a sound came from heaven like the rush of a mighty wind, and it filled all the house where they were sitting. And there appeared to them tongues as of fire, distributed and resting on each one of them. And they were all filled with the Holy Spirit and began to speak in other tongues, as the Spirit gave them utterance. (Acts 2:1-4)

On the Jewish feast of Pentecost, fifty days after the Resurrection of Christ, Jerusalem was filled with pilgrims from nearly every nation–from Persia, Rome, Arabia, North Africa, and all around the Mediterranean. The Apostles were all gathered in one place, most likely still fearing persecution. Just as Christ promised before he ascended to Heaven, the Holy Spirit descended upon them, anointing the Church for her mission of evangelization of the world.

On Pentecost, the Father and the Son sent the Holy Spirit, the Third Person of the Blessed Trinity, to complete and perfect that which Jesus Christ had begun:

> By his coming, which never ceases, the Holy Spirit causes the world to enter into the "last days," the time of the Church, the Kingdom already inherited though not yet consummated. (CCC 732)

Immediately following the Holy Spirit's descent, the Apostles began to preach the crucified and risen Christ with great power and authority (Acts 2:5-47). They were given the gift of tongues and found themselves miraculously speaking to the multitude, each hearing in his own tongue from among the languages spoken by the many pilgrims present in Jerusalem for Pentecost (Acts 2:8-11). St. Peter, responding to skepticism that the disciples were "filled with new wine" (Acts 2:13), addressed all who were present. He proclaimed the special calling of the Jews in God's plan of salvation for the world, used the Old Testament writings as proof of Christ's fulfillment of the prophets and the Law, and, like St. John the Baptist, called his hearers to repentance. St. Peter invited Jesus' new followers to be forgiven of their sins through the reception of Baptism.

> Peter said to them, "Repent, and be baptized every one of you in the name of Jesus Christ for the forgiveness of your sins; and you shall receive the gift of the Holy Spirit." (Acts 2:38)

Many converts came to the Faith through this first proclamation at Pentecost:

> Those who received his word were baptized, and there were added that day about three thousand souls. And they devoted themselves to the apostles' teaching and fellowship, to the breaking of bread and the prayers. (Acts 2:41-42)

The annual celebration of this feast is an opportunity to recall all that took place at the first Pentecost, whereby the Apostles were empowered with the strength of the Holy Spirit to preach Christ in word and in the heroic witness of martyrdom. Pentecost marks the enduring presence of the Holy Spirit in the Church that enables Christians to announce the truth of Christ's Gospel. It also shows that Christ will live in his Church throughout all ages.

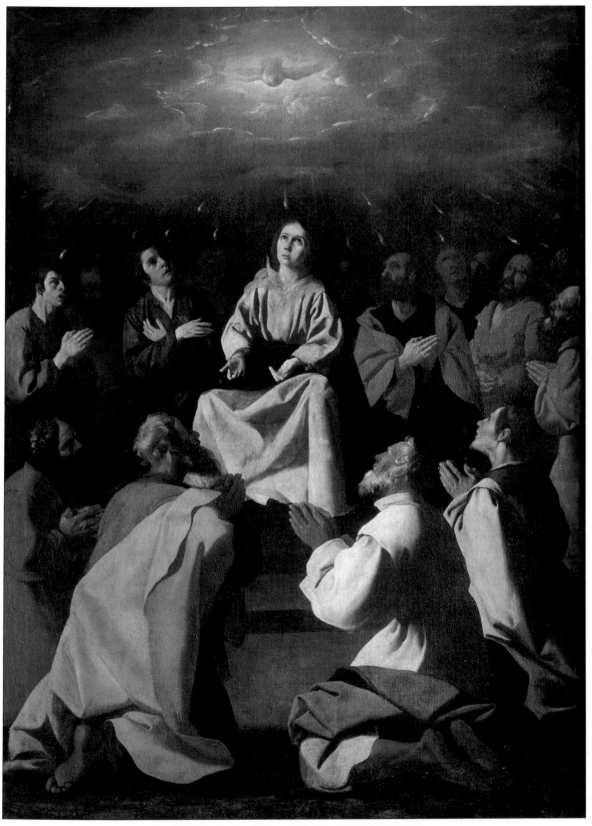

Pentecost marks the enduring presence of the Holy Spirit in the Church.

THE EARLY SPREAD OF CHRISTIANITY

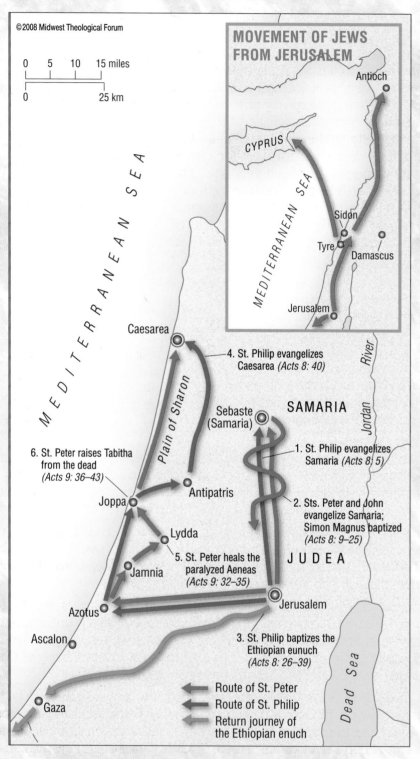

©2008 Midwest Theological Forum

0   5   10   15 miles

0   25 km

MOVEMENT OF JEWS FROM JERUSALEM

Antioch

CYPRUS

MEDITERRANEAN SEA

Sidon

Tyre

Damascus

Jerusalem

MEDITERRANEAN SEA

Caesarea

4. St. Philip evangelizes Caesarea (Acts 8: 40)

River

Plain of Sharon

SAMARIA

Sebaste (Samaria)

Jordan

1. St. Philip evangelizes Samaria (Acts 8: 5)

6. St. Peter raises Tabitha from the dead (Acts 9: 36–43)

Antipatris

Joppa

2. Sts. Peter and John evangelize Samaria; Simon Magnus baptized (Acts 8: 9–25)

Lydda

5. St. Peter heals the paralyzed Aeneas (Acts 9: 32–35)

Jamnia

JUDEA

Azotus

Jerusalem

Ascalon

3. St. Philip baptizes the Ethiopian eunuch (Acts 8: 26–39)

Dead Sea

Gaza

Route of St. Peter
Route of St. Philip
Return journey of the Ethiopian enuch

PART IV

The Church

What is the Church exactly? The Scriptures teach that the Church is the Body of Christ and the Temple of the Holy Spirit (cf. Eph 1: 22-23). The English word "church" etymologically comes from a Greek word meaning "thing belonging to the Lord," which applied originally to the church building. The Latin word *ecclesia* derives from another Greek word that means "assembly" or "congregation" The origins of these two words help to illustrate the many meanings the word "church" evokes for followers of Christ. This section will briefly look at the meaning of the Church, her aim, nature, names that have been employed to better understand her, and, finally, her four marks.

The *Catechism of the Catholic Church* states that, "The Church is both the means and the goal of God's plan: prefigured in creation, prepared for in the Old Covenant, founded by the words and actions of Jesus Christ, fulfilled by his redeeming cross and his Resurrection, the Church has been manifested as the mystery of salvation by the outpouring of the Holy Spirit. She will be perfected in the glory of heaven as the assembly of all the redeemed of the earth (cf. Rv 14: 4)" (CCC 778).

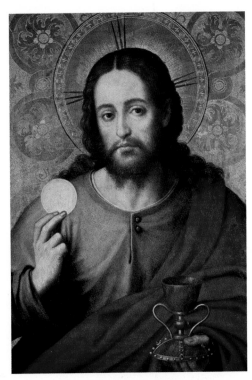

The Church forms the Mystical Body of Christ.

Willed by the Father, the Church founded by Jesus Christ enjoys the presence and guidance of the Holy Spirit. It is through the Church that God carries out his plan of salvation for all people. The teaching authority and sanctifying power of the Church serve as a means to bring all men and women to greater union with God, and with each other as well.

The groundwork for the Church was already being laid down when God made a covenant with the Jewish people. After this time of preparation in the Old Testament was completed, Jesus instituted the Church. The Church's foundation, goal, and fulfillment is in Jesus Christ. Through the Church, Jesus Christ unites himself with all men and women.

The Church has two dimensions: visible and spiritual. The Church is a visible, hierarchical society that is present in the world, just like any other organization or society. Unlike other societies, the Church has a spiritual dimension. The governing and teaching authority of the Church enjoys perennial guidance from the Holy Spirit. Moreover, she is the Mystical Body of Christ, a spiritual community, imbued with the healing and sanctifying power of God's grace.

The Church is made up of God's people, a people "born" into his family through faith in Christ and Baptism. The term "People of God" is taken from the Old Testament, in which God chose Israel to be his chosen people. Christ instituted the new and eternal covenant by which a new priestly, prophetic, and royal People of God, which is the Church, participates in the mission and service of Christ (cf. CCC 761, 783 at the end of this chapter). The Head of this people is Jesus Christ, and they enjoy the dignity and freedom of being sons and daughters of God, who dwells within their hearts.

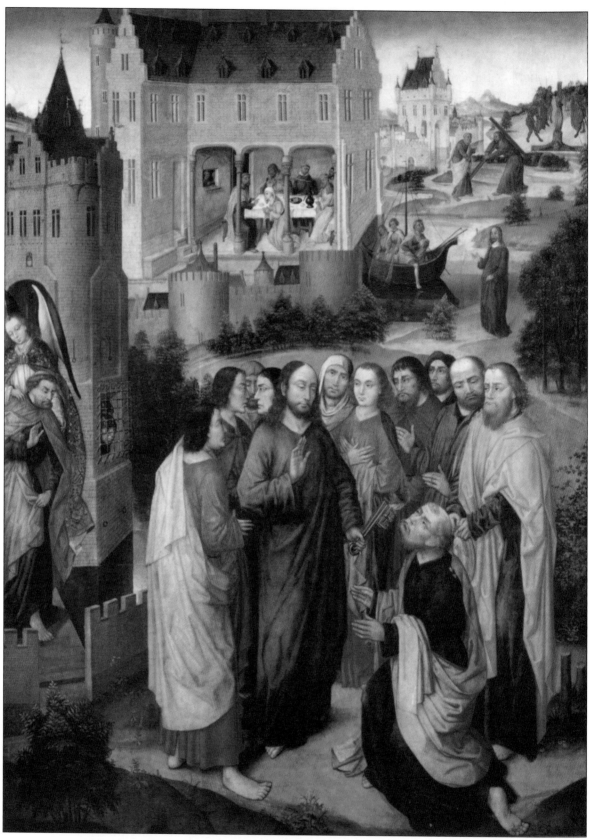

The Church is built upon the foundation of the Apostles. The hierarchy of the Church can be traced back to the Apostles.

This people is governed by the Christ's new commandment: to love each other as Christ loves them. By living this commandment, the People of God bring the hope of salvation to the world until the Kingdom of God is fully established and perfected at the end of time.

The Founder of the Church spoke of an intimate communion between himself and his people: "He who eats my flesh and drinks my blood abides in me, and I in him" (Jn 6:56). The Church, through the work of the Holy Spirit, forms the Mystical Body of Christ. This phrase likens the Church to the human body. The Church is united to Christ as a body is attached to a head. Analogous to a spousal relationship, the people of God are joined to Christ as a bride to her spouse.

The human soul is that which animates the human body; indeed, it is what makes it a living body and not a corpse. In a similar way, the Holy Spirit gives life to the Mystical Body of Christ, the Church. Thus the Holy Spirit, as the soul of the Church, is its source of unity and life.

The Church in her spiritual dimension reflects both a human and divine reality. As Christ's Spouse, she enjoys a divine component in her teaching and sanctifying power. Further expressions of her divine aspect are the Church's charism of infallibility and her durability until the end of time. Nothing will prevail over the divinely instituted Church. At the same time, her members are in constant need of purification in order to achieve holiness.

The Nicene Creed includes four marks that correspond to the Catholic Church founded by Christ. Throughout the course of history, these four marks have always served as the litmus test for the authenticity of the one, true Church.

THE CHURCH IS ONE

The Church acknowledges one God in Whom she professes one Faith. All Catholics adhere to the same teachings regarding the creed, sacraments, and morals. Lastly, they all recognize the authority of the pope as Supreme Pastor of the universal Church.

THE CHURCH IS HOLY

The Founder is holy, the means to salvation is holy, and the aim of the Church's teaching and sacraments is the holiness of its members. Those who live by the Church's teachings in their entirety become holy. Heroic sanctity even to the point of martyrdom has marked the life of some of the faithful throughout the centuries.

THE CHURCH IS CATHOLIC

The word "catholic" means "universal." The universality of the Church includes all ages, all races and nationalities, and every time period. Moreover, all the good traits of every culture are reflected in the teachings of the Catholic Church.

THE CHURCH IS APOSTOLIC

The Church is built upon the foundation of the Apostles. The hierarchy of the Church can be traced back to the Apostles. For this reason, the bishops are known as the successors of the Apostles, and the teaching of the Church finds its source in the very teachings of the Twelve Apostles governed by St. Peter.

PART V

The Apostles

The word "apostle" comes from the Greek *apostolos*, a form of *apostellein*, meaning "to send away." Thus, an apostle is literally "one who is sent." The designation traditionally refers to the twelve men chosen by Jesus during the course of his public ministry to be his closest followers. They were the pillars of his Church and were to be sent to preach the Good News to all the nations. Matthias, the Apostle chosen after the Resurrection to replace Judas Iscariot, as well as Sts. Paul of Tarsus and Barnabas, also enjoyed the status of Apostles, even though they did not hold that title during Christ's public ministry.

THE CALL OF THE TWELVE

The Twelve Apostles included fishermen, a tax collector, and friends and relatives of Jesus. Upon hearing Christ's call, these men left their former lives and dedicated themselves to following him. Matthew's Gospel relates the story of the call of the first four Apostles:

> As he [Jesus] walked by the Sea of Galilee, he saw two brothers, Simon who is called Peter and Andrew his brother, casting a net into the sea; for they were fishermen. And he said to them, "Follow me, and I will make you fishers of men." Immediately they left their nets and followed him. And going on from there he saw two other brothers, James the son of Zebedee and John his brother, in the boat with Zebedee their father, mending their nets, and he called them. Immediately they left the boat and their father, and followed him. (Mt 4:18-22)

St. Luke's Gospel relates that Jesus selected the Twelve from among his disciples after a whole night of prayer during his public ministry:

> In these days he [Jesus] went out into the hills to pray; and all night he continued in prayer to God. And when it was day, he called his disciples, and chose from them twelve, whom he named apostles; Simon, whom he named Peter, and Andrew his brother, and James and John, and Philip, and Bartholomew, and Matthew, and Thomas, and James the son of Alphaeus, and Simon who was called the Zealot, and Judas the son of James, and Judas Iscariot, who became a traitor. (Lk 6:12-16)

Mark 3:13-19 and Matthew 10:1-4 also contain similar passages. It is worth noting that all three accounts begin by naming St. Peter as the first Apostle, and they end by identifying Judas Iscariot as the traitor. The selection of the Twelve Apostles coincides with the twelve tribes of Israel, over which they would sit in judgment (cf. Mt 19:28; Lk 22:30).

Besides being the first ones sent directly by Christ to all the world, the Apostles were characterized by another singular quality. They were the first witnesses of Christ's life, message, and Resurrection. Before Pentecost, the Apostles wished to restore their number to twelve, because Judas Iscariot had committed suicide. In the book of Acts, St. Peter says:

> One of the men who have accompanied us during all the time that the Lord Jesus went in and out among us, beginning from the baptism of John until the day when he was taken up from us – *one of these men must become with us a witness to his resurrection.* (Acts 1:21-22) [emphasis added]

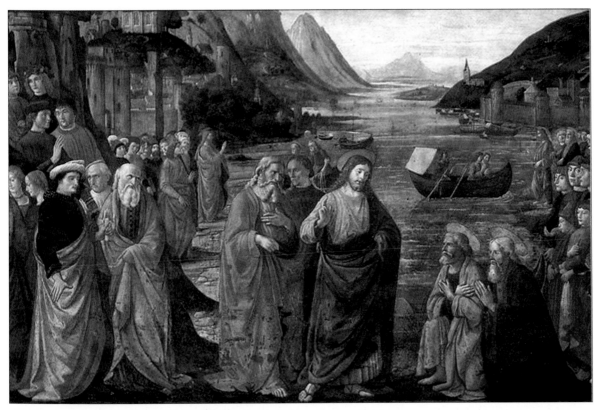

"Follow me, and I will make you fishers of men." (Mt 4:19)

The mission of the Apostles therefore consisted in introducing to the world Jesus' message of salvation through their teaching and witness of Christ's love. It was through the profound influence of the Holy Spirit that the Apostles could build and extend Christ's Church throughout the world.

THE APOSTOLIC TRADITION AND THE OFFICE OF BISHOP

The title "Apostle" is preeminent among all others because the Apostles, with St. Peter as their head, received teachings and instructions directly from Christ. They were personally chosen by Christ during his earthly life and empowered by the Holy Spirit to launch the first evangelization with faith and courage.

> "In order that the full and living Gospel might always be preserved in the Church the apostles left bishops as their successors. They gave them 'their own position of teaching authority'" (DV 7 § 2; St. Irenaeus, *Adv. haeres.* 3, 3, 1: PG 7, 848; Harvey, 2, 9). Indeed, "the apostolic preaching, which is expressed in a special way in the inspired books, was to be preserved in a continuous line of succession until the end of time" (DV 8 § 1). (CCC 77)

The Apostles continued Christ's ministry of preaching, healing, and exorcising demons. After his Resurrection, Jesus commanded the Apostles to spread the Gospel to every corner of the world (cf. Mt 28:16-20). They had received instruction with respect to the meaning of the Scriptures directly from Jesus and were the ultimate authority on the meaning of Christ's message. Upon the completion of their own earthly journeys, they passed on their priestly powers and mission to their successors through the office of bishop. A bishop is a successor of the Apostles who has received the fullness of Christ's priesthood. The Church has successfully transmitted the Apostolic Tradition down through the line of bishops, and she will continue to do so until Christ returns.

THE CONVERSION OF ST. PAUL

Saul was a pious Jew, well educated in the Law under the tutelage of a Pharisee and renowned doctor of the Law by the name of Gamaliel. Saul firmly believed, as a righteous and devout Jew, that the Law was the sacred covenant between God and his people and that the early Church posed an acute threat to that covenant. The idea that Jesus Christ was the messiah professed by the early Church deviated from the kind of messiah that was so long expected in Jewish tradition. Therefore, Saul would certainly see the early Church as dangerous to the integrity of the Jewish faith. He dutifully set out to persecute the followers of Christ.

After threatening the early Church throughout Jerusalem, Saul set out on a journey to Damascus to continue suppressing the Church. The Acts of the Apostles tells in detail what happened to Saul during his journey:

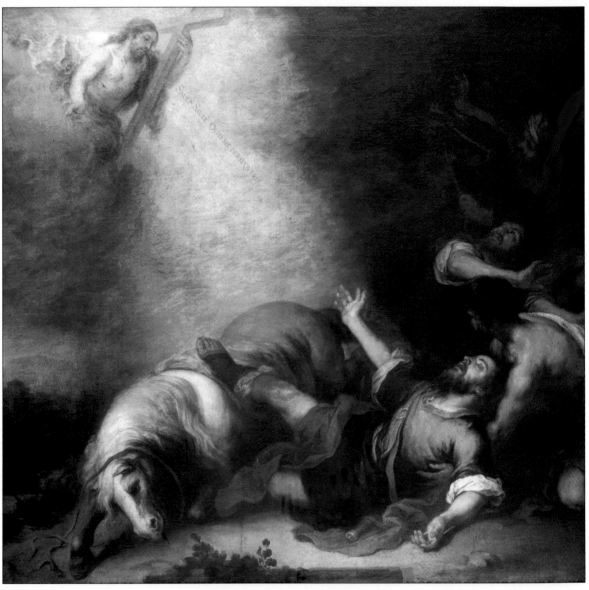

St. Paul's conversion, one of the Church's great ironies, shows how Christ even calls sinners to lead his Church.

As he journeyed he approached Damascus, and suddenly a light from heaven flashed about him. And he fell to the ground and heard a voice saying to him, "Saul, Saul, why do you persecute me?" And he said, "Who are you, Lord?" And he said, "I am Jesus, whom you are persecuting; but rise and enter the city, and you will be told what you are to do." The men who were traveling with him stood speechless, hearing the voice but seeing no one. Saul arose from the ground; and when his eyes were opened, he could see nothing; so they led him by the hand and brought him into Damascus. And for three days he was without sight, and neither ate nor drank. (Acts 9:3-9)

As he waited in Damascus, blind and troubled by the event that had befallen him, Saul was visited by a disciple of Christ named Ananias, who, through a vision, was instructed by the Lord to seek out Saul and restore his sight. The Lord told Ananias that this man, who had done great evils to the early Church, "is a chosen instrument of mine to carry my name before the Gentiles and kings and the sons of Israel" (Acts 9:15). Ananias listened to the Lord, sought out Saul, and laid his hands on him and spoke: "Brother Saul, the Lord Jesus who appeared to you on the road by which you came, has sent me that you may regain your sight and be filled with the Holy Spirit" (Acts 9:17). Immediately Saul miraculously recovered his sight and was baptized. Filled with the Holy Spirit, "in the synagogues immediately he proclaimed Jesus, saying, 'He is the Son of God'" (Acts 9:20). St. Paul's conversion, one of the Church's great ironies, shows how Christ even calls sinners to lead his Church. St. Paul (his Roman name, as he was known soon after his conversion) became one of Christianity's greatest evangelizers, traveling and spreading the Gospel throughout the Roman world. The Feast of the Converstion of St. Paul is commemorated January 25.

AN INTERLUDE: THE CONVERSION OF CORNELIUS AND THE COMMENCEMENT OF THE MISSION TO THE GENTILES

The early Jewish Christians, though persecuted by the Jewish community, still considered Christianity a part of the Jewish tradition. They still followed Jewish laws and customs, though they had begun to incorporate many of Christ's teachings into their religious worship and practice. Acceptance of Christ as the awaited messiah did not, in their minds, sever them from their Jewish heritage. One particular Jewish law created a major problem in the formation of the early Church.

Jewish Law forbade Jews "to associate with or to visit [Gentiles]" (Acts 10:28). However, the Apostles remembered how Christ reached out to all people during his life. They understood that Christ's message and salvation are universal. How, if bound by Jewish laws, were the members of the early Church to spread the Word of God to non-Jews? How could a Gentile be baptized into a Church whose traditional law forbids any interaction with people foreign to that tradition?

The Acts of the Apostles relates the story of the Roman centurion Cornelius, a "devout and God-fearing" Gentile in Caesarea. An angel of God came to him in a vision and told him to send for Simon Peter in Joppa. St. Peter at this time also had a vision:

He saw the heaven opened, and something descending, like a great sheet, let down by four corners upon the earth. In it were all kinds of animals and reptiles and birds of the air. And there came a voice to him, "Rise, Peter; kill and eat." But Peter said, "No, Lord; for I have never eaten anything that is common or unclean." And the voice came to him again a second time, "What God has cleansed, you must not call common." This happened three times, and the thing was taken up at once to heaven. (Acts 10:11-16)

As the vision faded, the men sent by Cornelius arrived to where St. Peter was staying. The meaning of the vision was clear to St. Peter: he must open the Church to the Gentiles, who were, by Jewish standards, considered unclean. He accepted the emissaries, and the next day traveled with them to Caesarea to visit Cornelius.

Upon meeting St. Peter, Cornelius explained to him that he had been told in a vision to send for him, and he told St. Peter that he would listen to all that the Lord had commanded him. Guided by the Holy Spirit, St. Peter took up the task of bringing the Gentiles into the Church. He said to Cornelius:

> Truly I perceive that God shows no partiality, but in every nation any one who fears him and does what is right is acceptable to him. You know the word which he sent to Israel, preaching good news of peace by Jesus Christ (he is Lord of all)....He commanded us to preach to the people, and to testify that he is the one ordained by God to be judge of the living and the dead. To him all the prophets bear witness that every one who believes in him receives forgiveness of sins through his name. (Acts 10: 34-36, 42-43)

Then St. Peter and the Jewish Christians with him witnessed the outpouring of the Holy Spirit upon Cornelius and those Gentiles with him. They were amazed to see the Gentiles receive the Holy Spirit as they had, and St. Peter agreed to have them baptized. Recognizing the severe implications of the event, St. Peter went to Jerusalem to explain to the Jewish Christians this recent episode. At first, they were outraged and objected to such dealings with the Gentiles. However, when they had heard the full story, including the descent of the Holy Spirit upon the Gentiles, "they were silenced. And they glorified God, saying, 'Then to the Gentiles also God has granted repentance unto life'" (Acts 11:18). Through the power and guidance of the Holy Spirit, the Church was now ready to include the entire world in her mission.

ST. PAUL, "APOSTLE OF THE GENTILES"

Unlike most of the other Apostles, St. Paul was well educated in the Jewish Law, and enjoyed an intelligent command of Sacred Scripture. His unique gifts and background were well suited to God's plan for his role as the "Apostle of the Gentiles."

St. Paul was a brilliant writer and theologian. Scripture contains thirteen of his epistles (Romans, 1 and 2 Corinthians, Galatians, Philippians, Colossians, 1 and 2 Thessalonians, 1 and 2 Timothy, Titus, Ephesians, and Philemon). In his writings, St. Paul refers to his missionary work, mostly in the cities of Asia Minor, and lays out the first written and highly developed theology of the Church. Most of his letters are believed to have been written in the 50s, prior to the writing of the earliest Gospel. They are thus the oldest writings in the New Testament.

St. Paul's profound writings would become central in the development of the Church's teaching up to this very day as he formed a theology out of the Gospel message. St. Paul particularly delved into the doctrines of the Cross, the Mystical Body of Christ, the power of grace, and the value of charity. The letters to the Romans and 1 and 2 Corinthians are central texts that especially reveal St. Paul's theological thought. His writings serve not only as sound theological sources, but also as invaluable historical references to the early Church. Reading his epistles, one cannot help but marvel at St. Paul's profound insights into Christ's Gospel and his indomitable determination to spread that Gospel to others.

THE COUNCIL OF JERUSALEM (AD 49/50)

St. Peter's experience with Cornelius unfortunately did not completely resolve all the issues involved in extending the apostolic mission to the Gentiles. Questions remained whether the Gentiles who

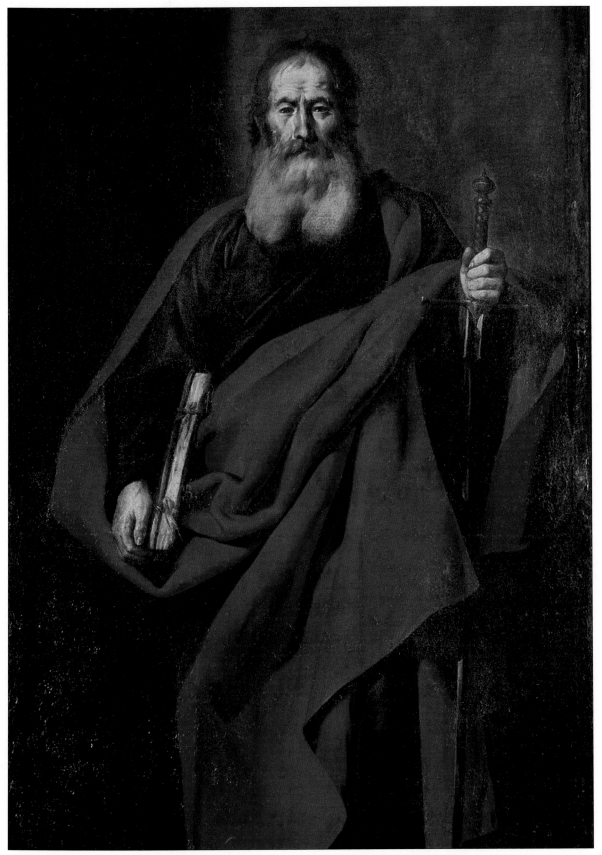

St. Paul, Antonio del Castillo; Cordoba Museum of Fine Arts, Cordoba, Spain; Archivo Oronoz

THE TRAVELS OF ST. PAUL

St. Paul's tireless and intrepid missionary work spread the Christian Faith far beyond the borders of Palestine and across most of the Roman Empire, founding some of the earliest and most prominent early Christian communities along the way. By some estimates, St. Paul's travels totaled well over 10,000 miles and brought him to Jerusalem, to every corner of Asia Minor, into Arabia, across Macedonia and Greece, to Eastern Europe, Rome, and many scholars believe he may have traveled as far as Spain.

Along the way, he found many eager disciples, but he also found many enemies among both the Jews and Gentiles. He endured many dangers and sufferings along the course of his travels. He describes some of his experiences in 2 Corinthians 11:24-25: "Five times I have received at the hands of the Jews the forty lashes less one. Three times I have been beaten with rods: once I was stoned. Three times I have been ship-wrecked; a night and a day I have been adrift at sea." St. Paul was driven out of many cities by mobs. He narrowly escaped death several times, as when he sneaked out of Damascus in a basket to avoid the guards at the gate (cf. Acts 9:23-25). Other times, he did not escape, as in Lystra where a mob caught him, stoned him until they thought he was dead and dragged him out of the city (cf. Acts 14:19).

St. Paul was fearless in his apostolate despite his physical shortcomings. There are several accounts of what St. Paul looked like. Even in his own words, he writes that his "bodily presence is weak" (2 Cor 10:10). Other early Christian accounts coincide in saying that he was short, broad-shouldered, bow-legged, and balding. He also had big eyes, a rather long nose, a thick, grayish beard and closely-knit eyebrows.

St. Paul also spent a good deal of time in prison. He was arrested in Philippi, and again later in Jerusalem, after which he spent a two-year stint in Caesarea, and two more years on house arrest in Rome. He was finally martyred in Rome around the year AD 64 by beheading. Tradition holds that when he was beheaded, his head bounced three times, and each time it hit the ground a fountain miraculously sprang up.

ST. PAUL'S FIRST JOURNEY, ca. AD 46-48

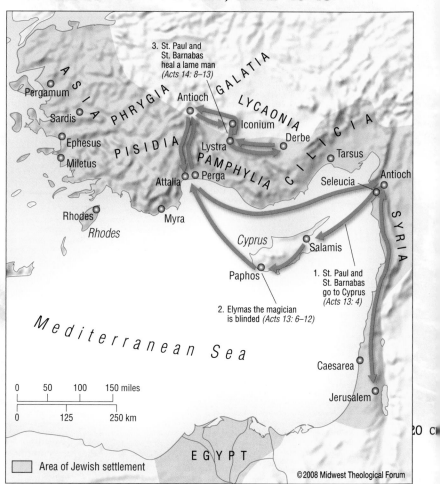

ST. PAUL'S SECOND JOURNEY, ca. AD 49-52

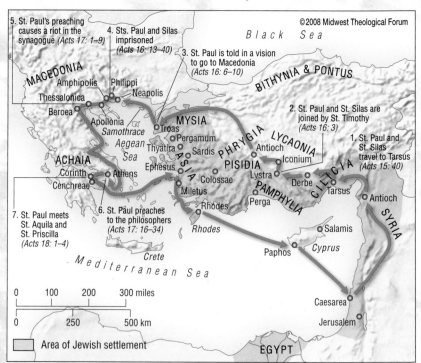

ST. PAUL'S THIRD JOURNEY, ca. AD 53-57

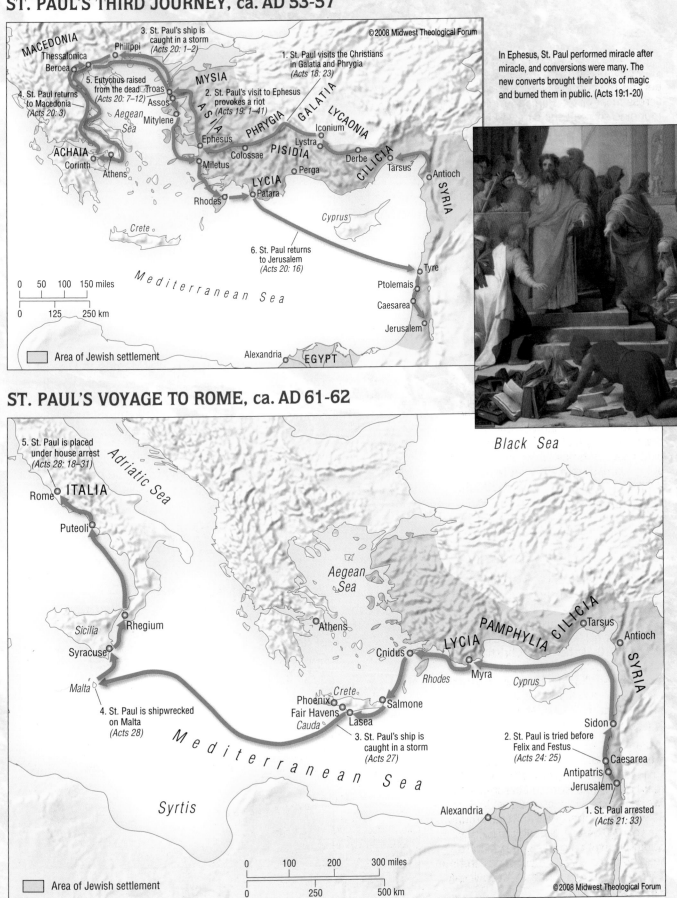

©2008 Midwest Theological Forum

MACEDONIA

Thessalonica
Beroea
Philippi

3. St. Paul's ship is caught in a storm *(Acts 20: 1–2)*

1. St. Paul visits the Christians in Galatia and Phrygia *(Acts 18: 23)*

5. Eutychus raised from the dead *(Acts 20: 7–12)*
Troas
Assos

4. St. Paul returns to Macedonia *(Acts 20: 3)*

MYSIA

2. St. Paul's visit to Ephesus provokes a riot *(Acts 19: 1–41)*

A S I A

Aegean Sea
Mitylene

PHRYGIA

GALATIA

LYCAONIA

Iconium

Ephesus

Lystra

ACHAIA
Corinth
Athens

Miletus
Colossae

PISIDIA

Derbe

CILICIA
Tarsus

Perga

Antioch

LYCIA

SYRIA

Rhodes
Patara

Cyprus

6. St. Paul returns to Jerusalem *(Acts 20: 16)*

Crete

Mediterranean Sea

0 50 100 150 miles

0 125 250 km

Tyre
Ptolemais
Caesarea
Jerusalem

Area of Jewish settlement

Alexandria
EGYPT

In Ephesus, St. Paul performed miracle after miracle, and conversions were many. The new converts brought their books of magic and burned them in public. (Acts 19:1-20)

ST. PAUL'S VOYAGE TO ROME, ca. AD 61-62

5. St. Paul is placed under house arrest *(Acts 28: 18–31)*

Adriatic Sea

Black Sea

Rome ITALIA
Puteoli

Aegean Sea

Rhegium
Sicilia

Athens

PAMPHYLIA

CILICIA
Tarsus

Antioch

Syracuse

LYCIA

Cnidus

Myra

Malta

Rhodes

Cyprus

SYRIA

4. St. Paul is shipwrecked on Malta *(Acts 28)*

Crete
Phoenix
Fair Havens
Lasea
Cauda

Salmone

Sidon

2. St. Paul is tried before Felix and Festus *(Acts 24: 25)*

3. St. Paul's ship is caught in a storm *(Acts 27)*

Caesarea
Antipatris
Jerusalem

M e d i t e r r a n e a n   S e a

Syrtis

Alexandria

1. St. Paul arrested *(Acts 21: 33)*

0 100 200 300 miles

0 250 500 km

Area of Jewish settlement

©2008 Midwest Theological Forum

converted to Christianity also had to observe the Mosaic Law, including dietary laws and the law requiring circumcision. Jewish Christians understood that Christ was the fulfillment of the Jewish law and therefore wanted to recognize both traditions.

St. Paul had established Christian communities in Asia Minor on the premise that faith in Jesus Christ implied freedom from the Jewish Law. In his epistle to the Galatians, St. Paul defended the New Law of grace against other early Christians who advocated the necessity of observing the Old Law. St. Paul knew that the authority of the Church lay in Jerusalem, and so St. Paul and his pupil Barnabas journeyed back to the holy city to reconcile the matter with the other Apostles and Church leaders.

In Jerusalem, some Pharisees who had converted argued that Gentiles must observe the Mosaic Law. There was much debate, and finally St. Peter addressed the council:

> You know that in the early days God made choice among you, that by my mouth the Gentiles should hear the word of the gospel and believe. And God who knows the heart bore witness to them, giving them the Holy Spirit just as he did to us; and he made no distinction between us and them, but cleansed their hearts by faith. Now therefore why do you make trial of God by putting a yoke upon the neck of the disciples which neither our fathers nor we have been able to bear? But we believe that we shall be saved through the grace of the Lord Jesus, just as they will. (Acts 15:7-11)

St. Peter, speaking with his authority as head of the Church–supported by St. James, the leader of the Church in Jerusalem–made the definitive statement on this issue. The Gentiles were to adhere to the following guidelines: to avoid eating the meat and blood of animals sacrificed to idols or from animals that had been strangled, and to refrain from unlawful marriage (cf. Acts 15:29). The dietary laws, circumcision, and other aspects of the Law would not be imposed upon the Gentiles.

The Council of Jerusalem, the first council among many more in the Church's long history, settled the question between the Jewish Christians and the Gentile converts regarding the observance of the Law. Councils would become an important means in understanding the position of the Church. A council is an authorized gathering of bishops, guided by the Holy Spirit, to discuss ecclesiastical matters with the aim of passing decrees on the themes under discussion. In Jerusalem, St. Paul sought and won permission to preach Jesus Christ crucified and resurrected without forcing circumcision and the formal observance of the Law on the new Gentile converts. St. Paul's teachings on the New Law and Faith, coupled with the conclusions of the Council of Jerusalem, further distanced the early Church from its Jewish foundations.

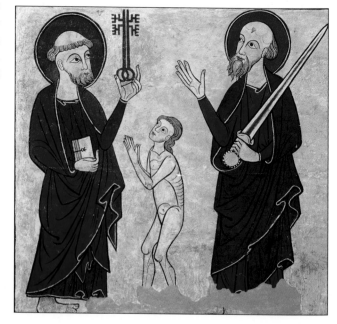

At the first Council of Jerusalem, St. Peter made the definitive statement on the issue of whether Gentiles must observe Mosaic Laws.

MISSIONARY ACTIVITIES OF THE APOSTLES

The Apostles were witnesses to the Resurrection of Jesus Christ and sent by him to preach the Gospel to all the world. These Jewish men, most of them uneducated–

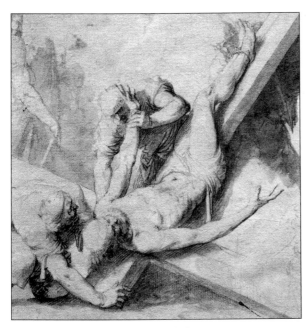

The martyrdom of St. Peter

St. Paul being the notable exception – soon came to be regarded by the Roman authorities as a menace to the state.

According to tradition, all the Apostles except St. John, who was miraculously spared, died as martyrs for the Faith. Around the year 64, **St. Peter** was crucified in Rome, upside down at his request, saying that he was not worthy to die right side up as Jesus did. The details of St. Peter's death in Rome have long been attributed to the "*Quo vadis?*" tradition. During persecutions, all groups seek to protect their leadership. As St. Peter was leaving Rome during Nero's persecution in AD 64, he is said to have met Christ along the road, asking Him: "*Domine quo vadis?*" ("Where are you going, Lord?") Christ replied, "I am coming to be crucified again." By this St. Peter understood that he should return to the city and suffer martyrdom.

St. Paul also spent his last days in Rome. After working for many years in Palestine and Asia Minor, St. Paul was arrested in Jerusalem and eventually sent to the imperial city for trial. It is unclear whether his dream of evangelizing Spain was ever realized. It is believed that St. Paul, like St. Peter, died in Rome between the years AD 62-65. Crucifixion, the cruelest form of execution, was reserved only for non-citizens and criminals; St. Paul, who was a Roman citizen, was beheaded outside the walls of Rome. Sts. Peter and Paul, the two Apostolic cornerstones of the Church – the first pope and the Church's greatest missionary – share June 29 as their feast day.

St. Andrew, the brother of St. Peter, is mentioned twice in the Gospels (cf. Mt 4:18-20; Jn 1:35-42), and the bishop and Church historian Eusebius (AD 260-340) recorded that Andrew's missionary activities took him to Scythia (modern day Ukraine and Russia). His last journeys took him through Byzantium and Greece to Patros, where the governor of Patros crucified Andrew on an X-shaped cross. According to tradition, his last words were, "Accept me, O Christ Jesus, whom I saw, whom I love, and in whom I am; accept my spirit in peace in your eternal realm." His feast is celebrated November 30, and he is the patron of Scotland, Greece, and Russia.

Sts. James and **John**, the sons of Zebedee, were, like Sts. Peter and Andrew, simple fishermen. Jesus exhorted them to place the highest importance in serving others, as they both sought to rank first in his kingdom (cf. Mt 20:20-28; Mk 10:35-45). St. James "the Greater," along with Sts. Peter and John, formed the inner circle among the Twelve, and they witnessed the raising of the daughter of Jairus (cf. Mk 5:35-43; Lk 8:41-56), the Transfiguration (cf. Mt 17:1-13; Mk 9:2-13; Lk 9:28-36), and the agony in the garden of Gethsemane (cf. Mt 26:36-46;

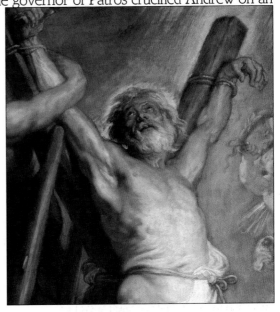

The martyrdom of St. Andrew

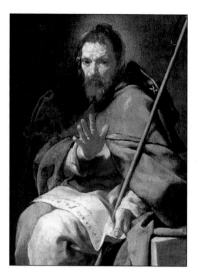
St. James "the Greater"

Mk 14:32-42). Herod Agrippa had St. James beheaded AD 44, and he thereby became the first of the Twelve to give his life for the Master (cf. Acts 12:2). St. James's feast day is celebrated on July 25.

St. John, according to tradition, authored the fourth Gospel, the Book of Revelation, and three of the Catholic Epistles. He is mentioned numerous times in the New Testament: willing to drink with Christ and his brother St. James the cup of suffering (cf. Mt 20:20-28), imprisoned with St. Peter and summoned before the Sanhedrin (cf. Acts 3:1, 11, and 4:1-21), and going with St. Peter to Samaria (cf. 8:14-25). St. John appears numerous times in the fourth Gospel under the title of the "Beloved Disciple," which tradition supports (cf. Jn 1:35-40, 13:23, 19:26, 20:2-8, and 21:7). During the reign of the Roman Emperor Domitian, St. John was exiled to the island of Patmos off the Turkish coast, where he wrote the book of Revelation. A Latin legend held that Domitian attempted to kill St. John by placing him in a cauldron of boiling oil *ante portam Latinam* ("before the Latin Gate") leading out of Rome to the Roman province of Latium. St. John walked away unharmed. His feast day is celebrated on December 27.

St. Bartholomew is mentioned only in the Synoptic Gospels (cf. Mk 3:18, Lk 6:14, and Mt 10:3) and in Acts 1:13. Some have suggested that Bartholomew may have been Nathanael, the one whom St. Philip brought to Jesus (cf. Jn 1:43-51). The name "Bartholomew" means simply "son of Tomai," and it is quite possible that this Apostle had another, personal name. St. Bartholomew made the journey to preach the Gospel in and around Persia–an arduous expedition from Palestine in the first century AD According to tradition, St. Bartholomew was martyred in Armenia where he was flayed alive. His feast day is on August 24.

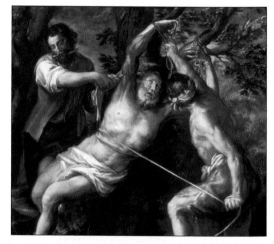
The martrydom of St. Bartholomew

According to ancient tradition, **St. Matthew**, one of the Twelve, is also the author of the Gospel with the same name. According to the early Church historian Eusebius, St. Matthew's apostolic mission was directed to the Jews. His Gospel is the only one written in Aramaic, and tradition holds that it was written thus in order to accommodate the Jewish people. It is interesting to note that he corroborates many details of Christ's life and words with Old Testament quotations. Before Christ called him to be his Apostle, St. Matthew was a tax collector who, according to the Gospels of Sts. Mark and Luke, went by the name of Levi. Jesus told St. Matthew to follow him, and then sat and ate with St. Matthew and other tax collectors and sinners that St. Matthew had invited. Some Pharisees criticized Jesus for his association such people, and Christ responded, "Those who are well have no need of a physician, but those who are sick. Go and learn what this means, 'I desire mercy, and not sacrifice.' For I came not to call the righteous, but sinners" (Mt 9:12-13). The same story appears in Sts. Mark and Luke. St. Matthew's name, *Mattai*, means "gift of God" in Aramaic. The feast day for St. Matthew is celebrated on September 21.

St. Thomas, also known as "Doubting Thomas," is listed as one of the Twelve in all four of the Gospels. He also appears in three prominent places in St. John's Gospel. A doubtful but zealous man, St. Thomas

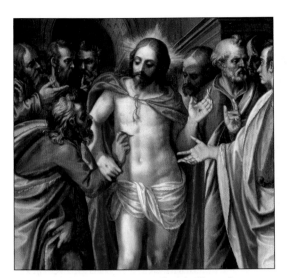

St. Thomas is also known as "Doubting Thomas."

urged the other disciples to follow Jesus and die with him upon hearing that he was going to visit the dead Lazarus (cf. Jn 11:16). An eager but apprehensive St. Thomas asked Jesus how the disciples should know the way to the Father's kingdom, to which Jesus replied, "I am the way, and the truth, and the life; no one comes to the Father, but by me" (Jn 14: 6); and, finally, a doubtful St. Thomas appears in the account of Christ's Resurrection appearances to the disciples in the locked room (cf. Jn 20:19-28). Sources such as Eusebius (cf. *Church History* 3.1) claim that St. Thomas evangelized the Parthians in present day Iran and Turkmenistan, while others, derived from the apocryphal, Gnostic book, *Acts of Thomas*, suggest that he established the Church in India and was martyred there. The Malabar Christians of India claim St. Thomas as their evangelizer. When the Portuguese explorers arrived in India in the fifteenth century they found, to their amazement, a very old Christian community, traditionally tracing its founding back to St. Thomas. His feast day is on July 3.

Very little is known about **St. James**, the son of Alphaeus, often referred to as "James the Less" in order to distinguish him from St. James, the son of Zebedee. After Pentecost, St. James became the head of the Church in Jerusalem and presided over the Council of Jerusalem. He shares his feast day with St. Philip on May 3. **St. Philip** is listed in the Synoptic Gospels and in the Acts of the Apostles, but only the Gospel of St. John provides any details. Christ called St. Philip, who in turn brought Nathanael to Christ (cf. Jn 1: 43-51). St. Philip was present at the miracle of the multiplication of the bread and fish (cf. Jn 6: 5-7), and he presented a group of Greeks to Jesus in John 12: 20-26. Finally, St. Philip also asked Jesus to show the Father to the Twelve (cf. Jn 14: 8-11).

St. Judas, brother of "James the Less," is listed as an Apostle in Lk 6:16 and Acts 1:13; he is referred to as "Judas (not Iscariot)" in Jn 14:22. St. Judas is also referred to as Thaddeus in Mk 3:18 and Mt 10:3, and it is believed that this was meant to further distinguish him from Judas Iscariot. He is sometimes called Judas Thaddeus, and in English speaking countries, St. Judas is typically known by the name of Jude. St. Judas is the patron of lost causes, and he authored the Epistle of St. Jude. St. Simon the Cananean, also known as "the Less" and "the Zealot," shares a feast day with St. Judas on October 28. An apocryphal source, The Passion of Simon and Jude, describes the martyrdom of both of these men in Persia.

Judas Iscariot betrayed Christ to the Jewish authorities as recorded in Mk 14:10-11 and 14:43-44. His motive is unclear; financial gain may have played a role, as it did when Judas criticized the woman who anointed Jesus with ointment (cf. Mt 26:6-13). Jesus spoke harshly of the man who betrayed him: "Woe to that man by whom the Son of man is betrayed! It would have been better for that man if he had not been born" (cf. Mt 26:24). Judas's fall serves as a warning that even the graces given to Christ's Apostles – and the familiar friendship of Jesus himself – may be of no avail if one is unfaithful and does not believe.

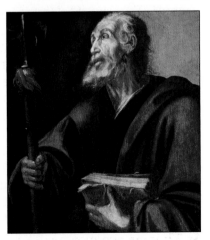

St. Judas Thaddeus

PART VI

Beliefs and Practices: The Spiritual Life of the Early Christians

The beliefs and practices of the early community of Christians took some time to develop – Christ did not leave his Church with a fully developed theology and disciplinary practice. Rather, these emerged through centuries of theological, philosophical, cultural, and historical development under the guidance of the Holy Spirit in and through the institution of the Church. From the Church's inception, the eternal truths present in Christ's teaching were passed on and unfolded within a living and changing body of practicing believers. As the early Christians reflected on the Gospel message and integrated it into their daily lives, the early tradition of Church teaching began to take shape and express itself especially in the liturgy.

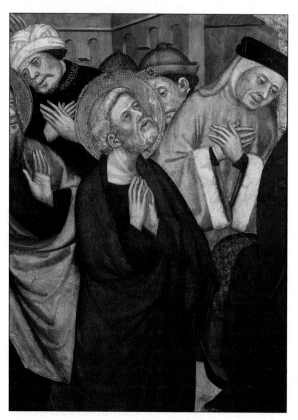

BAPTISM

> Go therefore and make disciples of all nations, baptizing them in the name of the Father and of the Son and of the Holy Spirit. (Mt 28:19)

> Truly, truly, I say to you, unless one is born of water and the Spirit, he cannot enter the kingdom of God. (Jn 3:5)

Jesus was baptized by St. John the Baptist with a baptism of repentance (cf. Mt 3:13-17). But it was Jesus who instituted the Sacrament of Baptism in the Holy Spirit (cf. Jn 3:22; Mk 1:8), instructing his disciples to do the same (cf. Jn 4:2; Mt 28:19). By this sacrament, a believer is forgiven of original and personal sin, begins a new life in Christ and the Holy Spirit, and is incorporated intothe Church, the Body of Christ (CCC 977, 1213).

In the first years after the Resurrection, adults who wanted to convert to the Faith were baptized freely. As Christianity grew, a more structured program of instruction preceding Baptism evolved. Catechumens ("the instructed," from the Greek katēkhein, "to instruct"), those adults seeking admission to the Church, met over a long period of time, normally two to three years, for instruction before being baptized. The lengthy process provided time for the catechumen to learn the message of the Gospels and to develop a strong foundation in the faith. Though one might imagine that there existed a high level of enthusiasm and zeal among prospective believers at a time so soon after Christ had walked the earth, one must keep in mind that these were often times of great persecution, which could easily

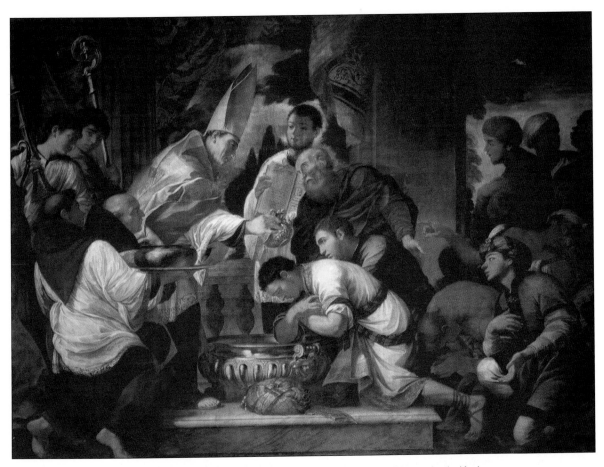

In the first years after the Resurrection, adults who wanted to convert to the Faith were baptized freely.

overwhelm a believer with a burgeoning but poorly grounded faith. The catechumens waited to be baptized at the Easter Vigil on the night of Holy Saturday or on the Saturday before Pentecost.

The practice of baptizing infants became more common during the third century, and by the early Medieval period, the practice of infant Baptism was universal. There is also evidence that it may have started prior to the third century, in the time of the Apostolic Fathers. St. Justin Martyr refers to Christians who had "from childhood been made disciples" (cf. Apologies 1.15). In the third century document written by Hippolytus (AD 170-236), Apostolic Tradition (21), the Baptism of children is discussed. Tertullian (AD 160-225) disagreed with the practice of infant Baptism (though he did not deny its validity). In order to avoid the danger of anyone profaning his Baptism during his youth, Tertullian argued that the baptized ought to be old enough to understand the sacrament. Origen (AD 185-254) claimed that the practice of infant Baptism was clearly recommended, and supported it since original sin ought to be wiped away as soon as possible.

The beauty and value of baptizing infants is that original sin is forgiven and the child is incorporated into the Mystical Body of Christ. Baptismal character imprinted on the soul renders the infant a child of God who now shares in the priesthood of Christ called the common priesthood. Lastly, this sacrament confers upon the child a special grace through which he may grow more fully in Christ. Prior to the twentieth century, even in the industrialized nations, many babies and women died during childbirth, and many children died afterwards from diseases that had no known cure. Infant Baptism secures the great gift of forgiveness and salvation from God and commits the family to raising the child in a Christian way.

Baptism has always been administered immediately when the recipient is in danger of death. In such a case, any baptized or non-baptized person can administer the sacrament. During the persecutions there were cases of non-believers administering Baptism to converts as they made their way to the place of torture and execution. These baptisms were valid because they utilized the Trinitarian formula and intended to follow the mind of the Church. There were also cases of catechumens who were martyred before receiving the Sacrament of Baptism. From the earliest times, the Church taught that those who died for the Faith received the graces of Baptism through their martyrdom, which is called Baptism of Blood.

> The Church has always held the firm conviction that those who suffer death for the sake of the faith without having received Baptism are baptized by their death for and with Christ. This Baptism of blood, like the desire for Baptism, brings about the fruits of Baptism without being a sacrament. (CCC 1258)

AGAPE AND THE EUCHARIST

> I received from the Lord what I also delivered to you, that the Lord Jesus on the night when he was betrayed took bread, and when he had given thanks, he broke it, and said, "This is my body which is for you. Do this in remembrance of me." In the same way also the cup, after supper, saying, "This cup is the new covenant in my blood. Do this, as often as you drink it, in remembrance of me." For as often as you eat this bread and drink the cup, you proclaim the Lord's death until he comes. (1 Cor 11: 23-26)

The Agape ("love" in Greek) refers to an early Christian religious meal that was at first closely related to the celebration of the Eucharist and often preceded this celebration. The close connection did not last long, however, because of the Eucharistic abuses that arose from its proximity to the Agape. St. Paul criticizes these abuses in his first letter to the Corinthians:

> When you meet together, it is not the Lord's supper that you eat. For in eating, each one goes ahead with his own meal, and one is hungry and another is drunk. What! Do you not have houses to eat and drink in? Or do you despise the church of God and humiliate those who have nothing? (1 Cor 11: 20-22)

In order to avoid impiety and denigration of the Eucharistic celebration, the Agape was soon celebrated in the evenings. Records of the Agape, however, are few, and the practice generally did not last long, except in some smaller and more isolated churches.

The ritual of the Mass developed gradually over time. The beginning of the ceremony included readings from the Bible, singing of the psalms and hymns, common prayers, and a collection for the poor. (Keep in mind, though, that even if the official Canon of Sacred Scripture was not set until the fourth century, many, including Tertullian, St. Irenæus, and St. Clement of Alexandria held the four Gospels as inspired.) Finally came the Liturgy of the Eucharist, which formed the high point of the liturgical celebration. In the earliest years, fixed prayers did not exist. Rather, the celebrant gave thanks in his own words before praying the Institution Narrative and Consecration. The Consecration, which comprises the actual words of Christ, was already written down in the earliest letters of St. Paul (cf. 1 Cor 11: 23-26) in the AD 50s.

The Eucharist, literally meaning "thanksgiving," was, and is, the central act of Christian worship, and it consisted in consuming the Sacrament of Holy Communion, the Body and Blood of Christ. All of the early documents from this period indicate that the early Christians considered Christ truly present in the Eucharist under the appearance of bread and wine, attested by many of the Fathers of the Church, including Sts. Cyril of Jerusalem, John Chrysostom, Gregory of Nyssa, Cyril of Alexandria, Ambrose, Augustine, Justin Martyr, and

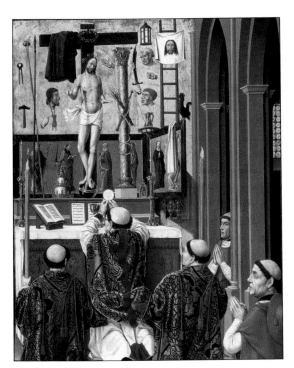

John of Damascus. This corresponds to the teaching of the Church based on the New Testament accounts. For instance, St. John Chrysostom teaches, "It is not man that causes the things offered to become the Body and Blood of Christ, but he who was crucified for us, Christ himself. The priest, in the role of Christ, pronounces these words, but their power and grace are God's. This is my body, he says. This word transforms the thing offered" (Prod. Jud. 1: 6: PG 49, 380). Likewise St. Ambrose says, "Be convinced that this is not what nature has formed, but what the blessing has consecrated. The power of the blessing prevails over that of nature, because by the blessing nature itself is changed….Could not Christ's word, which can make from nothing what did not exist, change existing things into what they were not before? It is no less a feat to give things their original nature than to change their nature" (De myst. 9, 50; 52: PL 16, 405-407).

CHURCHES

For the earliest celebrations of the Mass, people gathered together in private homes and in the catacombs, especially during periods of persecution. Some of the Roman emperors permitted Christians to build churches, especially at the beginning of the second century. Renewed persecutions, however, left most of these structures destroyed. It was not until the Edict of Milan (AD 313), when Emperor Constantine began a building program favorable to the Christians, that Roman architectural designs like the basilica were transformed into Christian churches.

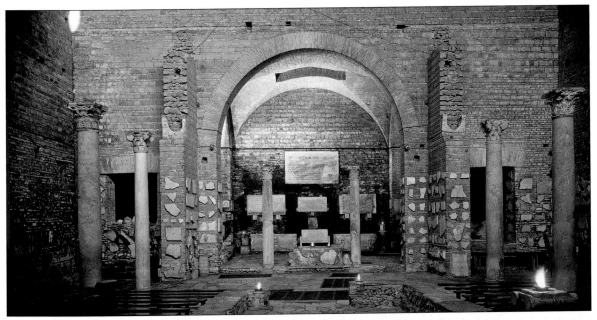

Basilica of St. Nereus, Domitilla Catacombs, Rome, Italy

THE CATACOMBS

Catacombs were an important gathering place for early Christians in certain areas. A catacomb is an underground series of tunnels, chambers, and tombs that were dug by Christians and served as burial places, shrines, and places of worship during the first few centuries after Christ. The most famous Christian catacombs are those found outside of Rome, but catacombs have also been discovered throughout Italy, France, and Northern Africa.

There are over sixty different catacombs scattered along the outskirts of Rome, and together they account for hundreds of miles of underground tunnels, and they are estimated to have held almost two million graves. The catacombs of St. Callixtus are among the most impressive. These catacombs are four stories deep, include about 12 miles of tunnels and galleries, and in them were buried 16 popes and dozens of martyrs!

The catacombs are made up of long narrow tunnels with several rows of rectangular niches on each side, called "loculi." Corpses would usually be wrapped in a shroud and laid in the **loculi**. Then, the **loculi** would be sealed with a marble slab or with tiles. The tombs would often be adorned with inscriptions of the person's name or a short prayer, as well as religious symbols. There were also small rooms called **cubicula** that served as family tombs, and larger rooms called crypts where the tombs of prominent figures, such as popes or martyrs, were converted into small churches.

Most of the catacombs were begun in the second century and initially were merely burial places. Christians shunned the Roman practice of cremation and preferred burial because of their belief in the resurrection of the body. This desire to be buried together showed the strong sense of community in the early Church. Although they were never actually used as hiding places during times of persecution, the catacombs did serve as places of refuge for baptisms and the celebration of the Eucharist. In the privacy of the catacombs, Christians could worship openly, and express themselves in prayer and religious art.

As the persecutions continued, martyrs were given places of honor in the catacombs. The tombs of the martyrs became popular places of prayer where Christians would ask for the martyrs' intercession. The catacombs were continually expanded and used for burial through the fifth century AD. Eventually, they were abandoned and forgotten, only to be rediscovered in the sixteenth century. Ever since that time, they have remained popular pilgrimage sites for Christians to find inspiration and learn about the early Church.

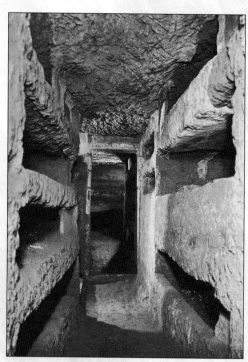

THE EARLY GROWTH OF CHRISTIANITY

CHRISTIAN COMMUNITIES BY AD 100

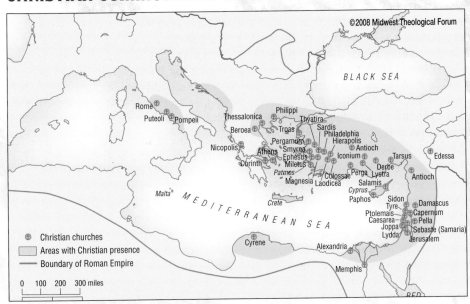

©2008 Midwest Theological Forum

BLACK SEA

Rome
Puteoli Pompeii
Thessalonica
Philippi
Beroea
Thyatira
Troas
Sardis
Philadelphia
Hierapolis
Pergamum
Nicopolis
Smyrna
Antioch
Athens
Ephesus
Iconium
Tarsus
Edessa
Corinth
Miletus
Patmos
Derbe
Perga Lystra
Antioch
Magnesia
Colossae
Salamis
Laodicea
Cyprus
Crete
Paphos
Sidon
Damascus
Malta
Tyre
Capernum
MEDITERRANEAN SEA
Ptolemais
Pella
Caesarea
Sebaste (Samaria)
Joppa
Cyrene
Lydda Jerusalem
Alexandria
Memphis
RED

⊕ Christian churches
▢ Areas with Christian presence
— Boundary of Roman Empire

0   100   200   300 miles

CHRISTIAN COMMUNITIES BY AD 300

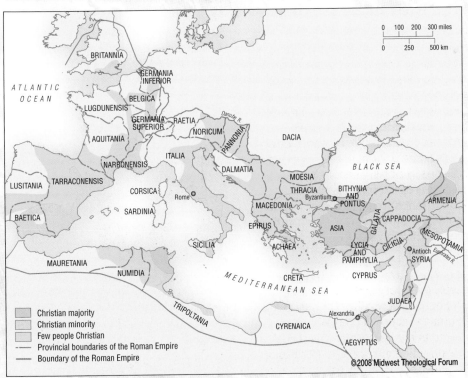

0   100   200   300 miles
0   250   500 km

BRITANNIA
GERMANIA INFERIOR
ATLANTIC OCEAN
BELGICA
LUGDUNENSIS
GERMANIA SUPERIOR RAETIA
Danube R.
AQUITANIA
NORICUM
PANNONIA
DACIA
NARBONENSIS
ITALIA
DALMATIA
MOESIA
BLACK SEA
LUSITANIA
TARRACONENSIS
CORSICA
Rome
THRACIA
BITHYNIA AND PONTUS
Byzantium
ARMENIA
BAETICA
SARDINIA
MACEDONIA
CAPPADOCIA
SICILIA
EPIRUS
ASIA
GALATIA
ACHAEA
LYCIA AND PAMPHYLIA
CILICIA
MESOPOTAMIA
Antioch Euphrates R.
SYRIA
MAURETANIA
NUMIDIA
CRETA
CYPRUS
TRIPOLITANIA
MEDITERRANEAN SEA
JUDAEA
Alexandria
CYRENAICA
AEGYPTUS

▨ Christian majority
▧ Christian minority
▢ Few people Christian
–·– Provincial boundaries of the Roman Empire
— Boundary of the Roman Empire

©2008 Midwest Theological Forum

HOLY DAYS

For the early Christians, Wednesdays and Fridays were days of fasting and penance. Though Friday was chosen because it was the day that Christ suffered and accomplished his redemptive sacrifice, it is not clear why Wednesday was also reserved for fasting and penance. Some traditions hold that this was the day that Judas conspired with the chief priests to betray Jesus.

The Jewish Sabbath lasted from sundown on Friday until sundown on Saturday. Christians at first kept the Jewish Sabbath (day of rest), but Sunday quickly replaced Saturday as the holiest day of the week because it represented both the day on which Jesus rose from the dead and the day on which Pentecost occurred. Sunday was reputed to be the first day of creation and it followed that the first day of "re-creation" would be recognized as well. Celebrating the Lord's Day on Sunday also provided convenient cover for Christians during the persecutions because it was observed by pagans as their holy day as well. By the end of the first three centuries, the practice of celebrating Mass on Sundays had taken root.

Feast days also developed throughout the years. The Feast of Epiphany, for example, was celebrated in many separate places in the West before the fourth century. St. John Chrysostom introduced this feast in the East.

CHRISTIAN SYMBOLS

The cross was the most widespread and enduring of all Christian symbols, since it expresses the entirety of the Christian Faith. By the early third century, the practice of making the Sign of the Cross was deeply rooted in the Christian world; Tertullian refers to Christians as "devotees of the cross." The Sign of the Cross took various forms over the centuries, from tracing the cross over the forehead, mouth, and heart to the common sign used to today. In the Eastern Church, people touch their first three fingers together while blessing themselves to symbolize the Trinity.

Another widespread and ancient Christian symbol is the fish. Among the earliest Christians, the fish for a time may have held even greater significance than the cross. It is an ancient symbol, long predating Christianity, and it became a universal Christian symbol for Christ. It recalls the multiplication of loaves and fishes, as well as Christ's appearance to the seven disciples after the Resurrection at the end of St. John's Gospel. The principal reason for its widespread popularity was that the Greek for fish, **ichthys**, can also be an acrostic for the Greek phrase, **Iesous CHristos THeou Yios Soter**, which, as a declaration of the central tenet of the Christian Faith means, "Jesus Christ, Son of God, Savior."

Often appearing with the fish was the symbol of the anchor. Like the fish, it is an ancient symbol of pre-Christian origins, and it long symbolized safety. The early Christians adopted the anchor and developed its significance from safety to hope. It was often paired with the ship—as a ship is kept from drifting by its anchor, so is faith kept from drifting by hope. The anchor also served the role of an esoteric depiction of the cross—easily recognized by Christians, but not by non-believers.

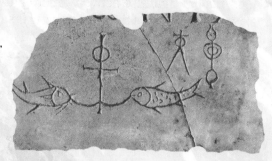

A carving on a tombstone in the early fourth century catacomb of St. Domatilla depicts the fish symbol combined with the cross-like anchor symbol.

THE PAPACY

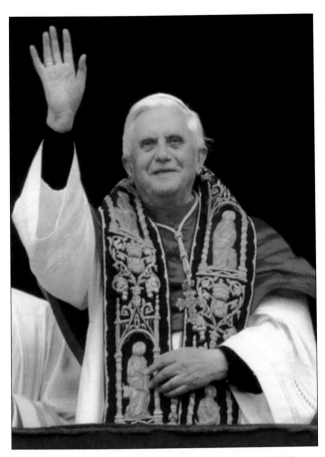

Pope Benedict XVI was elected the 265th "Vicar of Christ" on April 19, 2005.

Christ made St. Peter the head of his Church (cf. Mt 16:13-23, Jn 21:15-17), the first pope, the Vicar of Christ, conferring upon him the responsibility and supreme authority of guiding the Church after Christ's departure. There are clear historical sources that indicate that the authority of the Bishop of Rome was recognized and regarded as the supreme authority in all Church matters from the very beginning. The First Epistle of Pope St. Clement I (AD 88-97) demonstrates the recognized authority of the papacy as he settled controversies that were disrupting the Church in Corinth. The Epistle to the Romans written by St. Ignatius of Antioch (ca. AD 35-ca. 107), who was appointed Bishop of Antioch by St. Peter himself, affirms the deferential obedience to the authority of the Bishop of Rome. Similarly, St. Irenæus's writings stressed the importance of the traditional structures in the Church, such as the papacy.

Two popes during the first five centuries of Christendom were especially instrumental in the development of the papacy's ecclesiastical and jurisdictional powers. Pope St. Leo I (d. AD 461) explicitly tried to centralize Church governance based on the Bishop of Rome's preeminence. The city of Rome at the time of Pope St. Leo I was dwindling in size and importance. Political power had shifted east to Byzantium. But even as Rome's political significance and temporal power diminished and nearly vanished while at the same time the patriarchs of Constantinople and Alexandria were growing in political importance, the Church Councils still deferred to the pope in Rome before acting on a decision.

Pope St. Gelasius I (d. 496) also actively asserted the primacy of the Roman pontiff and seems to have been the first to have used the title "Vicar of Christ" to denote his divine authority, especially as he battled against a number of heresies in the East. From the eighth century, the title "Vicar of Christ" began to be employed by the popes in addition to being used by bishops, kings, judges, and priests. Many of the early popes used the title "Vicar of St. Peter"; nevertheless, at the time of Pope Innocent III in the thirteenth century, "Vicar of Christ" became used by the pope exclusively.

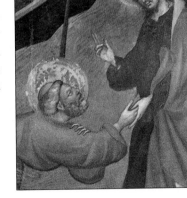

The Gospel reading at the Inauguration Mass for Pope Benedict XVI on April 25, 2005 was John 21:15-19. "…'Simon [Peter], son of John, do you love me?'…'Lord, you know everything; you know that I love you.' Jesus said to him, 'Feed my sheep.'… And after this he said to him, 'Follow me.'"

THE EPISCOPACY

As with the papacy, from the beginning the Church held the office of bishop to be of great importance. The bishops, as successors to the Apostles, were responsible for shepherding and guiding the flock in the various–and often dangerous–cities and situations in which Christians found themselves. The bishops baptized, offered up the Holy Sacrifice of the Mass, celebrated weddings, ordained priests, and engaged themselves in all of the sacramental work of the Church.

St. Ignatius of Antioch, of whom more will be said in the following chapter, wrote in his Epistle to the Smyrnaeans the following with regard to the importance of the bishop: "Wherever the bishop shall appear, there let the multitude [of the people] also be; even as, wherever Jesus Christ is, there is the Catholic Church" (Epistle to the Smyrnaeans, VIII). St. Ignatius was the first to use the term "Catholic Church."

PRIESTHOOD

The word "priest" is a contraction of the Greek word presbyteros that is normally translated as "presbyter." In the early Church, the presbyters were the church elders. The full understanding of the priesthood, as minister of Divine worship and of the Eucharistic sacrifice subordinate to the bishop to whom he has sworn canonical allegiance, developed over the centuries. However, there is evidence that as early as the second century there were already many priests being ordained to offer up the Sacrifice of the Mass.

The earliest extant ordination rites come from St. Hippolytus's (ca. AD 170 - ca. 236) Apostolic Tradition, as well as the fourth century Apostolic Constitutions.

THE SCRIPTURES

During the earliest centuries of the Church, the Canon of the Bible was certainly not intact as one integral whole as it is in its present form. Many of the books that would later come to comprise much of the Canon of the Old Testament, such as the five books of the Pentateuch, were long held to be canonical by the Jewish tradition. Other books, such as Tobit and Wisdom, would be accepted through the course of the formation of the Catholic Canon. Many books of the New Testament, such as St. Matthew's gospel and most of St. Paul's epistles, were from the earliest times universally accepted; others, such as Revelation, required more time.

By the early third century, the universally accepted books of the New Testament canon were the following: the four Gospels, thirteen of St. Paul's Epistles, Acts, Revelation, 1 and 2 Peter, and 1, 2, and 3 John. After much discussion among various Church authorities including Origen, Eusebius, St. Athanasius, and St. Jerome, a definitive Canon was declared at a large synod in AD 382 in Rome. Though it took a few more years for churches in Africa and Gaul to accept the canon, by the end of the first decade of the fifth century, the Western Church possessed the complete Canon of the New Testament. The Church in the East, though it had not made nor recognized any formal statement concerning the Canon of the New Testament, generally accepted what the West had affirmed, except for some lingering disputes over the legitimacy of the book of Revelation. The Canon of the Old Testament took longer to be officially determined, though for many centuries St. Jerome's Vulgate was taken as standard for ecclesiastical usage. Finally, in 1546 at the Council of Trent, the Church made its final definitive statement concerning the Canon of Scripture.

The issue of the Scriptures and the establishment of the Canon are very important. In contrast to what the Reformation would falsely teach, the early Church never considered the Scriptures as authoritative apart from their interpretation by the Church through her hierarchy. Indeed, without this perennial guidance by the Holy Spirit, the Church's leadership would not have the wisdom to judge whether a particular book was divinely inspired or apocryphal (a work of literature with scriptural pretensions that is not divinely inspired), there would be no Bible as it exists. The Church, under the guiding grace of the Holy Spirit, over many centuries of careful deliberation and prayer, authoritatively determined those inspired texts that would form the Bible.

The Old Testament writings played a significant role in the early Christian community. Though the Church lifted the burden of the Old Law's requirements, the books of the Old Testament were understood to be still authoritative. Christ fulfilled the Old Testament prophecies regarding the messiah. The Old Testament told the important story of how God established his covenant with the chosen people. The early Christians often sang the Psalms, especially in the liturgy and when they were being led to martyrdom.

The Scriptures, though obviously very important, were never seen as a record and interpretation of everything that Jesus and the Apostles did. It is the Tradition of the Church expressed in early Christian literature, liturgical practices, and statements of the Church that clarify and interpret Scripture. Sacred Scripture is a vital and central part of a broader tradition.

SEXUAL ETHICS: ABORTION AND CONTRACEPTION

The Church Fathers and early Christian thinkers universally rejected the practices of abortion and infanticide, which were both prevalent in Roman society. They also rejected the use of contraception. Such writers and thinkers included the author of the Didache, Clement of Alexandria, Tertullian, St. Ambrose, St. John Chrysostom, St. Jerome, and St. Augustine.

Abortion and infanticide violently reject the dignity of the human person and violate the fifth commandment: "You shall not kill" (Ex 20:13). The Church has always held this to be the case. Jesus never spoke directly about either of these topics, but Jewish law and Jesus' teaching concerning the

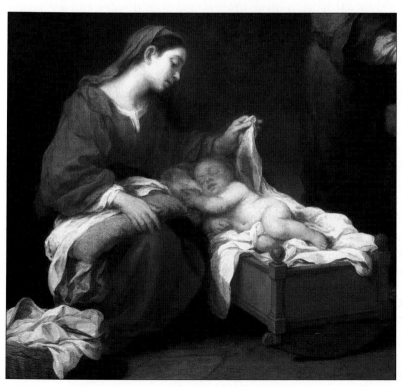

Abortion and infanticide violently reject the dignity of the human person.

sacredness of human life and the love of neighbor led the early Church to embrace this teaching. Christ "gives [his Apostles and their successors] a share in his own mission. From him they receive the power to act in his person" (CCC 935).

The Church Fathers taught that procreation within Matrimony is good and blessed, and that it is one of the intrinsic purposes of sexual intercourse. Artificial prevention of this possibility denigrates both the act and the subjects of the act. Even ancient Greek philosophy saw contraception as an unnatural violation since it destroys the possibility of one of the natural ends of sexual relations.

PART VII

Important Writings of the Early Christian Period

APOLOGISTS

> Always be prepared to make a defense to any one who calls you to account for the hope that is in you. (1 Pt 3:15)

Apologetics (from the Greek apologia, meaning "defense") is a branch of theology that purports to defend and explain the Christian religion. The history of apologetics is as old as the history of the Church and can be divided into four historical periods, each with its particular struggle. The first, which concerns this section, dates from the dawn of Christianity to the collapse of the Roman Empire in AD 476. The three great opponents facing Christianity at this time were Judaism, Gnostic heresies, and the various pagan religions throughout the Roman Empire.

Though the title "apologist" refers to anyone who writes an apologetic work, there was a group of early Church Fathers collectively known as Apologists. Writing mainly during the second and third centuries, these men composed some of the greatest Christian literature. The Apologists include St. Aristides, St. Justin Martyr, Tatian, Athenagoras, St. Theophilus, Minucius Felix, and Tertullian. Due in significant part to their work, Christianity had begun to gain more converts from among the educated and elite classes. Most of the writers were not trained theologians, but rather writers with an audience consisting of the public and the emperor with his immediate subordinates.

As previously mentioned, early Christianity found itself attacked by both the Jewish and pagan traditions. For the majority of the Jews at this time, the burgeoning Christian religion, which claimed its roots in the ancient and holy tradition of Israel, denigrated and desecrated Judaism, the Law, and the God of Abraham. In claiming fulfillment of the Mosaic Law, Christianity rejected the need for circumcision and other practices. Christ, the poor, common, humble teacher who was brutally executed beside two thieves, was far from the concept of a messiah so long expected by the Jews. The apologetic writings to the Jews focused on these issues.

The most important aim of apologetic work at this time was to address the pagan culture of the Roman Empire. Roman culture – from its literature and philosophy to its commercial and agricultural activities, from the political sphere to mundane, everyday habits – was imbued with paganism. Pomp, power, and glory of the Empire and its gods dominated the popular mind, and Christianity did not at all fit into this framework. The Christians worshiped in secret, rejected the gods of the land, and refused to follow imperial mandates concerning required sacrifices and venerations. Christians were met first with suspicion and superstition, which soon degenerated into fear and mistrust. The Agape and the celebration of the Eucharist soon were rumored to be orgies and obscure cannibalistic rites, and the Christians became known as enemies of the state. Thus, there was a great need for apologetic writings that explained the practices and beliefs of Christianity to the Roman pagan culture, as well as writings that made a case for the benign and even benevolent presence of Christians in the Empire. Particular attention was given to how Christianity forms exemplary citizens, and how it was a bulwark of the state rather than a cancerous tumor of disloyalty. Even as these writings addressed those issues, they also made clear and persuasive arguments concerning both the spiritual poverty of paganism and the promise of eternal life and happiness in Christ.

THE DIDACHE

The Didache (Greek meaning "teaching"), variously known as The Doctrine of the Twelve Apostles and The Lord's Teaching through the Twelve Apostles to the Nations, is a short exposition concerning Christian morals, doctrine, and customs that was most likely composed in the first century. Its sixteen chapters cover Christian moral life, Baptism, fasting, prayer, the Eucharist, and the developing Church hierarchy.

The author, exact date, and location are unknown, but many of the early Church Fathers, such as St. Clement of Alexandria, Eusebius of Caesarea, and St. Athanasius, used this text as a reference, and some even sought its admittance to the Canon of Scripture. Lost to scholars for centuries, it was finally rediscovered in 1873 by Philotheos Bryennios, a Greek Orthodox bishop.

TERTULLIAN

Tertullian (ca. AD 160 - ca. 225) was born in Carthage around AD 160. He was the son of a Roman centurion and received a sound education through his studies of Roman law. He eventually wrote numerous works, mostly apologetic, in both Latin and Greek (though the Greek works have been lost). He converted from Roman paganism to Christianity sometime in the middle of his life, and from that point on, Tertullian worked to demonstrate with compelling argumentation and rhetoric that the Christians posed no threat to the Roman Empire, but rather were a great asset to it. His writings were highly polemical and brilliantly witty–he did not take any pains to avoid vexing his Roman audience in his defense of the Faith. Tertullian's versatility in explaining and defending the Catholic Faith won for him the title "Father of Latin Theology."

At the beginning of the third century, Tertullian joined the heretical Montanist sect and definitively broke from the Church a few years later. Although his writing then turned against certain doctrines of the Church, he was never a consistent Montanist. The sect supported a rigorous form of Christianity that refused forgiveness for certain "irremissible" sins, especially those of a sexual nature. This particular sect also believed in periodic overwhelming outpourings of the Holy Spirit through Montanist prophets and prophetesses. Tertullian, picking and choosing which tenets of Montanism he thought important, eventually formed his own small following before he died.

ST. HIPPOLYTUS AND THE APOSTOLIC TRADITION

St. Hippolytus (ca. AD 170 - ca. 236) was an important writer and Father of the Church of the late second and early third centuries. Even though he was probably the most important theologian in the Roman Church during the third century, his importance was forgotten in the West for some time, perhaps because of his extensive use of Greek.

Though most of Hippolytus's voluminous corpus has been lost, his two most important works, The Refutation of all Heresies and The Apostolic Tradition, have survived, in part. The latter work describes the passing down of the Faith of the Apostles from generation to generation and provides insight into the rites of ordination, Baptism, and the Eucharist during the third century. The Eucharistic Prayer found in The Apostolic Tradition became the basis for the second Eucharistic Prayer in the 1970 Roman Missal, which was published as part of the intended reforms of the Second Vatican Council.

PART VIII

Martyrdom as the Greatest Testimony to Christianity

Behold, I send you out as sheep in the midst of wolves;
so be wise as serpents and innocent as doves. (Mt 10:16)

From as early as the first century, Christians, in the face of both Jewish and Roman opposition, found that they had to be prepared to die for Christ. Those who did actually lose their lives quickly became the most venerated of all saints. An entire theology developed around the martyrs that recognized their importance in the history of the Church.

The vast majority of martyrs were average, everyday people who naturally worried about the pain and suffering that they would endure; this worry was often mitigated by the solidarity of fellow Christians. Before being martyred the early Christians would exchange the kiss of peace, and were often described as dying with a tremendous bearing of peace and joy.

The word "martyr" comes from the Greek word martyros, meaning "witness." A martyr bears witness to Christ as the Way, the Truth, and the Life. In the early Church, as today, the actions and words of the martyrs strengthened and edified other Christians. Even in the last moments of their lives, in which the crowds often took sadistic pleasure, martyrs often led the assembled crowds along the path of conversion by giving the supreme witness of loving fidelity to Christ. The serenity, joy, and faithfulness with which the martyrs accepted their deaths deeply affected some of the people, such as the magistrates and the executioners, who witnessed their deaths.

Christians understood martyrdom as an honor and a privilege since it was a direct participation in the sufferings of Christ. The victims were sustained by Christ in their dreadful suffering and they saw martyrdom as the surest means to sanctity and entrance into Heaven. The entire Christian community viewed martyrdom as a grace and a gift, though Christians were not supposed to seek out martyrdom because of the obligation to practice and preserve one's life. Through martyrdom the three theological virtues of faith, hope, and charity would reach unparalleled dimensions. The next chapter will explore many of the early persecutions and their causes, as well as the stories of some of the most renowned martyrs.

CONCLUSION

St. John was the last of the Apostles to die, and with his death public revelation ended. Since Christ is the culmination of God's direct revelation to his people, possession of the Deposit of Faith and its interpretation corresponds to the Apostles who were the Lord's closest followers and witnesses to his life. The teachings of the Apostles initiated the body of living truths called the Tradition of the Church, which began with their preaching and instruction. During their lifetimes, the Apostles transmitted their episcopal power and authority to their first successors. The generation succeeding that of Jesus Christ's contemporaries already had a keen notion of this Tradition and of its bishops' direct link to the Apostles. From the earliest times, the successors of the Apostles have been given the duty to protect and transmit Christ's teaching as it was taught and interpreted by the first Apostles.

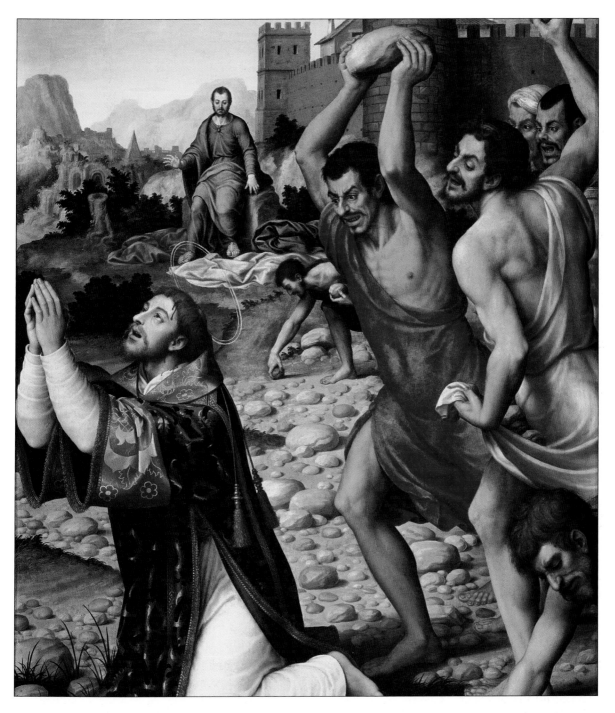

The early Christians, by their tremendous faith in Jesus and imitation of his life, transformed the Roman world and its values. The decadent Roman culture, with its basis in the law of power, was supplanted by a culture based on Christ's new commandment: "Love one another; even as I have loved you" (Jn 13: 34). Guided by the Holy Spirit, the Church grew as an institution and a community of believers united as the Mystical Body of Christ. Ordinary people from all walks of life carried out a peaceful revolution that spread from person to person through the simple living witness to the richness of Christ's kingdom, even in the face of terrible persecution and horrific death.

VOCABULARY

AGAPE

Literally "love." The Agape was an early Christian religious meal that was at first closely related to the celebration of the Eucharist and often preceded this celebration.

APOCRYPHAL

A work of literature with scriptural or quasi-scriptural pretensions which is not genuine, canonical, or inspired by God.

APOLOGIST

Generally, one who writes a work in order to defend and explain the Christian religion. The title also refers specifically to a group of Church Fathers who wrote during the second and third centuries in the Roman Empire.

APOSTLE

The word "apostle" comes from the Greek *apostolos,* a form of *apostellein,* meaning "to send away." An apostle is literally "one who is sent." Refers to the twelve men chosen by Jesus during the course of his public ministry to be his closest followers, as well as Sts. Matthias, Paul of Tarsus, and Barnabas, who were chosen after Jesus' Resurrection.

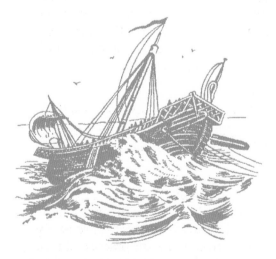

The Roman grain ship that St. Paul traveled on carried 276 men. Midships was a high mast, usually of cedar wood, and near the prow was a smaller one for hoisting a small sail. Two large oars were used to steer. On the deck was a wooden hut for the helmsman which was also used as a temple of worship containing an idol.

APOSTOLIC TRADITION

Refers to the passing of the Faith of the Apostles from generation to generation. Hippolytus's work of the same name illustrated the principle by preserving the rites of ordination, Baptism, and the Eucharist used during the third century. The Eucharistic Prayer found in The Apostolic Tradition became the basis for the second Eucharistic Prayer in the 1970 Roman Missal, which was published as part of the intended reforms for the Second Vatican Council.

BAPTISM

This first Sacrament of Initiation, instituted by Jesus, unites the believer to Christ. In this sacrament, a believer is forgiven of original and personal sin, and thus begins a new life in Christ and the Holy Spirit, and is incorporated into the Church, the Body of Christ (cf. CCC 977, 1213).

BISHOP

A bishop is a successor of the Apostles who has received the fullness of Christ's priesthood.

CATECHUMENS

Literally "the instructed." Those adults seeking admission to the Church after having met over a long period of time for instruction before being baptized.

CHURCH

In the Scriptures, the Church is described as the Body of Christ and the Temple of the Holy Spirit (cf. Eph 1: 22-23). The English word "church" etymologically comes from a Greek word meaning "thing belonging to the Lord," which was applied originally to the church building. The Latin word *ecclesia* derives from another Greek word that means "assembly" or "congregation." Willed by the Father, the Church was founded by Jesus Christ and enjoys the presence and guidance of the Holy Spirit. It is through the Church that God carries out his plan of salvation for all people. The teaching authority and sanctifying power of the Church serve as a means to bring all men and women to greater union with God and with each other as well.

VOCABULARY

CHURCH HISTORY

The history of the Church is the record of the life of Jesus, the actions of men, and the guiding light of the Holy Spirit acting in the Church. This history began with the initial evangelization of the Apostles, and the narrative about Christ's kingdom on earth is forged as the Church interacts and responds to every culture and historical situation.

COUNCIL

An authorized gathering of bishops, guided in a unique way by the Holy Spirit, to discuss ecclesiastical matters with the aim of passing decrees on the themes under discussion.

DEPOSIT OF FAITH

Deposit of Faith, that is the heritage of Faith contained in Sacred Scripture and Tradition, handed on in the Church from the time of the Apostles.

THE *DIDACHE*

From the Greek meaning "teaching," a first century treatise concerning Christian morals, practices, and ministry. Its sixteen chapters cover Baptism, fasting, prayers, the Eucharist, and the developing Church hierarchy among the early Christians.

EUCHARIST

Literally meaning "thanksgiving," was, and is, the central act of Christian worship. It consists in consuming the Sacrament of Holy Communion, the Body and Blood of Christ.

ICHTHYS

An acrostic for the Greek phrase Iesous Christos Theou Yios Soter, which is a declaration of the central tenet of the Christian Faith meaning "Jesus Christ, Son of God, Savior." The acrostic itself spells the word "fish" in Greek.

INFANT BAPTISM

The practice of baptizing infants that became more common during the third century and became universal by the early Medieval period. It remained the common practice for all western Christians until the Reformation in the sixteenth century.

MARTYRDOM

Being killed for one's Faith. Christians understand martyrdom as an honor and a privilege since it is a direct participation in the sufferings of Christ.

MARTYRDOM

The supreme witness given to the truth of the Faith by bearing witness even unto death.

PAPACY

The Vicar of Christ as instituted by Jesus who holds the responsibility and supreme authority for guiding the Church.

PENTECOST

Pentecost celebrates the descent of the Holy Spirit upon Mary and the Apostles fifty days after the Resurrection.

PEOPLE OF GOD

Those "born" into the Church through faith in Christ and Baptism. The term "People of God" is taken from the Old Testament in which God chose Israel to be his chosen people. Christ instituted the new and eternal covenant by which a new priestly, prophetic, and royal People of God, the Church, participates in the mission and service of Christ.

PRESBYTER

From the Greek word presbyteros for "priest," which is a contraction of the Greek. In the early Church, the presbyters were the church elders.

SIGN OF THE CROSS

The act of tracing the cross down from the forehead with the finger to the breast and then from left to right across the breast. By the early third century, the practice of making the Sign of the Cross was deeply rooted in the Christian world.

STUDY QUESTIONS

1. When did Jesus send the Holy Spirit to guide the Church?

2. Who is the cornerstone of the Church?

3. Who is Christ's vicar on earth?

4. What is Church history?

5. What are two basic components of the history of the Church?

6. Who were Simeon and Anna?

7. What was the "Slaughter of the Innocents"?

8. What is the inaugural event of Jesus' public ministry?

9. What was the teaching of the New Law?

10. What effects did the Holy Spirit have upon the Apostles at Pentecost?

11. What laid the groundwork for the Church?

12. What are the four marks of the Church?

13. What sets the Apostles apart from other early members of the Church?

14. What does the Greek root of the word "apostle" mean?

15. Who are the successors to the Apostles?

16. Who was the famous Jewish teacher under whom St. Paul studied?

17. To which city was Saul going when he met Jesus Christ?

18. How was Saul physically impaired after his encounter with Jesus?

19. Who healed Saul?

20. What is the significance of Cornelius's conversion?

21. Why was it important that St. Peter received this message from God first?

22. Who was the author of the oldest texts in the New Testament and when were they written?

23. Why did Jewish Christians criticize St. Peter?

24. When and why was the Council of Jerusalem called?

25. What was the outcome of the Council of Jerusalem?

26. Why was St. Paul beheaded instead of being crucified like Sts. Peter and Andrew?

27. Which Apostle was exiled to the island of Patmos after allegedly having survived being put into a vat of boiling oil?

28. Who was St. Jude?

29. What are some of the advantages of infant Baptism?

30. Where were the earliest Masses celebrated?

31. Which two days of the week did the earliest Christians keep holy as days of fasting and penance? (Hint: It was not Sunday.)

32. Why did Christians come to observe Sunday as the holiest day of the week?

33. What does the term "Vicar of Christ" mean?

34. What is the value of the episcopacy?

35. From what word does the word "priest" derive?

36. When was the canon of the New Testament declared in the West?

37. Who is the authentic interpreter of Sacred Scripture?

38. What did the early Christians think about abortion and infanticide?

39. What was the goal of the Apologists?

40. The word "martyr" means "witness." To whom do martyrs bear witness?

PRACTICAL EXERCISES

1. How was Jesus' life authentically human? How was it divine? Cite specific examples from the Gospel.

2. Why is Pentecost one of the most important feast days in the liturgical year? What does it mean that the Holy Spirit "dwells" in the Church?

3. The Gospel is an account of Jesus' calling of the Apostles. How did Jesus convince these total strangers to give up everything and go follow him after meeting him only for the first time? In small groups, write a brief skit in which you try to use Jesus' words to convince someone in today's society to come and follow him.

4. What kind of men were the Apostles? What does their social status, education, and personality demonstrate about how Jesus calls people to live a Christian life?

5. Protestants accept the principle of sola scriptura, Scripture alone, as the primary basis for authority. The Catholic position is that the Church alone interprets the Scriptures. Discuss why the Catholic position makes more sense historically.

FROM THE CATECHISM

766 The Church is born primarily of Christ's total self-giving for our salvation, anticipated in the institution of the Eucharist and fulfilled on the cross. "The origin and growth of the Church are symbolized by the blood and water which flowed from the open side of the crucified Jesus" (*LG* 3; cf. Jn 19:34). "For it was from the side of Christ as he slept the sleep of death upon the cross that there came forth the 'wondrous sacrament of the whole Church'" (*SC* 5). As Eve was formed from the sleeping Adam's side, so the Church was born from the pierced heart of Christ hanging dead on the cross (cf. St. Ambrose, *In Luc.* 2, 85-89: PL 15, 1666-1668).

889 In order to preserve the Church in the purity of the faith handed on by the apostles, Christ who is the Truth willed to confer on her a share in his own infallibility. By a "supernatural sense of faith" the People of God, under the guidance of the Church's living Magisterium, "unfailingly adheres to this faith" (*LG* 12; cf. *DV* 10).

890 The mission of the Magisterium is linked to the definitive nature of the covenant established by God with his people in Christ. It is this Magisterium's task to preserve God's people from deviations and defections and to guarantee them the objective possibility of professing the true faith without error. Thus, the pastoral duty of the Magisterium is aimed at seeing to it that the People of God abides in the truth that liberates. To fulfill this service, Christ endowed the Church's shepherds with the charism of infallibility in matters of faith and morals. The exercise of this charism takes several forms:

891 "The Roman Pontiff, head of the college of bishops, enjoys this infallibility in virtue of his office, when, as supreme pastor and teacher of all the faithful – who confirms his brethren in the faith – he proclaims by a definitive act a doctrine pertaining to faith or morals....The infallibility promised to the Church is also present in the body of bishops when, together with Peter's successor, they exercise the supreme

FROM THE CATECHISM Continued

Magisterium," above all in an Ecumenical Council (*LG* 25; cf. Vatican Council I: DS 3074). When the Church through its supreme Magisterium proposes a doctrine "for belief as being divinely revealed" (*DV* 10 § 2), and as the teaching of Christ, the definitions "must be adhered to with the obedience of faith" (*LG* 25 § 2). This infallibility extends as far as the deposit of divine Revelation itself (cf. *LG* 25).

1231 Where infant Baptism has become the form in which this sacrament is usually celebrated, it has become a single act encapsulating the preparatory stages of Christian initiation in a very abridged way. By its very nature infant Baptism requires a post-baptismal catechumenate. Not only is there a need for instruction after Baptism, but also for the necessary flowering of baptismal grace in personal growth. The Catechism has its proper place here.

1233 Today in all the rites, Latin and Eastern, the Christian initiation of adults begins with their entry into the catechumenate and reaches its culmination in a single celebration of the three sacraments of initiation: Baptism, Confirmation, and the Eucharist (cf. AG 14;

CIC, cann. 851; 865; 866). In the Eastern rites the Christian initiation of infants also begins with Baptism followed immediately by Confirmation and the Eucharist, while in the Roman rite it is followed by years of catechesis before being completed later by Confirmation and the Eucharist, the summit of their Christian initiation (cf. CIC, cann. 851, 2 ; 868).

2271 Since the first century the Church has affirmed the moral evil of every procured abortion. This teaching has not changed and remains unchangeable. Direct abortion, that is to say, abortion willed either as an end or a means, is gravely contrary to the moral law:

> You shall not kill the embryo by abortion and shall not cause the newborn to perish (Didache 2, 2: SCh 248, 148; cf. Ep. Barnabae 19, 5: PG 2, 777; Ad Diognetum 5, 6: PG 2, 1173; Tertullian, Apol. 9: PL 1, 319-320).

> God, the Lord of life, has entrusted to men the noble mission of safeguarding life, and men must carry it out in a manner worthy of themselves. Life must be protected with the utmost care from the moment of conception: abortion and infanticide are abominable crimes (GS 51 § 3).

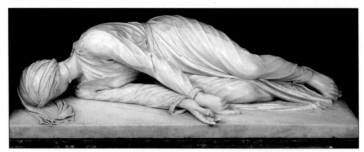

This sculpture of St. Cecilia makes us all eternal witnesses to her faith and martyrdom. It was commissioned by Cardinal Sfondrato, who had opened her tomb in 1599. Tradition holds that this incredible figure represents the position in which St. Cecilia's body was found. On her neck can be seen the three marks of the axe blows that ended her life in the name of Christ.

Persecution Of The Way And Heresies

The complex and often troubling relationship between the Church and the state is one that began in the Roman Empire, and still remains with us today.

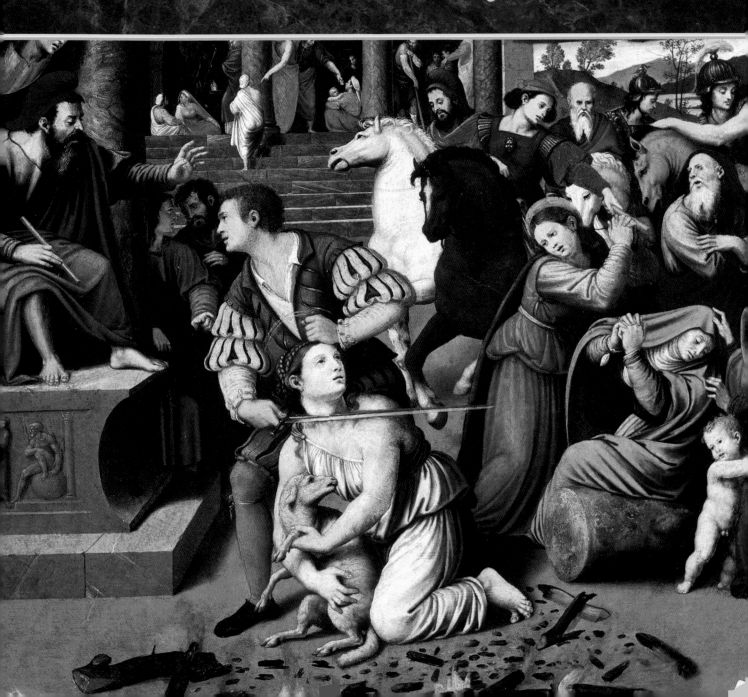

CHAPTER 2

Persecution Of "The Way" And Heresies

In the earliest years, the Christians referred to the Faith as "the Way" (cf. Acts 9:2 and 19:9). Living the Way required a life of integrity according to the commandments and counsels of the Gospels and a strong commitment to become a disciple of Christ. Although living the Way is always difficult and requires much sacrifice, the early Christians especially suffered in the pursuit of its ideals.

Many thousands of early Christians lost their lives during three hundred years of persecutions in the Roman Empire. There are numerous accounts of martyrs from this period, many of whom were priests and bishops of the early Church. Scores of lay men and women from all walks of life comprised the majority of the martyrs. When reading the accounts of the martyrs, it is hard not to be shaken by the brutality with which they were killed. It is important, however, to understand the reasons behind their persecution and to focus upon the courage shown by so many otherwise ordinary men and women. These martyrs lived with their families, had normal occupations in life, and were simply devoted to Christ. Despite the tremendous pressure put on them by the emperors to renounce their Faith, the early Christians remained faithful to the teachings of Jesus.

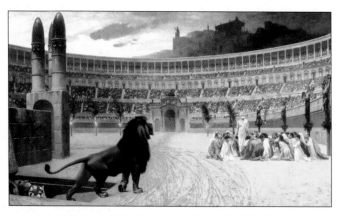

Last Prayers of the Christian Martyrs by Jean-Léon Gérôme

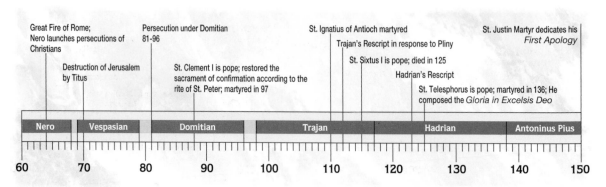

PART I

The First Roman Persecutions

The earliest Christians had suffered persecution at the hands of the Jews, but the Roman Empire for a time did not trouble itself with what appeared to be merely a small group of schismatic Jews. As the early Church grew and distanced itself from the Jewish tradition, the Roman Empire began to view these early Christians as enemies of the empire who, through their disregard for some imperial institutions and traditions, were seen as a breeding ground for corruption and discord within the empire. Soon, periodic imperial persecutions, many of which were incredibly brutal, became a normal part of the life of an early Christian.

THE FIRST PERSECUTION
UNDER EMPEROR NERO (AD 64)

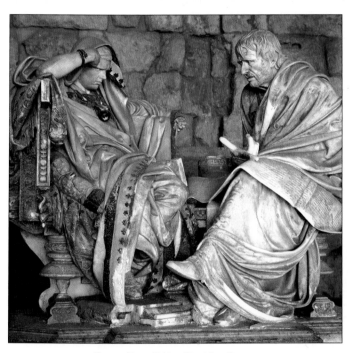

Emperor Nero with his noble advisor, Seneca.

The Emperor Nero (AD 37-68, emperor AD 54-68) was a figure of immense cruelty, psychological sickness, and paranoia. Even the Roman historical tradition portrays him as a tyrant. The stepson of Emperor Claudius and the nephew of Emperor Caligula (infamous for his depravity and psychosis), Nero was the last of the Augustinian line. His rule began in AD 54 at the age of seventeen, and for a time, things ran smoothly. The noble Stoic Seneca was an advisor to Nero and had been his tutor when Nero was young. By the year AD 59, however, Nero's evil character had clearly emerged. He murdered his mother, and then renounced and slandered his own wife, Octavia, before having her beheaded. In AD 65, Nero forced Seneca to commit suicide.

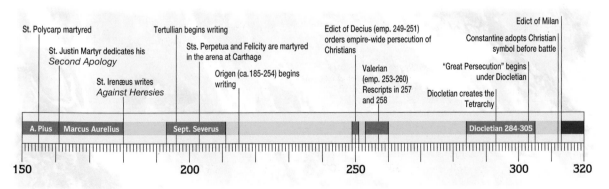

St. Polycarp martyred

St. Justin Martyr dedicates his *Second Apology*

St. Irenæus writes *Against Heresies*

Tertullian begins writing

Sts. Perpetua and Felicity are martyred in the arena at Carthage

Origen (ca.185-254) begins writing

Edict of Decius (emp. 249-251) orders empire-wide persecution of Christians

Valerian (emp. 253-260) Rescripts in 257 and 258

Edict of Milan

Constantine adopts Christian symbol before battle

"Great Persecution" begins under Diocletian

Diocletian creates the Tetrarchy

| A. Pius | Marcus Aurelius | | Sept. Severus | | | | | Diocletian 284-305 | |

150　　　　　　200　　　　　　250　　　　　　300　　320

Early on the night of July 19, AD 64, fire broke out near the Circus Maximus and engulfed the city of Rome for nine straight days. The fire raged throughout the city, and consumed the lives and the property of members of every Roman class.

Immediately, the rumor began to circulate that Nero had started the fire. The reason behind this rumor was Nero's announced intention to seize private property in the center of Rome in order to build an expansive new palace, later called the Domus Aurea (House of Gold). The rumor told of Nero taking delight in watching Rome burn while he read his own poetry. The famous saying, "Nero fiddled while Rome burned," originates from this rumor.

Nero provided emergency shelter to victims, and quickly sought to remove suspicion from himself by falsely accusing the Christians of starting the fire. He tortured several Christians, elicited from them forced confessions, and then ordered large numbers of other Christians to be arrested. The Roman historian Tacitus writes that when it became clear to everyone that Nero's accusations against the Christians were wildly implausible, he charged them with "hating the human race" (Annals, XV, 44).

Although Nero's first persecution of Christians was limited to the city of Rome proper, its egregious brutality remains unquestioned. St. Clement of Rome, the third pope, relates that Christians were first taken across the Tiber to an arena on Vatican hill called Nero's Circus, where St. Peter's Basilica now stands. They were then sewn into animal skins and distributed throughout the gardens. Next Nero released hungry mastiff dogs into the gardens, which hunted down and ate the trapped Christians. Other Christians were martyred in an assortment of awful ways in the Circus Maximus. Finally, in perhaps the greatest example of the emperor's cruelty, Nero coated hundreds of live Christians with pitch and resin and then set them on fire to provide light for him as he passed through his gardens and along the city streets at night.

Nero was the first to declare Christianity unlawful, and sought to punish all believers with death under his principle *Christiani non sint* (Let the Christians be exterminated)..

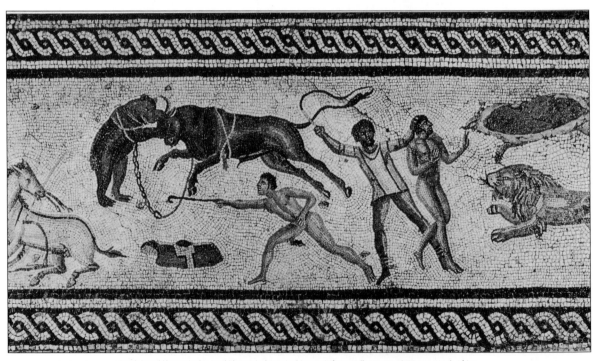

Death by wild beasts in the Amphitheater is shown in this mosaic from a villa near Leptis Magna, North Africa.
The crowd would roar *"Salvum lotum"* (well washed) at the blood-bath.

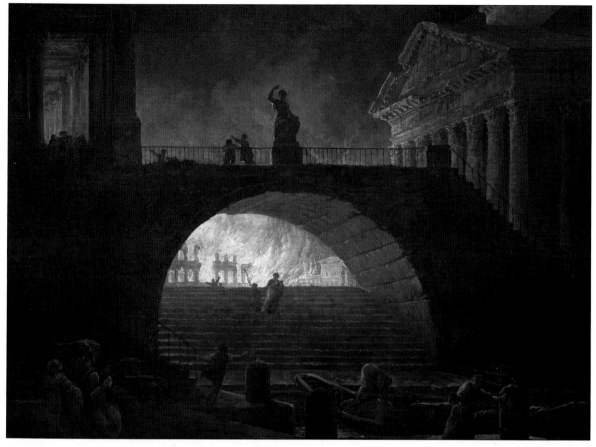

The fire raged throughout the city, and consumed the lives and the property of members of every Roman class.

PERSECUTION UNDER EMPEROR DOMITIAN, "LORD AND GOD"

Domitian (AD 51-96) served as emperor beginning in AD 81. An effective and hard-working ruler, Domitian took particular interest in directing military campaigns and securing the patronage of the army. He had good cause to curry the favor of the army, for his relationship with the Roman Senate was less than ideal. He is reported to have opened his letters to the Senate with the words, "Our lord god orders that this be done." He also habitually referred to himself in the third person as Dominus et Deus ("Lord and God"). As the years passed, Domitian became pathologically suspicious of conspirators and once quipped, "No one believes in a conspiracy against an emperor until it has succeeded."

Domitian was particularly intent on stopping the spread of Christianity from the lower classes to the aristocracy, which included members of his own family. When the Emperor murdered his cousin, an office-holding Christian, he set in motion a conspiracy against him (his wife Domitia possibly being one of the conspirators) that culminated in his assassination.

Despite the fact that growing numbers of patricians began to convert to Christianity, all believers remained subject to heavy impositions placed upon them by the empire. Domitian levied a special tax only on Christians and Jews to pay for a new temple dedicated to Jupiter, and Pope St. Clement I speaks of "misfortunes and catastrophes" in the Roman community because of persecution.

PART II

"The Five Good Emperors"
(AD 96-180)

The five emperors that followed Domitian have been called "The Five Good Emperors" because of their skill in leading the Empire. They are Nerva, Trajan, Hadrian, Antoninus Pius, and Marcus Aurelius. These emperors generally enjoyed the support of the army, senate, and the people, and were certainly much more stable than either Caligula or Nero. They worked to secure the existing borders of the Roman Empire and even expanded them.

While these five emperors were good for the Empire's interests, they were not necessarily supportive of Christianity. Although the first four of these emperors were more moderate than Nero, they by no means halted the persecution of Christians.

TRAJAN'S RESCRIPT (AD 112)

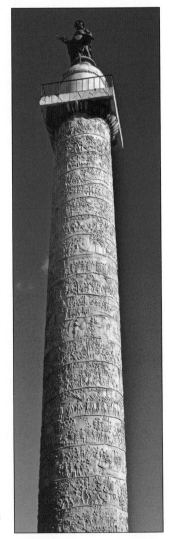

Trajan (ca. AD 53-117) began to rule in AD 98. His nearly twenty year reign is considered to be one of the most excellent in the empire's history. With respect to Christianity, Trajan took what he deemed to be an enlightened and balanced approach. A letter from one of his governors, Pliny the Younger (ca. AD 61-ca. 112), asked for Trajan's advice concerning the persecution and punishment of Christians. According to both Nero and Domitian, Christians were to be summarily executed, and Pliny had executed Christians out of a sense of responsibility. Pliny made it clear to Trajan that Christians by this time existed across all strata of society, and lived in rural as well as urban areas. Pliny posed four questions to Trajan: whether anonymous denunciations of Christians were to be pursued; whether the age of Christians should be taken into consideration in determining their punishment; whether Christians who denied their faith publicly should be allowed to live; and whether the profession of Christianity itself, apart from the crimes associated with the practice of the Faith, was sufficient to warrant execution.

Trajan's response to Pliny offered a nuanced, though definite, policy for handling Christianity. Trajan decreed that if Christians renounced their faith and offered sacrifice to the Roman gods, they would be allowed to live in spite of their past Christian life. Furthermore, Trajan declared that anonymous denunciations were not to be pursued. Nevertheless, anyone denounced openly who admitted his status as a Christian was to suffer death. Trajan's decision thus confirmed that the profession of Christianity was itself a crime, but clarified under what conditions it could be prosecuted.

Trajan's Column is made from a series of 18 colossal Luna marble drums, each weighing about 40 tons, and is exactly 100 Roman feet (30 meters) high. The frieze winds around the shaft 23 times and contains over 2,500 figures. Inside the column, a spiral staircase of 185 stairs provides access to a viewing platform at the top. Originally, a gilded bronze statue of Trajan crowned the top of the column. In 1588, Pope Sixtus V replaced it with a statue of St. Peter.

Trajan's Rescript still left Christians with an awful choice: death or apostasy. While Trajan did seek to remedy the gross abuses of the legal system that were often used in the persecution of Christians, in the end, he upheld the principle first attributed to Nero: Christiani non sint.

ST. IGNATIUS, BISHOP OF ANTIOCH

St. Ignatius (ca. AD 50-ca. 107) was likely the third Bishop of Antioch, after Sts. Peter and Evodius, and he is thought to have listened at the feet of St. John the Evangelist. Because of his close association with Sts. Peter and John, St. Ignatius is an Apostolic Father, i.e., one of those saintly figures who had direct contact with the Apostles, and consequently his writings are considered especially authoritative. In fact, St. Ignatius's letters are considered the most important documents which link the Twelve Apostles with the early Church.

Little is known of St. Ignatius's life up to his arrest during the reign of Trajan for being a renown-ed Christian bishop. Under a guard of ten soldiers, he traveled to Rome to meet a martyr's death. Along the way he was happily received by the Christian communities of the day, and it was during this time that St. Ignatius carried on a correspondence with the various churches of Asia Minor and the bishop of Smyrna, St. Polycarp.

In these letters, known as the Seven Epistles, St. Ignatius makes clear his ardent desire for martyrdom, going so far as to ask the Christians not to intervene with the pagan officials to save his life. Instead, he wrote, "I am God's wheat, and I am ground by the teeth of wild beasts, that I may be found Christ's pure bread" (Epistle to the Romans, IV.1).

St. Ignatius denounced all heresy and schism, and he singled out the episcopacy in the Church as a bulwark against false belief and as a means of unity with Christ. Without bishops, St. Ignatius asserted, neither Matrimony nor celebration of the Eucharist were possible. Indeed, St. Ignatius counseled the early Christians to remain "aloof" from the heretics who "confess not the Eucharist to be the flesh of our Saviour Jesus Christ, which suffered for our sins, and which the Father, of His goodness, raised up again" (Epistle to the Smyrnaeans, VII). The Eucharist, St. Ignatius wrote, is "the bread that is the flesh of Jesus Christ, this flesh which has suffered for our sins." St. Ignatius elaborated on the Incarnation, Passion, death, and Resurrection of Christ.

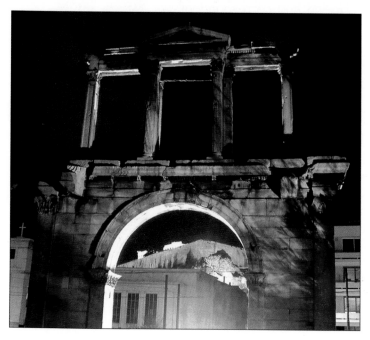

St. Ignatius was also the first person to use the term "Catholic Church," which he again linked to the episcopacy. Finally, St. Ignatius supported the primacy of the papacy, and advocated deference to the Bishop of Rome.

Upon his arrival in Rome, St. Ignatius was martyred in the Coliseum. St. Ignatius was led out in front of a great crowd and was fed to lions. His feast day is celebrated on October 17.

The Hadrian Arch in Athens was built by Hadrian in AD 131 as part of a wall separating the old and new cities. On the side facing the Acropolis is the inscription, "This is Athens the former city of Theseus." The side facing the new city reads, "This is the city of Hadrian and not of Theseus."

HADRIAN'S RESCRIPT (AD 123/124)

The Emperor Hadrian succeeded Trajan in AD 117 and served until his death in AD 138.

In religion, Hadrian promoted the cult of the gods and designed a special temple built for Venus and Roma in the Roman Forum. Hadrian banned circumcision among the Jews, and planned to turn Jerusalem into a Roman colony called Aelia Capitolina. The Jews responded by revolting under their leader Bar Kokhba in AD 132. After this revolt was suppressed in AD 135, the Jews were forbidden to enter Jerusalem.

In AD 123/124 Hadrian answered the request of Serenus Granianus, Proconsul of the Province of Asia, who wanted the emperor's advice on how to handle the often violent crowds intent on murdering Christians and inquired whether they should be prosecuted for simply being Christian.

In his official response, or rescript, Hadrian emphasized the primacy of the rule of law over mob action. Furthermore, he ordered that Christians could only be prosecuted for actual violations of the common law, not just for professing Christian belief. If an accuser made false accusations, then the accuser himself was to be punished. Accordingly, under Hadrian, Christians enjoyed a relative amount of toleration, although there was no official codification of such toleration.

ST. POLYCARP, BISHOP OF SMYRNA

St. Polycarp (ca. AD 69 - ca. 155) suffered martyrdom during the long and peaceful reign of Roman Emperor Antoninus Pius (AD 86-161, emperor AD 138-161). St. Polycarp spent much of his life defending orthodox Catholic belief against various heresies. He is an important link to the Apostles and a great number of Christian writers who lived toward the end of the second century. Along with St. Ignatius and Pope St. Clement I, St. Polycarp is one of the most important Apostolic Fathers. He was a friend and correspondent of St. Ignatius. Only one of St. Ignatius's letters to St. Polycarp has survived.

After traveling to Rome to discuss the date of Easter with Pope St. Anacletus, St. Polycarp returned to Smyrna (modern Izmir, Turkey). Shortly thereafter he was arrested during a pagan festival and charged with being a Christian. The letter "Martyrium Polycarpi" (The Martyrdom of Polycarp) was written by someone of the church in Smyrna to the church in Philomelium, and relates the details of St. Polycarp's martyrdom.

The governor wished to save St. Polycarp, and asked him to curse Christ in public so that his life could be spared. St. Polycarp refused to renounce Christ and was sentenced to be burned alive. The executioners, impressed by St. Polycarp's courage, honored his request to be tied to the stake, rather than fastened with spikes. Once the fire began, St. Polycarp remained unharmed from the flames. Finally, an executioner killed St. Polycarp with a sword. The Church celebrates his feast day on February 23.

THE COLISEUM

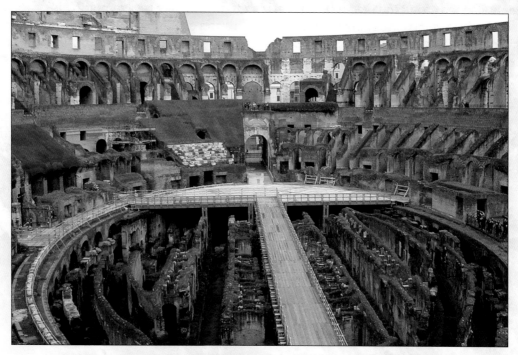

The Coliseum's "Door of Death" and the skeleton of cages and cells which were located under the stadium floor.

The Coliseum of Rome remains both a tribute to the brilliant engineering of the ancient Romans and a witness of their gruesome entertainments and disregard for human life. The construction began around AD 72 under Emperor Vespasian and was completed by the Emperor Domitian. The Coliseum was originally known as the Flavian Amphitheater.

In its heyday, the building boasted a number of technological wonders. It featured a cooling system made from a large canopy suspended by ropes over the audience that provided shade and created a breeze. Underneath the stadium floor, there were cells to house wild beasts, condemned criminals, and trained gladiators. These "entertainers" could enter the arena through dozens of elevators or trap doors.

Although the standard forms of entertainment were executions, fights between various animals, between men and animals, and, of course, the famous gladiatorial combats fascinated the Romans. During the emperor Titus's hundred-day festival celebrating the Coliseum's inauguration, contests pitted bears, buffalo, elephants, rhinoceri, lions and other wild animals against each other and against armed or unarmed men.

It is possible that some Christians were condemned ad bestias in the Coliseum, but it is more likely that they were killed in the circus Flaminius, the Gaianum, the Circus of Hadrian, the Amphitheatrum Castrense, or the Stadium of Domitian.

Gladiatorial combats were finally outlawed in 404, largely due to the influence of Christianity, and the Coliseum quickly became a site of pilgrimage. Indeed, it remains standing today, preserved as a testament to those great sacrifices made by Christians during the dark days of persecution.

EMPEROR MARCUS AURELIUS, THE PHILOSOPHER-KING

Marcus Aurelius (AD 121-180) was a favorite adopted son of Emperor Hadrian. Upon the death of Emperor Antoninus Pius, Marcus Aurelius ascended the throne in AD 161. Marcus Aurelius was an ardent Stoic, and philosophy was the central focus of his life. When he died, Marcus Aurelius's book Meditations was found on his person. Marcus Aurelius's Meditations is a thoughtful and moving work that reflects the profound discipline of a Stoic's life. He exemplified Stoicism's ideal of living free from passion, unmoved by joy or grief, and submitting without complaint to unavoidable fate.

Marcus Aurelius adhered to Trajan's Rescript, outlawing Christianity and persecuting the Christians. He reinstituted the practice of anonymous denouncements, and did not hesitate to kill Christians when it served the empire's interests. Many of the persecutions undertaken during Marcus Aurelius's reign, however, originated not directly from the emperor, but from angry provincial mobs and the governors who were meant to hold them in check. Allowing mobs to kill Christians was an effective way of diffusing their anger, which otherwise might turn against the empire itself. Marcus Aurelius's attitude towards any new religion was generally disdainful. If the new sect excited the people, the emperor was willing to respond with strong punishments.

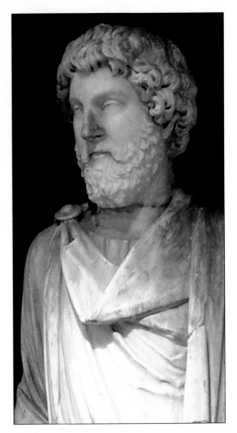

Emperor Marcus Aurelius

ST. JUSTIN MARTYR

St. Justin Martyr (ca. AD 100 - ca. 165) was one of the most famous martyrs to die under the persecution of Marcus Aurelius. Born of pagan parents in Shechem in Samaria in Palestine, Justin studied philosophy from his early youth, and converted to Christianity in his thirtieth year. Tradition has it that Justin was walking along the sea one day and met a mysterious old man whom he had never seen before. The old man began talking to Justin and convinced him that true knowledge of God could not come only from philosophy, but must be supplemented by reading the revealed word of the prophets. After his conversion, Justin continued studying philosophy and became an excellent apologist for the Faith.

Justin worked tirelessly during the Roman persecutions to defend the Church against those pagans who falsely accused her. Justin respected philosophy, but saw that its truths were mere shadows compared to Christ's teachings.

In his First Apology, which he addressed to Emperor Antoninus Pius and his two adopted sons, Marcus Aurelius and Lucius Verus, Justin provides important descriptions of the rituals for the celebration of Baptism and the Eucharist. The Second Apology was addressed to the Roman Senate just after Marcus Aurelius became emperor in AD 161. Shortly thereafter Justin and six others were denounced as Christians. When they refused to sacrifice to the gods, they were beheaded.

St. Justin Martyr's feast day is celebrated on June 1.

PART III

Later Persecutions and the Edict of Milan

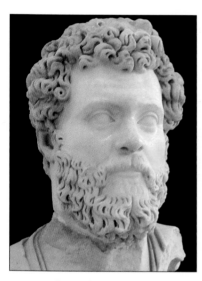

Emperor Septimus Severus

The reign of Emperor Septimus Severus (emperor AD 193-211) was characterized by warfare in Britain and Mesopotamia. By this time the military played an ever-increasing role in the selection of the emperor and the elimination of his enemies. Severus issued a decree in AD 202 declaring that circumcision and Baptism were to be forbidden. This threatened not only Christians, but Jews as well. Another round of persecutions followed, which were concentrated mainly in Syria and Africa.

ST. IRENÆUS, BISHOP OF LYON

St. Irenæus (ca. AD 130 - ca. 200) was a disciple of St. Polycarp, and is believed to have come from Smyrna. Although a native of Asia Minor, St. Irenæus served as Bishop of Lyon, and is regarded as the preeminent figure of the early Church in Gaul. Irenæus devoted much of his energy to combating heresies, especially Gnosticism. In his defense of orthodoxy, St. Irenæus emphasized key elements of the Church: the episcopacy, Sacred Scripture, and Tradition. He spoke explicitly of the importance of recourse to the Church's tradition, even though Christianity was still very much in its infancy. He argued, "If the revelation of God through creation gives life to all who live upon the earth, much more does the manifestation of the Father through the Word give life to those who see God" (St. Irenæus, Adversus hæreses, IV.20.7).

St. Irenæus's writings are of special interest given the way they systematically describe the origin and history of each heresy before contrasting its false claims with Catholic teaching. St. Irenæus's work is still necessary and helpful to scholars seeking an in-depth look at early theological disputes. The most famous of these works is the Adversus haereses, also known as the Refutation of Gnosticism.

St. Irenæus subsequently became the Bishop of Lyon in 178, and held the office for approximately twenty-five years. According to tradition, St. Irenæus was martyred during the reign of Emperor Septimus Severus. His feast day is celebrated on June 28.

THE EDICT OF DECIUS (AD 250)

After the reign of Septimus Severus, Christians enjoyed relative peace for about fifty years. Emperor Alexander Severus (emperor AD 222-235) even permitted Christians to own property and build churches. However, in the second half of the third century the empire entered into a troubling political period. In a short span of just forty-six years (AD 238-284), there were eighteen legitimate emperors, and many others who sought illegitimate ascendance. Most of these emperors ruled for a brief time before meeting with a violent end.

Emperor Decius (emperor AD 249-251) reigned for only three years, but he inaugurated the first empire-wide persecution of Christians. Other emperors had limited their directives, horrible as they may have been, to the city of Rome or to specific provincial communities. Decius, however, who believed that the survival of the empire depended upon the restoration of the old pagan cults, sought to extirpate Christianity from the empire.

Decius assumed control of the Roman Empire at a precarious point in its history. The empire was threatened both by the army, which essentially controlled the emperor, and by external enemies, specifically Germanic hordes who constantly attacked along the eastern frontier. Faced with such a bleak political situation, Decius sought to reinvigorate the empire's strength and unity through a return to the ancient religious practices of the state.

Since Christianity called for ultimate allegiance to Christ and not to the state, Decius saw this as incompatible with his plan. In his view, Christianity, which by that time was the religion of roughly one-third of the Roman Empire, was in part the cause of the divided empire.

Emperor Decius promulgated an edict of extermination against the Christians. Anyone suspected of being Christian had to present him or herself before the local magistrate and offer a simple sacrifice to prove he or she had given up the Faith. Those Christians who offered sacrifice to the pagan gods were known as sacrificanti; those who burned incense to the pagan gods were called thurificati. Certificates, purchased at a price from officials, stating that the bearer had already offered sacrifice to the gods were also available. Christians who purchased these certificates were called libellatici.

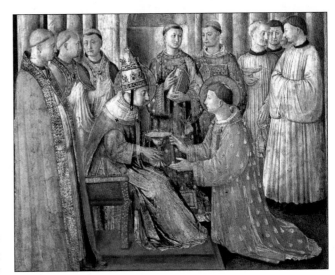
Pope St. Sixtus II ordains St. Lawrence

Decius ordered the arrest of all known Christians who failed to appear before the magistrate or who could not produce a certificate. Christians who refused to renounce their faith were sent into exile or put to death, and all of their property was confiscated.

The Church's loss was two-fold in these times: she lost those faithful Christians who were martyred during the persecutions, and she lost those unfaithful Christians who committed apostasy. Apostasy is the willful denunciation of the Faith in its entirety.

The persecutions of Decius unfortunately resulted in many apostates, and the leaders of the Church at this time had difficult decisions to make regarding the status of apostates and their possible re-entry into the community of believers. The most rigorous factions of the Church denied that the lapsi–Christians who formally renounced their faith, offering sacrifices to pagan gods–could be readmitted. The popes decided that with long penances, the lapsi would be allowed to return. The controversy surrounding these lapsi gave rise to the Novatianist schism. The Roman presbyter Novatian led a "rigorist" faction, declaring that those who had renounced the Faith (the lapsi) could never be re-admitted into the Church.

ORIGEN: THEOLOGIAN AND BIBLICAL EXEGETE

Origen (ca. AD 185-ca. 254) was the most prolific writer and important theologian and biblical exegete in the eastern part of the Empire. Origen was an Egyptian who spent much of his life working and teaching in Alexandria. His father was martyred during a persecution in AD 202, and Origen later became the head of the first Catechetical School in Alexandria. This institution combined instruction in Catholic doctrine with an investigation into the sciences and philosophy, and in some ways might be considered the first Catholic university.

During the persecution of the Emperor Decius, Origen was taken into custody in AD 250. For approximately two years, he was brutally tortured. Origen, however, held fast to his faith, inspiring many with his zeal. He was eventually released and lived for several more years, but his broken body quickly gave out.

It is estimated that Origen wrote between two and five thousand different tracts, nearly all of which are lost. However, one of his chief works, "De principiis," survives. In addition to his many scholarly writings, Origen is considered to have initiated the concept of the homily.

POPE ST. SIXTUS II AND DEACON ST. LAWRENCE

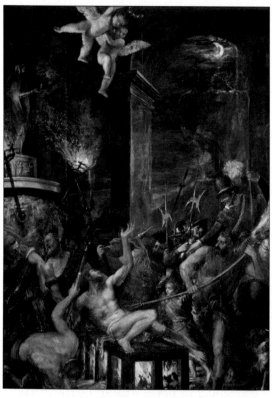

The Martyrdom of St. Lawrence.
"I am roasted enough on this side; turn me around."

Emperor Valerian ruled from AD 253 to 260, and during this time issued two rescripts, one in AD 257 and one in AD 258. The rescript of AD 257 forbade Christians from meeting in public places and from celebrating the Eucharist in the catacombs. The rescript of AD 258, however, was harsher. Under this rescript, issued because of political pressure, bishops, priests, and deacons were immediately executed, and Christians of rank were removed from their offices and often sold into slavery.

In the days of Valerian's second rescript, Pope St. Sixtus II was apprehended while celebrating Mass with seven deacons, one of whom was St. Lawrence. Pope St. Sixtus and six of the deacons were beheaded on the spot, but Lawrence was spared for the time. The authorities demanded that he bring the Church's treasure to them, and sent him to get it. When he returned a short time later, Lawrence brought with him a group of poor people – the Church's treasure. In response, the Roman authorities sentenced Lawrence to be roasted alive on a gridiron. Tradition holds that as he burned, Lawrence told the judge, "I am roasted enough on this side; turn me around."

PERSECUTIONS UNDER DIOCLETIAN

Born in Dalmatia (modern-day Croatia), Diocletian rose through the ranks of the Roman army to serve with the emperor's guards during the Persian campaign. When Numerian was murdered in AD 284 the army made Diocletian the new emperor. Like his predecessors Decius and Valerian, Diocletian desired to unify the empire. He used his organizational prowess to this end, eventually crushing the Persian Empire and ending the crisis of the third century.

Diocletian spent much of his first ten years as emperor battling the barbarians on the German and Persian frontiers. This diversion initially inclined the early Church historian Eusebius to praise Diocletian's clemency toward Christians. But in AD 303, with the barbarians defeated, Diocletian turned his attention to the Church. On February 23 a new edict was issued at Nicomedia and The Great Persecution began. Christian Churches were destroyed; books were burned. The palace at Nicomedia was set ablaze prompting additional edicts. For the next ten years, until Constantine's defeat of Maxentius at the Milvian Bridge on AD October 28, 312, and the "Edict of Milan" in 313, the Christians throughout the Empire were imprisoned, tortured, forced to offer sacrifices to pagan gods, and martyred according to the changing fortunes of the Imperial rulers.

FOUR EDICTS

Though he was superstitious, Diocletian was initially tolerant of Christianity, and even admired some of its adherents. Maximian and Galerius, on the other hand, were wary of the religion and pressed Diocletian to eradicate it for the good of the empire. At their request, Diocletian issued four edicts. These edicts resulted in the worst of all the persecutions the Christians suffered under the Romans. Diocletian's first edict commanded the destruction of churches and the burning of the Scriptures, as well as banning all Christian gatherings. Those who opposed this law faced execution or enslavement.

The succeeding edicts were applied only in the east by Galerius and Diocletian. The second edict sanctioned the imprisonment of the clergy. The third edict demanded pagan sacrifice from the clergy. Finally, the fourth edict demanded sacrifice from every Christian, not just the clergy. This last edict resulted in the deaths of many thousands of Christians who refused to offer pagan sacrifice. Constantine the Great later commented that if the Romans had slain as many barbarians as they had slaughtered Christians during the reign of Diocletian, there would be no barbarians left to threaten the safety of the Empire.

THE CHURCH TRIUMPHS

Due to his failing health, Diocletian abdicated on May 1, AD 305, and he convinced Maximian to step down as well. Galerius remained in power in the East, and Constantius took over control of the

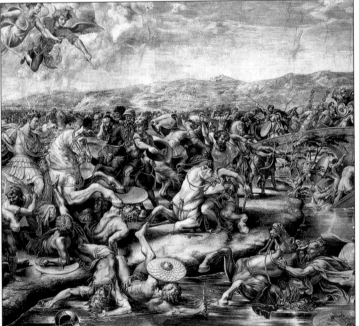

West. Constantius was succeeded by his son Constantine in AD 307.

Constantine was friendly with the Christians, although he was not one himself, but Galerius continued the persecution in the East until just before his death. In AD 311, however, Galerius was stricken with an eastern form of leprosy that left his body crippled and decrepit. He confessed and whimpered in utter terror that his sickness was the divine retribution of the Christian God. On April 30, AD 311, Galerius issued an edict admitting the failure of his policy with regard to the Christians. He then instituted the free exercise of the Christian religion as long as Christians obeyed the law and promised to pray for the emperor

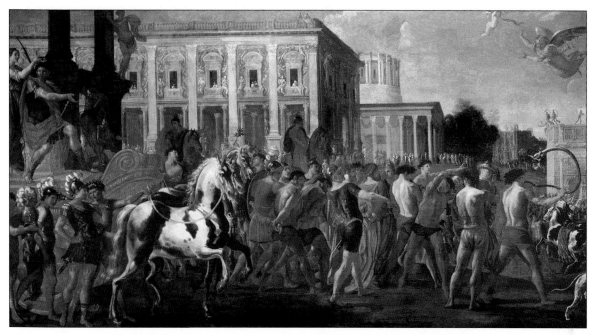

Constantine sought unity in his empire, and he saw that Christianity was a religion likely to provide such unity.

and the empire. Galerius's edict was also adopted in the West. Thus the last and greatest persecution begun under Diocletian gave way to a tentative peace.

Upon the death of Galerius, a complex struggle for power ensued. Maxentius, who was Maximian's son and who now controlled Italy, sought to defeat the army of Constantine and gain control of the Western empire. Constantine, who was well aware of Maxentius's intentions, decided to attack Rome. At the Milvian Bridge, just outside the city, the two armies met.

Before engaging in battle, Constantine claimed that he had looked above the sun and saw the symbol of the cross inscribed with the words in hoc signo vinces ("in this sign you will conquer"). After this vision, Constantine instructed his soldiers to put this sign on their shields. With crosses etched into Roman shields, Constantine's army met Maxentius in battle. Though Maxentius's forces were said to have been four times greater, Constantine won the Battle of Saxa Rubra, securing his rule over the West. Maxentius drowned near the Milvian Bridge.

After his victory against Maxentius, Constantine declared that the Christian God had favored him, and that he intended to stay in this God's good graces. He immediately restored the property of the Church, and began aiding in the construction of churches. In Rome the Arch of Constantine commemorated his victory, and his statue was placed in the city. In one hand the statue held the Labarum, the standard of the cross, with the inscription, "Through this saving sign have I freed your city from the tyrant's yoke."

THE EDICT OF MILAN (AD 313)

Constantine met with the only other living caesar, Licinius, in Milan in AD 313. Together they issued the Edict of Milan. This edict restored all property taken from the Church by the empire, and it granted Christians the freedom to practice their religion. The Edict of Milan represented a milestone for the early Christians and the Catholic Faith. It legitimized a religion that had been outlawed since Nero's decree in AD 64, and solidified the presence of Christianity in the public square.

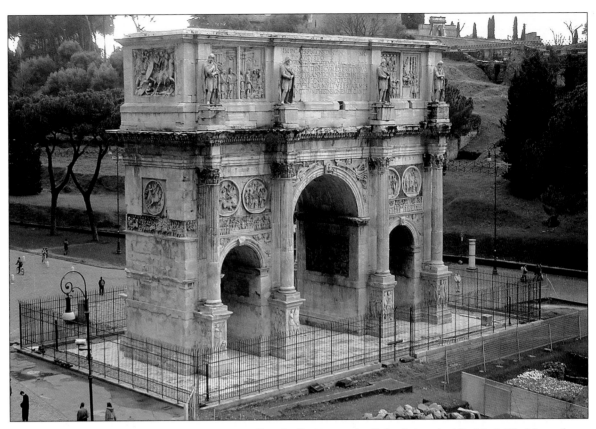

In Rome, the Arch of Constantine commemorated his victory over Maxentius. His statue was placed in the city. In one hand, his statue held the Labarum, the standard of the cross, with the inscription, "Through this saving sign have I freed your city from the tyrant's yoke."

It would be remiss not to mention the clear political motives that were at least partly responsible for the Edict of Milan. Like many Roman rulers before him, Constantine sought unity in his empire, and he saw that Christianity was a religion likely to provide such unity. In this, Constantine followed the regular practice of using religion to support political ends. However, it would be ridiculous to suppose that for Constantine, Christianity was nothing but a tool for the state. He is known to have prayed daily, and to have received instruction in the Faith until he was formally received into the Church, penitent and hopeful, receiving the Sacrament of Baptism on his deathbed.

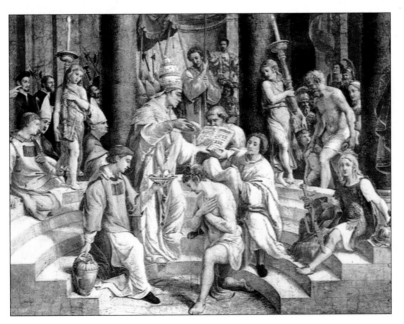

The Baptism of Constantine
by Giovan Francesco Penni

Constantine received instruction in the faith and was formally received into the Church.

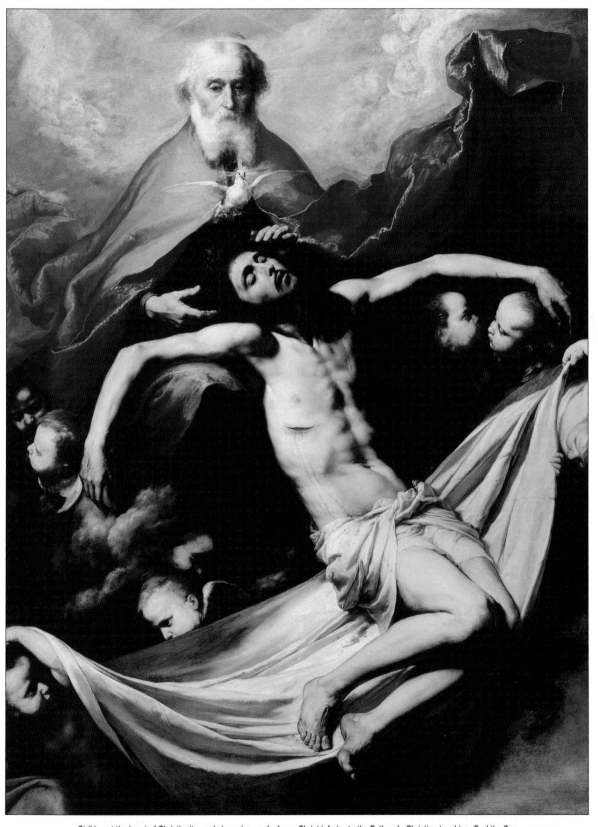

Striking at the heart of Christianity, early heresies made Jesus Christ inferior to the Father. In Christian teaching, God the Son, the Logos, is the Second Person of the Blessed Trinity, a person in the Divine Nature, and therefore equal to God the Father.

PART IV
Early Heresies

The persecution of Christians in the fourth and fifth centuries was followed by a series of heresies that rocked the emerging Church down to her foundations. Given the gravity and widespread effect of these early heresies, it would seem that nothing less than divine intervention guided the growing Church through these trials, along her road of survival and growth.

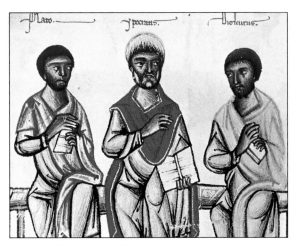

Almost from the beginning, Christian thinkers used the tools of Greek philosophy to help explain Christian truths.

From almost the very beginning, many Christian thinkers welcomed the Greek philosophical tradition, and used the tools of Greek philosophy to help explain Christian truths. St. Paul preached at the Areopagus in Athens – though with limited success – and the Apologists utilized philosophy in explaining Christianity to intellectuals and the ruling classes of the Empire.

A dizzying array of heresies and schismatic leaders confronted the Church following the Edict of Milan (313). Over the course of the third to fifth centuries, popes and bishops led the Church through a number of ecumenical councils, addressing each new controversy, and consequently developing a rich theological tradition. This would become the greatest age of heresy until the advent of Protestantism in the sixteenth century, and these heresies were not restricted to a circle of academics but rather affected the entire populace. The random observer may see here confusion and arbitrary decisions; the believer sees the Holy Spirit guiding and directing the Church to protect, define, and promulgate the truths about the Person of Jesus Christ and God's plan for the Church.

What exactly is heresy? St. Thomas Aquinas defined heresy as "a species of unbelief, belonging to those who profess the Christian faith, but corrupt its dogmas" (STh II-II, 11, 1, r.). Heresy must be distinguished from other forms of unbelief, namely, the unbelief of other religious traditions such as Judaism or any of the various pagan religions. Orthodox (meaning "right teaching" in Greek) Catholicism derives from the Deposit of Faith (the sum of all truths revealed in Scripture and through Tradition, and entrusted to the care of the Church). Heresy, on the other hand, derives from this same source, i.e., from belief, but denies or alters some part or parts of the Deposit of Faith.

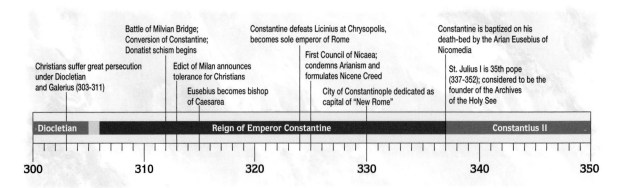

Christians suffer great persecution under Diocletian and Galerius (303-311)

Battle of Milvian Bridge; Conversion of Constantine; Donatist schism begins

Edict of Milan announces tolerance for Christians

Eusebius becomes bishop of Caesarea

Constantine defeats Licinius at Chrysopolis, becomes sole emperor of Rome

First Council of Nicaea; condemns Arianism and formulates Nicene Creed

City of Constantinople dedicated as capital of "New Rome"

Constantine is baptized on his death-bed by the Arian Eusebius of Nicomedia

St. Julius I is 35th pope (337-352); considered to be the founder of the Archives of the Holy See

Diocletian	Reign of Emperor Constantine	Constantius II

300 — 310 — 320 — 330 — 340 — 350

GNOSTICISM

The word "Gnosticism" is derived from the Greek word gnosis (knowledge). The name refers to one of the principle tenets of this multifaceted heresy, namely, that salvation may be achieved through knowledge. There were many forms of Gnosticism (many whose origins predate Christianity), and therefore it is difficult (if not impossible) to encapsulate them into one coherent system. In the second century, Gnosticism, which had eastern origins and influences from Persia and India, very successfully perverted the meaning of Christianity and its symbols. Gnosticism co-opted the Old and New Testaments for some of the contents of the Gnostic religions and to give some particular Gnostic teachings a certain authority.

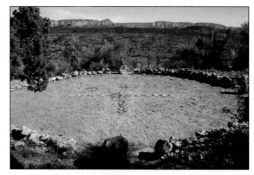

A Coptic image of Pisces.

As mentioned above, Gnosticism is a blanket term for a very broad and complex group of beliefs. Despite these complexities, it is possible to delineate some of Gnosticism's fundamental points. Gnostic beliefs held that a secret knowledge regarding God and the origin and destiny of man had been given to a select few. Its worldview pitted the Demiurge, the creator god of the material and visible world, against the remote and unknowable Divine Being. The Demiurge was of lesser stature than the Divine Being, from whom the Demiurge had originated through a series of emanations. The Gnostics claimed that the Demiurge was the author and ruler of the created world. Being material and imperfect, the created world would naturally have an antagonistic and inferior relationship to the spiritual, perfect world of the Divine Being. Thus, the spiritual Divine Being is the agent of goodness, and the Demiurge, the author of the material world, propagates evil in the world.

A divine spark, belonging to the Divine Being, could, however, be found among some people in the created order. The redeemer, sent from the Divine Being, came in order to release the sparks trapped in the bodies so they might return to the Divine Being. This was only possible if the individuals understood the secret knowledge of the redeemer's teaching and practiced the appropriate Gnostic rituals.

In Gnosticism's view, Judaism was a false religion that worshiped the wrong god, the Demiurge, who is evil. Instead of trying to free the divine spark from its evil material confines, Judaism mistakenly affirmed the material world as good.

Gnosticism rejected the Church's teaching regarding both Christ's human and divine nature. According to

A contemporary New Age medicine wheel in Arizona.

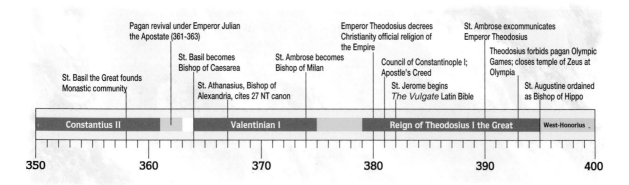

Pagan revival under Emperor Julian the Apostate (361-363)

Emperor Theodosius decrees Christianity official religion of the Empire

St. Ambrose excommunicates Emperor Theodosius

St. Basil becomes Bishop of Caesarea

St. Ambrose becomes Bishop of Milan

Theodosius forbids pagan Olympic Games; closes temple of Zeus at Olympia

St. Basil the Great founds Monastic community

St. Athanasius, Bishop of Alexandria, cites 27 NT canon

Council of Constantinople I; Apostle's Creed

St. Jerome begins *The Vulgate* Latin Bible

St. Augustine ordained as Bishop of Hippo

| Constantius II | | Valentinian I | | Reign of Theodosius I the Great | West-Honorius |

350   360   370   380   390   400

Gnostic thought, Jesus did not have a human nature; for a human nature, being materially bound, is naturally evil. Instead, he was a good divine being whose purpose, as the Gnostic redeemer, was to bring the secret knowledge (gnosis) and make it known to man. They believed that Jesus came as the representative of the supreme Divine Being. This Jesus did not inhabit a human body, nor did he die on the cross. Instead, the spirit of the divine being was present in Jesus temporarily, Jesus' body was only an apparition, and his spirit left his "body" before he was put to death on Calvary. In Gnosticism's cosmological view, a divine being could never have suffered the humiliation of death, let alone death on a cross.

Generally, a Gnostic religion holds the following beliefs:

1. Matter is a corruption of spirit, and thus the world is corrupt;

2. Man must seek through knowledge to overcome this fallen state and return to God; and

3. God has made this possible by sending a savior (usually held to be Jesus).

The principle involved here of finding the light within oneself through a pagan ceremony is the essence of the New Age movement in contemporary times. As will be seen in this chapter, the Church has witnessed a staggering range of heresies and schisms in her two-thousand year history. Many of the false teachings that appeared in the Medieval period, during the Reformation, and even in the contemporary world are not new, but, rather, the reemergence of ancient heresies under fresh guises.

MARCIONISM (144-400s)

Marcion (d. ca. AD160) founded his heretical movement very early in the life of the Church, and it lingered well into the fifth century in the West and for centuries longer in the East.

Marcion adapted important ideas from Gnostic beliefs to form his own theology. From Gnosticism he took the idea of the Demiurge, whom he identified as the jealous, revengeful God of the Old Testament. The Jewish God, the Demiurge, is the God of the Law. In opposition to this cruel God of the Law, Marcion heralded the God of Jesus Christ, the true God, sent to bring about the demise of the Demiurge. The God of Jesus Christ is the God of Love who has no connection with the Law. Jesus' teaching was taken from the true God. His Passion and death came about through the machinations of the evil Creator God of the Old Testament. This dualism of Law and Love is the main thesis of Marcion's system.

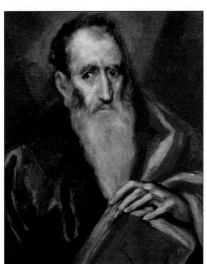

Marcion recognized only St. Paul (above) as a legitimate Christian authority.

Marcion recognized only St. Paul as a legitimate Christian authority because of his teaching regarding freedom from the Law. The Apostles, in Marcion's view, did not fully understand the mission of Christ being blinded by Judaism and its Creator God. Therefore, only ten of St. Paul's Epistles and a modified version of the Gospel of St. Luke (any Jewish influence was removed) were given canonical status in Marcionism. Marcion was either not aware of the Pastorals – other epistles of the New Testament – or rejected them outright. This canon reflected Marcion's attempt to free the New Testament from Jewish influence.

Unwittingly, Marcion helped the development of the Catholic Church's canon of Sacred Scripture. Partially in reaction to Marcion's flawed and incomplete group of inspired texts, the Church gradually determined the canon: the official, inspired writings of the New Testament.

MANICHÆISM (250s -1000s)

Manichæism was probably the most elaborate and polished branch of Gnosticism. Its founder, Mani (ca. 216-276), was born in Persia. He developed this particular brand of Gnosticism in Persia and India during the third century until he was eventually condemned to death by the Persian emperor Bahram I. Accounts of his death conflict – some report that he died in prison, others that he was crucified, flayed, and his skin stuffed with straw and hung upon the gates of the city. Despite his condemnation, by the fourth century Manichæism had spread to Rome and was already deeply rooted in North Africa.

Manichæism continued the age-old dualist cosmology involving the conflict between darkness and light. This heresy stated that Satan had managed to steal light particles and place them in the brains of humans. The goal of Manichæism was to share the secret knowledge which liberates this light so it could return to its original source. Mani understood himself as just another spiritual leader in a long line of leaders that included the Jewish prophets, Jesus, and Buddha, all of whom showed the path to true freedom. The ritual acts of Manichæism also incorporated the movements of the cosmic bodies – the Sun, the Moon, and stars – also points of light. The "hearers" and the "elect" comprised the two groups in the sect. The latter group was comprised of the authentic followers of Mani.

Manichæism borrowed heavily from the Scriptures, especially from the writings of St. Paul. Mani incorporated many of St. Paul's arguments and imagery to support his own teaching concerning the struggle between darkness and light.

Followers of Manichæism adhered to a strict form of asceticism, and it is here that one understands part of the appeal of Gnostic and other heretical teachings. In the Roman world of lax morals, Christianity required faithfulness to a demanding moral life as inspired by Jesus. Manichæism and other movements attempted to out-perform Christianity in terms of their moral rigor. If Christianity required fasting, Gnostic groups would require tougher and longer fasts. Manichæism also drew adherents by its intellectual appeal. St. Augustine, for instance, drawn by the philosophical bases of the heresy, was a fervent adherent of Manichæism for nine years.

MONTANISM (156 - 200s)

Montanism was an apocalyptic movement founded by Montanus in Phrygia (Asia Minor, modern day Turkey) following what he said were private revelations made to him. Montanus worked closely with two female prophets, Prisca and Maximilla. Montanus's central principle was that the new, heavenly kingdom was about to begin in Pepuza, a small town in Phrygia (the exact location of this town is lost to history); he knew this because of the outpouring of the Holy Spirit upon him. Montanism also held that Christians who had fallen from grace could never be redeemed. Because Montanus and his followers believed they were directly inspired by the Holy Spirit, they rejected the authority of the Church.

The movement also appeared in North Africa, where its most famous adherent was the Christian thinker Tertullian, who rejected Catholic Christianity after having been one of its greatest apologists for many years. In its African form, Montanism placed a high value on the ascetical life. It forbade second marriages, enacted stricter fasting disciplines than the Church, and rejected flight from persecutions.

Montanism is rightly understood as one of the first apocalyptic movements in Christianity that claimed to supersede the Church because of its direct inspiration by the Holy Spirit. Its expectation of the New Jerusalem on earth in Pepuza is also unique.

DOCETISM (30s-100s)

Docetism, yet another Gnostic heresy rising from the presupposition of the corrupt nature of matter, maintained that Jesus was not truly human and did not actually suffer the pain of crucifixion and death. The name of the heresy derives from the Greek word dokesis, meaning appearance or semblance. It often taught that someone else (e. g., Judas Iscariot or Simon of Cyrene) miraculously switched places with Christ just before the crucifixion and suffered death in Christ's place. Many of the Apologists, including St. Ignatius of Antioch, wrote at length against this belief.

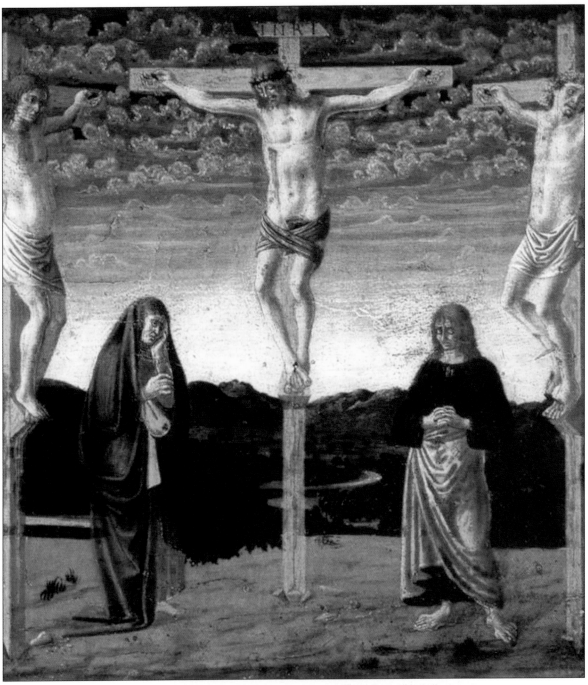

Docetism held that the human form of Jesus as well as his crucifixion was an illusion.

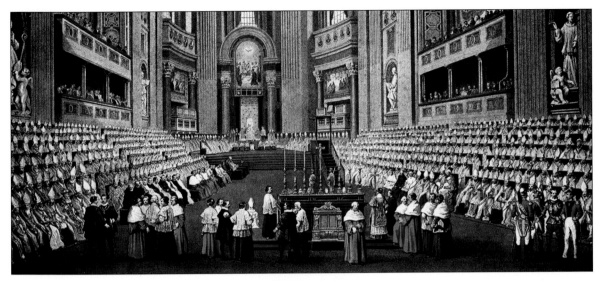

First Vatican Council 1869-1870

PART V

The Ecumenical Councils

In order to meet the challenges posed by the various heresies, the Church convened several ecumenical councils, the first being the First Council of Nicaea, in 325. Altogether, there have been twenty-one ecumenical councils throughout the history of the Church (the Second Vatican Council, 1962-1965, being the most recent). The first six councils addressed the various Christological heresies that have been examined in this chapter in an effort to provide a true theological answer to the question, "Who is Jesus Christ?" The word "ecumenical" comes from the Greek word oikoumene, meaning "the whole inhabited world." Ecumenical Councils bring bishops under the leadership of the pope together from all over the world to discuss central issues of the Church.

Current canon law in the Church grants the power to convene a council only to the papacy. The pope governs the council and he alone has the power to accept or reject the decrees passed by it. If the pope should die during a council, as happened during the Second Vatican Council in the 1960s, the council is halted until the election of a new pope, who then decides whether to continue the council as well as the selection of the topics it considers.

Besides ecumenical councils, members of the Church hold a number of other types of councils. What distinguishes an ecumenical council is that it convenes all the bishops of the world, and its teachings are regarded as having the highest authority. An ecumenical council's definitions regarding tenets of faith and morals are held to be infallible, if infallible pronouncements are the intentions of the pope and the bishops. Furthermore, the resolutions and conclusions of an ecumenical council must always be approved by the Supreme Pontiff.

The first seven councils are recognized by both East and West. However, Eastern Orthodox Christians do not recognize the ecumenical nature of any of the councils held in the West after 787 because they did not participate. At the time of the Reformation, the mainline Protestant bodies recognized at least the special status of those first seven councils, though later Protestant churches often gave no special recognition to them.

ECUMENICAL COUNCILS

COUNCIL NAME	YEAR	CONCERN OF COUNCIL
1 Nicaea	325	Arianism and the Nicene Creed
2 Constantinople I	381	Divinity of the Holy Spirit
3 Ephesus	431	Nestorianism and Mary as Mother of God
4 Chalcedon	451	Monophysitism (specifically the Eutychian form)
5 Constantinople II	553	The Three Chapters Controversy: Nestorianism, Monophysitism, and imperial-papal relations
6 Constantinople III	680-681	Monothelitism; admonished Pope Honorius I
7 Nicaea II	787	Iconoclasm
8 Constantinople IV	869-870	Photian Controversy: potential East-West schism; deposed Patriarch Photius
9 Lateran I	1123	Investiture Controversy; simony; clerical celibacy
10 Lateran II	1139	Arnold of Brescia's (twelfth century heretic who condemned all clerical material possession) teaching and criticism of the Church; put an end to papal schism
11 Lateran III	1179	Process for papal elections (only cardinals); condemned Albigensianism and Waldensianism
12 Lateran IV	1215	Transubstantiation of the Eucharist; annual Penance; suppression of Albigenses; crusades
13 Lyon I	1245	Deposition and excommunication of Emperor Frederick II; crusades
14 Lyon II	1274	Healing of the Great Schism with Constantinople
15 Vienne	1311-1312	Suppression of the Knights Templar
16 Constance	1414-1418	Great Schism of the papacy; condemnation of Jan Hus
17 Basel-Ferrara-Florence	1431-1445	Reform and union with the East
18 Lateran V	1512-1517	Reform of the Church, especially discipline (failed)
19 Trent	1545-1563	Protestantism and reform
20 Vatican I	1869-1870	Papal infallibility; condemnation of various errors
21 Vatican II	1962-1965	Renewal of the Church in the modern world

PART VI

The Church Fathers

A number of great and holy leaders arose to lead the Church, explain the Faith, and meet the unique challenges posed by the different heresies. They are known as the Church Fathers. The Church Fathers shared the following characteristics: orthodoxy in doctrine, holiness, notoriety, and antiquity. The title "Church Father" is not conferred by the Church; it is simply a traditionally held title. While no definitive list exists, the Church Fathers are typically divided into two groups: Latin (West) and Greek (East) Fathers. The Golden Age of the Church Fathers was from 320 to 461. St. Isidore of Seville (ca. 560-636) in the West and St. John of Damascus (ca. 655-ca. 750) in the East are generally regarded as the last significant Church Fathers.

The study of the Church Fathers and their many writings is known as patristics. The writings of the Fathers provide a unique opportunity to learn and appreciate the wealth of the earliest Christian tradition. Because of their proximity to the teachings of the Apostles, the Fathers' clarification and interpretation on Scripture will always serve as a standard reference point for Church teaching.

A Doctor of the Church (*Doctor Ecclesiæ*) is a specific title granted by the Pope to those whose development of theology and personal sanctity are exemplary. This tradition began in the Medieval period and continues into the present. There are more than thirty Doctors of the Church. In 2012 Pope Benedict XVI named St. John of Avila, a sixteenth-century Spanish priest, and St. Hildegard of Bingen, a twelfth-century German nun, to the ranks of Doctors of the Church. A complete list of the thirty-five Doctors of the Church appears on page 431.

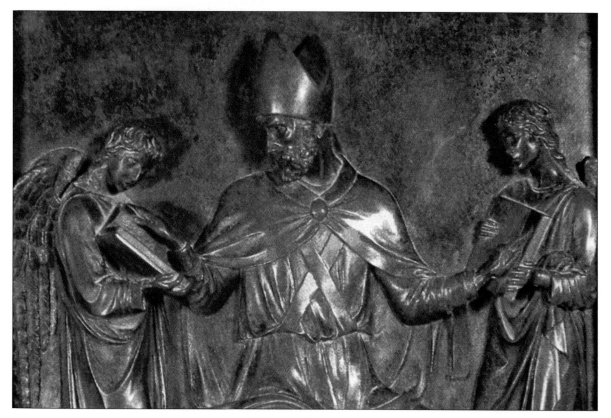

St. Ambrose of Milan (ca. 339-97)

ST. AMBROSE OF MILAN

St. Ambrose of Milan (ca. 339-97) was born in Trier, Germany, close to the frontier with the barbarians. He was the son of the Praetorian Prefect for Gaul. St. Ambrose studied law, became a lawyer, and eventually governor, based in Milan. Upon the death of Milan's Arian bishop around 373, the people clamored for St. Ambrose to succeed him. Though from a Christian family, St. Ambrose was only a catechumen, and he initially resisted accepting the office. Eventually, he acceded and was soon baptized, ordained, and installed as bishop.

St. Ambrose was a zealous defender of the Church's independence from the state. He both counseled and, at times, condemned decisions of the emperors. St. Ambrose supported Emperor Gratian's decision to remove the Altar of Victory, a powerful symbol of pagan influence on the Republic and Empire, from the Senate house in Rome. Later, he threatened Emperor Valentinian II with ecclesiastical sanction if he restored it. In 388 St. Ambrose forbade Theodosius from rebuilding a synagogue that had been destroyed in a riot in Callinicum.

St. Ambrose took a courageous stand against Emperor Theodosius in 390, excommunicating and forcing him the emperor to make public penance for slaughtering 7000 village people in Thessalonica that year. (The people of Thessalonica had assassinated one of Theodosius's generals after he imprisoned their favorite charioteer.) Having been barred from even entering the Church by St. Ambrose, let alone receiving Holy Communion, the emperor prostrated himself in the form of a cross in normal clothes in the vestibule just like any other penitent of the time. After eight months of penance and public prayer, St. Ambrose finally pardoned the emperor.

As Bishop of Milan, St. Ambrose became an ardent opponent of the Arian heresy, as well as a renowned preacher. St. Ambrose encouraged monasticism, facilitated theological exchanges with the East due to his knowledge of Greek, and incorporated hymns into the liturgy, a number of which he composed in Latin. His feast day is celebrated on December 7.

ST. JEROME

St. Jerome (ca. 345-420) led a very interesting life. Born in Strido in Dalmatia, near Aquileia, St. Jerome traveled and lived throughout Italy, Gaul, northern Africa, the Holy Land, and Constantinople. His two enduring passions were the ascetical life and scholarship.

St. Jerome spent four to five years in the Syrian desert leading an ascetical life with companions, and while there he learned Hebrew, which would prove vital for his future work of translating Scripture into Latin. St. Jerome never stopped advocating or living a penitential life even when he lived in cities. From 382 to 385 St. Jerome served as a secretary to Pope St. Damasus I. After 386 he spent the last years of his long life in Bethlehem as the head of a new monastery where he continued his scholarship.

Being of a cantankerous and passionate character, St. Jerome, with righteous indignation, was known to insert himself and his sharp pen into the important issues and heresies of his day. Nevertheless, his most important work was undoubtedly the translation of the Bible from the original sources into Latin, known as the Vulgate, which is still the normative text in the Church today. With the Vulgate, the Scriptures were for the first time brought into a uniform translation for the people of the Western Empire. The name Vulgate comes from the Latin vulgus, "common," as it was written in the common language of the people of the day. St. Jerome translated the Old Testament from Hebrew, the Psalms from the Greek Septuagint (the Greek version of the Old Testament). He translated the New Testament from Greek and revised what had been already translated into Latin. His feast day is celebrated on September 30.

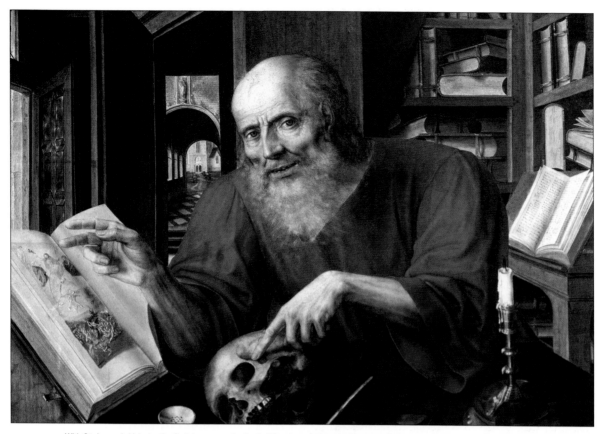

With St. Jerome's Vulgate, the Scriptures were for the first time brought into a uniform translation for the people of the Western Empire.

TRANSLATIONS OF THE BIBLE

It is widely believed that St. Jerome's Vulgate translation is most faithful because he had access to manuscripts of the original languages that no longer exist. The Douay-Rheims (1582-1609) translation into English was based upon the Vulgate.

The issues involved in translating are manifold, and deeply affect the text that is produced. A high school student who reaches a certain proficiency in a foreign language understands that the different ways ideas and issues are understood in one language are not necessarily the same as in another. Obviously, the process becomes even more crucial in translating a text, such as the Bible, on which people will ground their religious faith. The Church teaches that the books of the Bible are divinely inspired, and that even those books written in different ages by different authors in several languages enjoy the status of God's Word. This issue would become particularly important at the time of the Reformation, but St. Jerome had already set the standard for translation of the Bible with his Vulgate.

Other approved Catholic translations into English use the original sources, including the Jerusalem Bible and the New American Bible (NAB), the latter of which has become the standard translation for American liturgies today, except for the Gospels.

The Revised Standard Version (RSV) translation, which was compiled from 1946-1952, is based upon the King James Bible, otherwise known as the Authorized Version (1611). Though based on the Protestant King James Bible, the RSV was given Church approval when it also included the deuterocanonical texts, those books of the Old Testament that the Orthodox and Catholic

Churches recognize, but which the Protestants do not. (Protestants refer to these books as the Apocrypha.) The RSV was the first ecumenical Bible produced with Catholic, Protestant, Orthodox, and Jewish scholars. The RSV has been lauded for the beauty of its English usage and idiom, and has been used as the source for biblical quotations in this text. There is a Catholic edition with all the deuterocanonical books as well.

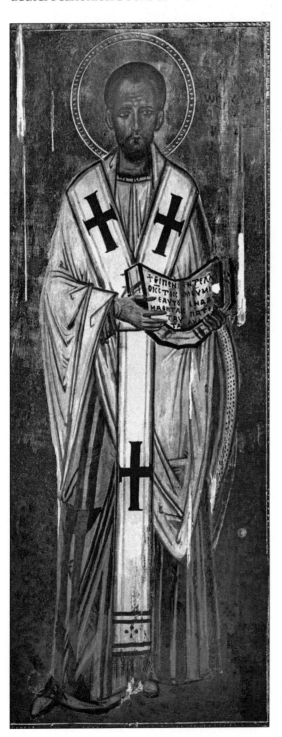

ST. JOHN CHRYSOSTOM, THE GOLDEN MOUTHED

St. John Chrysostom (ca. 347-407) was an outstanding preacher and commentator on the Bible. He studied law in Antioch, as well as theology under Diodorus, the future bishop of Tarsus. Thus, Chrysostom studied in the influential Antiochene school and became well versed in Greek scholarship and classical culture.

In 386 he was ordained a priest in Antioch, where he became such a renowned preacher that he earned the name "Chrysostom," meaning "golden-mouthed." His many sermons capture the deep spiritual meaning of biblical texts, without excluding their literal sense. In addition, St. John Chrysostom combined this biblical meaning with a real-world, practical application to the Christian life. He also wrote the celebrated treatise On the Priesthood, a work that discusses the importance and duties of a priest.

Against his wishes, the emperor named him Patriarch of Constantinople in 398. St. John Chrysostom criticized the prevailing moral laxity in Constantinople, including that of the imperial family. Very forthright and direct in his declaration of the truth, he repeatedly clashed with the Empress Euodoxia, who twice had St. John Chrysostom removed from his position as patriarch and banished. He quickly returned from his first period of exile, and the Empress feared some great punishment from Heaven. Shortly thereafter, in 404, even though he enjoyed the firm support of the people of Constantinople, Pope St. Innocent I, and the western Church, St. John Chrysostom was banished again by Euodoxia. This time, he was exiled to the area around Antioch, and then the Roman province of Pontus. While there, he was forced into a death march despite his already failing health, and died in 407. His feast day is celebrated on September 13.

PART VII

Heresies of the Fourth and Fifth Centuries

The fourth and fifth centuries saw a golden age in the history of the Church. Persecutions had ceased, and it was during this time that there emerged some of the greatest leaders the Church had ever seen. The newfound freedom from the fear of persecution allowed for a greater outward expression of ideas in the Church. This not only paved the way for great theological and doctrinal developments, but it also opened the door for new heresies and for one of the most serious crises in the history of the Church. Moreover, this same freedom of Christian expression and practice made it possible for the entire hierarchy of the universal Church to meet in ecumenical councils in response to

these heresies. The pronouncements of these councils over the course of the fourth and fifth centuries comprised the Church's teaching on Trinitarian and Christological belief. These first councils owe their success in significant part to many of the Church Fathers, who displayed an imposing intellectual acumen, exceptional leadership qualities, and extraordinary sanctity.

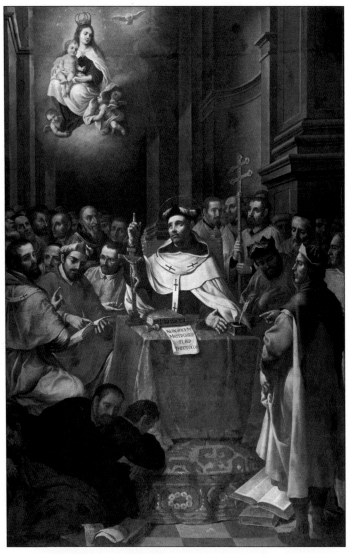

St. Cyril of Alexandria. Employing the language of Cyril, the Alexandrian school gave special status to the divinity of Christ and the unity of his person.

Among the many causes of these heresies, inaccurate interpretations of the Gospels coupled with imprecise philosophical explanations played a significant role. The intervention of the Church led to the development of a theology that was firmly rooted in the true meaning of the Gospel. The principle Christian teaching about the Incarnation–the belief that God the Son became man–raised essential questions regarding the Person of Christ. The Church Fathers made an effort to explain the mysteries of Faith with an accurate terminology. After the Church gave an authoritative answer, those groups who nevertheless adhered to false teaching were known definitively as heretics. A heretic is a baptized person who deliberately and obstinately disavows a revealed truth of established Church dogma.

CHRISTOLOGICAL HERESIES
ARIANISM (Fourth Century)

Arius (ca. 250-336) was a priest in Alexandria who studied in Antioch. He was an extremely charismatic individual and attracted huge crowds of listeners and devotees on account of his intellectual and rhetorical gifts. He was ordained a priest in 310 and became a pastor of a parish in Alexandria. His study of Origen and Neo-Platonism together with his familiarity with Gnosticism prepared the way for his erroneous interpretation of Christ's relation to the Father.

Using Neo-Platonism and scriptural passages, Arius claimed that Jesus Christ is neither God nor equal to the Father. For example, certain passages of the Gospel of St. John clearly maintain that Christ was sent by the Father and only did the will of the Father. Arius erroneously interpreted passages such as these to mean that Christ was not equal to the Father.

Nevertheless, Arius argued that Christ was an exceptional creature and was raised to the level of "Son of God" because of his heroic fidelity to the Father's will and his sublime holiness. Neo-Platonic thought held that God is a radically transcendent supreme "being" whose nature is incommunicable. This belief is certainly consistent with Christianity. However, the neo-Platonic God was absolutely One, and neo-Platonists could not conceive that anything emanating from the One could be equal to the One. This is at the root of the Arian heresy and its denial of Christ's divinity. This issue of the relationship between God the Father and God the Son was resolved by the Church, as is well addressed in the Athanasian Creed: "He is equal to the Father in his divinity, / but inferior to the Father in his humanity" (n. 31). Christ, according to his divine nature, is equal to the Father, and, according to his human nature, he is inferior to the father. It would take a few centuries to surmount all the theological difficulties connected to Arianism.

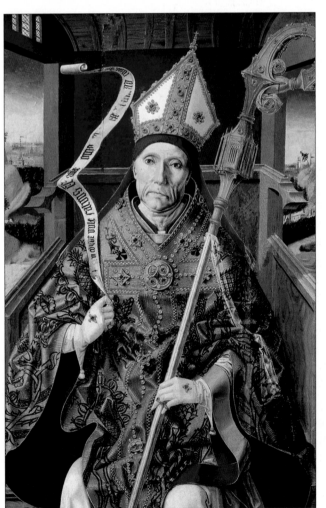

Arius reduced Jesus Christ to the status of a creature of the Father, although above every creature in dignity and perfection. The Son of God, the logos, was created before the world began and served as a vehicle to bring the rest of creation into existence. This heresy was an extremely serious threat to Christianity because the rejection of Christ's divinity invariably leads to a rejection of virtually all of the Church's central tenets, especially her doctrine on the Trinity and the Redemption. For this reason, Arius was responsible for ushering in the greatest doctrinal crisis that the Church would experience until the sixteenth century.

St. Athanasius marshaled the necessary orthodox forces to defeat the Arian heresy in the Church.

THE COUNCIL OF NICAEA

St. Athanasius (ca. 296-373) marshaled the necessary orthodox forces to defeat the Arian heresy in the Church. His task was not easy, but St. Athanasius was a persistent and fearless man who would not be silenced. When almost the entire Eastern Church had fallen to the Arians, St. Athanasius still raised his voice to testify to the truth. Even after at least five forced exiles, he was not deterred. The process by which the Church determined her own teaching regarding the divinity of Christ took time, and it was a road with many twists and turns.

The Emperor Constantine pushed for a General Council at Nicaea in 325. He was anxious to promote unity in the Empire through a general adherence to Christianity, which was then divided over Arianism. Constantine even paid for the traveling expenses of the western Bishops to secure their involvement and resolve the problem promptly. At the Council of Nicaea, Constantine opened the first session and played the important role of peacemaker between the two factions, Arian and Catholic, though it is doubtful that he understood all the subtleties involved in the discussions on the divinity of Christ.

This was the first of the great ecumenical councils that would be convened over the next few centuries to deliberate, pray, and make pronouncements about the beliefs of the Church in light of contemporary heresies. The ecumenical councils of the first eight centuries are held in the greatest esteem because they brought together bishops from the entire Christian world, East and West. The Council of Nicaea opened with 250 bishops present and ended with 318.

This First Ecumenical Council of Nicaea (325) was especially meaningful since only twelve years prior, the Roman Empire had granted toleration to Christianity after nearly 300 years of persecutions. There were many bishops in attendance who bore physical scars that they had suffered for their Faith during the persecutions under Diocletian, the worst of all the persecutions.

At the beginning of the council, the pope led and guided the councils in their deliberations through his legates. In the case of the Council of Nicaea, Pope St. Sylvester I was too old and infirm to travel. Bishop Hosius of Cordova, Spain, represented Pope St. Sylvester I, who happened to be a close friend of the emperor.

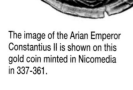

The image of the Arian Emperor Constantius II is shown on this gold coin minted in Nicomedia in 337-361.

St. Athanasius proposed a statement of Catholic belief regarding the divinity of Christ that included the Greek term homoousios (Latin, consubstantialis), which means "of the same essence or substance." The outcome was the Nicene Creed, the first solemn declaration of Catholic teaching which proclaimed more fully the central truths of Christianity.

The Church, through her teaching and interpretative role under the guidance of the Holy Spirit, is the final arbiter of all such matters regarding the terminology used for her statements. Two camps emerged from the Council of Nicaea: the homoousians (meaning "identical ousia" and representing the orthodox position), and the homoiousians (meaning "similar ousia" and representing the Arian position). Though the council concluded with the Nicene Creed, Arianism still lingered in various forms of Semi-Arianism, and later on re-emerged.

All but two Bishops signed the Nicene Creed, and these two were exiled by the emperor, who supported the creed. The Arian camp included Eusebius of Nicomedia (not to be confused with the Eusebius of Caesarea who wrote the first history of the Church, Ecclesiastical History), an important bishop who was favored by Constantine's sister Constantia. Though Eusebius of Nicomedia signed the Nicene Creed, he had only signed under pressure from the emperor, and he was exiled within months for giving aid and support to the Arians.

Emperor Constantine, however, reversed course in 328 and permitted Eusebius of Nicomedia and Arius to return. Leaders of the Nicene party who supported the orthodox position were then forced into exile. This included St. Athanasius, who fled in 336 from his diocese in Alexandria to Trier. In 336 the emperor decided that Arius would be recognized as the bearer of the orthodox position, when Arius suddenly died in Constantinople.

A dizzying array of councils was convened in the East and West over the next twenty-five years. When the councils functioned freely, they chose the Nicene Creed. However, when they operated under duress (the bishops were at times threatened with exile or torture), the bishops – even Bishop Hosius, and St. Hilary of Poitiers – sometimes signed Arian statements (Hosius was beaten and whipped when he was one hundred years old, and Pope Liberius, also in old age, was forced into exile). When these bishops returned to their dioceses from the forced councils, they would renounce the heresy and profess the Nicene Creed.

When Emperor Constantine died in 337, the Arian Eusebius of Nicomedia, who had become the patriarch of Constantinople, baptized him on his deathbed. Of Constantine's three sons, one was Arian and the other two were orthodox Catholic.

Joint synods, one in the West and one in the East, were convoked in 359 at Seleucia and Ariminum under the emperor's influence, and they approved an Arian statement. It was at this time that St. Jerome made his famous statement at the apparent triumph of Arianism: "The whole world groaned and marveled to find itself Arian."

This heretical triumph was short-lived. Emperor Constantius died in 361, and the Council of Paris affirmed the Nicene Creed. The Semi-Arians returned to the Catholic fold after seeing the threat that Arianism posed. After a short term of exile imposed upon him by Emperor Julian the Apostate, St. Athanasius returned to Alexandria, where he labored for the remaining six years of his life among his people. During his lifetime St. Athanasius wrote many books and tracts in defense of the Nicene Creed and against Arianism. The Council of Constantinople (381) reaffirmed the Nicene Creed, which was St. Athanasius's life-long work. His feast day is celebrated on May 2.

THE NICENO-CONSTANTINOPOLITAN CREED

I believe in one God, / the Father almighty, / maker of heaven and earth, / of all things visible and invisible. / I believe in one Lord Jesus Christ, / the Only Begotten Son of God, / born of the Father before all ages. / God from God, Light from Light, / true God from true God, / begotten, not made, consubstantial with the Father; / through him all things were made. / For us men and for our salvation / he came down from heaven, / and by the Holy Spirit was incarnate of the Virgin Mary, / and became man. / For our sake he was crucified under Pontius Pilate, / he suffered death and was buried, / and rose again on the third day / in accordance with the Scriptures. / He ascended into heaven / and is seated at the right hand of the Father. / He will come again in glory / to judge the living and the dead / and his kingdom will have no end. / I believe in the Holy Spirit, the Lord, the giver of life, / who proceeds from the Father and the Son, / who with the Father and the Son is adored and glorified, / who has spoken through the prophets. / I believe in one, holy, catholic and apostolic Church. / I confess one Baptism for the forgiveness of sins / and I look forward to the resurrection of the dead / and the life of the world to come. Amen.

The Niceno-Constantinopolitan Creed is recited as the Profession of Faith on most Sundays immediately following the homily in the Mass. Bear in mind that the exact wording of the creed is important because of its theological complexity, opposition to heresy, historical continuity, and the unity that it provides throughout the Church.

The Nicene and Niceno-Constantinopolitan Creeds represent an area of agreement and unity for both East and West as the summation of the work of the first two ecumenical councils. A number of the Reformation era churches also recognize its authority, particularly the Lutheran and Anglican churches.

ST. HILARY OF POITIERS: "THE ATHANASIUS OF THE WEST"

St. Hilary of Poitiers (d. ca. 375-367/8) was a Latin Church Father during the period of the Arian heresy, and the leading Latin theologian of his day. St. Hilary ardently defended orthodox teaching against the Arians, and for this he is often called the "Athanasius of the West." Rather than merely condemning all heretics without exception, St. Hilary tried to explain to some (especially many of the Semi-Arians who were moving toward reconciliation with the Catholic Church) that often many of their disagreements were merely semantic and that the ideas were actually the same. The author of many brilliant theological texts, St. Hilary was named a Doctor of the Church by Pope Bl. Pius IX in 1851; his feast day is celebrated on January 13.

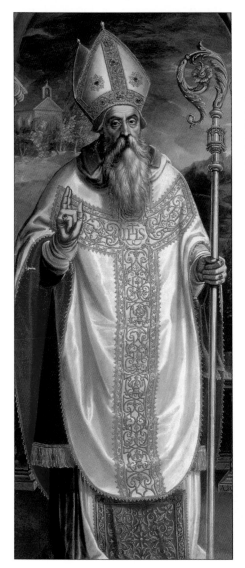

THE THREE CAPPADOCIANS

St. Basil the Great

St. Basil the Great (ca. 330-379) looms over Eastern Christianity as St. Augustine does in the West. He settled at Neocaesarea in 358, where he lived as a hermit while working with St. Gregory of Nazianzus in spreading the faith. St. Basil's ascetical life set the example for the structure and spirit of Eastern monasticism. Unlike in the West, monasticism in the East never fractured into new orders and rules but has remained together as an organic whole under St. Basil's Rule.

As the Bishop of Caesarea, St. Basil encountered opposition from the emperors and other churchmen regarding Arianism. He remained a staunch defender of orthodoxy against the heresies of his time. His work as Bishop of Caesarea extended beyond the intellectual realm of theological debate. St. Basil worked tirelessly for clerical rights, and he saw to it that his priests were rigorously and properly trained. As leader of a great diocese, he strove to care for the material and spiritual needs of the Christian laity. In one of his most important acts as Bishop, a system of hospitals and social service institutions was built up to serve the poor.

Finally, the Divine Liturgy of St. Basil was authored by him. It was the chief liturgy of the Eastern Churches, though in successive centuries the Divine Liturgy of St. John Chrysostom became more widely celebrated outside Lent. The Divine Liturgy of St. Basil has also greatly influenced the composition of Eucharistic Prayer IV as in use in the Roman Missal of the Catholic Church. His feast day is celebrated on January 2.

St. Gregory Of Nazianzus, "The Theologian"

St. Gregory of Nazianzus (329/30-389/90), like St. Basil, enjoyed the benefits of a philosophical education at Athens. He has often been given the title "The Theologian" because of his writings and teachings. Like St. Basil, he led a rigorous ascetical life and was elevated to the episcopacy at Sasima around 372.

Also like St. Basil, St. Gregory devoted much of his theological writing to the topic of the Holy Spirit. His Five Theological Orations expound upon the third Person of the Trinity.

St. Gregory played an important role at the Council of Constantinople in 381. Through his preaching in the city, he helped to bring the Arians back to the Nicene Faith. The emperor even appointed him Patriarch of Constantinople, but St. Gregory served less than a year before returning to his native Cappadocia. He shares his feast day with his life-long friend St. Basil on January 2.

St. Gregory Of Nyssa

St. Gregory of Nyssa (ca. 330-ca. 395), the younger brother of St. Basil, planned an ecclesiastical career after a short time as a rhetorician. Deeply opposed to the Arian beliefs, St. Gregory was forced into exile by the Arian Emperor Valens, a fate common to many of his brother bishops who espoused the Nicene Creed.

St. Gregory utilized neo-Platonic philosophy in his theological work, which served as an important tool for his teaching. He also defended the popular title *Theotokos* for Mary. *Theotokos* is Greek for "Mother of God" (literally, "the one who gave birth to God"). His feast day is celebrated on March 9.

APOLLINARIANISM (ca. 360-381)

Apollinaris (ca. 310-390) ardently supported orthodox positions, especially against the Arians, but his unguided fervor led him into heresy. Originally from Beirut and raised to the episcopacy around 360, he was a close friend of St. Athanasius.

Though he affirmed that Christ had a human body, Apollinaris denied the existence of a human mind and will in Christ as a misguided defensive measure against Arianism. Therefore, it would follow that Christ did not live a complete human life as a man. This is incompatible with the Church's teaching that Christ is true God and true man. Beginning with councils in Rome from 374-380, Apollinarianism was declared erroneous. The Second Ecumenical Council of Constantinople (381) specifically condemned this heresy, and the state prohibited adherence to it as well.

NESTORIANISM (ca. 351- ca. 451)

Nestorius became the Patriarch of Constantinople through the intervention of Emperor Theodosius II in 428. In an attempt to escape Apollinarianism, Nestorius maintained that Christ was the unity of a divine Person and a human person in an effort to emphasize his full divinity and full humanity. He attempted to eliminate the title *Theotokos* (bearer of God) to avoid falling into Apollinarianism. The term *Theotokos* had always before been used in orthodox circles, and it was gaining acceptance in popular culture as a devotion to Mary. (In 1969 Pope Paul VI declared the feast of *Theotokos* (Mary, Mother of God) to be observed in the West on January 1, a holy day of obligation.) Nestorius professed that though Mary was the Mother of Christ, she was not the Mother of God. Nestorius defended his rejection of this Marian title by his doctrine that Jesus Christ is the result of the union of two separate persons, one man and one God.

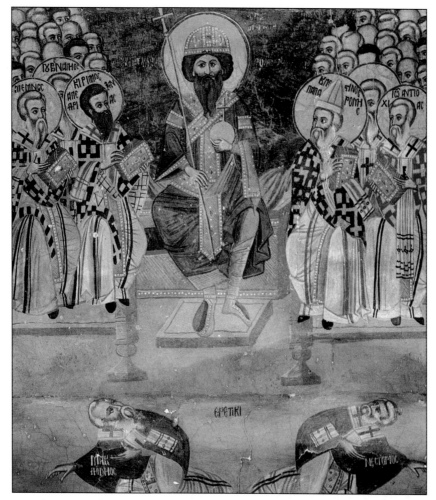

This 16th century fresco in a Cyprus church shows Emperor Theodosius II exiling Nestorius and another heretic during the Third Ecumenical Council at Ephesus in 431.

The orthodox position taught that Jesus Christ is one Person with two natures, human and divine. St. Cyril of Alexandria described the relationship of the two natures as the Hypostatic Union, a doctrine that was formally accepted by the Church at the Fourth Ecumenical Council of Chalcedon (451). The Definition of Chalcedon was a declaration of Catholic teaching that reaffirmed the Nicene and Niceno-Constantinople Creeds and rejected Nestorianism.

St. Cyril and Pope St. Celestine rejected as heretical the teachings of Nestorius in August 430 at a council in Rome. Pope St. Celestine also charged St. Cyril with the task of dealing with the Nestorian heresy. Legates delivered to Nestorius, the Patriarch of Constantinople, a set of twelve anathemas on December 7, 430. Nestorius was asked to repudiate his teachings within ten days.

Since Nestorius did not recant, Emperor Theodosius II called the Third Ecumenical Council at Ephesus (431) the following summer, where the council condemned Nestorius's teachings and declared Mary as the true Mother of God (*Theotokos*). The emperor accepted its decision, and Nestorius was removed as patriarch and sent to a monastery. So overjoyed were the people over this pronouncement that they carried the council fathers on their shoulders in great jubilation. In 435, the emperor ordered Nestorius's books to be burned, and in 436 Nestorius was banished to Egypt where he died.

MONOPHYSITISM (400s - 600s)

Monophysitism claimed that there is only one nature in Christ, and not two, as the definition of the Council of Chalcedon (451) would state. The name is derived from the Greek monos (alone, single) and physis (nature) that together mean "only one nature." It was a way of preserving the theological teaching of Christ's Divinity – the human nature of Christ would be "incorporated" into the Divine Nature. This particular heresy took on a various number of forms and attracted those who rejected the two-nature definition given at Chalcedon.

One of these erroneous doctrines was Eutychianism, initiated by Eutyches. Eutyches (ca. 378-454) was the head of an important monastery in Constantinople. He held that there was only one nature in Christ after the Incarnation, and he denied that Christ's humanity was identical with that of a man. For Eutyches, Christ's nature had the unique quality of being joined to the Divine Nature. He claimed that the human nature of Christ was, as it were, absorbed into the Divine Nature as a drop of water is absorbed into an ocean. His friendship with the influential eunuch Chrysaphius at the court of the emperor seems to have offered him some protection, as well as a hearing before Pope St. Leo the Great, before his teaching was finally condemned at the Fourth Ecumenical Council of Chalcedon (451).

Pope St. Leo was steeped in the heretical challenges threatening the Church. His support was sought by all sides involved in the Monophysite controversy. At the Council of Chalcedon (451), whose primary task was handling Monophysitism, St. Leo's legates spoke first, and his Tome (449) was accepted as the orthodox position by the ecumenical council. It declared that Jesus Christ was the God-man, one Person with two natures. Thereafter it was said, "Peter has spoken through Leo."

POPE ST. LEO THE GREAT

Pope St. Leo I (d. 461) consolidated papal power through a variety of means based upon Jesus Christ's strong endorsement of the papacy transmitted through the New Testament. (Mt 16:18: "You are Peter, and on this rock I will build my church.") With the firm conviction of God's will and authority behind the Chair of St. Peter, he secured a rescript from Emperor Valentinian III that acknowledged papal jurisdiction in the West.

St. Leo also took very bold positions vis-à-vis the barbarian invaders, which will be discussed in more detail in the following chapter. His leadership regarding the heresies of the time and dealings with the barbarians, as well as his administration in the Church earned St. Leo the title "the Great." His pontificate gave great moral authority and prestige to the papacy.

St. Leo's writings in Latin have been lauded for their clarity and precision, particularly at a time when the response to heresies required the use of precise language. St. Leo did not speak Greek and had to rely on translations to communicate with the East. This absence of a common language contributed to a strained relationship between the West and the East. In addition to being considered a Father of the Church, St. Leo has also been given the title Doctor of the Church, and his feast day is celebrated on November 10.

MONOTHELITISM (600s)

Monothelitism is the doctrine that professes the existence of only one will in Christ but still maintains that he has two natures. The name is derived from the Greek monos (alone, single) and thelos (one who wills). This heresy originated not with a churchman, but with the emperor. The tenets of Monothelitism were proposed in 624 as part of a conciliatory document to reconcile the Monophysites with the Church. Emperor Heraclius supported the document. Heraclius's predecessor, Emperor Justinian I, had deeply wounded the unity of the Empire by persecuting the Monophysites, and Heraclius sought to repair that damage. He thought that Monothelitism would help to maintain unity.

Patriarch Sergius of Constantinople approved the formula, though Sophronius (ca. 560-638), the Patriarch of Jerusalem, opposed it. Patriarch Sergius then wrote to Pope Honorius to clarify the matter. The pope approved of Sergius's handling of the matter and used the term "one will" in his reply, which the patriarch and emperor then quoted in the official document of Monothelitism known as the Ecthesis in 638. Two subsequent councils at Constantinople in 638 and 639, though not ecumenical, accepted the Ecthesis for the Eastern Church. The local councils confirmed that Patriarch Sergius had successfully won over a number of the Monophysites.

However, the next three papal successors to Honorious – Severinus, John IV, and Theodore I – all condemned Monothelitism and the Ecthesis. The Sixth Ecumenical Council of the Church (680-681) – the third at Constantinople – condemned the heresy and even anathematized Pope Honorius.

Pope Honorius's use of the term "one will" in an unguarded letter has often been cited as an example of papal fallibility. However, his private reply to a concern of only the Eastern Church does not meet the conditions for infallibility. In this case the pope did not define a doctrine for the entire, universal Church, nor was it the pope's intention to descend into theological details on the "wills" in Christ. He could very well have meant simply that Christ's will was in faithful conformity with the will of His Father. The incident does indicate, once again, that the other churches, even the patriarch in Constantinople, would appeal to the papacy to settle theological questions.

DOGMATIC AND SACRAMENTAL HERESIES

DONATISM (311-411)

Donatism rejected the validity of sacraments celebrated by priests and bishops who had formerly betrayed their faith. This schism in the Church in Africa began around 311 when Bishop Caecilian of Carthage was ordained by Bishop Felix of Aptunga, who had been a traditor during Diocletian's persecution. (A traditor was any early Christian who renounced the Christian Faith during the Roman persecutions.) The Donatists rejected the validity of Bishop Caecilian's ordination because of the sin of being a traditor. The heresy gets its name from Donatus, who was a bishop elected in opposition to the legitimate one.

Moreover, the Donatists claimed that the Church of the saints must remain holy and free from sin and even from those who have sinned. Sinful priests and bishops, the Donatists maintained, were incapable of validly celebrating the Sacraments. Indeed, the Donatists re-baptized persons who joined them because they did not consider the Sacrament valid except in their own circle. The Donatists went so far as to identify the true Church with only themselves.

St. Augustine was their chief opponent. He developed the Catholic position that Christ is the true minister of every Sacrament, even if the person celebrating the Sacrament is in a state of sin. St. Augustine separated the issue of worthiness on the part of the priest from the validity and efficacy of the Sacrament.

The Donatists were finally suppressed by the state in 411, though they were never fully defeated until Islam destroyed the Church in Africa in the seventh and eighth centuries.

PELAGIANISM (late 300s - 431)

Pelagianism advocated a theological position in which man can be redeemed and sanctified without grace. Specifically, it denied the existence of original sin as well as its transmission into the human family. According to this opinion, the sacraments are superfluous since salvation and holiness could be solely achieved through mere human endeavor.

This heresy was started by Pelagius, an English monk, who attracted several other defenders of these positions. They included Celestius and Julian of Eclanum; the latter engaged St. Augustine in a bitter and protracted debate that ended only with the death of St. Augustine in 430.

Pelagius and Celestius were repeatedly condemned at two councils in Carthage and Milevis in 416, and they were eventually excommunicated by Pope St. Innocent I (410-17). The Council of Carthage of May 1, 418 issued a teaching that adopted St. Augustine's positions on the Fall and original sin, which subsequently became the teaching of the Church. Emperor Honorius denounced the Pelagians on April 30, 418.

Nothing is known of what became of Pelagius, but Celestius appealed to Nestorius for support in 429 with the hope of gaining favor with Pope St. Celestine I. The Council of Ephesus (431) condemned Pelagianism yet again. Though this heresy still had some following in Britain, it eventually died out. However, the issues surrounding the Fall, original sin, and grace reappeared during the Middle Ages and again at the time of the Reformation (sixteenth century).

ST. AUGUSTINE OF HIPPO

St. Augustine (354-430) was perhaps the greatest Father of the Church. He fulfilled many roles: pastor, penitent, monk, preacher, bishop, teacher, and theologian. He is one of the greatest theologians of the Catholic Church. For almost a thousand years, he was the dominant figure in Catholic thought. No other theologian rivaled St. Augustine's importance until the thirteenth century when St. Thomas Aquinas would make his mark.

Born in Thagaste in Northern Africa (modern Souk-Ahras, Algeria) to a pagan father and a Christian mother, St. Monica, St. Augustine lived a dissolute life for many years before coming to the Faith. St. Augustine received a good education in the Latin classics and in rhetoric, though his Northern African accent was often mocked in Rome.

The intense attractions of both lust and heresy proved to be very powerful for St. Augustine. For this reason, even after more than a thousand years, his conversion story has not lost its appeal. He once prayed, "Lord, give me chastity and continence, but not yet" (Confessions, Book VIII.VIII). At 17 he cohabitated with a woman, and they later had a son, Adeodatus, who died in 389. Around the age of 20, St. Augustine also became deeply involved with the heresy of Manichæism.

Around the year 375, St. Augustine taught rhetoric in Thagaste. In 383 he moved to Rome and eventually Milan, where he continued his teaching career. St. Augustine was under tremendous stress not long after arriving in Italy: he lost his belief in Manichæism, and he separated from his mistress after many years of being together. It was at this same time, however, that he found great intellectual stimulation through a deeper introduction to neo-Platonic philosophy and the moving and edifying preaching of St. Ambrose.

In July 386, St. Augustine had a conversion experience while in a garden in Milan. He heard a voice from a young boy singing, "Tolle et lege," ("Take and read"). St. Augustine obeyed, picked up the Scriptures, and turned to a passage without looking. In Romans 13:13 he found in St. Paul's words comfort and direction for his life: "Let us conduct ourselves becomingly as in the day, not in reveling and drunkenness, not in debauchery and licentiousness, not in quarreling and jealousy."

St. Augustine resolved at this time to convert to the Catholic Faith and to abandon his sinful life and embark upon the road to holiness. From this point on, St. Augustine lived a life that is summarized by his constant affirmation: "Our hearts are restless until they rest in Thee, O Lord" (Confessions, Book I.I).

At the Easter Vigil on Holy Saturday of 387, St. Augustine and his son Adeodatus were baptized by St. Ambrose, but misfortune followed swiftly. In 388 his mother St. Monica, who had prayed for her son's conversion her entire life, died, and Adeodatus died the next year.

Then St. Augustine returned to Thagaste, where he established a monastic community dedicated to prayer and penance. In 391 he was seized by the people on a visit to Hippo Regius and ordained a priest by Bishop Valerius. By 395 he had been ordained to the episcopacy and became coadjutor for Valerius, and subsequently succeeded Valerius as Bishop of Hippo. St. Augustine's ordination and elevation to the office of bishop were very controversial, especially in view of his former life.

St. Augustine's writings are voluminous. They include a wide range of themes that delve into almost every conceivable issue of the time. Not only does he address the heresies of his day – the Manicheans, Donatists, Pelagians, and Arians – he also defends Christianity from pagan attackers who blamed the religion for Rome's enfeeblement and collapse. St. Augustine's two most important works are the Confessions and City of God, the latter of which was his answer to the pagan charges and the barbarian invasions. Confessions is St. Augustine's autobiography of his life and conversion.

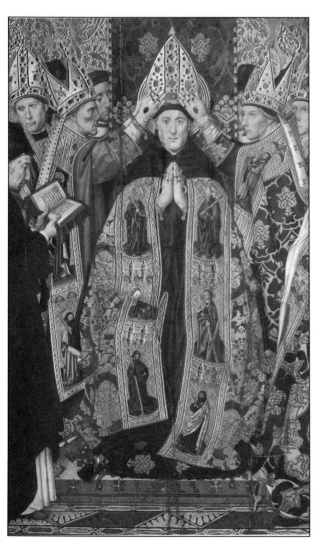

St. Augustine's ordination and elevation to the office of bishop were very controversial.

St. Augustine's spirit for the ascetical life is found throughout his rule. A number of monastic orders adopted his rule beginning in the eleventh century. They include the Augustinian Canons, the Augustinian Hermits and Friars, the Dominicans, and the Servites, as well as the Visitation and Ursuline nuns.

Though St. Augustine was born shortly after the Edict of Milan (313), he lived in a tumultuous age for the Church and for Roman society. Intransigent heresies tore at the unity of the Church, and the Empire was well along the path to oblivion in the temporal order. As St. Augustine lay dying in Hippo, the Vandals were destroying the city, and other Germanic tribes were invading throughout the Roman Empire. The entire temporal, social, and economic order that St. Augustine knew was abruptly ending. St. Augustine set the theological tone in the West, and his philosophy and theology dominated Christian thought for some eight hundred years, until the thirteenth century, when Scholasticism and St. Thomas Aquinas would emerge, enriching the philosophy and theology of St. Augustine.

St. Augustine's feast day is celebrated on August 28.

PART VIII

PART VIII

Christianity: Official Religion of the Roman Empire

CONSTANTINE'S ASCENDANCY

Constantine and Licinius ruled the Empire after the Edict of Milan (313), though Licinius was not faithful to his promised religious toleration. Around 321 Licinius began a persecution directed at the bishops and clergy, and in 324 he openly declared war against Constantine. Licinius was defeated, thus making possible religious toleration throughout the Empire.

Constantine increasingly supported Christianity as the years passed. Through law and his own actions, he set the tone: priests and churches were freed from taxation, individual churches were permitted to receive donations, work on Sunday was forbidden, and crucifixion as a state form of execution was ended. Constantine himself withdrew from participation in the pagan rites and ceremonies to which the emperors had always been connected.

Constantine's other great influence was to found the city of Constantinople on the site of the Greek city of Byzantium in 330. On May 11, 330 the city was officially dedicated under Christian and pagan rites. Constantinople was dedicated to the protection of Mary under the title of *Theotokos.* The city's natural defenses protected it for over a thousand years until it fell to the Ottoman Turks in 1453.

After Constantine moved the capital of the Empire to Byzantium along the Bosporus Straits in 330, economic, cultural, and linguistic power shifted. The ruling city of the Roman Empire did not speak Latin but Greek. Byzantium, as the new Eastern Empire came to be known, was wealthier and more heavily populated and looked upon Italy and the West as backward and poor. During that period, knowledge of the Greek language was becoming less common in the West, adding to the cultural breach between East and West. Not until the Renaissance did the West take a renewed interest in Greek and the access to the great body of ancient knowledge it provided.

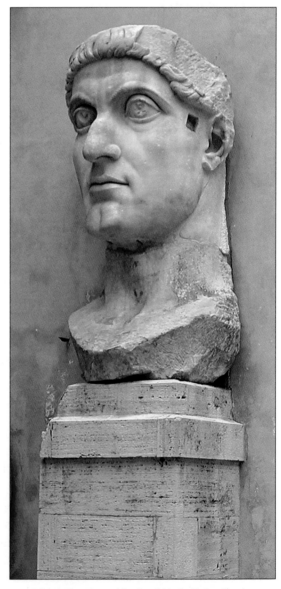

Constantine was proclaimed a saint by the Eastern Church, and is known as "the Great" in the Western Church.

JULIAN THE APOSTATE

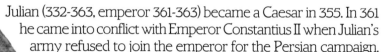

Julian (332-363, emperor 361-363) became a Caesar in 355. In 361 he came into conflict with Emperor Constantius II when Julian's army refused to join the emperor for the Persian campaign. Civil war was averted only because Constantius died of natural causes. Julian was then immediately promoted by the military to the imperial throne.

The title "Apostate" (one who willingly renounces his faith) has been given to Julian because, though he was baptized a Christian, as emperor he tried to de-emphasize Christianity. Julian did not persecute the Christians, but he sought to re-establish paganism on equal footing with Christianity and to strip Christianity of the special benefits that Constantine the Great and his successor had granted.

The Christogram symbol (Chi-Rho), which Constantine carried into his battle with Maxentius, appeared on Roman coins after the Edict of Milan (313).

Julian took several steps to achieve these ends. He pushed to re-establish pagan worship throughout the Empire, and this included the development of an elaborate pagan liturgy and organized his pagan religion in imitation of the Church's ecclesiastical and sacramental structures. Julian himself lived a very ethical life, to which he was committed in order to raise the moral tone of pagans in the Empire. The curriculum in the Empire's schools was paganized. Julian revoked the financial exemption and benefits that had been given to the Church by his predecessors. He wrote many tracts in support of paganism and in opposition to Christianity and imposed harsh sentences on his subjects because of their faith. Finally, Julian generated great confusion in the Church when he permitted exiled heretical bishops to return.

Julian also had to deal with the Persian threat. On June 26, 363, he was struck by an arrow while on a campaign in Mesopotamia, and he died the same day.

Julian had been viewed in a negative way in much of the Empire, especially in the East where the largest numbers of Christians dwelt. Succeeding emperors moved to progressively reduce paganism to oblivion, and to re-grant the special status of Christianity. Jovian (emperor 363-364), the immediate successor to Julian, returned to Christianity the rights Julian had stripped from it.

THEODOSIUS I THE GREAT (379-395)

Theodosius I cemented the union between the Church and State with his 391 decree declaring Christianity the official religion of the Empire. Heresy became a legal offense before the state, pagan sacrifice was outlawed, and, essentially, all other forms of paganism as well. Clearly, this was a watershed moment in the history of the Church. Within eighty years Christianity emerged from the worst persecution it had ever known to official toleration under the Edict of Milan and finally to the status of official religion of the Empire.

Being a persecuted minority forced Christians to rely authentically on their faith and to forge deep bonds of solidarity. Now these same values of sacrifice and love were officially being taken up by the State. If carried out correctly, the situation provided the Church with an extraordinary possibility to evangelize the Empire and others outside of it. However, an established religion can also find its voice and values co-opted. In any case, given the historical circumstances of that era, it seems that a close connection between Church and State was necessary.

CONCLUSION

The early Church was often perceived as a small segment of Judaism, beginning after the Resurrection of Jesus. She then suffered through a long period of intermittent, though intense, persecution, and, finally (and quite remarkably), she emerged as an imperially sanctioned religion in AD 313. The first three hundred years of the Church's history were tumultuous, although they contain many lessons that remain perennially applicable. The martyrs of the early Church are emulated today by many Christians who live in cultures that are as hostile to Christianity now as was Rome two-thousand years ago. The lives of martyrs such as Sts. Ignatius of Antioch remain quite relevant to Christians then as well as today, who share in the communion of saints. The complex and often troubling relationship between the Church and the state is one that began in the Roman Empire, and still remains today. Lastly, the structure of the episcopacy and the importance of Tradition for resolving theological disputes both found expression in the many writings of Apostolic Fathers like Sts. Ignatius of Antioch and Irenæus.

The Church experienced a moment of freedom and hope with the Edict of Milan in 313, but this by no means meant that the situation in the Church was relaxed over the next two centuries. The Church was convulsed by one theological controversy after another, any number of which threatened to destroy the Faith. Only the providential leadership of the popes, the Church Fathers, and the ecumenical councils under the influence of the Holy Spirit guided the Church through the treacherous waters of heresy that threatened to sink her at any time. The proclamation of Christianity as the official religion of the Empire in 391 by Theodosius I the Great inaugurated a new era in Christianity, one filled with the promise of evangelization, as well as with the dangers of temporal meddling in the affairs of the Church.

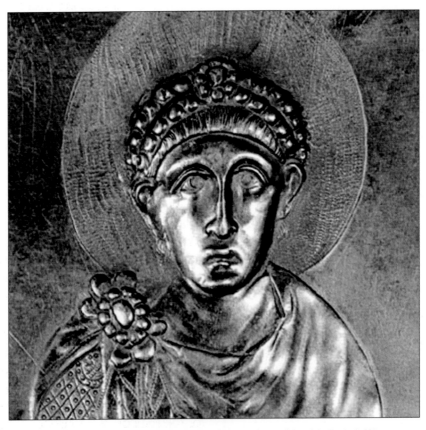

Emperor Theodosius I the Great declared Christianity the official religion of the Empire in 391.
Above: The image of Theodosius I the Great embossed on a 4th century silver plate.

VOCABULARY

ANATHEMA
A ban solemnly pronounced by ecclesiastical authority and accompanied by excommunication

ANOMOEANS
From the Greek anhomoios, meaning "dissimilar," this sect of Arianism stressed an essential difference between the Father and Son in the Trinity.

APOLLINARIANISM
Founded by Apollinarius in the fourth century, this heresy denied the existence of a human mind and will in Christ.

APOSTASY
Apostasy is the willful renunciation of the Faith in its entirety.

APOSTATE
A person who denies the Faith altogether.

APOSTLES' CREED
A statement of belief of the Apostles based upon the New Testament. It is derived from a baptismal creed used especially in Rome known as the Old Roman, and it is therefore associated particularly with the Church of Rome.

ARIANISM
Third and fourth century heresy founded by the Alexandrian priest Arius. It denied Jesus' divinity, claiming that Jesus is neither God nor equal to the Father, but rather an exceptional creature raised to the level of "Son of God" because of his heroic fidelity to the Father's will and his sublime holiness.

CAESAROPAPISM
Refers to the dual role of head of State and leader of the Church in which the temporal ruler extends his own powers to ecclesiastical and theological matters. The Church in the East, influenced by the growing power of the patriarch of Constantinople at the hands of the emperor, tended to accept a role for the Church in which it was subservient to the interests of the State.

CHRYSOSTOM
Moniker of St. John Chrysostom meaning "golden mouthed," it refers to the saint's extraordinary preaching skills.

CHURCH FATHERS
Great, holy leaders who have come forward to lead the Church, explain the Faith, and meet the unique challenges posed by different heresies.

DEMIURGE
Gnostic creator god of the material world.

DOCETISM
Derived from the Greek word dokesis, meaning appearance, this Gnostic heresy maintained that Jesus did not die on the cross but was spared by someone else who took his place.

DOCTOR OF THE CHURCH
Doctores Ecclesiae, a specific title given by the pope to those whose development of theology and personal sanctity are exemplary.

DOKESIS
Greek word for appearance. Referred to heresy which claimed Jesus only appeared to die on the Cross.

DONATISM
Heresy that rejected the sacraments celebrated by clergy who had formerly betrayed their faith.

ECUMENICAL COUNCIL
Derived from the Greek word oikoumene, meaning "the whole inhabited world," Ecumenical Councils bring bishops and others entitled to vote from all over the world to discuss central issues of the Church. They are presided over by the pope and issues decrees which, with the approval of the pope, bind all Christians.

FILIOQUE
Latin word meaning "and the Son," it is used to express the double procession of the Holy Spirit from the Father and the Son. St. Augustine's discussion on the relationship of the Father, Son, and Holy Spirit laid the essential groundwork for the addition of the Filioque clause to the Nicene Creed in the Medieval period.

GNOSTICISM

Derived from the Greek word gnosis ("knowledge"), the name refers to one of the principle tenets of this multifaceted heresy, namely, that salvation may be achieved through knowledge. In the second century, Gnosticism, which had eastern origins and influences from Persia and India, very successfully perverted the meaning of Christianity and its symbols. To prove its authenticity, Gnosticism co-opted the Scriptures, the Old and New Testaments, and erected an entirely new cosmological structure that challenged the intent of Christianity.

HERESY

The refusal to accept one or more truths of the Faith which are required for Catholic belief. It is a species of unbelief belonging to those who profess the Christian Faith, but corrupt its dogmas.

HERETIC

A person who denies one or more doctrines of the Faith.

HOMOEANS (SABELLIANS)

From Greek homoios, meaning "similar," this Scriptural purist party rejected the use of the word homoousios at the Council of Nicaea because it was not used in the Bible.

HOMOOUSIOS

Greek word meaning "of the same substance."

INFALLIBLE

Free from error. Ecumenical Councils' definitions on Faith and morals are considered free from error, or infallible, if that is the intention of the pope and bishops in union.

LOGOS

An ambiguous Greek word with a multitude of meanings that include: word, account, meaning, reason, argument, saying, speech, story and many more. The Gospel of St. John utilizes the word's complex meaning, referring to the Person of Jesus, the Son of God and a member of the Blessed Trinity, as the logos.

MANICHÆISM

Heresy founded by Mani in the 3rd century. An elaborate form of Gnosticism, it involved the relationship between light and darkness, believing that through rituals and sharing their knowledge believers could regain the light stolen by Satan and hidden in the brains of men, thus freeing the light to return to its original source. Manichæism heavily borrowed from the Scriptures, especially from the writings of St. Paul. Mani incorporated many of St. Paul's arguments and imagery to support his own teaching concerning the struggle between darkness and light.

MARCIONISM

Founded by Marcion in the second century, he borrowed the Gnostic idea of a Demiurge, calling this force the jealous and vengeful God of Law. According to Marcionism, the God of Jesus Christ, the true God, has no law and is sent to bring about the demise of the Demiurge. He renounced all Jewish influence on the Church, believing that the God of the Old Testament was the evil Demiurge.

MONOPHYSITISM

From the Greek monos, meaning "alone," and physis, meaning "nature," this heresy claimed that there is only one nature in Christ and that His human nature is "incorporated" into the Divine Nature.

MONOTHELITISM

Heresy claiming that Christ has two natures but only one will.

MONTANISM

Founded by Montanus in the second century, he believed that due to an outpouring of the Holy Spirit upon him, he knew that a new, heavenly kingdom was imminent. One of the first apocalyptic heresies, his followers lived a very austere life rejecting second marriages and flight from persecution.

VOCABULARY Continued

NEO-PLATONISM
School of philosophy which held that the logos was a created being, not the Supreme Being. Platonic philosophies, in general, viewed the material world as less perfect than the world of ideas. Thus, besides denying Christ's true divinity, many early Platonic heresies greatly deemphasized Christ's humanity, if not openly denying it.

NESTORIANISM
Founded in the fourth century by Nestorius, the Patriarch of Constantinople, this heresy maintained that Christ was both human and divine but was not himself fully human or fully divine. Instead, he believed that Christ was a union of two men, one human the other divine.

PELAGIANISM
Heresy denying original sin and the need for grace in man's salvation. According to this heresy, the sacraments are superfluous since salvation and holiness can only be achieved through human endeavor.

THEOTOKOS
Literally "bearer of God," often translated "mother of God." Used since the early centuries of the Church, this title of Mary was defended by the Council of Ephesus in 431.

TRAJAN'S RESCRIPT
Policy for handling Christians in the Roman Empire which stated that Christians who renounced their faith and offered sacrifice would be allowed to live. Those who did not renounce their faith would suffer death.

VULGATE
First translation of the Bible from its original languages into Latin by St. Jerome.

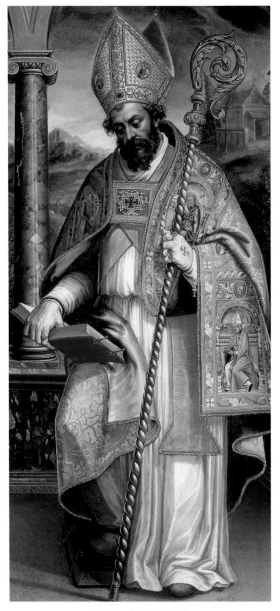

St. Athanasius (ca. 296-375)

STUDY QUESTIONS

1. Where in the Bible is Christianity referred to as "the Way"?

2. If it is true that Nero set the fire in Rome on July 19, what was his ultimate motivation? How did the Christians prove to be expedient political tools?

3. Summarize Trajan's Rescript. How does it differ from the previous law of Nero?

4. What does St. Ignatius have to say about the importance of the episcopacy?

5. How did Hadrian's Rescript (AD 123/124) improve the situation for Christians?

6. How did the Roman emperor Septimus Severus threaten both Judaism and Christianity?

7. St. Irenæus was an important leader in which region of the empire? (This is of particular interest because he came from the Greek-speaking east.)

8. Summarize Diocletian's Four Edicts.

9. What is the famous story about how Constantine won the Battle at Saxa Rubra?

10. Discuss the importance of the Edict of Milan (AD 313).

11. What were the guiding premises of Gnosticism?

12. What role did asceticism play in Manichaeism and other Gnostic heresies?

13. Who has the power to start, change, and end an ecumenical council?

14. Who is a "Church Father" and what are the five characteristics of a Church Father?

15. How and why did St. Ambrose stand up to the very powerful emperor Theodosius in 390?

16. For what is St. John Chrysostom best known?

17. What was Arianism, and why was Arianism such a threat to Christianity?

18. Who convened the Council of Nicaea in 325 and what was the council's outcome?

19. Under what circumstances was it said of Pope St. Leo I that "Peter has spoken through Leo"? What does this statement really mean?

20. How did Pope St. Leo I increase papal power?

21. How did St. Augustine answer the challenges posed by Donatism?

22. Describe St. Augustine's background. Why would his ordination as bishop have been particularly controversial with the Donatists?

23. What do the words "tolle et lege" mean, and what is their significance in St. Augustine's life?

24. What topics did St. Augustine address in two of his best-known works, Confessions and City of God ?

25. When and by whom was Christianity declared the official religion of the empire?

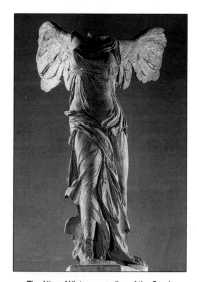

The Altar of Victory, a replica of the Greek "Winged Victory of Samothrace," was the ultimate symbol of Roman supremacy. The Altar was a "majestic female standing on a globe, with expanded wings, and a crown of laurel in her outstretched hand."

PRACTICAL EXERCISES

1. During the Columbine school massacre in 1999, one of the shooters asked a young female student if she was a Christian. When she answered "Yes, I believe in God," he executed her. Can you imagine a situation where your faith could be so dramatically tested?

2. How do the presence of martyrs in a culture lead to conversions to the Faith?

3. How could effective apologists like St. Justin Martyr be of great help to the Catholic Church today? What issues would a modern apologist tackle? To whom would the defense be addressed?

4. Check out a local bookstore's religion and philosophy sections. How many books on "finding the light inside yourself" or other New Age movement texts did you find? Why do you think so many people have turned to the New Age movement? What is the difference between these "self-help" solutions and the way of life offered in the example of Christ?

5. What might be some reasons why the pope has authority over the ecumenical councils? If another ecumenical council were called today, what do you think would be the topics for discussion?

6. Think of reasons and examples of how the union of the secular and spiritual powers might cause conflict between the Church and the state.

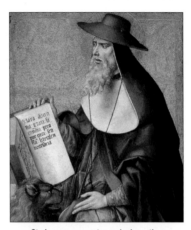

St. Jerome never stopped advocating or living a penitential life.

FROM THE CATECHISM

465 The first heresies denied not so much Christ's divinity as his true humanity (Gnostic Docetism). From apostolic times the Christian faith has insisted on the true incarnation of God's Son "come in the flesh" (cf. 1 Jn 4: 2-3; 2 Jn 7). But already in the third century, the Church in a council at Antioch had to affirm against Paul of Samosata that Jesus Christ is Son of God by nature and not by adoption. The first ecumenical council of Nicaea in 325 confessed in its Creed that the Son of God is "begotten, not made, of the same substance (homoousios) as the Father", and condemned Arius, who had affirmed that the Son of God "came to be from things that were not" and that he was "from another substance" than that of the Father (Council of Nicaea I (325): DS 130, 126).

1173 When the Church keeps the memorials of martyrs and other saints during the annual cycle, she proclaims the Paschal mystery in those "who have suffered and have been glorified with Christ. She proposes them to the faithful as examples who draw all men to the Father through Christ, and through their merits she begs for God's favors" (SC 104; cf. SC 108, 111).

2089 Incredulity is the neglect of revealed truth or the willful refusal to assent to it. "Heresy is the obstinate post-baptismal denial of some truth which must be believed with divine and catholic faith, or it is likewise an obstinate doubt concerning the same; apostasy is the total repudiation of the Christian faith; schism is the refusal of submission to the Roman Pontiff or of communion with the members of the Church subject to him" (CIC, can. 751: emphasis added).

FROM THE CATECHISM Continued

2473 Martyrdom is the supreme witness given to the truth of the faith: it means bearing witness even unto death. The martyr bears witness to Christ who died and rose, to whom he is united by charity. He bears witness to the truth of the faith and of Christian doctrine. He endures death through an act of fortitude. "Let me become the food of the beasts, through whom it will be given me to reach God" (St. Ignatius of Antioch, Ad Rom. 4, 1: SCh 10, 110).

2474 The Church has painstakingly collected the records of those who persevered to the end in witnessing to their faith. These are the acts of the Martyrs. They form the archives of truth written in letters of blood:

Neither the pleasures of the world nor the kingdoms of this age will be of any use to me. It is better for me to die [in order to unite myself] to Christ Jesus than to reign over the ends of the earth. I seek him who died for us; I desire him who rose for us. My birth is approaching… (St. Ignatius of Antioch, Ad Rom. 6, 1-2: SCh 10, 114).

I bless you for having judged me worthy from this day and this hour to be counted among your martyrs.…You have kept your promise, God of faithfulness and truth. For this reason and for everything, I praise you, I bless you, I glorify you through the eternal and heavenly High Priest, Jesus Christ, your beloved Son. Through him, who is with you and the Holy Spirit, may glory be given to you, now and in the ages to come. Amen (Martyrium Polycarpi 14, 2-3: PG 5, 1040; SCh 10, 228).

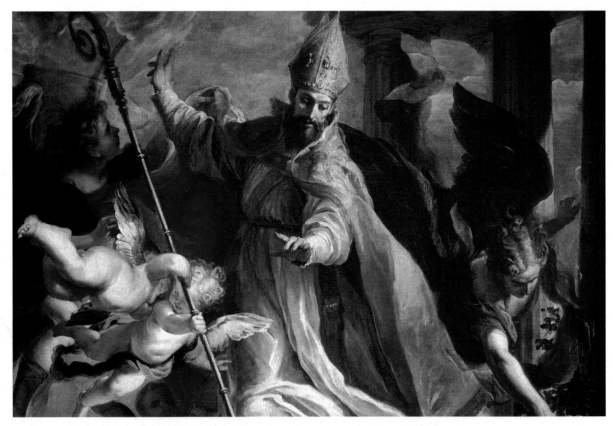

The Triumph of St. Augustine, Claudio Coello; Prado Museum, Madrid, Spain; Archivo Oronoz

CHAPTER 3

Light In
The Dark Ages

Throughout all of the insecurity, one institution remained firm: the Church. Amid the darkness, the Church held up the powerful light of Christ.

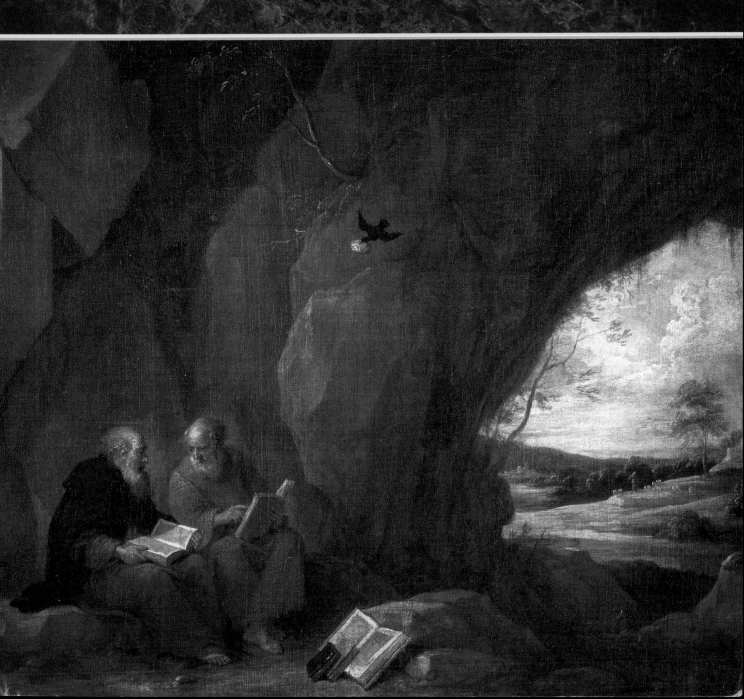

CHAPTER 3

Light In The Dark Ages

As St. Augustine waited for death in Hippo, Vandals beset the city. The collapse of the Roman Empire during the fifth century inaugurated a period of decline in the West as the old world passed away, and confusion reigned as the basis for a new order had yet to come. Throughout all of the insecurity, one institution remained firm: the Church. She continued to spread the Gospel message while providing continuity in an uncertain time. Regardless of the transitoriness of any age, the Church proclaims a message of trust in the life and light of Christ amid trials and tribulations and promises eternal life after death. Amid the darkness, the Church holds up the powerful light of Christ.

The great evangelizers of this period were fervent in their faith in Jesus and his Church, and hoped for everyone, including the different pagan peoples, to share in this spiritual and moral treasure of Christianity. These heralds of Christ not only wanted to prepare their people for everlasting life, but also wanted to spread the benefits of a more civilized society and higher human culture.

PART I

The Collapse of the Roman Empire

The collapse of the Roman Empire resulted in a crisis that took the early Church by surprise. The Church now had to dissociate herself from the fallen Empire, which was assumed would last forever. Throughout the decline of the Roman Empire and the rise of monasticism, the Holy Spirit inspired and strengthened the Church for the next great wave of evangelizing activity among the German tribes. By the time the different groups in Europe had converted in the eleventh century, Christianity had spread to virtually the entire European continent.

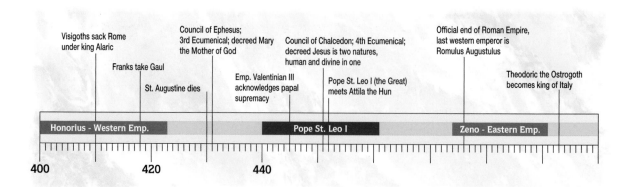

Timeline:
- Visigoths sack Rome under king Alaric
- Franks take Gaul
- St. Augustine dies
- Council of Ephesus; 3rd Ecumenical; decreed Mary the Mother of God
- Emp. Valentinian III acknowledges papal supremacy
- Council of Chalcedon; 4th Ecumenical; decreed Jesus is two natures, human and divine in one
- Pope St. Leo I (the Great) meets Attila the Hun
- Official end of Roman Empire, last western emperor is Romulus Augustulus
- Theodoric the Ostrogoth becomes king of Italy

Honorius - Western Emp. | Pope St. Leo I | Zeno - Eastern Emp.

400   420   440

THE FALL OF ROME (476)

Historians do not have an official date for the fall of Rome, but sometime during the fifth century, the West collapsed. In 410, Alaric, king of the Visigoths, sacked Rome. Odoacer (sometimes Odovacar), chieftain of the Heruli, who served as a mercenary in Rome, led a revolt and overthrew the last western emperor in 476. Soon after, the Ostrogoths, united under Theodoric, invaded Italy in 489 and overthrew Odoacer by 493. The last ten western emperors rarely sat for more than a few years on the throne before they were deposed by invading barbarians.

The moral situation from the fifth through eighth centuries was grim as the former Roman order crumbled. The Roman Empire was not yet completely Christianized when the barbarian invasions injected a foreign and often violent character into the culture. The concept of human rights was unfamiliar to many Romans as well as to the invading barbarian tribes.

The absence of academic pursuits among the Germanic Franks quickly undermined the great Greco-Roman tradition of learning and culture. Thus, the fall of Rome brought about a dramatic and immediate collapse in intellectual activity throughout the former empire of the West. Classical literature was lost, Latin deteriorated, and illiteracy became the norm. The loss of literacy particularly affected the Church because most people could no longer read the Scriptures. The Church remained the only locus of intellectual activity. Academic training was limited to priests and religious studying the Scriptures and theology. The long Greco-Roman tradition of philosophical inquiry came to a halt.

In addition to the collapse of education, the vibrant economy of the empire entered a period of decline as well. Roads became unsafe. People lived in fear and distress, and crime increased. As production and commercial activity declined, the cities and towns began to shrink. Consequentially, the former empire dissipated into a rural society of isolated towns and villages.

With the disappearance of the Roman Empire, the Church had the important task to adapt herself to a dramatic cultural change. The Church's organization reflected the ways and customs of the Empire. The governing structure of the Church was modeled after the rule and territorial division of the Empire. Christians had assumed, as had the Roman emperors, that the destiny of Christianity was permanently intertwined with the Empire, especially after Theodosius I made Christianity the official religion in 379. The Barbarian invasions helped the Church realize that she was not wedded to the Roman Empire and had to adapt to a significant cultural shift.

THE GERMANIC TRIBES

The mission of the Church is to bring the Good News to all peoples. This effort invariably involves Christianizing cultures and at the same time adapting insofar as possible to these

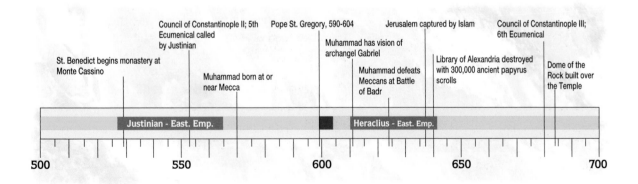

Council of Constantinople II; 5th Ecumenical called by Justinian

Pope St. Gregory, 590-604

Jerusalem captured by Islam

Council of Constantinople III; 6th Ecumenical

St. Benedict begins monastery at Monte Cassino

Muhammad has vision of archangel Gabriel

Muhammad born at or near Mecca

Muhammad defeats Meccans at Battle of Badr

Library of Alexandria destroyed with 300,000 ancient papyrus scrolls

Dome of the Rock built over the Temple

Justinian - East. Emp.

Heraclius - East. Emp.

500   550   600   650   700

cultures. With the advent of the barbarian invasions, the Church was now called to extend her messages to the Germanic tribes who were different in many ways from the citizens of the previous Roman civilization.

The culture of the Germanic tribes is complicated and multi-faceted, by no means unified, although they shared the same family of languages. They were the second largest Northern European group after the Celts, who had been such powerful warriors that they had settled as far south as Austria and even managed to sack Rome in 390. After settling down, they developed into a peaceful people engaged in agrarian life. By the time of the Germanic invasions, the Celts had been long conquered by the Romans or were being taken over by the advancing Germanic tribes.

Ever occupied with the difficult task of defending the vast borders of the Empire, the Roman legions had battled the barbarians for some time but were never able to conquer them in their own territory. For three centuries the barbarians pushed to enter into the Empire, but the Romans used whatever advantage they could to stop them. They did, however, invite many of the tribes to settle along the frontier in Roman territory. The Romans intermittently battled the barbarians to keep them out and settled them along the frontier in exchange for conscripts for the Roman legions. The peaceful settlement of some tribes also helped to bolster the Empire's lagging population.

Over time, the Roman legions were Germanized to such an extent that the army remained Roman in name only. This influx of Germanic soldiers afforded a great opportunity given the obvious vulnerability of the Roman Empire. That the Roman army no longer consisted primarily of Romans – as the Germanic tribes eagerly desired the conquest of new territory – partially explains the fall of Rome.

It was only a matter of time before the Germanic barbarians would score a number of military victories against the Romans which would lead to their ultimate defeat. It was common for the tribes to arrive in waves, only to be supplanted by succeeding tribes. In 378, the Visigoths defeated the Byzantine army at the Battle of Adrianople, and by December 406, many tribes had crossed the Rhine to settle in Gaul. With the border of the Empire penetrated, Gaul soon fell to the Visigoths, led by Alaric. Soon thereafter Rome fell on August 24, 410, and was pillaged for four days.

Of the different tribes that merit mention here, the two branches of Goths – Visigoths and Ostrogoths – were first to invade the empire. Alaric, as mentioned above, was the Visigoth leader who led the invasion of the Italian Peninsula. Later, the Visigoths were pushed into the Iberian Peninsula by the Franks, where they remained until Spain fell to the Muslims in the eighth century. Theodoric led the Ostrogoths who occupied the Italian Peninsula, replacing the Visigoths. Ostrogoth rule would end with their defeat in 536 by Byzantine forces.

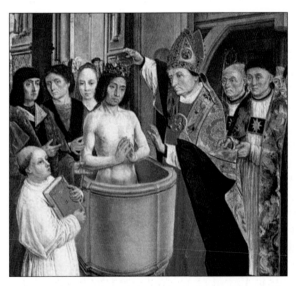

The baptism of the leader of the Franks, Clovis. Under his leadership, the Franks were the first Germanic tribe to convert to Christianity.

The Franks – a name meaning "fierce" or "bold" – were a Germanic people who settled in Gaul late in the third century. They are the ancestors of modern France and, under the leadership of the great chieftain Clovis, were the first Germanic tribe to convert to Christianity (497). A more detailed account of the conversion of the Franks appears in the following chapter.

The Alemanni (meaning "All Men") were another Germanic people. They settled south of the Main River in central Germany around 260 before moving later to Alsace and Switzerland.

The Burgundians arrived on the Main River around 250. They established a capital at Worms before being defeated by the Romans in 436.

The Lombards lived along the Elbe and began advancing toward the Danube by the middle of the second century. Eventually they settled in the Roman province of Pannonia (eastern Austria and western Hungary, bounded on the north and east by the Danube River) before finally migrating to Italy in the sixth century.

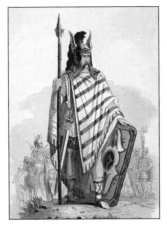

German Barbarian Chief

The Vandals were the most ruthless of the Germanic tribes. Beginning in 406 they attacked Gaul before moving to Spain and then to North Africa. The Vandals were so fierce and committed such atrocities that the word "vandal" is still used in English today. They were also relentless persecutors of the Church.

ATTILA THE HUN
MEETS POPE ST. LEO THE GREAT (452)

As the Empire was struggling to control the invading Germanic tribes, a new unforeseen threat to both the Romans and the barbarians emerged from the Far East in the first half of the fifth century. The Huns, a powerful nomadic people of unknown ethnic origins, swept west from northern China and had crossed into the Volga valley by the end of the fourth century. They were ferocious and ruthless fighters, and by 432 they had established themselves in the Eastern Empire, forcing tribute from Emperor Theodosius II. By 451, the Huns had invaded Gaul and threatened the heart of the Western Empire.

Attila (d. 453), "the Scourge of God," succeeded to joint kingship over the Huns with his brother in 433. Not long after, his brother died (perhaps murdered by Attila), and Attila for the first time successfully united the Hunnish hordes under one rule. He was a tremendously brave warrior, a skilled diplomat, and a keen military strategist. He was also ruthless–if he discovered that a Hun had served the Romans as a mercenary soldier, he ordered his crucifixion. Earlier in his life, he had been held as a hostage in Rome where he learned Latin and discovered Rome's weaknesses. His ambition was to establish an Asiatic empire with himself as emperor. He did succeed, but the empire collapsed after his death.

After having successfully united the hordes, Attila moved west, began engaging the Romans in the 440s, and invaded Gaul. With relentless swiftness, Attila's Huns devastated Gaul and continually augmented their army with each military victory. Finally, in 451, an allied army of Romans and Visigoths defeated Attila on the Plains of Chalons, forcing Attila back across the Rhine.

Defeated in Gaul, Attila turned his sights south to Italy. Beginning in 452, his Huns ravaged northern Italian cities and towns. As they drew closer to Rome, Pope St. Leo the Great went to meet him. In one of the great mysteries of history, it remains unknown exactly what words Pope St. Leo used to dissuade Attila from attacking Rome. Attila is said to have come upon a procession of priests, deacons, and acolytes singing hymns and psalms. At the end of the procession there was an old man sitting on a horse praying intensely. Attila asked him, "What is your name?" The old man replied, "Leo the Pope." In an unprecedented move, Attila did not attack Rome, and he withdrew entirely from Italy. Attila died shortly thereafter, and his empire, divided among his sons, soon disintegrated. This confrontation with Pope St. Leo in a certain sense changed the course of history. The pope was able to repeat the same success in 455 when he convinced the leader of the Vandals, Genseric, not to burn Rome, and spare the lives of the people.

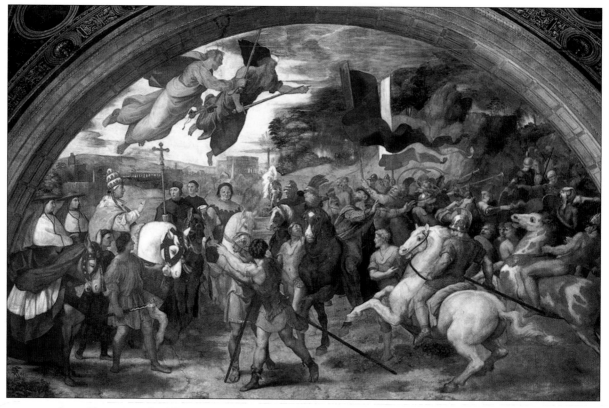

In one of the great mysteries of history, it remains unknown exactly what words Pope St. Leo used to dissuade Attila from attacking Rome.

HISTORICAL INTERPRETATION OF THE GERMANIC INVASIONS

It took some time for the Church to digest the historical significance of the Germanic invasions, and what they meant for her mission of evangelization. Over time, several concrete ideas emerged.

Primarily, the Church recognized that Christianity was universal. The Faith needed to be communicated as much to the Germanic tribes as it was in previous centuries to the Greco-Roman world. Christianity was meant to incorporate everyone, and this would be emphatically reinforced in the future when the Church was presented with opportunities to evangelize the Americas, Africa, Asia, and Australia.

Though the Church was identified with the Roman Empire for four centuries and adopted its governmental structures (dioceses), customs, language, and laws, the Church now began a monumental shift, civilizing and evangelizing the Germanic peoples.

The effort to reach out to the Germanic tribes was no small task. The German character was very different from the Greco-Roman one: the Germans were less philosophically and theologically inclined, placed less emphasis on order, culture, organization, and law. In effect, most of what the Church learned and developed within the context of Roman culture had to be radically altered in order to work with the Germanic populace without changing the essential doctrines of the Catholic Faith. Through monasticism the Church found access to these people. Monasticism had established itself firmly by the end of the fifth century, by which time the Roman Empire had been reduced to a mosaic of kingdoms ruled by Germanic chieftains.

THE BARBARIAN INVASIONS, 4TH AND 5TH CENTURIES

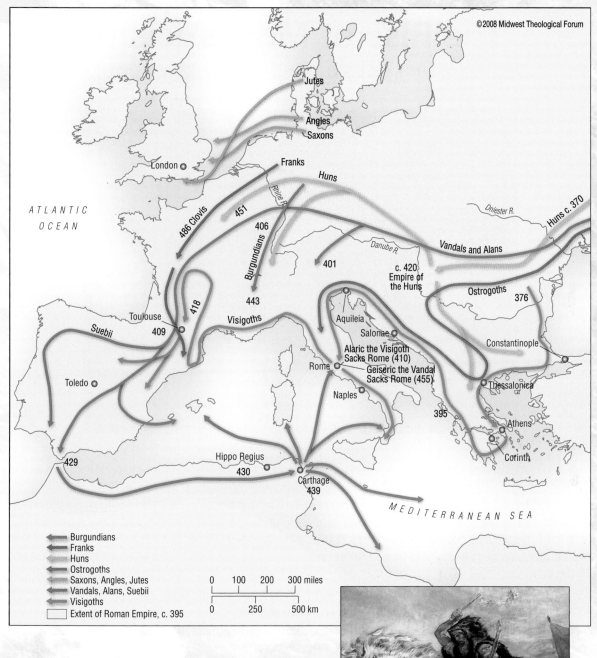

©2008 Midwest Theological Forum

Jutes

Angles
Saxons

Franks

Huns

ATLANTIC
OCEAN

Dniester R.

Huns c. 370

London

Rhine R.

486 Clovis

451

406
Burgundians

Danube R.

Vandals and Alans

401

c. 420
Empire of
the Huns

Ostrogoths

376

418

443

Toulouse
409

Visigoths

Aquileia

Salonae

Constantinople

Suebii

Alaric the Visigoth
Sacks Rome (410)

Toledo

Rome

Geiseric the Vandal
Sacks Rome (455)

Thessalonica

Naples

395

Athens

Corinth

Hippo Regius

429

430

Carthage
439

MEDITERRANEAN SEA

Burgundians
Franks
Huns
Ostrogoths
Saxons, Angles, Jutes
Vandals, Alans, Suebii
Visigoths
Extent of Roman Empire, c. 395

0   100   200   300 miles

0   250   500 km

The Germanic tribes began pressing on the Roman frontier in the early fourth century as the Huns steadily pushed west from Mongolia and China.

It is reported that the Huns' imposing physical appearance shocked the people of the Roman Empire.

With relentless swiftness, Attila's Huns devastated Gaul, and Attila continually augmented his army by assimilating conquered Germanic tribes.

PART II

The Rise of Monasticism
THE FIRST APPEARANCE OF MONASTICISM

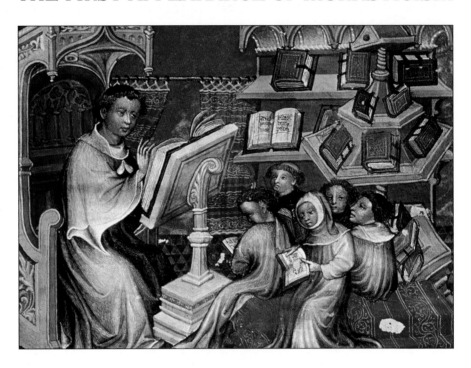

Monasticism is a way of life characterized by prayer and self-denial lived in seclusion from the world and under a fixed rule with professed vows. Monastic communities withdraw from the affairs of the world in order to seek God through asceticism and silence. Though monasticism is common to many of the world's religions, Christian monasticism is unique. Men and women who enter the monastic life seek to model themselves on Christ by dedicating themselves to a life of prayer and penance. Once the call from God has been recognized, the person makes a life-long commitment to the monastic life.

Monasticism started very early with St. Paul of Thebes (d. ca. 340) and St. Anthony (251?-356), both of whom lived lives of prayer and seclusion in Egypt. St. Paul of Thebes is held by tradition to be the first hermit; he had fled a persecution under the Roman Emperor Decius (AD249-51). St. Anthony indirectly influenced Western monasticism through his impact on St. Athanasius, who, during one of his exiles, wrote a celebrated biography of St. Anthony. St. Athanasius brought this book to Rome, and it would later serve as a handbook for Western monasticism.

St. Pachomius (ca. 290-346) found himself in a situation similar to many of the holy men and women in Egypt. He desired to withdraw from the world in order to be more united with God, but as word of his holiness grew, ordinary people sought him out in the desert to ask for intercessory prayers and guidance. His solitude disrupted, Pachomius instead allowed many to join him in his way of life, and he wrote an early form of monastic rule for his followers. His Rule influenced St. Basil the Great, St. John Cassian, and St. Benedict in their establishment of monastic orders. At the time of his death, St. Pachomius ruled over nine monasteries and convents in Egypt. His feast day is celebrated on May 9.

MONASTICISM AND THE EMERGENCE OF A NEW CHRISTIAN CULTURE

The rise of monasticism in the early Church proved vital for the spread of Christianity, the preservation of Greco-Roman writings, and the formation of a new Christian culture. For the Church, monasteries served a triple purpose: (1) they were a source of great spiritual strength; (2) they served as seminaries for priests and bishops; and (3) they functioned as centers of evangelization of the barbarian tribes through various forms of education.

The monasteries also had three major effects on Europe. The first effect was the recovery and evangelization of rural society. Up until the barbarian domination, a significant part of the population was concentrated in cities. However, as the cities began to depopulate and disintegrate, people scattered and clustered around landowners. As the former empire became more rural, forming pockets of isolated agricultural towns and villages, a new evangelizing force was called into play. Communities of monks and nuns spread into these farming areas to meet the spiritual needs of the people.

The second great effect of the monasteries on Europe was intellectual. Monasteries became the chief centers of learning until the rise of the great universities beginning in the thirteenth century. The barbarian invasions had dismantled the empire and with it intellectual and cultural centers of learning. Academic matters fell into neglect except among the monks who copied and retained the literary works of the Greco-Roman civilization. Monks meticulously copied manuscripts of texts in an age when it took months and years to copy a book by hand. Benedictine monasteries quickly established scriptoria (singular, scriptorium), large rooms in the monasteries set aside for the purpose of copying and maintaining texts. It could be said that the monasteries single-handedly saved Western culture during this dangerous period. If monasteries had not been established and become depositories for the great patrimony of Greek and Roman learning, it would have been lost. The oldest manuscripts of ancient Greece and Rome owe their survival to the Benedictine scriptoria.

The third effect was one of civilization. As a consequence of their work of evangelization, the monasteries had a great civilizing effect on these Germanic peoples. Attracted by the holiness and goodness of the monks and nuns, the tribes proved to be willing pupils in many practical disciplines. Through their agricultural work, the monks taught the barbarians, who were nomads, how to farm. Monks trained them in the skilled trades of carpentry, stone masonry, and ironwork as the monasteries were being erected. The monks infused a spiritual meaning into the act of work itself and thus taught the dignity of work as a form of adoration and emulation of Jesus Christ, who was also a worker.

Through its educational work, the monastery also taught the surrounding population how to read and write. The monks elevated them intellectually, which facilitated the development of a new culture expressed in a fusion of the old Greco-Roman tradition and a Germanic culture. Once a student at the monastery learned Latin, he was taught Sacred Scriptures, the writings of the Church Fathers, geometry, and music for the singing of the Divine Office. This emphasis on the Bible and the Church Fathers would plant deep Christian roots into this new people.

ST. BENEDICT:
THE "PATRIARCH OF WESTERN MONASTICISM"

Little is known about the early life of St. Benedict (ca. 480-ca. 547). He was born at Nursia, Italy, and educated in Rome, but eventually the moral decay of the city impelled him to withdraw to a cave in Subiaco to live the life of a hermit. As time passed, others joined him, and his reputation for sanctity spread.

St. Benedict gained a reputation as a miracle worker, which led people to seek him out for guidance. Finally, he founded twelve monasteries and placed a superior to head each one. He then began a thirteenth monastery at Monte Cassino around 529. It was there that he died some years later, and was buried in the same grave as his sister St. Scholastica. St. Benedict's feast day is celebrated on July 11 (formerly March 21), and St. Scholastica's feast day is celebrated on February 10.

The Rule of St. Benedict was adopted by virtually all monastic communities throughout the Medieval period. The Rule has been lauded for its spirit of peace and love, as well as its moderation in the ascetical life. For example, monks were to sleep between six to eight hours a night (with a siesta in the summer following lunch) and were to have a bed, pillow, and sufficient food. This was in stark contrast to the austerity of the Egyptian hermits, who prided themselves on a strict ascetical life that included sleep deprivation and little food as a means of furthering the quality of their spirituality.

The Rule essentially divides the schedule of the monk into four parts: chanting the Psalms and reciting prayers in community (four hours), private prayer and Scriptural reading (four hours), physical labor (six hours), and meals and sleep (ten hours).

According to the Benedictine model, the monastic life is lived in common. No one is allowed to own personal property, though the monastery itself may. The Rule made provision for an abbot, who holds virtually all power to govern the monastery. St. Benedict intended that the monastery would be a family and a self-sustaining community. Different monks had different tasks and functions, which were organized and distributed in such a way as to ensure self-sufficiency.

Even in the earliest years, Benedictine monks made vows of poverty, chastity, and obedience after undergoing a year-long novitiate. These vows are binding for life. A vow is a solemn promise made voluntarily by a person of reason, to practice a virtue or perform some specific good deed in order to accomplish a future good, viz., the individual's growth in the spiritual life.

POPE ST. GREGORY THE GREAT

St. Gregory (ca. 540-604) became pope in 590. A Church Father, he is considered the last of the traditional Latin Doctors. St. Gregory's papacy is often used as a marker for the beginning of the Medieval age, and certainly his papacy illustrates the noblest ideals of Medieval Christianity, as well as some of the tensions of his day.

St. Gregory was the son of a senator, a nobleman, and he played an important role in the civic affairs of the city of Rome. In 573 he became prefect for the police and a judge for criminal cases. After the death of his father (his mother Silvia and two aunts Tarsilla and Æmiliana were eventually canonized as saints), St. Gregory sold his properties and gave away his wealth in order to found seven monasteries and alleviate the plight of the poor. This was a common cultural phenomenon of the time among some of the nobility, a practice that was subsequently extolled as model Christian behavior in the Medieval Church. One of the monasteries was in Rome. Here St. Gregory became a regular monk, and he placed an abbot in charge, to whom he pledged obedience.

After several years of living the holy, austere life of a monk, the pope made St. Gregory one of the seven deacons of Rome. Around 579 Pope Pelagius II appointed him as the nuncio, the pope's personal ambassador, to the court in Constantinople. Though St. Gregory preferred to remain a simple monk, he deferred to the pope and went to Byzantium. Later St. Gregory returned to Rome and worked directly for Pelagius II, who died in 590.

Upon Pelagius's death, the Roman populace universally acclaimed St. Gregory as the new pope. Initially St. Gregory fled the city to avoid taking the office of St. Peter, but after intense soul searching, he relented to God's will.

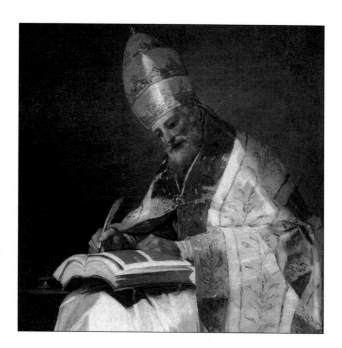

St. Gregory's missionary success, along with his continual support of the poor through the administration of the Church's estates, won for St. Gregory the title "the Great."

Though in weak health from the physical austerities he had imposed on himself as a monk, St. Gregory was a tireless worker, and he enjoyed the support of the people. He wrote many treatises and commentaries on Sacred Scripture, many of which have survived, as have over eight hundred of his letters. St. Gregory's greatest strength was his combination of humility and skillful administrative ability. He took the title *Servus servorum Dei* ("Servant of the servants of God"), which highlights the humble view of his position. He also helped to establish plainsong chant in the liturgical life of the Church, more commonly known as Gregorian Chant.

The Lombards began threatening Rome shortly after St. Gregory became pope. The Eastern emperor's exarch (an imperial representative) displayed no intention of preventing or averting a Lombard invasion; he simply remained idle in Ravenna. When St. Gregory received a threatening letter from the Lombard king Agiluf and then found him just outside the walls of Rome, he took action himself – without the consent or counsel of the exarch or emperor – and succeeded in achieving a separate peace in 592-593. This only lasted a short time, however, due to hostile actions of the hitherto idle exarch. Again working without the consent of exarch or emperor, St. Gregory finally made peace with the Lombards in 599. This peace was short-lived, but the brief warring eventually gave way to a peace that lasted throughout the remainder of St. Gregory's life. St. Gregory's actions demonstrate the growing temporal power of the popes and their care for Rome. It also marked the beginning of a rejection of the Eastern emperor's political power in the West. This instance only highlighted the fact that the Eastern emperors and the popes increasingly viewed each other as competitors.

St. Gregory's missionary initiatives included some of his most successful endeavors, more of which will be covered in the following chapter. For now, it is sufficient to recall the account of the conversion of St. Ethelbert and the Saxons in England. St. Gregory also influenced the Lombard princess Theodelinda, a Catholic, to marry the Lombard king Agiluf. Their children were raised Catholic and Theodelinda worked to build many churches. By the seventh century, the Lombards had converted to Christianity. St. Gregory's missionary success, along with his continual support of the poor through the administration of the Church's estates, won for St. Gregory the title "the Great." His feast day is celebrated on September 3.

THE EXTENT OF ISLAM BY AD 661

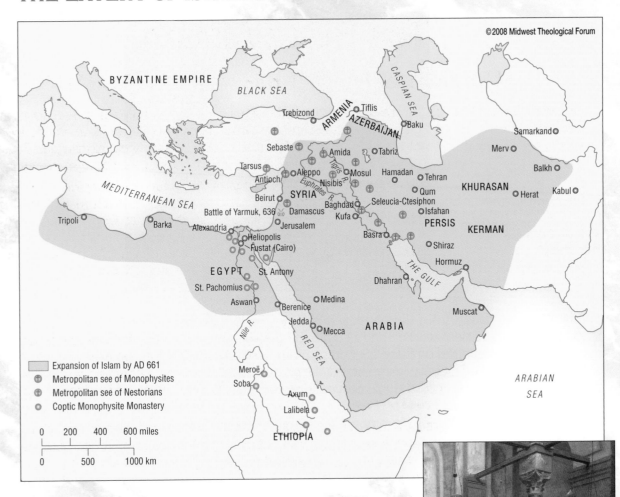

©2008 Midwest Theological Forum

Legend:
- Expansion of Islam by AD 661
- ⊕ Metropolitan see of Monophysites
- ⊕ Metropolitan see of Nestorians
- ◉ Coptic Monophysite Monastery

Scale:
0   200   400   600 miles
0   500   1000 km

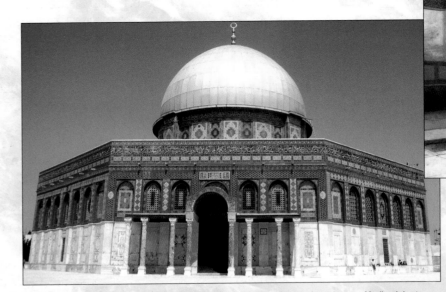

In 684 the Dome of the Rock was erected on the site of the Temple Mount in Jerusalem as a Muslim shrine to commemorate "the Night Journey" of Muhammad.

Muslims worship in a mosque.

PART III

The Rise of Islam

MUHAMMAD (ca. 570-632) AND THE KORAN

Muhammad was born near Mecca around 570. By the age of six he was an orphan, and an uncle took over his upbringing. He worked as a camel driver until he married a wealthy, widowed woman, Khadeejah, when he was twenty-five years old. He had six children, all of whom died except his daughter Fatima. Shortly thereafter, Muhammad decided to withdraw from the world to pursue a life of mystical prayer.

By the age of 30, Muhammad had become despondent. Pagan worship gave him no spiritual peace. He retired to a cave and around the year 612, he announced to his acquaintances that he had had a vision of the archangel Gabriel that called him to be the herald of Allah, the Jewish God. Muslims believe Muhammad's followers memorized and wrote down the exact words of these revelations, resulting in the Koran.. Thus, Muslims believe that the Koran (Arabic for "recitation") is not Muhammad's work but God's. The Koran is comprised of 114 chapters of sayings that Muhammad received.

THE SPREAD OF ISLAM

Islam's success in spreading and establishing a strong and long-lasting empire remains one of the most remarkable stories in history. Beginning in 634, the Muslims remained unstoppable for the next one hundred years. Within eighty years of Muhammad's death, Muslim territory already spread from the Indus River in India to parts of North Africa and southern Spain. Asia Minor and Europe, for the most part, were as yet unthreatened by Muslim expansion.

The spread of Islamic territory and faith went hand in hand. Believers were obligated by their religion to seek converts and wage a holy war to destroy unbelievers. With an excellent cavalry and light archery (learned from the Persians and Byzantines), the Muslim army became the best in the world. As the army expanded, Islam did as well.

Muslim forces began by defeating the Persians and sacking Jerusalem in 638. The fall of the city sent a shockwave throughout the East and West and would eventually prompt Christians to launch a counterattack to try to retake the Holy Land during the Crusades. Having taken Jerusalem, Muslims spread westwards sacking Christian Alexandria, also a great repository of one thousand years of Greek culture, in 643. With Alexandria taken, Muslims quickly spread throughout North Africa. By 698, all of North Africa was under Muslim rule. Six hundred years of North African Christianity, with its apologists, early Doctors of the Church, and martyrs, were destroyed. The Old Roman (Byzantine) Empire was reduced to an area not much larger than Greece.

In 711, Spain fell to the Muslims as well. The Muslims then crossed the Pyrenees and entered France where they were met in 732 by the Frankish chieftain Charles Martel, known as Charles "the Hammer." The subsequent battle, the Battle of Tours, marked the high water mark of the Muslim expansion into Europe. The Franks dressed in armor and stood firm before the hail of arrows. When the Muslims charged, their general was killed and the defeated army slinked back towards Spain. After their retreat to Spain, the Muslims never attempted any further advance into Europe through Spain. But the Muslims did remain in Spain for over 700 years, and it would not be until the *Reconquista* under the reign of Queen Isabella in 1492 that Spain would be completely liberated from Muslim domination.

In 717, the Muslim army laid siege to Christian Constantinople, but Emperor Leo III defeated them. The Muslims would attempt to breach the city again in 740 but would suffer a second defeat against Leo III. The emperor's successful defense against the Muslim forces established Byzantium's position as an eastern bulwark to the Muslim empire.

The Church's Work of Conversion

The work of conversion and assimilation into a Christian mindset would take many generations since the barbarians were generally uncivilized, bellicose peoples with little developed culture. Over the succeeding centuries, the Germanic tribes mixed with the Romans and adopted some aspects of the Greco-Roman culture. The great work of conversion and evangelization was the fruit of patient and dedicated labor of the monks.

The task before the Church was truly immense. The monks and bishops not only had to build the churches, monasteries, and institutions of the Church from scratch, but also had to raise the moral and cultural level of the tribes so they could be fully disposed to internalize the Gospel.

There were two forces at work during this period. First, missionaries emerged from those lands that were most recently evangelized–especially Ireland, England, and Germany. Secondly, Christian queens influenced their pagan husbands to convert to Christianity. The general population usually soon followed the conversion of their king.

PART IV

Conversion of France, the "Church's Eldest Daughter"

CONVERSION OF THE FRANKS

The Franks, unlike most of the other invaders, were not Christians (Arian, orthodox, or otherwise) when they settled Gaul (modern-day France) in 485. A bishop introduced the beautiful Burgundian princess St. Clotilda, a Christian, to the Frankish chief Clovis. Since Clovis was a pagan, St. Clotilda worked ceaselessly to obtain his conversion. Yet, the death of their first child and the near death of their second child strengthened Clovis's view that the Christian God was ineffective. Over the course of 496 and 497, Clovis and his troops battled the barbarian Alemanni. With defeat staring him in the face, Clovis promised the Christian God that if he won he would convert and be baptized.

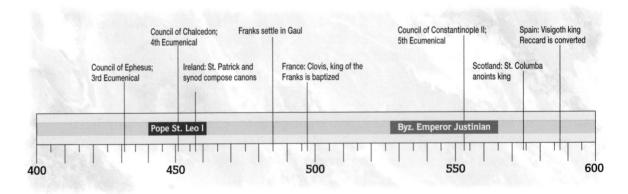

Council of Ephesus;
3rd Ecumenical

Council of Chalcedon;
4th Ecumenical

Ireland: St. Patrick and
synod compose canons

Franks settle in Gaul

France: Clovis, king of the
Franks is baptized

Council of Constantinople II;
5th Ecumenical

Scotland: St. Columba
anoints king

Spain: Visigoth king
Reccard is converted

Pope St. Leo I

Byz. Emperor Justinian

400   450   500   550   600

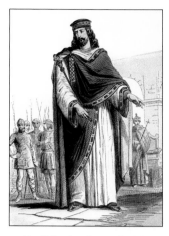

After his baptism, Clovis united Gaul.

At Tolbiac the Franks were triumphant, and in 497, Clovis was faithful to his promise.

Clovis presented himself to the church in Rheims to be baptized with three thousand of his troops. They were dressed in fur coats, wore long hair, and held their battle-axes in hand. Clovis disrobed and entered a pond, followed by his soldiers. Bishop Remigius pronounced the words of Baptism. By this act of Baptism, the Franks were the first of the Germanic tribes to embrace the Catholic Faith, thereby making France "the Church's eldest daughter."

After his Baptism, Clovis united Gaul by conquering neighboring Germanic tribes. Burgundy, an eastern province of France, was annexed. Part of this unity involved a fusion of the Greco-Roman culture with the German warrior culture. The descendants of Clovis were known as the Merovingian Dynasty, named after Meroveus, an ancestor of Clovis.

By the middle of the sixth century, all of Gaul–from the English Channel to the Pyrenees–was Christianized. Other than Gaul, only Italy, Ireland, and a small part of England made up the Church's faithful in the West. The rest of central and northern Europe remained to be evangelized.

PART V

Spain

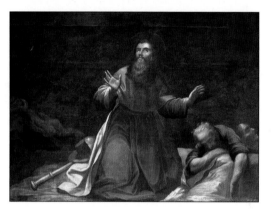

According to tradition, Spain received Christianity directly from the Apostles St. James the Greater and St. Paul.

Christianity arrived in Spain while still part of the Roman Empire. According to tradition, Spain received Christianity directly from the Apostles St. James the Greater and St. Paul, and from that time until the eighth century, Christianity flourished, despite much suffering under Roman persecution. By the middle of the fourth century, Spain enjoyed a stable hierarchy of bishops who periodically held councils to combat the heresies of that time.

In 711, the Muslim invaders began to sweep through Spain. Within three years, they had conquered the entire Iberian peninsula–a task which had taken the Roman legions nearly a century to accomplish. The Spanish peoples chose either to live under Muslim rule or to retreat to the most

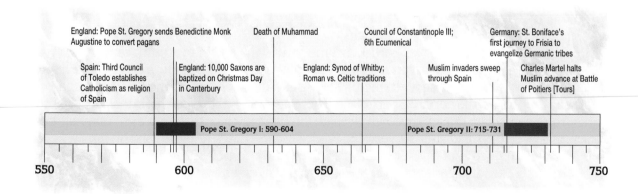

England: Pope St. Gregory sends Benedictine Monk Augustine to convert pagans

Death of Muhammad

Council of Constantinople III; 6th Ecumenical

Germany: St. Boniface's first journey to Frisia to evangelize Germanic tribes

Spain: Third Council of Toledo establishes Catholicism as religion of Spain

England: 10,000 Saxons are baptized on Christmas Day in Canterbury

England: Synod of Whitby; Roman vs. Celtic traditions

Muslim invaders sweep through Spain

Charles Martel halts Muslim advance at Battle of Poitiers [Tours]

Pope St. Gregory I: 590-604

Pope St. Gregory II: 715-731

550   600   650   700   750

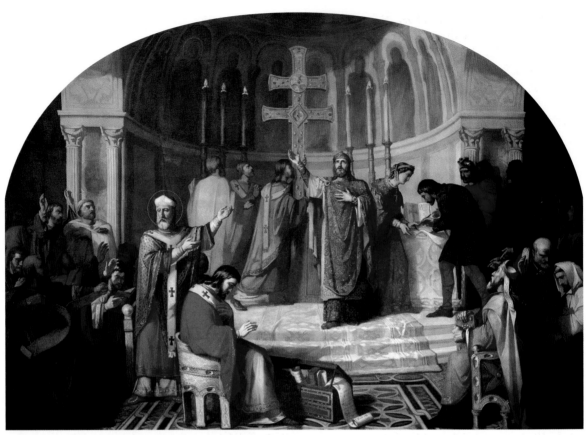

The Council of Toledo in 589 condemned Arianism and established Catholicism as the religion of Spain.

northerly provinces of Spain, mainly in Asturias, protected by the Picos de Europa, a mountain range in northern Spain. Those who chose to live under Muslim rule called themselves Mozarabs. Mozarabic Christians did not fare poorly at first; but, in the early ninth century, persecutions began. Years of struggle and slow re-conquest followed. Not until 1492, when the *Reconquista* (Spanish for "re-conquest") was complete, did Christians again rule all of Spain.

PART VI

The Conversion of the Celts

ST. PATRICK: THE "APOSTLE OF IRELAND"

A boy named Patricius (d. 493) was born sometime around the end of the fourth century. He was a Roman Briton and the son of a former Roman city official who had become a deacon in order to avoid taxation. When he was about sixteen, Irish pirates kidnapped him off the southwest coast of Britain and took him to the northwest of Ireland. There he lived the life of a slave in that foreign land, working as a herdsman. Prayer gave him strength (St. Patrick wrote that he prayed one hundred prayers in a given day), and after six years, St. Patrick escaped back to Britain and his family. Soon after his return, he wrote of a vision which called him back to Ireland to walk among its people again. This supernatural experience prompted him to begin his studies for the priesthood.

Sometime in the early 430s, St. Patrick, now a priest, was on the road back to Ireland with several clerics. He had been commissioned by Pope St. Celestine I to aid the Bishop of Ireland, Palladius; but somewhere on the road in Gaul they received the news of Palladius's death. As a consequence St. Patrick was consecrated as the new bishop immediately, and sailed to the north of Ireland. He was familiar with this area, which had not yet been evangelized by Palladius, who had confined his work to the southern regions. Within fifteen years, despite resistance from many of the Druid chieftains, the entire northern half of the island heard the Word of God, thousands were baptized, and consecrated religious communities were started. St. Patrick governed this new Christian community from his episcopal headquarters in Ultster. Humility, eloquence, and many miracles were St. Patrick's tools. He began working with bishops who arrived in the south in 439; and in 457, they met in a synod to establish laws and directives for the newborn Church in Ireland.

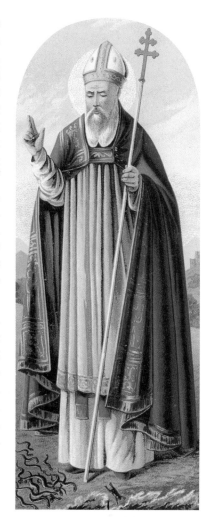

Within a generation of St. Patrick's work, the island had converted to the Faith. St. Patrick, being such a strong advocate of monasticism, promoted the foundation of many monasteries in Ireland. St. Patrick's most important written work is his Confessions, which he wrote in Latin in the period around 461 and 462. In it, he humbly describes his spiritual journey of conversion and faith. St. Patrick lived to an old age, and was fortunate enough to see the fruits of his labor. His feast day is celebrated on March 17.

IRISH MONKS: PROTECTORS AND PROMOTERS OF WESTERN CIVILIZATION

During the sixth and seventh centuries, the Irish monks enjoyed the height of their influence on Christian culture and the work of evangelization. In the early sixth century, the Irish monasteries were the most important centers of learning in all of Europe. The scriptoria and libraries in the Irish monasteries saved a great deal of the Greco-Roman literary tradition, even though Ireland was never colonized by the Romans. Through trade and the influx of some Greek monks, the Irish even gained a certain proficiency in the Greek language, which had virtually disappeared in the West.

Christianity among the Celtic peoples, which had developed separately from Roman Christianity, also had some unique features. For example, in Ireland there were no diocesan priests, but the only priests were from the ranks of the monks. In addition, the abbots exercised most of the governing power in the church in Ireland.

ST. COLUMBA: THE "APOSTLE OF SCOTLAND"

St. Columba (521-597) was an important evangelizer of northern Britain and Scotland, as well as the founder of a number of important monasteries in the Irish tradition. St. Columba had been preparing for the monastic life from an early age, and even before he left Ireland he is reputed to have founded monasteries in Durrow and Derry. St. Columba left Ireland and went to Scotland in 563.

On the isle of Iona, St. Columba built a monastery and set about evangelizing the Picts, a Celtic tribe with deep pagan roots. Successful in this, he continued his work throughout Scotland. A man of constant study and prayer, St. Columba is said to have written some 300 books, only two of which have survived. The Latin poem "Altus Prosator," a description of the Last Judgment in all its fury, is believed to have been written by him. In 574, St. Columba anointed the new Scottish king, which led to the eventual conversion of the Scottish population. His feast day is celebrated on June 9.

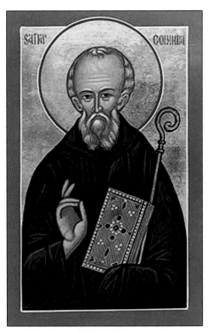

St. Columba

ST. COLUMBANUS AND THE IRISH ON THE CONTINENT

St. Columbanus (d. 615) is the most famous among a band of Irish monks who helped to evangelize the northern coast of France as well as Switzerland. He helped renew the spiritual life and discipline in areas where Christian practice was waning. He was a huge man, capable of killing a bear with his own bare hands. When leaving by boat for his missionary undertaking, he would just travel wherever the boat took him. In his last years, Columbanus worked in Switzerland and founded a monastery in the Italian Alps in a small town called Bobbio, near Genoa, in 612. In later years Bobbio became an important center of learning. He died there in 615. St. Columbanus's feast day is celebrated on November 23.

The Celtic spirituality that St. Columbanus helped to spread around Europe bore many lasting fruits. One such fruit of this spirituality was promotion of frequent sacramental Penance, which has become one of its greatest contributions to the Christian Faith. The practice of frequent Penance–at first limited to the Irish monks and those under their care–quickly became incorporated into the universal Church.

In the Roman tradition by the third century, a system of austere public penance had developed. Under it, the penitent was enrolled publicly with other penitents, with whom he committed himself to a rigorous and lengthy period (the length varied depending on the seriousness of the sin) of prayer, almsgiving, and severe fasting. Besides the strict spiritual regimen, there were two other unique aspects of this system that eventually led to this system's decline. The public penitential practice was understood as a second Baptism, and Baptism can be received only once. In addition, the individual was bound to life-long continence. For these reasons, many people delayed Penance until the approach of death given the obvious challenges connected to this sacrament during those first centuries.

For the Irish, Penance remained lengthy, severe, and public, but penitents were not officially enrolled with others, nor was reception of the sacrament limited to a single time, as with Baptism. Thus the promise of lifelong continence–a difficult task, even for the saints–was no longer a necessity. Hence, the nearly exclusively "deathbed" recourse to the Sacrament of Penance fell into decline. Eventually, absolution, which had previously been withheld until the completion of the public penance, was granted upon confession of sins, and Penance became a matter of private responsibility. To determine specific penances, the Irish monks made use of Penitential Books, books that listed various sins with the corresponding penance.

The Irish had a tremendous influence in bringing about the custom of frequent Penance. Not until 1215, at the Fourth Lateran Council, did the Church officially teach that every individual Christian was bound to make at least one private Penance each year if one were conscious of having committed mortal sin.

PART VII

The Conversion of England

It is not known exactly how the Celts in England were first evangelized during the era of the Roman Empire, but English bishops were already present at the Council of Arles (314) in France. The spread of Christianity suffered a tremendous setback as invading Angles, Jutes, and Saxons pushed the burgeoning Christian communities to the farthest western reaches of England. It was into this situation that St. Augustine of Canterbury and his brother monks were thrown in the late sixth century.

ST. AUGUSTINE OF CANTERBURY: THE "APOSTLE OF ENGLAND"

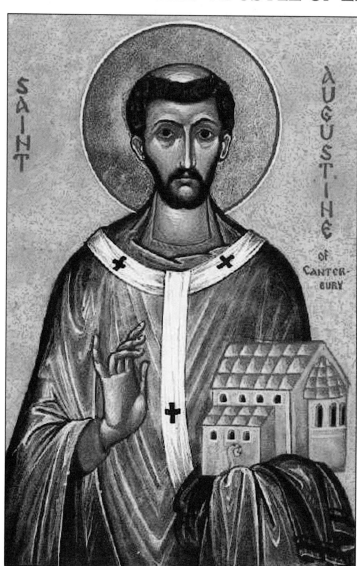

St. Augustine wearing his pallium.

St. Augustine of Canterbury, a giant in the Church's history of evangelization, brought the Catholic Faith to the pagan and violent Anglo-Saxons. St. Augustine was a Benedictine monk and prior of St. Andrew's monastery in Rome, one of the monasteries founded by Pope St. Gregory the Great, when he was asked by Pope St. Gregory himself to bring the Gospel message to England.

Perhaps the most salient aspect of Pope St. Gregory the Great's pontificate was his strong support for the conversion of the Anglo-Saxons, especially in England. During his service to his monastery as abbot in 585, before becoming pope, St. Gregory saw a group of blond, blue-eyed foreigners in the streets of Rome. He asked who they were, and an assistant told St. Gregory that the men were slaves, Angles from England. St. Gregory replied, "Non Angli, sed angeli" ("Not Angles, but angels"). St. Gregory never forgot the Angles, and he selected St. Augustine as his personal emissary and missionary to England when he became pope.

In 596 Pope St. Gregory sent St. Augustine with a group of forty other monks to travel by land through

Italy and France to reach England. In France the band of monks halted, and St. Augustine wrote a frantic letter to Pope St. Gregory that the monks were frightened by the frontier and heard appalling stories of the brutality of the barbarians in England. St. Augustine asked for permission to return to Rome, but Pope St. Gregory declined the request, and told the group to continue its mission.

Learning from historically tested experiences, St. Augustine tried to gain the favor of a king with a Christian wife. Ethelbert, the king of Kent had married Bertha, a Frankish princess, and the great-granddaughter of King Clovis. Bertha had remained Christian after her marriage to Ethelbert, but she had not attempted to influence her husband in the manner that her ancestors St. Clotilda and Ingund had influenced theirs. When St. Augustine and his monks arrived, Ethelbert, though he had heard of Christianity, was still pagan. He received the monks quite openly, but he did not convert immediately. He gave them freedom to preach the Catholic Faith and to win over as many willing converts as possible. Ethelbert also gave them a dwelling in Canterbury, his capital. Nevertheless, Ethelbert for some time remained set in his ways.

On Christmas Day in 597, more than ten thousand Saxons were baptized in Canterbury. Accounts conflict on precisely when Ethelbert was baptized–some say before that Christmas, some say four years later. Soon Christianity was rapidly spreading throughout England. St. Augustine was presented with a palace in Canterbury, which became the most important episcopal see in England. Monasteries quickly spread over the land, and St. Augustine ordered that all pagan temples be converted into Christian churches.

Pope St. Gregory named St. Augustine the Primate Bishop of England in 601 and sent him the pallium, a sign of authority and papal favor.

St. Augustine consecrated others to the episcopacy and sent them to other centers in England, including Rochester and London. Upon his death in the first decade of the seventh century, St. Augustine had secured such a strong foundation of Christianity that England would serve as a venue for a Christian renaissance in the early middle ages. His feast day is celebrated on May 27.

THE MISSION IN ENGLAND CONTINUES

An unrivaled string of missionaries and scholars emerged from England because of the vision, faith, and dedicated labor of Pope St. Gregory the Great and St. Augustine of Canterbury.

Through the missionary work of the Irish over the next several decades, the Catholic Faith became firmly established in England by 655, the year that the first native Englishman became Archbishop of Canterbury, St. Deusdedit.

South of the Thames River, Christianity of a more Roman tradition predominated due to the mission of St. Augustine. However, the Roman and Celtic traditions clashed, especially over the question of when to celebrate Easter. The Synod of Whitby (664), held in the kingdom of Northumbria in England, sought to reconcile the two divergent traditions. At the synod, St. Wilfrid (634-709), later Bishop of York, led the party that was pushing in favor of the Roman tradition. With this finally accomplished, the English accepted the Roman tradition's practice of the observance of Easter and the Benedictine form of monasticism. The Irish monks eventually withdrew to a Celtic monastery on the island of Iona and to other monasteries in Ireland proper.

Over time, the Church in England became especially united to the papacy. Of all the areas of Europe that had so far converted, England identified most closely with the Church of Rome. This set the stage for English missionary activity in Germany and the Low Countries, as well as for the development of scholarship in England through the emergence of many Benedictine monasteries. England became the strongest supporter of Benedictine monasticism.

ST. BEDE: THE "FATHER OF ENGLISH HISTORY"

St. Bede (ca. 673-735) was the most important Anglo-Saxon scholar of his time, and much of his scholarly work became standard subject matter in the Medieval curriculum. St. Bede represents the finest example of the role played by the English monasteries as centers of learning in the seventh and eighth centuries. This is especially remarkable when one considers that in 590, upon the ascension of Pope St. Gregory the Great to the throne of St. Peter, England was a pagan and unconverted land.

St. Bede was a dedicated and prolific scholar. St. Bede's guiding principle for all his scholarly works is expressed in the perennial question: How can one clearly communicate a particular body of knowledge to students? His works covered topics that included Latin grammar and poetry, astronomy and the tides, chronology, a biography of St. Cuthbert, commentaries on many books of the Bible, and history. His Ecclesiastical History of the English People places the Roman Catholic Church at the foundation of the development of English culture.

In his commentaries on the Bible, St. Bede preferred clear exposition and found no use for philosophical speculation. He based his spirituality and scholarship on the biblical-patristic tradition. Through the Scythian monk Dionysius Exiguus (fifth-sixth centuries), St. Bede did the mathematical computations for the BC/AD distinction, and his work utilized the Christian measurement of time and made it popular throughout Europe.

Within a century of his death, St. Bede was given the title "Venerable," and in 1899 Pope Leo XIII declared him a "Doctor of the Church." The title "Venerable" generally denotes a particular stage in the canonization process, but it can also simply refer to a person's holy life, as was the case with St. Bede. His feast day is celebrated on May 25.

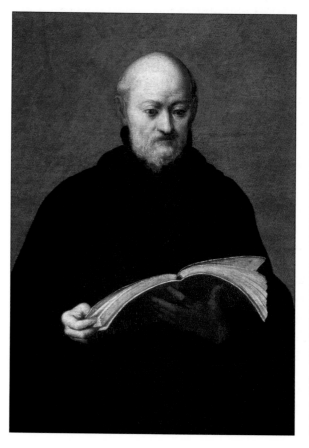

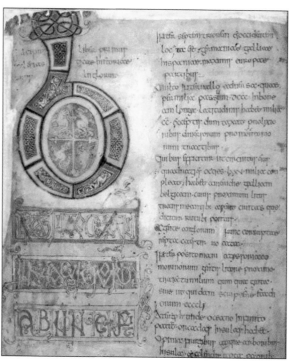

St. Bede's *Ecclesiastical History of the English People* places the Roman Catholic Church at the foundation of the development of English culture. The manuscript shown above is the front cover of this masterpiece completed in 731 which is the primary source of historical reference for this period.

PART VIII

The Conversion of Germany and the Low Countries

The conversion of the lands that have become Germany was a long and arduous task. Some of the small Roman cities, such as Cologne, were evangelized during the time of the Roman Empire. Beginning in the seventh century, English missionaries played a pivotal role in carrying on missionary activities, especially in northwest and central Germany, north of the Mainz River. Groups of Germanic tribes were still being converted along the Baltic Sea long after the beginning of the second millennium, even as the German church focused much of its energies on converting the Slavs.

ST. BONIFACE: THE "APOSTLE OF GERMANY"

St. Boniface (ca. 675-754) set the stage for a radical reshaping of the heart of Europe. Before his arrival on the continent, conversion efforts among the Germans had failed. Not only did St. Boniface succeed in converting the Germans, he also laid the foundation of a church based on a monastic model that would continue to flower for the next three centuries. He also revitalized the deteriorating practice of the Faith among the Franks.

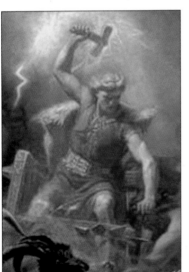

The pagan god Thor

St. Boniface was born with the name Winfrid, most likely somewhere in Wessex, England. Like St. Bede, he also entered a Benedictine monastery at the age of seven. By temperament he was unsteady, timid, and tended to discouragement and despair. However, St. Boniface matured into a brilliant pupil and eventually became a teacher and the head of the monastic school.

St. Boniface loved his homeland tremendously, but he discerned a call from God to leave England and evangelize the German people. Therefore, in 716 he left for Frisia to begin his work of evangelizing the Germanic tribes. Since the Frisians had received Catholic teachings of St. Willibrord with mixed results, St. Boniface hoped to bring the Frisians fully into the Church.

St. Boniface's tendency to discouragement seemed to have reappeared when he met formidable obstacles in Frisia over the next couple years. He researched the lives of the early Christians to see if any of the saints were exempt from suffering, and to his dismay he found no exceptions. St. Boniface struggled to be courageous and thus looked upon the most ferocious barbarians as his brothers.

His temptations towards despair were so great that St. Boniface felt compelled to consult with the reigning pope, St. Gregory II (715-32). St. Boniface believed that he had failed in his missionary efforts in Frisia, and he sought the pope's counsel: Should he return to England or persevere in Frisia? Pope St. Gregory II was so impressed with Winfrid's sanctity that he gave Winfrid a new Latin name, Boniface – from the Latin words Bona Facere, meaning "doer of good" – which symbolized his favor with the pope. By this action Pope St. Gregory II also made St. Boniface his personal papal legate to Germany.

Upon his return to Germany, St. Boniface turned his attention south of Frisia to Hesse and the conversion of the Hessians. On a second trip to Rome in 722, the pope consecrated St. Boniface to the episcopacy. Around 732 Pope St. Gregory III (731-741) sent the pallium to St. Boniface.

After he felled the Oak of Thor (Wata), the sacred tree of the pagans of Hesse, St. Boniface gained so much moral authority that he enjoyed a new-found freedom to establish a string of monasteries. Cutting down the tree brought many converts into the Church when the pagan people saw that Thor did not strike St. Boniface down with a thunderbolt. Out of the wood of the tree St. Boniface made a small chapel dedicated to St. Peter.

During a third trip to Rome in 736, St. Boniface was made Archbishop of Mainz. When he returned to Germany, St. Boniface founded many more monasteries, the most important of which was located in the city of Fulda (744). St. Boniface planned that the monastery at Fulda would serve as a center for conversion and spiritual renewal and a training facility for priests and missionaries.

It was St. Boniface's great dream to return to the mission land of his youth, Frisia. Though seventy-six years old, he set out from Mainz with fifty other monks and sailed down the Rhine to Frisia. There at Dorkum he and his comrades were martyred by the pagans. His body was returned to Fulda for burial.

St. Boniface converted German pagans, founded monasteries, established the ecclesiastical structure of the Church in Germany, and reformed the Church in the lands under Frankish rule. The religious fervor of the German monasteries that he founded in the eighth century was still robust in the tenth and eleventh centuries. Like their Irish and English counterparts before them, the German monasteries became important centers of learning with their libraries and scriptoria. They were aided, in part, by the privilegium that St. Boniface won for them from the papacy. With this papal privilege (privilegium) the monasteries were exempted from local diocesan control and answered directly to the papacy. St. Boniface's feast day is celebrated on June 5.

PART IX

The Conversion of the Slavs

STS. CYRIL AND METHODIUS: THE "APOSTLES OF THE SLAVS"

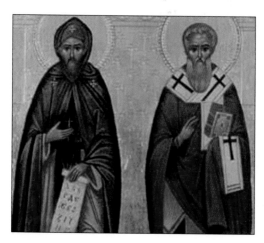

Two brothers, Sts. Cyril (827-869) and Methodius (826-885), were the first missionaries among the Slavs. They were from a senatorial Greek family in Thessalonica. Rather than continuing with their family's secular activities, St. Cyril (who originally bore the name Constantine) and St. Methodius entered the priesthood. St. Cyril, a man of great intellectual ability, joined the philosophy faculty at the university in Constantinople. St. Cyril then gave up a promising career in scholarship, and undertook a mission to the Khazars in south Russia. Then, in 863, Emperor Michael III commissioned the brothers as missionaries to Moravia (Slovakia).

The Glagolithic Alphabet							
✝	Ⰱ	ⰲ	ⰳ	ⰴ	Э	ⰶ	ⰷ
a	b	v	g	d	ε	ž	dz
Ⰹ	Ⰻ	Ⰺ	ⰼ	Ⰽ	ⰾ	ⰿ	Ⱂ
z	i	i	ǵ	k	l	m	n
Ⱁ	Ⱂ	ь	Ⱄ	ⱅ	Ⱆ	ф	Ⱒ
ɔ	p	r	s	t	u	f	x (kh)
Ⱁ	Ⱇ	ⱍ	ш	Ⱋ	Ⱓ	Ⱏ	Ⱏ
ɔ	ts	č	š	št	w/ə	i	y
Ⰰ	Ⱓ	Ⱔ	Ⱗ	Ⱘ	Ⱙ	ⱚ	Ⱛ
æ/e	yu	ę	yę	ǫ	yǫ	f	i/v

The brothers knew the difficult Slavic language quite well–Thessalonica was surrounded by Slavic settlements and was itself populated by a fair number of Slavs. Before their departure, St. Cyril developed the Glagolithic script for use with the Slavs. (The Cyrillic alphabet, which bears St. Cyril's name, is a later development of his original Glagolithic alphabet. Both alphabets are rooted in Greek.) Use of the Glagolithic script ceased and gave way to Cyrillic after the 1100s, except in Croatia, where it was used until around 1900.

During their missionary work, Sts. Cyril and Methodius used the vernacular Slavonic language for the celebration of the liturgy and translated the Bible into Slavonic, using the new Glagolithic alphabet. Though their innovative use of the vernacular proved a vital tool in reaching many people with Christ's message, German missionaries were offended by Sts. Cyril and Methodius's use of Slavonic instead of Latin in the liturgy, and denounced them to the pope as heretics.

In order to clarify the situation, Sts. Cyril and Methodius went to Rome for guidance from Pope St. Nicholas I (858-867). St. Nicholas died before their arrival, but Pope Adrian II (867-872), his successor, received them warmly in 868 and granted them permission to use Slavonic in the liturgy. St. Cyril made his final vows as a monk, but died in Rome before being able to return to Moravia. Pope Adrian II made St. Methodius Bishop of the Moravians, and St. Methodius continued his evangelizing mission.

In spite of papal support, St. Methodius was arrested by German missionaries and held in captivity for three years upon his return to Moravia. The Germans, who were harsh and forceful with the Slavs, scourged and denounced St. Methodius yet again. Pope John VIII eventually secured St. Methodius's release. The Holy Father reaffirmed the use of the Slavonic language, though he later distanced himself from St. Methodius's work, as did later popes because of miscommunication and political intrigue. Because later popes refused to recognize the use of Slavonic, many Slavs turned away from Rome to Constantinople.

By the time St. Methodius died in 885, all of Moravia was converted. In 1980 St. John Paul II named the brothers "Patrons of Europe." The feast day of Sts. Cyril and Methodius is February 14.

POLAND

Christianity most likely arrived in Poland in the tenth century through Moravian refugees who fled north to Poland during the Hungarian invasion. German monks were also intent on converting Poland. Though there was no organized Church, the presence of Christianity among the pagan Poles made the official transition smooth and peaceful. A Polish noble, Duke Mieszko (962-992) was the first Polish ruler to encourage his subjects to become Christian. He had married St. Dubravka, the daughter of Boleslaus I of Bohemia, and, consistent with the familiar model, it was under her Christian influence that Mieszko converted.

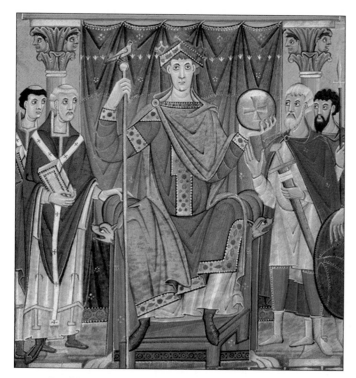

Otto III Enthroned. St. Adalbert became the confessor of the teenage Holy Roman Emperor Otto III. St. Adalbert made a deep impact on the young Otto III through his Christian example and teaching.

In 973 Duke Mieszko and St. Dubravka placed their seven-year-old son, Boleslav Chrobry the Brave, in the care of Otto II for his education. Duke Mieszko sent a locket of his son's hair to the pope to show that he considered his son to be under the special protection of the papacy. In 992 Mieszko placed all of Poland at the service of the Holy See, thus making Poland a vassal land of the popes. Thus began a unique relationship between the Polish people and the papacy – one that proved essential for the survival of the Polish people in the many difficult centuries ahead.

ST. VLADIMIR:
THE "APOSTLE OF THE RUSSIANS AND UKRAINIANS"

The story of the conversion of Russia is inseparable from the story of St. Vladimir (d. 1015). The life of the man responsible for the Christianization of Russia itself parallels the country's miraculous movement from barbaric paganism to Christianity. St. Vladimir then ruled all Russia (980) and lived a very typical pagan life – he had five wives and twelve children, he erected many idols and shrines to pagan gods, and he was a ruthless ruler.

He eventually set his sights on the Greco-Roman empire, and as he was planning his campaign, he began to take a slight interest in Christianity. St. Vladimir never stopped looking for ways to strengthen his rule, so much so that he even began to survey, compare, and contrast Islam, Judaism, and both Latin and Byzantine Christianity to see if any of these foreign religions would solidify his rule. St. Vladimir sent emissaries to investigate the three monotheistic faiths. The emissaries are said to have found both Islam and Judaism rather unedifying, though the Latin rite they thought suitable. During the Byzantine Divine Liturgy at Hagia Sophia in Constantinople, the emissaries "knew not whether they were in Heaven or on earth." They reported their findings to St. Vladimir, who was aware that his grandmother Olga had accepted this same Byzantine Christianity. Christianity had faintly entered his mind, though for purely utilitarian purposes.

The Byzantine emperor, Basil II, found himself in need of aid in the late 980s. He faced two internal rebellions, and St. Vladimir had suddenly appeared, dangerously close to Constantinople. The emperor finally made a military deal with St. Vladimir (St. Vladimir proposed the terms): the Russian would take Basil's sister Anna in marriage (or else he would march on Constantinople), and in return St. Vladimir would provide the hard-pressed emperor with 6,000 Viking warriors to put down the rebellions. The Byzantines were shocked that a pagan and virtual barbarian would dare to ask for the hand of a Byzantine princess in marriage. Basil had very few other options, and therefore agreed, but only on the condition that his sister would be marrying a Christian. As St. Vladimir was familiar with Christianity and had been considering Baptism, this condition proved to be no problem. Around 989 St. Vladimir was baptized, and he and Anna were married.

The conditions under which St. Vladimir came to be baptized and the situation of his entire life prior to that point certainly suggest that he merely assented to Basil's request, treating Baptism as a formality rather than as the sacrament of Faith. But the radical changes that followed upon St. Vladimir's Baptism instead suggest the powerful work of Grace moving in a man who truly understood Baptism and desired faith. No influential priest aided in his conversion, and his new bride was yet terrified of her new Viking husband, his lands, and his people. With the same deliberate and pragmatic will that had been previously aimed at building up a pagan kingdom, St. Vladimir then focused on living as a serious follower of Christ. He dismissed his five wives for Anna. He tore down the same idols and shrines he himself had erected years before, and he built churches in their places. He also established a number of monasteries and Christian schools. Zealously wishing to follow the examples in the Gospels, he threw huge banquets for the poor and even sent wagonloads of food to the sick who could not get to the banquets. St. Vladimir focused relentlessly on converting his people. The Christian Viking was still a Viking, and he made Baptism compulsory–though many were quite willing to be baptized. By the time of his death in 1015, St. Vladimir had firmly established the Christian Faith throughout Russia. His feast day is celebrated on July 15.

PART X

Byzantium

BYZANTIUM: THE LONG VIEW

From the fourth century into the eleventh century, the Church channeled her energies into the conversion of peoples on the European continent. However, this was only one aspect of the

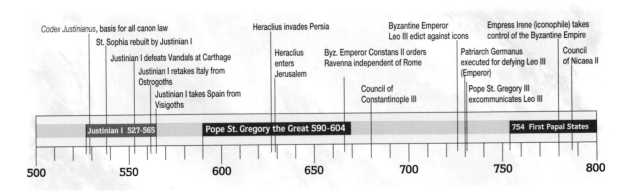

many challenges facing the Church. In the eighth and ninth centuries, a number of political and religious factors coalesced that proved to have important ramifications for Christianity. During these two centuries, the deep-rooted, growing divergence between East and West began to surface as the different languages, cultures, geography, and conceptions of political and religious power that had long divided the East and West became more acute. These two diverse cultures, born from the same sources but now separated by deep cultural differences, were yet united by the same sacramental Christianity. It proved, however, a fragile unity. The rise of the patriarchs and the question of papal supremacy, liturgical and disciplinal differences, the Iconoclastic Controversy, and other disagreements all pushed East and West towards a final confrontation.

Byzantium was at one time the most important center of political, religious, cultural, and economic activity in the world of the former Roman Empire. Constantine the Great founded the Byzantine Empire when he moved his capital to Byzantium, renaming it Constantinople and formally dedicating it on May 11, 330. The Empire lasted until May 29, 1453, when it fell to the Ottoman Turks. Byzantium lasted for more than eleven hundred years – longer than the combined duration of the Roman Republic and the Roman Empire which together lasted some nine hundred eighty-five years (taking 509 BC as the beginning of the Republic and AD 476 as the collapse of the Empire). Unlike the Republic and the Empire, Byzantium enjoyed the blessing of a wholly Christian orientation and development from its inception. Even though the capital was dedicated under both pagan and Christian rites, Constantine always heavily favored the Church, and, as mentioned previously, Emperor Theodosius I made Christianity the official religion of Byzantium in 379. The intricate theological disputes of the fourth and fifth centuries demonstrated a deeply Christian culture that marked the Empire even until its decline and fall.

The rise of Islam, however, proved to be a mortal enemy to the Eastern Empire. As Islamic expansion constantly loomed on the horizon in the Middle East, Africa, and Asia Minor as a powerful threat to the Empire's territorial integrity. Certain tenets of the Muslim faith prompted the Arabic people to raise a strong military force that had already conquered Byzantine lands by the seventh century, including three of the four great Eastern Christian patriarchates (Jerusalem, Antioch, and Alexandria). Islam remained a constant threat to the empire until finally, in the fifteenth century, Constantinople, and with it the remnants of the decaying Byzantine Empire, fell to the Muslim Ottoman Turks on May 29, 1453.

Constantinople was located on the tip of the Balkan Peninsula just across from Asia Minor along the narrow Bosporus Strait, which connects the Black Sea to the Mediterranean. The city was built on this triangular rocky promontory, surrounded by the sea on the northern, southern, and eastern borders. Emperor Constantine, Emperor Theodosius II, and later Emperor Anastasius I soon erected a series of formidable walls (Anastasius's walls were some forty miles long) along its western edge to complete the boundaries of the triangular city – an impressively secure military site that British warships were not capable of taking during the First World War, even with heavy bombardment.

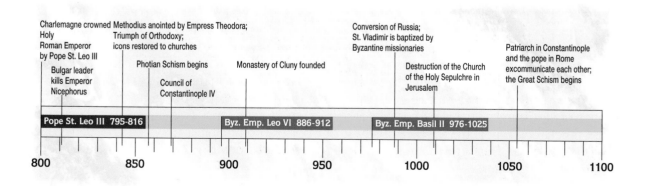

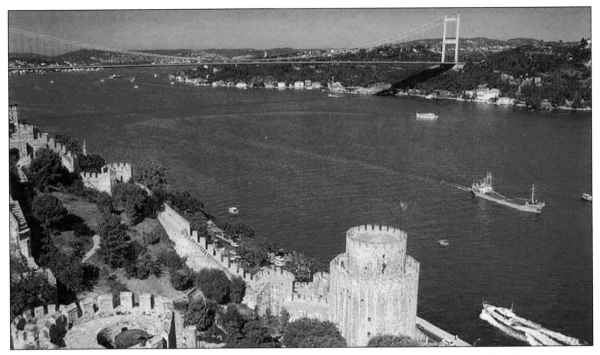

The Bosporus is a strait that separates the European part of Turkey from the Asian part and connects the Sea of Marmara with the Black Sea. Two bridges cross the Bosporus Strait. Due to the importance of the strait for the defense of Istanbul, the Ottoman sultans constructed a fortification on each side, the Anadoluhisari (1393) and the Rumelihisari (1451) shown above.

The Byzantines were Roman in their laws, Greek in their culture, and oriental in their habits. All of these traditions came together in Constantinople, which rose as a center of learning, art, and architecture. Hagia (or Saint) Sophia (the Church of "Holy Wisdom," dedicated to Christ), the cathedral of the patriarch of Constantinople, is still regarded as a wonder of Byzantine art and architecture. The riches of Byzantium likewise converged in Constantinople. The docks were crowded with exotic goods from all over the world–wood, grains, silks from Asia, spices, luxuriant clothing, and precious jewelry filled the markets.

BYZANTINE CHRISTIANITY

The numbers of Christians in Byzantium far exceeded those in Rome and the West. It must be remembered that all of the areas to which Christianity first took hold, such as Palestine and the cities of Asia Minor, were located within the boundaries of the Byzantine Empire; and Greek, the language of the East, was the original language of almost the entire New Testament.

Although Rome remained the location of St. Peter's successors, it no longer enjoyed the influence that it once had during the era of the Roman Empire. The pope continued to serve as the ultimate authority in the Church, but the intimate relationship between the emperor and the patriarchs of Constantinople would come to overshadow the authority of the papacy. Furthermore, the Church in the East developed along very different lines than the Church in the West. In the West, as the political structures of the Empire collapsed and missionary activity surged across Europe, the notion of the Church as universal began to take an even stronger form. This universal conception of the Church took root in the absence of any strong political communities to which Christians could attach themselves. Hence the Church came to be viewed as something that transcended all national boundaries or allegiances.

In the East, however, missionary activity, though equally successful, regularly culminated in the creation of national churches attached to specific political communities. Hence various eastern churches arose in partial concert and conflict with the imperial church of the Byzantine Empire. The burgeoning nationalism of some of these minor churches was strong enough to cause several schisms within the Eastern Church. The Eastern Church soon found itself ministering solely to its Greek subjects.

The political environment of the Eastern Empire also gave rise to a manner of rule called caesaropapism, in which the sovereign temporal ruler extends his authority to ecclesiastical and theological matters. To be sure, strains of caesaropapism could be detected as early as Constantine the Great, but the emperors who succeeded him only intensified their desire to have a hand in the governance of the Church. Such emperors appointed bishops and the Eastern Patriarch, directed the development of liturgical practices, and even aided in the recruitment of monks. In time, the increasing power of Eastern emperors put them into direct conflict with the authority of the papacy, paving the way for many contentious disputes and schisms.

MILITARY CAMPAIGNS

In 553/4 Justinian I led a campaign against the Vandals in northern Africa. The Vandals were disorganized and ill-equipped, but had, during the collapse of the West, overrun the northern shores of Africa. In addition to his desire to restore the empire, Justinian I was moved by the African bishops' pleas for help, as the Vandals were particularly harsh on Christians. Justinian I sailed five hundred ships carrying ten thousand infantry and five thousand cavalry against the Vandals and marched on Carthage, the Vandal stronghold. Justinian I took Carthage and captured the Vandal king Gelimer, bringing him as a prisoner to Constantinople, thus temporarily resuscitating the empire's presence in Africa.

Apart from his African campaign, Justinian I retook Italy (562) from the Ostrogoths after a long and expensive war, and secured most of Spain (555), capturing this land from the Visigoths. In all, by the time of Justinian I's death he had reconquered half of Europe as well as northern Africa.

CODEX JUSTINIANUS (529)

As part of his ambitious quest to restore the empire, Justinian I undertook the collection and systemization of all Roman law as it had developed from his earliest predecessors. Justinian I wanted to ensure a uniform rule of law throughout his growing empire, and sought to provide an ultimate reference for any legal question that might arise. The result, the Codex Justinianus, represents the highest achievement in classical legal scholarship. Justinian I's Codex is an important basis for the development of Canon Law – the law of the Church – as well as for civil law in all the countries of Europe.

HAGIA SOPHIA (538)

As wondrous and long-lasting as Justinian I's advancements in the arena of legal scholarship proved to be, his innovations in architecture were perhaps even more impressive. From Justinian I's patronage grew a unique style of architectural design, which is now called "Byzantine," and virtually all building in the West and East owes much to his influence. The most famous work built under his reign, the magnificent church of Hagia Sophia (Holy Wisdom) at Constantinople, is widely thought to be one of the most perfect buildings in the world.

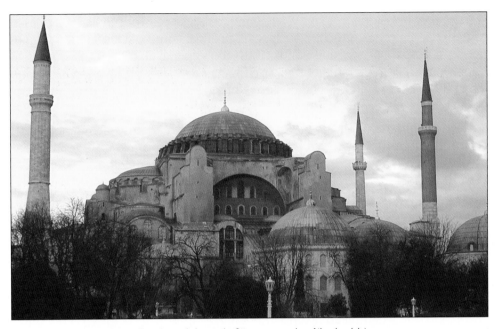

Hagia Sophia. The minarets belong to the Ottoman conversion of the church into a mosque.
Hagia Sophia remains one of the great achievements of world architecture. In it, every Byzantine saw the perfect church. "The church
is an earthly heaven in which the super-celestial God dwells and walks about." Germanos, Patriarch of Constantinople (715-730).

MONOPHYSITISM AND JUSTINIAN I

Monophysitism, or the belief that Christ possesses only one nature and that his human nature is "incorporated" into the divine nature, remained a prevalent and troubling heresy in Justinian I's time. His own wife, Theodora, had definite Monophysite sympathies, and her influence over Justinian I was not always for the best.

The notion of Christ's two natures present in one Divine Person was supposedly resolved at the Council of Chalcedon (451). There, it was to have been shown that the West–in the person of Pope St. Leo I–and the East–in the person of St. Cyril–were united in their understanding of Christ's Person. Unfortunately, controversy still remained. Many Eastern Christians felt that St. Leo's formulation of Christ's two natures did not truly square with St. Cyril's teaching on the same subject matter and represented a kind of creeping Nestorianism. This was the first council not recognized by any of the Churches of the Eastern Christian tradition (called "Old Oriental Churches").

Justinian I's desire was to reconcile the remaining Monophysites in the East with the Church. This in itself was laudable. Often, however, Justinian I's desire for such reconciliation, combined with his great love for his wife–who privately held Monophysite tendencies–proved disastrous for the Church. The case of Pope St. Silverius provides an apt example.

Pope St. Silverius was elected in 536 to succeed Pope St. Agapitus. However, Theodora wished that Vigilius, a Monophysite who had risen to great power in the Church, be made pope instead. Theodora and Vigilius conspired against Pope St. Silverius and forged documents proving his betrayal of the empire. Pope St. Silverius was deposed and sent into exile. Justinian I, largely because of his wife's influence, was unable to investigate fully the accusations leveled against St. Silverius. Hence the emperor's deference to his wife in this instance led to St. Silverius's continued exile and eventual death.

Justinian I's activity in ecclesiastical activities led to other abuses in the same vein, and constitutes the main flaw of his otherwise admirable reign.

PART XI

The Iconoclastic Controversy
(ca. 725-843)

ICONS

An icon is a flat, two-dimensional picture of Christ, the Virgin Mary, or one of the saints. Icons became numerous in the East beginning in the fifth century, and were used as aids for Christian acts of piety. Highly ritualized prayer before icons involving bowing and the lighting of incense became the norm among the Christian faithful. These practices, to a greater or lesser extent, remain in both the Western and Eastern Rites of the Church today. The general artistic style of icons reflects a certain mystical beauty of Christ the Savior and the saints. When rightly understood, the icon, by virtue of what is represented, is seen as an invitation to prayer and not as an object to be worshiped.

There are various explanations as to the rise of iconoclasm. The word "iconoclast" is the translation of the Greek word eikonoklastēs, which, as the compound of eikôn (image) and klan (to break), literally means "image breaker." Some scholars point to the influence of Judaism and Islam, which both proscribed the use of images in worship, to explain the rise of iconoclasm. Others argue that from the beginning of the Church, a latent strain of iconoclasm lay hidden below the surface, clouded over for a time by other, more pressing theological disputes.

In any case, many scholars agree that by the beginning of the eighth century, abuses of icons had sprung up among the faithful. Many people came to believe that icons held special powers. This devolved quickly into a kind of superstition, and worshipers often fixed their attention on the icon itself, rather than at the spiritual mysteries the icon was intended to represent. A kind of idolatry, forbidden by the First Commandment, emerged from this incorrect use of the icons. As a guard against such idolatry, the iconoclasts sought to destroy the icons, and, in their view, purify the practice of the Christian religion.

FIRST ICONOCLASM

EMPEROR LEO III, THE ISAURIAN (717-741)

Leo III's distrust of icons must be viewed in the context of the preceding centuries. Two or three centuries earlier, the Monophysite heresy had minimized or denied the humanity of Christ, and Manicheanism denied that Christ possessed corporeality. Although both heresies had already been condemned by the Church, remnants of heterodox belief had survived here and there. These specific heresies were aided by Islamic and Jewish influences upon Christian thought. In these other monotheistic religions, representations of God are definitively forbidden. The icons, which were representations of Christ in his full corporeality, thus came under fire from both sides. The Monophysites objected to the icons's portrayals of Christ as human; and those Christians allied with Muslims and Jews objected to the representation of any Person of the Godhead.

Aside from these theological pressures, political ones played a role as well. Leo III, like his Roman predecessors, desired a unified state, and one way of obtaining such unification was to secure a unity of religious belief. Hence it was in Leo's interest to persuade Muslims and Jews to convert to Christianity. He soon became convinced, however, that the chief impediment to their conversion was the Christian use of icons in liturgical practice. By discouraging the use of icons, Leo III thought to appease certain influential factions of Christians (those tending toward Monophysitism) and at the same time win over countless Jews and Muslims, thus consolidating his state.

Thus, in 726 Leo issued an edict declaring that all icons were occasions for idolatry and ordered their destruction. Pope St. Gregory II, Patriarch St. Germanus I of Constantinople, most bishops, and nearly all monks, immediately condemned Leo's edict. Leo wasted no time in combating his opponents, and forcibly deposed Patriarch St. Germanus I. Meanwhile, Pope St. Gregory II, after corresponding with Leo III regarding the icons, suddenly died in 731. Consequently, Leo's proscription of iconography remained in force, and when the Eastern monks refused to surrender their icons to the emperor, he unleashed a brutal persecution upon them. Many of the oldest Byzantine icons were destroyed, and hundreds of monks and nuns lost their lives in the icons' defense. Finally, Pope St. Gregory III, who succeeded Pope St. Gregory II, convened two councils in Rome in 731 that condemned Leo's actions, and then excommunicated him.

Nevertheless, Leo III remained obstinate. At his death in 741, iconoclasm was still in force in the East, and the Eastern Church was no longer in communion with Rome regarding this matter.

ST. JOHN OF DAMASCUS

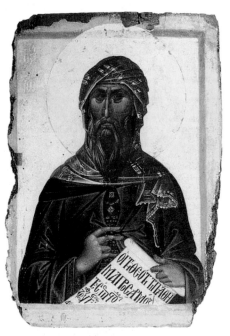

Greek icon of St. John of Damascus, early 14th century

A great defender of icons and their veneration was St. John of Damascus (ca. 655-ca. 750), also known as St. John Damascene. At a young age, St. John renounced his family wealth and became a monk near Jerusalem. During the years 726 to 730, St. John wrote the iconophile works in defense of Pope St. Gregory II against Leo III. (Iconophile – Greek for "lover of icons"–refers to support of the proper use of icons in Christian worship.) Aside from criticizing iconoclasm itself, St. John also decried imperial interference in ecclesiastical matters.

St. John's crowning work is the Fount of Wisdom, especially the section titled "De Fide Orthodoxa." In it, St. John explicates the teaching of the Greek Fathers on all the important doctrines of Christianity. Here St. John defends the use of icons by reference to the mystery of the Incarnation. In coming to the world as the God-man, Jesus Christ, God gave implicit permission for the depiction of Christ's human form in art. It would therefore follow that dignified and respectful representations of God would be praiseworthy.

Considered the last of the Eastern Church Fathers, St. John of Damascus was made a Doctor of the Church by Pope Leo XIII in 1890. He enjoys the same feast day in both the East and West, celebrated on December 4.

ICONOPHILE RECOVERY: THE SEVENTH ECUMENICAL COUNCIL: THE SECOND COUNCIL OF NICAEA (787)

Leo IV eased the persecutions of the monks, and did not enforce, though he did not repeal, his predecessors' iconoclast measures. Leo IV ruled only for a short while, and died in 780. Upon Leo IV's death, his wife, the Empress Irene, who was mother to the child heir, Constantine VI, took control of the empire. The Empress Irene had Catholic sympathies, and was secretly an iconophile. In a move to restore the icons, she persuaded Pope Adrian I to convene the Seventh Ecumenical Council, the second council at Nicaea (787). The chosen location was no accident. Empress Irene and the iconophiles hoped that those in attendance would be reminded of the First Ecumenical Council at Nicaea called by Constantine the Great, and would restore orthodoxy in the East.

The Council, just one month after convening, declared its acceptance of the veneration of icons in line with the papal position regarding their legitimacy. It then went on to distinguish between two types of adoration. An icon may be venerated through acts of respect and honor (Greek, dulia), since bowing, lighting lamps, or burning incense before the picture of a saint is honor paid for the person it represents, and not for the image itself. God alone is worthy of absolute adoration (Greek, latria). The Scholastic tradition in the West later solidified this distinction when it used the terms dulia to indicate the reverence due to creatures such as saints, and the term latria to indicate the absolute adoration due to God alone.

SECOND ICONOCLASM (815-843)

The Byzantine military staged a successful coup against the defunct Byzantine leadership under Michael I. The new emperor Leo V (775-820) sought to rehabilitate iconoclasm in Byzantium as a way of strengthening the influence and power of the military. For even though the recent Second Council of Nicaea had officially ended iconoclasm's status as a viable theological view, the heresy retained many adherents in the military and upper echelons of Byzantine society. Leo V, in propagating iconoclasm, hoped to solidify this base. As a result, both he and his two successors Michael II (emperor 820-829) and Theophilus (emperor 829-842) continued the iconoclast policy.

Leo V deposed the Patriarch of Constantinople, who clung to orthodoxy despite the emperor's threats, and in his stead appointed Theophilus, a patriarch friendly to him. This patriarch soon called a council with the aim of returning to the Council of Hiereia's (753) conclusions. When in the course of the council Leo V encountered a surprisingly strong resistance from the episcopacy, he revived the persecutions, which continued unabated until Theophilus's death in 842.

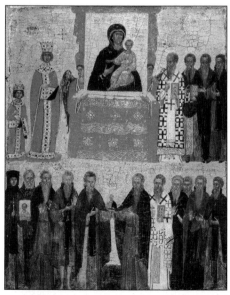

Icon of the Triumph of Orthodoxy, Constantinople, late 14th century. This icon depicts those who fought for Orthodoxy during the period of iconoclasm.

THE FEAST OF THE TRIUMPH OF ORTHODOXY (843)

It required another empress and regent, Empress Theodora, to reverse the new wave of iconoclasm and restore orthodoxy in the East. Theodora deposed the iconoclast Patriarch Theophilus of Constantinople, and in 843, put in his place Bl. Methodius, who had been tortured and imprisoned by Theophilus. Under Bl. Methodius, iconoclast bishops were deposed and replaced by orthodox iconophiles, and the first Sunday of Lent was named the Feast of the Triumph of Orthodoxy in order to celebrate the triumph of the icons. The Eastern Churches still celebrate this feast today.

Hence, in 843 – after more than one hundred years of controversy and schism – the barren walls of churches were again decorated with beautiful icons, and the orthodox practice of venerating icons was finally secure.

PART XII

The Rise of the Carolingians and an Independent Papacy

THE ORIGIN OF THE CAROLINGIAN LINE

Pepin the Short (741-767) was a Carolingian and the son of the famed Charles Martel, who had defeated the Muslims at Tours in 732. Pepin appeared to be a brute in his physical characteristics: short, broad-shouldered, and strong. However, he also had a keen intelligence and understanding of others. He combined these qualities with an extraordinary ambition for power.

Pepin solidified his position as the only heir to the Carolingian dynasty when his other brother became a monk. Pepin wrote to Pope St. Zachary requesting that he and his progeny be given kingship over the Franks, since it was they who retained actual power among the Franks. St. Boniface, who was the papal legate in the Germanic territories, successfully acquired Pope St. Zachary's permission to recognize the new Carolingian dynasty as the rightful rulers in central Europe, officially transferring power from the Merovingian Dynasty.

St. Boniface anointed Pepin king in 751, marking the beginning of a long and complicated allegiance between the Carolingians and the papacy in the West.

ESTABLISHMENT OF THE PAPAL STATES

Pope Stephen II (752-757), who succeeded St. Zachary, expected protection from Pepin the Short in exchange for the official papal support of the Carolingians. To reiterate the papacy's expectations, Pope Stephen traveled across the Alps into France to meet with Pepin. The Lombards were presently threatening Rome, and the Byzantines did not intend to protect Italy. Pope Stephen, aware that the Byzantines would not hesitate to abandon the papacy, sought to recruit Pepin's aid in the defense of Rome. On July 28, 754, the pope publicly anointed Pepin and his two sons – repeating with more pomp the consecration already performed by St. Boniface – and threatened to condemn anyone who disobeyed them. This consecration was designed to show that the Church could bestow secular authority to kings. Pepin in turn agreed to intervene on behalf of the pope before the Lombard ruler.

In the end, Pepin won Rome for the papacy, as well as securing Ravenna and Perugia. These lands would become known as the Papal States. For the first time in the history of the Church, the pope, who had always been a spiritual leader, became a sovereign one as well. This direct administration of temporal lands by the papacy would last until 1870, when Italy would unify itself as a nation-state.

The direct involvement of the papacy in the administration of a state was both advantageous and troublesome for the Church. On the one hand, it ensured that the papacy would enjoy independence from Byzantine emperors who wished to exert influence over the Church's ecclesiastical affairs. Hence, it made the ongoing missionary work and ecclesiastical organization more manageable for the Church hierarchy. Furthermore, the defined territory of the Papal States would also serve as a means of protection against the Lombards and other bellicose peoples. On the other hand, the kinds of temptations that always beset those in political power became suddenly relevant for those in authority. Because of this, some abuses arose in the Church which otherwise might have been avoided.

CHARLEMAGNE (REIGNED 769-814)

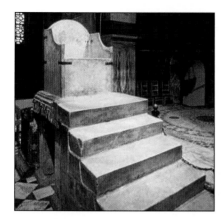

Charlemagne's simple throne in the Palace Chapel in the Aachen Cathedral chapel.

Charles, the son of Pepin, became after the death of his brother Carolman the inheritor of his father's kingdom. Charles ruled for a long period, many years of which were devoted to securing and expanding his kingdom. Although economically draining, his frantic military activity–he led at least fifty military campaigns–was not in vain. By the time of his death in 814, Charles had unified most of Western Europe under one Christian ruler.

Charles, known as "the Great" (in English, the French title "Charlemagne" is used; in Latin, Carolus Magnus), was the most powerful and charismatic ruler to emerge in the West since the days of the great Caesars. He was a powerful and ruthless warrior, as was his grandfather; but unlike his grandfather, he combined his military excellence with extraordinary political ability. No common warlord, Charlemagne knew both Latin and Greek, and had committed large parts of St. Augustine's City of God to memory. His interest in ecclesiastical and civil reforms did much for the growth of European culture. Centuries after his death European leaders and kings sought to emulate his reign.

Charlemagne's public policy was explicitly Christian. He drew from the laws of the Church (Canon Law) for his own civic legislation, and he considered the decrees of synods and councils to be lawfully binding for his subjects. Moreover, officials of the Church also served in Charlemagne's civil posts, and often acted as his diplomats. Charlemagne himself, in an effort to model his rule on the Person of Christ, built himself a throne without precious stones to signify the simplicity of Christ's Incarnation.

Providentially, Charlemagne acted in the best interests of the Church. He tried to reform the clergy, established new dioceses, and raised the necessary funds to support worship and the priests. In order to maintain control over his empire, Charlemagne appointed missi dominici, civil servants who were investigators. Their responsibility was to enter all the different parts of the empire and provide reports on the civil and religious life of particular areas.

A devout Catholic, Charlemagne rigorously observed his times for prayer and fasting, and attended many liturgical ceremonies. In addition, he sang in the choir and read the Bible daily.

CHARLEMAGNE'S RELATIONSHIP TO THE PAPACY

The Lombards, who had been defeated under Pepin, again threatened Rome in July of 773. Pope Adrian I (772-795) sought Charlemagne's aid, and in response Charlemagne and his troops routed the invading

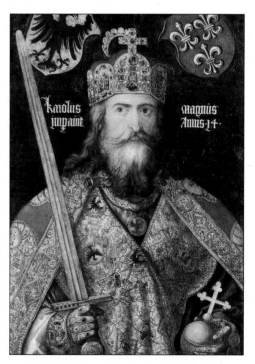

This portrait of Emperor Charlemagne by Albrecht Dürer portrays him with a divine, iconic countenance. He is shown with the robe, crown, sword and orb used in the actual coronation, which were sketched from the originals by Dürer.

Lombards. As Charlemagne marched into Rome on Easter the following year, he received a hero's welcome. Three doors of St. Peter's were opened wide to receive Charlemagne, and upon entering, he prostrated himself before the pope. Adrian granted the title "Patrician of Rome" to Charlemagne and renewed the papacy's alliance with the Franks. Charlemagne subsequently made himself king of the Lombards, and thus became the first ruler to unite all the Germanic kingdoms.

CHARLEMAGNE CROWNED EMPEROR (800)

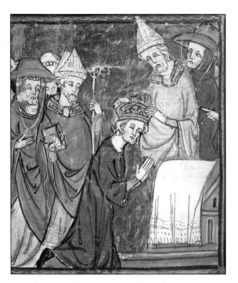

Pope St. Leo III crowned Charlemagne emperor during the Christmas day Mass at St. Peter's Basilica in 800. This crowning, which sources say took Charlemagne by surprise, was not just a reaffirmation of Charlemagne's title as "King of the Franks and Lombards" which he had held for some years, it now made him a Roman Emperor. The new imperial title given by the pope placed Charlemagne's Carolingian empire in a direct line of descent from the old Roman Empire. Charlemagne's crowning by the pope meant that the Germans were finally incorporated into Roman civilization.

The actions of Pope St. Leo III and Charlemagne infuriated the Byzantine emperors. Since the Byzantine emperors still considered themselves the rightful imperial rulers of Western Europe, they viewed the papacy's actions with contempt. In place of Byzantine rule, which they traced to Constantine the Great, the West was now ruled by a person whom they considered a barbarian. At first Byzantium refused to recognize the legitimacy of this newly formed empire, but because of Charlemagne's power and influence, they eventually recognized him, referring to him as the Basileus (king) of the West.

THE CAROLINGIAN RENAISSANCE

The years before Charlemagne's rule had decidedly been years of decline in the West. Political instability and corruption led quickly to an intellectual collapse, and when Charlemagne assumed office, the study of theology and literature–so rich in the East–was absent in large part in the continental West. Further, Latin had so deteriorated that it was rendered almost unintelligible to a listener from Classical Rome. One of Charlemagne's most enduring legacies was to combat this cultural decay by emphasizing the importance of education and artistic excellence in his political vision. He commanded that every monastery and parish had to have a school.

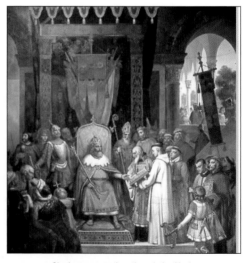

Charlemagne receives the scholar Alcuin at his palace in Aachen, Germany.

Because of Charlemagne's insistence, the clergy of the Church were better instructed in classical and biblical texts than they had been for several hundred years. This improved literacy led to a renewed enthusiasm for the Catholic Faith and the rich, profound literature connected with it, thus paving the way for a new wave of missionary activity.

THE EMPIRE OF CHARLEMAGNE, 768-814

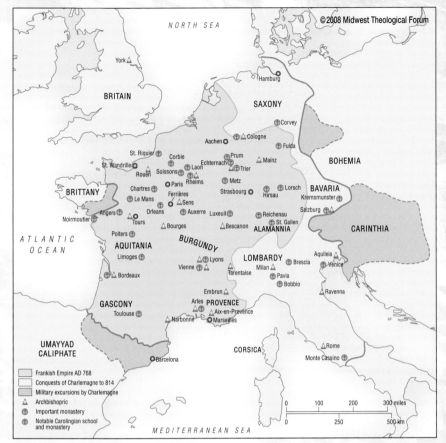

©2008 Midwest Theological Forum

NORTH SEA

York

BRITAIN

Hamburg

SAXONY

Corvey

Aachen · Cologne
Fulda

St. Riquier · Corbie · Prum
St. Wandrille · Laon · Echternach · Mainz
Rouen · Soissons · Trier
Chartres · Rheims · Metz · Lorsch
Le Mans · Paris · Ferrières · Strasbourg · Hirsau
Angers · Orleans · Sens · Auxerre · Luxeuil · Reichenau · Salzburg
Noirmoutier · Tours · Bourges · Bescanon · St. Gallen
Poitiers · BURGUNDY · ALAMANNIA

BRITTANY

BOHEMIA

BAVARIA
Kremsmunster

CARINTHIA

ATLANTIC OCEAN

AQUITANIA
Limoges · Lyons · LOMBARDY · Brescia
Vienne · Tarentaise · Milan · Venice
Bordeaux · Pavia
Embrun · Bobbio
GASCONY · Arles · PROVENCE · Ravenna
Toulouse · Aix-en-Provence
Narbonne · Marseilles

Aquileia

UMAYYAD CALIPHATE

CORSICA

Rome
Monte Cassino

Barcelona

	Frankish Empire AD 768
	Conquests of Charlemagne to 814
	Military excursions by Charlemagne
△	Archbishopric
⊕	Important monastery
⊕	Notable Carolingian school and monastery

0 100 200 300 miles
0 250 500 km

MEDITERRANEAN SEA

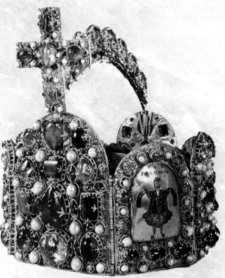

Above: The Imperial Crown of the Holy Roman Empire, the "Crown of Charlemagne," is crafted of gold, cloisonné enamel, precious stones, and pearls. Eight hinged plates form the octagonal body of the imperial crown. Four plates bear pictorial representations from the Old Testament in cloisonné enamel, and four plates have precious stones and pearls. The twelve precious stones on the brow plate correspond to the number of the Apostles. The twelve stones on the neck plate refer to the breast-plate of the Jewish high priest and are engraved with the names of the twelve tribes of Israel.

THE GREAT SCHISM, 1054

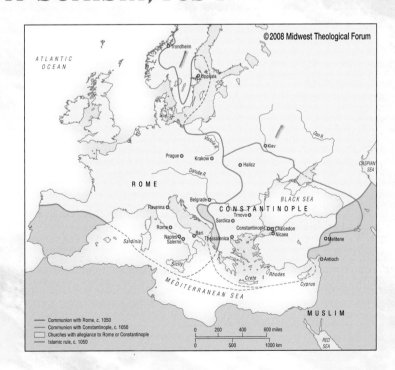

©2008 Midwest Theological Forum

ATLANTIC OCEAN

Trondheim

Uppsala

Prague · Krakow · Kiev
Vistula R. · Halicz
Danube R. · Don R.
CASPIAN SEA

ROME

Belgrade
Ravenna · BLACK SEA
CONSTANTINOPLE
Rome · Sardica · Trnovo
Bari · Thessalonica · Constantinople · Chalcedon
Naples · Nicaea
Salerno · Melitene
Sardinia
Antioch
Sicily · Crete · Rhodes
Cyprus

MEDITERRANEAN SEA

MUSLIM

	Communion with Rome, c. 1050
	Communion with Constantinople, c. 1050
	Churches with allegiance to Rome or Constantinople
	Islamic rule, c. 1050

0 200 400 600 miles
0 500 1000 km

RED SEA

PART XIII

The Great Schism

The final shattering of communion between East and West in 1054 is one of the saddest chapters in the history of the Church. Though the seed of division had already been planted with the founding of Constantinople in the fourth century, alienation intensified during the ninth century because of both the Iconoclast controversy and Charlemagne's rise in power. By the eleventh century, the East and West were held together by only the most tenuous of relationships, and the slightest event was likely to separate them.

THE EMERGENCE OF DIFFERENCES

Aside from the subtleties of theological disputes and the many misunderstandings that arose, the growing distance between East and West also owed much to their different conceptions of Church government and hierarchy. It may be helpful to present a brief account of this difference.

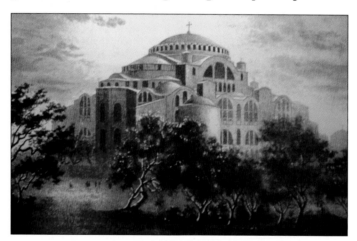

An artist's concept of Justinian I's Church of Holy Wisdom in ca. 538.

The Bishop of Rome, the pope, had a dual jurisdiction in the Church: the Latin West, centered in Rome, as well as the universal Church. As Constantinople grew in power over successive centuries, it tightened its grip around the other ancient eastern centers of Christianity at Antioch, Alexandria, and Jerusalem. After the doctrinal statements at the Ecumenical Council of Chalcedon in 451, these were recognized along with Rome as especially ancient and important centers of Christianity.

For both political and theological reasons, however, the Christians of the East tended to minimize the pope's status as chief shepherd of the Church. Eastern Christians seldom referred to him except in extreme cases, often during a difficult dispute in the Church, at which point he was often sought out to settle the dispute. From very early on—for varying reasons covered in this chapter—Eastern believers allied themselves more closely with their own national patriarchs than with the successor of St. Peter.

In addition to this, caesaropapism, expressed in the symbiotic relationship between the patriarch of Constantinople and the eastern emperor, was also a cause of tension. The patriarch crowned the emperor, and in turn the emperor made an oath to protect the Church and preserve the Faith. Thus, the patriarch of Constantinople often acted as a very important government official in the bureaucracy of imperial administration in the East, and the emperor, in turn, often acted as a very high-ranking member of the Church's body.

Finally, the relationship of the religious to the laity in the East was very different from that in the West. In the West the monasteries and convents worked together with the surrounding populations to teach them the rudiments of agrarian life along with the fundamentals of Christianity. In the East the monks were more secluded, if not more learned, and had little contact with the outside world whatsoever, thus limiting their influence.

LITURGICAL PRACTICES OF THE EASTERN CHURCHES

There are two basic kinds of Eastern Churches: Orthodox and Catholic. Whereas the Eastern Orthodox Churches are not in communion with Rome, a number of Orthodox Churches have reunited with Rome at various times during the last millennium. These are called Eastern Uniate (from *union*) Churches or Eastern Catholic Churches. Though some theological differences divide them, the Orthodox and Uniate Churches share the same liturgical and devotional practices.

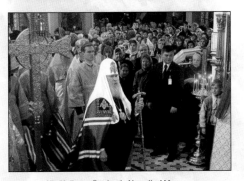

His Holiness Patriarch Alexy II of Moscow and Russia celebrating the Divine Liturgy, 2003.

The liturgy practiced in both the Eastern and Western (Roman) Churches is ultimately based on the liturgical practices of the Apostles and Fathers of the Church. Because Greek was the common language and culture of the Roman Empire in the first century, it was no surprise that liturgical practices in the early Church were essentially Greek. The liturgy of the Eastern Churches has always been conducted in the vernacular; a good example of this may be found in the story of Sts. Cyril and Methodius, who translated the Bible and liturgical texts into the native language of the Slavs (see chapter 6). Over time, however, the liturgy of the West incorporated more Latin (Roman) customs, whereas in the lands east of the Mediterranean Sea, the liturgy remained Greek.

Music in the Eastern Churches is divided into two main traditions: Byzantine and Russian. Byzantine music—generally sung *a cappella*—is based on modes developed by the Greeks before the time of Christ. Mixed with elements of Jewish chant and psalmody, this music sounds foreign and unfamiliar to westerners. Russian music is based on Byzantine but developed in the seventeenth century under Polish influence. Most Russian liturgical music employs western scales, making it incorporable with German, French and Italian musical traditions.

One of the basic differences between West and East is the sign of the cross. In the Eastern Churches, the tradition is retained of bringing together the thumb, forefinger, and middle finger whereas the other two are pressed against the palm. This is a symbolic reminder of the three Persons of the Triune God and the two natures of Christ. In addition, the horizontal "beam" of the cross is traced from right to left. For blessing, a bishop or priest joins his thumb, ring, and little fingers while forming a cross with the other two.

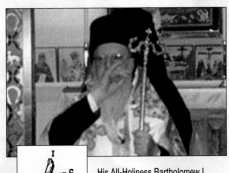

His All-Holiness Bartholomew I, Patriarch of Constantinople, blessing the congregation.

In the Eastern Church's blessing the fingers form the shape of the Greek letters "IC XC," the abbreviation in Greek for Jesus Christ.

THE *FILIOQUE* CONTROVERSY

Beginning at a local council, the Third Council of Toledo in 589, the words "and the Son" (Latin, Filioque) were added to the Niceno-Constantinopolitan Creed. By 800 this formulation of the creed was standard throughout the Frankish empire of Charlemagne.

This addition was meant to clarify a theological point. The Niceno-Constantinopolitan Creed could be read to attribute the procession of the Holy Spirit from the Father but only through the Son, though this was not what that creed intended. The Niceno-Constantinopolitan Creed was developed in opposition to those who denied that the Holy Spirit proceeded from the Father. The Niceno-Constantinopolitan Creed, then, did not deny that the Holy Spirit proceeded from the Son as well as the Father; it just failed to mention it explicitly. So the new Toledo creed merely clarified what was already an ancient belief in both East and West, namely, that the Holy Spirit proceeded from the Father and the Son.

The Patriarch of Constantinople steadfastly refused the addition to the creed, even though historical evidence suggests that most of the Greek Fathers believed in the Holy Spirit's double-procession from the Father and the Son. Eastern scholars argue that the Catholic Church violated the Council of Chalcedon's (449) injunction not to change the creed, but it is accepted all around that the addition of Filioque amounts to a clarification rather than an alteration intended to improve or change belief. Nonetheless, the Greeks did not accept Filioque even when it was imposed upon them during two councils aimed at healing the Great Schism (Councils of Lyon [1274] and of Florence [1439]), and have not accepted it to this day.

THE PHOTIAN SCHISM (857-867)

In 857, Patriarch Ignatius of Constantinople refused a high government official, by the name of Bardas, Holy Communion on the Feast of the Epiphany because of rumors regarding an adulterous affair. Bardas's reaction, and Ignatius's determination interpreted as insolence, convinced emperor Michael III to depose Ignatius in 858.

In Ignatius's place, Emperor Michael III elevated Photius (ca. 810-895) to Patriarch of Constantinople. Photius, though a layman, was a brilliant and ambitious scholar. He was quickly ordained and ushered into the patriarchate.

When Ignatius refused to step aside, Michael III and Photius wrote obsequious letters to the Pope, requesting that he send legates to Constantinople to handle the situation. Pope St. Nicholas I (858-867) sent two legates who were promptly bought off by Michael and Photius. The legates settled the dispute in favor of Photius and returned to Rome with the intention of convincing the Pope of their decision. When the Pope discovered their treachery, he excommunicated them. He, then in 862, wrote letters to both the emperor and Photius claiming that his legates had exceeded their authority and that Ignatius was to be reinvested as Patriarch. In 863 another council in Rome voided the settlement in Constantinople. Photius and all his appointments in the Church were denied recognition.

This infuriated the emperor. He wrote the Pope demanding that the matter be reexamined. The Pope agreed in 865 to look at the case again. During this time Photius remained silent, but carried out the duties of his office. In 867, however, Photius rejected the presence of Latin missionaries in Bulgaria, which he considered the missionary territory of Constantinople. In addition, Photius charged the papacy with tampering with the Nicene Creed through its use of the Filioque clause, and tried to stir a popular uprising against Rome.

The year 867 marked a turning point in the dispute. Pope St. Nicholas I died, and Michael III and Bardas were assassinated during a revolution in Constantinople. The new emperor Basil I desired reconciliation with the new pope, Adrian II, and at the Eighth Ecumenical Council, Constantinople IV (869-870), Photius was removed. Ignatius was reinstated but continuing tension over Bulgaria and the Filioque kept hard feelings of the schism alive. When Pope Adrian II denied the institution of a patriarchate in Bulgaria, King Boris of Bulgaria chose Constantinople as the spiritual center for his people. In 870 Ignatius began consecrating bishops for Bulgaria in disobedience to the pope, and this renewed hostilities between Rome and the East.

Ignatius died in 877, and Photius, who had spent the intervening years building a strong base of support, once again became patriarch. The Holy See could not but recognize his appointment, for even though he was an unqualified candidate for the patriarchy, the position was, this time, legitimately open. Once reinstated, Photius renewed his campaign against Rome, excommunicating the entire Latin Church for their liturgical irregularities and their alteration of the creed of 451. Although many Eastern bishops realized the error of Photius's ways, he possessed so much power among the people, whom he had turned against Rome, that it was impossible to resist him. Photius finally was forced into a second, and final, resignation upon the ascension of the new emperor Leo VI in 886. The East remained in communion with Rome for the next two hundred years, but Photius's dissension had struck deep roots among the Greek people and would resurface later, during the Great Schism.

THE GREAT SCHISM (1054)

The final split between the eastern and western Churches came in the year 1054. In the Great Schism all of the tension that had developed over the previous centuries came to a head. The doctrinal dispute over the Filioque, the crowning of Charlemagne as emperor of the West in 800, the issues of authority raised in the Photian schism, and the reforming tendencies under the leadership of the papacy in the West all came into focus. In addition, Byzantium had increased its military strength, and wanted to achieve a greater degree of independence from the West. These circumstances combined to shatter the thousand-year communion between East and West.

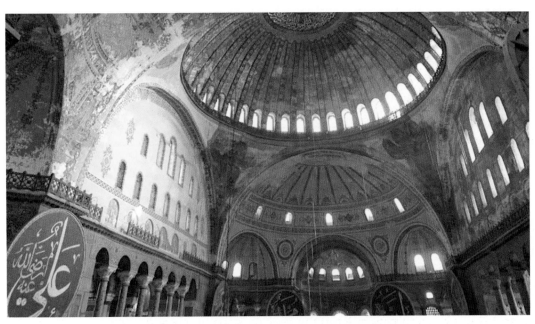

Interior and dome of Hagia Sophia, Istanbul (formerly Constantinople).
In this magnificent location Cardinal Humbert, on July 16, 1054, laid down upon its altar a bull of excommunication
from Pope Leo IX, which would have a negative impact on the Christian world that has lasted for centuries.

PATRIARCH MICHAEL CERULARIUS

Before being appointed patriarch, Michael Cerularius (1043-1058) had lived in seclusion in a monastery in the East. Many, though not all, Eastern monasteries had been decidedly influenced by Photius's dissent. When Cerularius became patriarch, his anti-Latin sentiments came out into the open, and the target of his attack was the papacy, which he regarded with disgust.

Patriarch Michael Cerularius objected to many Western practices that differed from the East. In particular he objected to a celibate priesthood, the Saturday fast, the use of unleavened bread in the Mass, beardless priests, eating meat with blood, and omitting the alleluia during Lent.

The patriarch was so disenchanted with the West that he closed Latin parishes in Constantinople. When consecrated hosts from Latin churches were trampled upon, Cardinal Humbert in the West translated this as a Greek attack on the Latin Church and Pope Leo IX (1049-1054). Cardinal Humbert was entrusted with the papal reply that would prove disastrous.

Cardinal Humbert made it plain to the patriarch that it is impossible to excommunicate the Pope, and that the Pope holds primacy in the Church, even over patriarchs. Patriarch Cerularius is said to have replied: "If you venerate my name in a single church in Rome, I will venerate your name in all the churches in the East." The papal response came in the form of an ultimatum: "Either be in communion with Peter or become a synagogue of Satan." Henceforth the patriarch deleted the Pope's name from all liturgies.

Two papal legates, Cardinal Humbert and Frederick of Lorraine, the latter of whom would later become Pope, were sent to Constantinople. Neither possessed much diplomatic skill, and because of their arrogance, Patriarch Cerularius was able to turn the population of Constantinople against them.

THE ACTUAL SCHISM

On July 16, 1054, Cardinal Humbert attended the Divine Liturgy at Hagia Sophia in Constantinople. There he denounced the patriarch for refusing papal authority. Upon the high altar in Hagia Sophia, Cardinal Humbert laid a document excommunicating Patriarch Cerularius. Humbert and Frederick then left the cathedral and shook the dust from their shoes outside.

Technically, however, the two legates did not have the authority to excommunicate in the Pope's name because Pope Leo IX had just died.

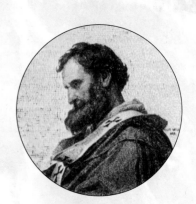

The Eastern Emperor Constantine IX wanted to heal the rift, especially since he needed military help from the West against the Normans. In response to his call for reconciliation the patriarch incited riots; the emperor, not wanting to face a civil war, backed down from his position. The documents of excommunication were burned by the patriarch, and a council in Constantinople declared on July 24, 1054 that the Latins had perverted the faith. Patriarch Michael Cerularius had returned excommunication for excommunication.

Pope Stephen IX (X) was Pope for only eight months, 1057-1058. His original name was Frederick of Lorraine, one of the two papal legates sent to Constantinople by Pope Leo IX to confront Patriarch Cerularius. The results from that journey in 1054 precipitated the final split between the eastern and western churches. He continued his position as abbot of Monte Cassino during his short reign as Pope. An ardent reformer, he was advised by Peter (St.) Damian, Cardinal Humbert and Hildebrand who would become Pope St. Gregory VII.

Since that time, the Patriarch of Constantinople has been known as the "Ecumenical Patriarch" of the East, and in Eastern tradition is regarded as the "first among

CONTEMPORARY EFFORTS TO HEAL THE SCHISM

While schisms are easily made, they can be very difficult to heal. Unfortunately, misunderstandings and disputes have caused seemingly permanent damage and weakened the Church to this very day. St. John Paul II realized this, and made great efforts to reach out to the Eastern Orthodox Church by opening dialogue that may, someday, ultimately heal this ancient schism. In an unprecedented visit to Greece in May 2001, the pope addressed the Orthodox Archbishop and Holy Synod in Athens. An excerpt of the pope's address sheds light on his mission and goal to heal the Schism:

"Finally, Your Beatitude, I wish to express the hope that we may walk together in the ways of the kingdom of God. In 1965, the Ecumenical Patriarch Athenagoras and Pope Paul VI by a mutual act removed and cancelled from the Church's memory and life the sentence of excommunication between Rome and Constantinople. This historic gesture stands as *a summons for us to work ever more fervently for the unity which is Christ's will.* Division between Christians is a sin before God and a scandal before the world. It is a hindrance to the spread of the Gospel, because it makes our proclamation less credible. The Catholic Church is convinced that she must do all in her power to 'prepare the way of the Lord' and to 'make straight his paths' (Mt 3:3); and she understands that this must be done in company with other Christians—in fraternal dialogue, in cooperation, and in prayer. If certain models of reunion of the past no longer correspond to the impulse towards unity which the Holy Spirit has awakened in Christians everywhere in recent times, we must be all the more open and attentive to what the Spirit is now saying to the Churches (cf. Rv 2:11)"

(John Paul II, "Holy Father Asks Pardon for Past Sins," *L'Osservatore Romano,* Weekly Edition in English, no.19, May 9, 2001, p. 5).

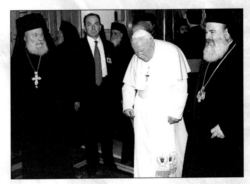

St. John Paul II in Athens in 2001.

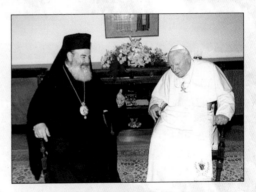

St. John Paul II in Syria in 2001.

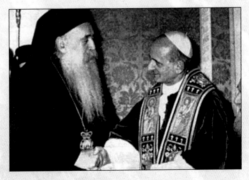

Patriarch of Constantinople Athenagoras meets with Pope Paul VI in 1964.

among the eastern patriarchs. On December 7, 1965, before the closing Mass of the Second Vatican Council, Pope Paul VI and Patriarch Athenagoras of Constantinople participated in a show of reconciliation. In a joint declaration they expressed regret over the mutual excommunication of Patriarch Cerularius and the papal legate Cardinal Humbert in 1054.

CONCLUSION

In this tumultuous period, the Church made the transition from existing within the Roman Empire to surviving amidst the Germanic invasions. However, the Church did not merely survive. Rather, she set about a proactive mission of the evangelization of Germanic tribes, facilitated largely by the rise of monasticism. The chapter relates the stories of the men and women who brought the Gospel message to all corners of Europe. Though beset by great challenges, the steadfast labors of these holy monks, nuns, kings, queens, and soldiers under the guidance of the Holy Spirit brought a new unity to the West after the fall of the Empire.

At the core of her mission in the world, the preaching and spreading of the Gospel is one of the Church's chief responsibilities. Through the many challenges that this period of evangelization posed, the Church remained focused on expanding the message of Christ to all who would listen. Not until the Spaniards and the Portuguese arrived in the Americas late in the fifteenth century would Christianity again experience such growth among new peoples. At the same time that the West was the beneficiary of this great work of evangelization, tensions began to mount between Christianity in the West and Christianity in the East. Seemingly irreconcilable differences drove the two traditions farther apart, despite great efforts to improve the situation. During this period two distinct forms of Christianity came into being. While the East turned violently onto itself in the Iconoclastic Controversy, the West developed its first unity under the leadership of the Franks and the popes. However, the communion between East and West was shattered in the Great Schism that has separated, to this day, the two traditions with the same sacraments. From the perspective of the Catholic Church, the major difference between Eastern and Western Christianity primarily involves the teaching authority and jurisdiction of the papacy established by Christ through his Apostle St. Peter.

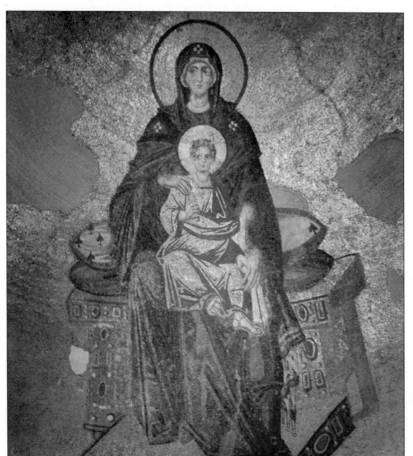

Mosaic in the apse of Hagia Sophia in Istanbul (Constantinople), dedicated by Photius on March 29, 867 as the first new mosaic after the period of iconoclasm.

Photius's celebratory oration, Homily XVII, is one of the key documents in Byzantine art history.

"For though the time is short since the pride of the iconoclastic heresy has been reduced to ashes, and true religion has spread its lights to the ends of the world,…this too is our ornament."

VOCABULARY

ALLAH
Arabic word for God.

BONIFACE (BONA FACERE)
Latin for "doer of good" and the name given to St. Boniface, the missionary to Germany who set the stage for a radical reshaping of the heart of Europe.

CAESAROPAPISM
System in which the temporal ruler extends his own powers to ecclesiastical and theological matters. Such emperors appointed bishops and the Eastern Patriarch, directed the development of liturgical practices, and even aided the recruitment of monks.

CANTERBURY
The most important episcopal see in England in the sixth century and the site of St. Augustine's mission to England.

CODEX JUSTINIANUS
Compiled under Emperor Justinian I, the codex was the collection and systemization of all Roman law as it had developed from his predecessors put together for the purpose of legal uniformity throughout the empire. It is the basis for canon law as well as the civil law throughout Europe.

DIOCESE
A territorial division of the Church, adapted from the Roman Empire.

DULIA AND LATRIA
Two types of adoration whose distinction was drawn at the seventh Council of Nicaea. An icon may be venerated through acts of respect an honor, called dulia, but God alone is worth of absolute adoration, known in Greek as latria.

ECUMENICAL PATRIARCH
Title adopted by the Patriarch of Constantinople.

FILIOQUE
Latin meaning "and the Son," this was first added at the Third Council of Toledo (589) to the Niceno-Constantinopolitan Creed to clarify that the Holy Spirit proceeded from both the Father and the Son. Later, the Patriarch of Constantinople and the bishops of the East refused the addition, thus contributing to the Great Schism.

GLAGOLITHIC SCRIPT
Based on the Greek alphabet, it was developed by St. Cyril to aid his mission to the Slavic peoples.

GREAT SCHISM
The final split between the eastern and western Churches in the year 1054.

HAGIA SOPHIA
Most famous example of Byzantine architecture, it was built under Justinian I and is considered one of the most perfect buildings in the world.

HERMIT
One who, for religious motives, has retired into solitary life, especially one of the early Christian recluses. Derived from the Greek word erēmia, meaning "desert," it is also known as eremitical life.

HUNS
A powerful nomadic people of unknown ethnic origin who invaded Europe ca. 375.

ICON
A flat, two-dimensional picture of Christ, the Virgin Mary, or one of the saints which is used as an aid for Christian acts of piety. The general artistic style of icons reflects a certain mystical beauty of Christ the Savior and the saints. When rightly understood, the icon, by virtue of what is represented, is seen as an invitation to prayer.

ICONOCLASM
Thoughts or deeds of an iconoclast. Refers to periods in history when a large number of iconoclasts were present.

ICONOCLAST
From the Greek word eikonoklastēs meaning "image breaker," iconoclasts saw icons as occasions of idolatry and sought to destroy

VOCABULARY Continued

them and purify the practice of the Christian religion. They were condemned at the second council of Nicaea in 787.

ICONOPHILE
Greek for "lover of icons," this term refers to those who defend and promote the proper use of icons in Christian worship.

ISLAM
Arabic for "submission," the faith of the prophet Muhammad, it traces its roots back to Abraham, Hagar and Ishmael.

KORAN
Arabic for "recitation," this is the holy book of the Muslim faith, written by Muhammad, and containing all of the writings that Muhammad claimed he was told by the archangel Gabriel under God's direction.

LATRIA
See dulia.

MONASTICISM
A way of life characterized by asceticism and self-denial lived more or less in seclusion from the world and under fixed rule and vows. Monastic communities withdraw from the affairs of the world in order to seek God through asceticism and prayer.

MONOPHYSITISM
Heresy claiming that there is only one nature in Christ and that His human nature is "incorporated" into the Divine Nature.

MOZÁRABES
Spanish people who chose to live under Arab rule after the Muslim invasion of Spain in 711.

PAPAL STATES
Lands around Rome, Italy, won by Pepin on behalf and given to the papacy, making the pope a sovereign as well as spiritual leader. The Papal States were ruled by the pope from 754 to 1870.

SCRIPTORIUM
Large room in a monastery dedicated to the copying and maintaining of texts.

SERVUS SERVORUM DEI
Latin for "servant of the servants of God," this title was adopted by Pope St. Gregory the Great.

VOW
A solemn promise made voluntarily by a person of reason, to practice a virtue or perform a specific good deed in order to accomplish a future good which is better than its contrary.

STUDY QUESTIONS

1. Describe conditions in the Roman Empire during the fifth century when the empire collapsed.

2. What was the key for the Church in converting the Germanic tribes?

3. How did the Germanic invasions change the Christian attitude in the fifth century?

4. How is Christian monasticism unique?

5. What was a common problem of the early hermits in Egypt?

6. What were the three major effects of the monasteries on Europe?

7. What are the chief qualities that lend the Rule of St. Benedict to harmonious religious life?

8. What three vows were accepted by the Benedictines?

9. In what ways was Pope St. Gregory I (the Great) an historical marker?

STUDY QUESTIONS Continued

10. What was Pope St. Gregory I's background?

11. What title did Pope St. Gregory I use during his papacy, and what title did he reject for the Patriarch of Constantinople. What did these titles imply?

12. Why is France known as the "Church's eldest daughter"?

13. Who is known as the "Apostle of Ireland," and what is his background?

14. How did Irish monasteries protect and promote Western civilization?

15. Who was the "Apostle of Scotland"?

16. When did the Church finally implement the Sacrament of Penance in the form recognized today? How often are Catholics required to go to Penance?

17. How is it known that English Christianity existed at least before 314?

18. Who was the "Apostle of England"?

19. What was the most important episcopal see in England?

20. Who is the "Father of English History" and what important contribution did he make with regard to the calendar?

21. Who is the "Apostle of Germany," and how did he shape the heart of Europe?

22. The monastery of which city became the most important in all of Germany?

23. How did the conversion of the Slavs cause tension?

24. Who were the "Apostles of the Slavs," and what were their backgrounds?

25. Why did many Slavs later turn against the Catholic Church in favor of Constantinople?

26. What German city was made an archdiocese specifically for the formation of missionaries for the Slavs?

27. Describe the geography of the location for Constantinople.

28. What was Emperor Justinian I's great ambition?

29. How is an icon not a violation of the first commandment?

30. What were the results of Emperor Leo III's forbiddance of icons?

31. What was St. John of Damascus's basic argument in support of icons?

32. What happened to Emperor Nicephorus, and how did this help to inaugurate the Second Iconoclasm?

33. What was the significance of the relationship between the papacy and the Frankish king?

34. How did the Papal States come into existence?

35. Who was Charlemagne, and how did he help the Church?

36. When was Charlemagne crowned emperor by Pope St. Leo III?

37. Define the Carolingian Renaissance.

38. What was the Photian Schism?

39. What were some practices that Cerularius disliked in the Latin Church?

40. What did the Eastern emperor think about the schism?

PRACTICAL EXERCISES

1. Why is it easy to understand why many Christians thought that the Second Coming was close at hand when the Roman Empire collapsed? Can you think of other times in history when conditions also seemed to be right for the Second Coming?

2. The "Dome of the Rock" was built in 684 over the site of the former Jewish temple in Jerusalem. What psychological impact might this have had upon Jews?

3. The Rule of St. Benedict, written in the sixth century, is still used by Benedictines and a number of other monastic communities today. Its focus on a simple life of prayer and work and its adaptability to different circumstances have been credited with the Rule's enduring to the present day. Find a copy of the Rule and comment on any two of its chapters. What is contained within each of your two chosen chapters? Why are these topics important to cenobitical life? How might following these chapters of the Rule help a monk get to Heaven?

4. The introduction mentions bias against missionaries. Respond to someone who said the following: "Missionaries cause destruction. They find native peoples, and then force western conceptions of God on them. Christian missionaries destroy the families and culture of natives, who have been living just fine without Christianity."

5. What are three ways that every Christian today can evangelize?

6. Discuss Sts. Cyril and Methodius and the trials which they faced. How did their methods exemplify the Church's respect for different cultures?

7. By the end of the twentieth century, practically every nation discussed in this chapter has suffered in its practice of Christianity after the effects of materialism, communism, and war. For example, in the states within the former East Germany, more than seventy percent of the people are not baptized. What do you think might be the effects of the loss of faith in these European cultures? How might things be changed?

8. Bible churches and even some of the Reformation era churches claim that by the presence of statues and icons, the Catholic Church violates the First Commandment. What arguments would you give, for example, that veneration of a statue of Mary is not idol worship?

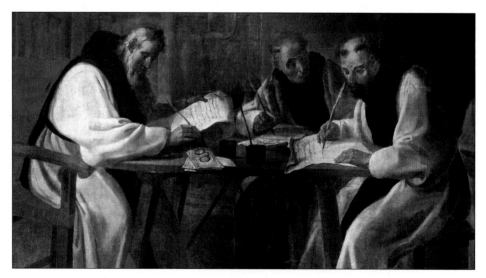

Once a student at the monastery learned Latin, he was taught Sacred Scriptures,
the writings of the Church Fathers, geometry, and music for the singing of the Divine Office.

FROM THE CATECHISM

817 In fact, "in this one and only Church of God from its very beginnings there arose certain rifts, which the Apostle strongly censures as damnable. But in subsequent centuries much more serious dissensions appeared and large communities became separated from full communion with the Catholic Church – for which, often enough, men of both sides were to blame" (UR 3 § 1). The ruptures that wound the unity of Christ's Body – here we must distinguish heresy, apostasy, and schism (cf. CIC, can. 751) – do not occur without human sin:

> Where there are sins, there are also divisions, schisms, heresies, and disputes. Where there is virtue, however, there also are harmony and unity, from which arise the one heart and one soul of all believers (Origen, Hom. in Ezech. 9, 1: PG 13, 732).

818 "However, one cannot charge with the sin of the separation those who at present are born into these communities [that resulted from such separation] and in them are brought up in the faith of Christ, and the Catholic Church accepts them with respect and affection as brothers.... All who have been justified by faith in Baptism are incorporated into Christ; they therefore have a right to be called Christians, and with good reason are accepted as brothers in the Lord by the children of the Catholic Church" (UR 3 § 1).

819 "Furthermore, many elements of sanctification and of truth" (LG 8 § 2) are found outside the visible confines of the Catholic Church: "the written Word of God; the life of grace; faith, hope, and charity, with the other interior gifts of the Holy Spirit, as well as visible elements" (UR 3 § 2; cf. LG 15). Christ's Spirit uses these Churches and ecclesial communities as means of salvation, whose power derives from the fullness of grace and truth that Christ has entrusted to the Catholic Church. All these blessings come from Christ and lead to him (cf. UR 3), and are in themselves calls to "Catholic unity" (cf. LG 8).

849 The missionary mandate. "Having been divinely sent to the nations that she might be 'the universal sacrament of salvation,' the Church, in obedience to the command of her founder and because it is demanded by her own essential universality, strives to preach the Gospel to all men" (AG 1; cf. Mt 16:15): "Go therefore and make disciples of all nations, baptizing them in the name of the Father and of the Son and of the Holy Spirit, teaching them to observe all that I have commanded you; and Lo, I am with you always, until the close of the age" (Mt 28:19-20).

850 The origin and purpose of mission. The Lord's missionary mandate is ultimately grounded in the eternal love of the Most Holy Trinity: "The Church on earth is by her nature missionary since, according to the plan of the Father, she has as her origin the mission of the Son and the Holy Spirit" (AG 2). The ultimate purpose of mission is none other than to make men share in the communion between the Father and the Son in their Spirit of love (cf. John Paul II, RMiss 23).

851 Missionary motivation. It is from God's love for all men that the Church in every age receives both the obligation and the vigor of her missionary dynamism, "for the love of Christ urges us on" (2 Cor 5:14; cf. AA 6; RMiss 11). Indeed, God "desires all men to be saved and to come to the knowledge of the truth" (1 Tm 2:4); that is, God wills the salvation of everyone through the knowledge of the truth. Salvation is found in the truth. Those who obey the prompting of the Spirit of truth are already on the way of salvation. But the Church, to whom this truth has been entrusted, must go out to meet their desire, so as to bring them the truth. Because she believes in God's universal plan of salvation, the Church must be missionary.

FROM THE CATECHISM Continued

916 The state of consecrated life is thus one way of experiencing a "more intimate" consecration, rooted in Baptism and dedicated totally to God (cf. PC 5). In the consecrated life, Christ's faithful, moved by the Holy Spirit, propose to follow Christ more nearly, to give themselves to God who is loved above all and, pursuing the perfection of charity in the service of the Kingdom, to signify and proclaim in the Church the glory of the world to come (cf. CIC, can. 573).

922 From apostolic times Christian virgins (cf. 1 Cor 7:34-36) and widows (cf. John Paul II, Vita consecrata 7), called by the Lord to cling only to him with greater freedom of heart, body, and spirit, have decided with the Church's approval to live in the respective status of virginity or perpetual chastity "for the sake of the Kingdom of heaven" (Mt 19:12).

925 Religious life was born in the East during the first centuries of Christianity. Lived within institutes canonically erected by the Church, it is distinguished from other forms of consecrated life by its liturgical character, public profession of the evangelical counsels, fraternal life led in common, and witness given to the union of Christ with the Church (cf. CIC, cann. 607; 573; UR 15).

2502 Sacred art is true and beautiful when its form corresponds to its particular vocation: evoking and glorifying, in faith and adoration, the transcendent mystery of God – the surpassing invisible beauty of truth and love visible in Christ, who "reflects the glory of God and bears the very stamp of his nature," in whom "the whole fullness of deity dwells bodily" (Heb 1:3; Col 2:9). This spiritual beauty of God is reflected in the most holy Virgin Mother of God, the angels, and saints. Genuine sacred art draws man to adoration, to prayer, and to the love of God, Creator and Savior, the Holy One and Sanctifier.

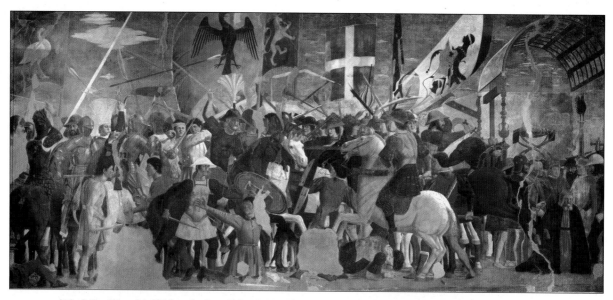

At the Battle of Nineveh in 627, Byzantine forces led by Flavius Heraclius Augustus, Byzantine emperor from 610 to 641, defeated the Persian forces of King Chosroe. Heraclius took for himself the title of *Basileus,* the Greek word for "emperor," and that title was used by the eastern Roman emperors for the next 800 years. Heraclius also discontinued the use of Latin as the empire's official language, replacing it with Greek. Although the empire called itself Roman throughout the rest of its history, it was in reality a Hellenic empire from Heraclius onward.

Collapse, Corruption, And Reform In Europe And The Church

This period contained some of the worst scandals in the history of the Church. In response, saintly priests, monks and nuns brought about some of the most important reforms in Christian history.

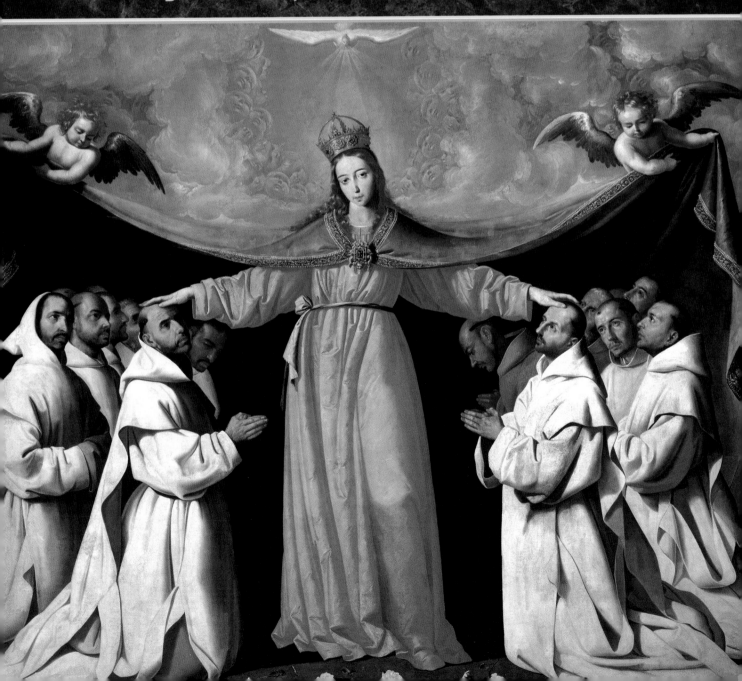

CHAPTER 4

Collapse, Corruption, And Reform In Europe And The Church

The end of Charlemagne's reign in 814 marked the end of a delicate, but nonetheless satisfactory, balance of power in Western Europe between the Papal States on the one hand and their Frankish protectors on the other. Although Charlemagne involved himself excessively in ecclesiastical affairs, he never lost his respect for the proper autonomy of the Church, and even when he interfered, he retained a pious and respectful attitude toward her spiritual mission. Further, Charlemagne's steel will and heavy hand proved more than a match for the Roman nobility who, well before the emperor's reign, had pestered the Church with intrigue and conspiracies. But upon Charlemagne's death these different Roman factions returned more powerfully than ever. The papacy was, by this time, a very lucrative and strategic state office to hold. Sadly, the Holy See was often viewed as a political pawn to be seized and used by anyone with the power to do so. Thus three parties, as it were, struggled for the control of the papacy: leaders within the Church herself, the Roman nobles, and the Holy Roman Emperors (successors of Charlemagne). This period, lasting roughly from 814 to 1046, contains some of the worst scandals that have ever visited the Church. At the same time, this period also contains the most important ecclesiastical reformations since the earliest days of Christianity. These reforms were launched and implemented by many saintly priests, monks, and nuns. Where sin and corruption abounded among corrupt bishops and abbots, grace abounded all the more in such saints as Pope Nicholas I, Cyril and Methodius, Pope Gregory VII, and the many anonymous holy monks of Cluny, France.

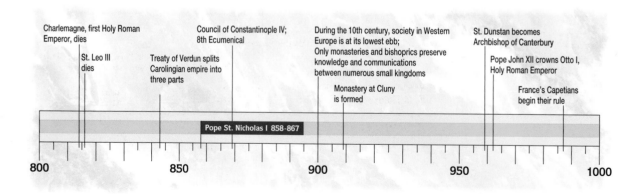

Charlemagne, first Holy Roman Emperor, dies

St. Leo III dies

Treaty of Verdun splits Carolingian empire into three parts

Council of Constantinople IV; 8th Ecumenical

During the 10th century, society in Western Europe is at its lowest ebb; Only monasteries and bishoprics preserve knowledge and communications between numerous small kingdoms

Monastery at Cluny is formed

St. Dunstan becomes Archbishop of Canterbury

Pope John XII crowns Otto I, Holy Roman Emperor

France's Capetians begin their rule

Pope St. Nicholas I 858-867

800   850   900   950   1000

PART I

The Carolingian World Collapses

Charlemagne died in 814 and was succeeded by his son, Louis the Pious (814-830). Louis, though well-intentioned, lacked the political talent and strength of his father. Upon his death, he would make one of his worst mistakes by dividing the kingdom among his three sons: Lothar, who would become emperor, Charles, and Louis the German.

For a time, his sons jockeyed for power before signing the Treaty of Verdun in 843. This treaty divided the Carolingian empire into a western kingdom including France (Charles), a middle kingdom that stretched from the Low Countries to northern Italy (Lothar), and an eastern kingdom comprised of Germany (Louis). The middle kingdom, lacking true geographical or ethnic borders, collapsed immediately. Parts of it were brought into the German kingdom later in the tenth and eleventh centuries. Other parts, such as Alsace-Lorraine, became the objects of centuries-long conflict between France and Germany.

Simultaneous with the destruction of Carolingian unity was the influx of a new breed of invaders. Christian Europe, which under Charlemagne had defended and expanded its existing borders, came under attack from three different fronts after his death. The Saracens (Muslims) pressed from the south and advanced as far as Rome, the Vikings pressed from the north, attacking Paris, and the Slavs and Magyars advanced from the east.

THE RISE OF FEUDALISM

As the Carolingian authority collapsed, a new system of organization emerged throughout western society. First, the Carolingian empire broke down into about fifty duchies, which spread across France and Italy and throughout Germany. Because few of these duchies were strong enough to protect all those living under their domain, eventually even smaller communities formed themselves around towns or monasteries. These communities built castles or fortifications and usually allied themselves around one lord.

This emergent system, known as feudalism, is most simply understood as a contractual system between the king and his vassals (wealthy, landowning lords) and the remainder of the population, which included common villagers, farm-workers, and even religious. Though a relatively simple arrangement, feudalism came to organize the politics, economy, and social life throughout Medieval Europe. Ownership of land accorded one rights, but it also accorded one duties, and this held both

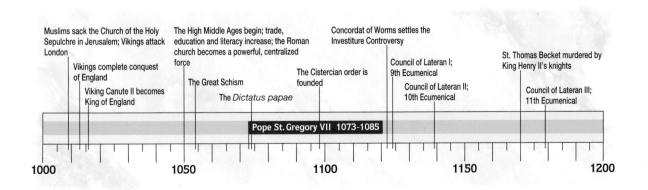

Muslims sack the Church of the Holy Sepulchre in Jerusalem; Vikings attack London

Vikings complete conquest of England

Viking Canute II becomes King of England

The High Middle Ages begin; trade, education and literacy increase; the Roman church becomes a powerful, centralized force

The Great Schism

The *Dictatus papae*

Concordat of Worms settles the Investiture Controversy

Council of Lateran I; 9th Ecumenical

Council of Lateran II; 10th Ecumenical

The Cistercian order is founded

St. Thomas Becket murdered by King Henry II's knights

Council of Lateran III; 11th Ecumenical

Pope St. Gregory VII 1073-1085

1000   1050   1100   1150   1200

INVASIONS OF EUROPE, 7TH TO 10TH CENTURIES

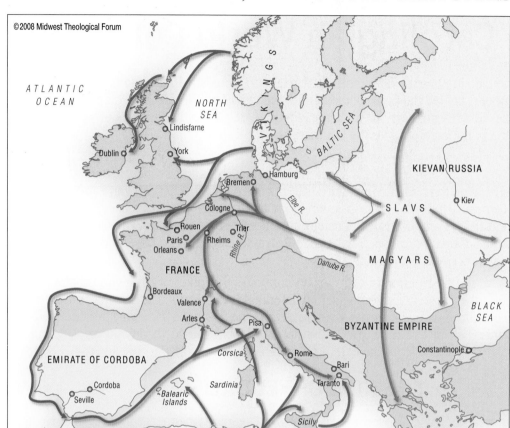

©2008 Midwest Theological Forum

ATLANTIC OCEAN

NORTH SEA

VIKINGS

BALTIC SEA

KIEVAN RUSSIA

Lindisfarne

Dublin

York

Bremen

Hamburg

Kiev

Cologne

Elbe R.

SLAVS

Rouen

Trier

Paris

Rheims

Rhine R.

Orleans

FRANCE

Danube R.

MAGYARS

Bordeaux

Valence

Arles

Pisa

BLACK SEA

Corsica

Rome

BYZANTINE EMPIRE

Constantinople

EMIRATE OF CORDOBA

Cordoba

Sardinia

Bari

Taranto

Seville

Balearic Islands

Sicily

MUSLIMS

Tunis

Kairouan

MEDITERRANEAN SEA

Western Christendom	Slav expansion, to 700
Eastern Christendom	Viking invasions, 8th and 9th centuries
Pagan lands	Magyar invasions, 10th century
Islamic empire	Muslim invasions, 9th and 10th centuries

0   100   200   300 miles

0   250   500 km

for secular and religious landholders. Therefore, in return for the lord's military protection against foreign or domestic foes, his vassals (those who were under his rule) would pay him in labor or services. Some of his vassals would have to serve in his army. There were, of course, different levels of vassals. Some were landowners themselves, who chose to ally themselves around a more powerful lord. Others, by far the majority, were serfs, who barely enjoyed any freedom since they were completely tied to the land and lord they were serving. A feudal kingdom was a vast pyramid of such arrangements, with many levels of lord and vassals at the apex of which stood the king and his attendant dukes.

FEUDALISM AND THE CHURCH

In exchange for protecting the Church, some secular rulers demanded control over episcopal appointments. This was nothing new. Both Charlemagne and the Eastern emperors claimed the right to appoint bishops, but this right was always held in check by a strong, central Church. Now, with the papacy under the thumb of the emperor and Roman nobility, and the precarious political situation of the region, some of these rulers took it upon themselves to become the ultimate authorities of the Church. This exaggerated secular interference in ecclesiastical affairs spawned two terrible abuses in the Church: nepotism and simony. Nepotism is the appointment of family members to important positions of authority; and simony, in this context, is the selling of ecclesiastical offices by either secular or spiritual rulers. Many lords believed they could distribute ecclesiastical offices just as they would secular ones. For instance, it was not uncommon for a powerful lord either to sell a bishopric to the highest bidder or to install his own son as bishop.

On the ecclesiastical side, bishops and abbots often received extra income from royal benefices that was distinct from the income of their community. Even more scandalously, several bishops and abbots were known to have married and had children. Many of these bishops and abbots then bequeathed to their eldest son their own ecclesiastical title! These abuses were more destructive to the work of the Church than the violence hurled at the people of God during the time of the Roman persecutions. Hence, when reform came to the Church (as it soon would), monastic and episcopal abuse, in the form of nepotism and simony, was one of the first issues to be addressed.

THE VIKING INVASIONS

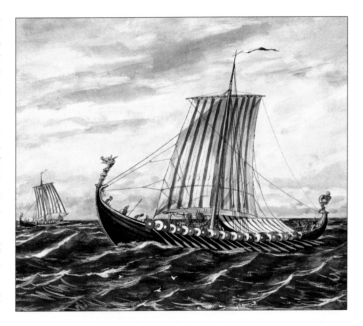

Besides the internal decay of monastic life in these centuries, a very real external threat helped thwart for some time any effective monastic reform. This threat materialized in the figures of the Norsemen, or Vikings, who originated in Scandinavia and, beginning in the late eighth century, wreaked havoc on Europe for nearly three hundred years. The Vikings were not a centrally governed empire, like Persia or Byzantium; rather, they were small bands organized and led by local chieftains. The Norsemen, originating in Norway, concentrated their attacks upon England, Ireland, and Scotland. Those from present day Denmark hit nearly every major European city.

Carolingian Europe was poorly equipped to handle the Viking invasions. The factions that took hold after the death of Charlemagne were too busy fighting among themselves to mount a reliable defense against these foreign invaders. The Vikings instilled overwhelming dread in the Christians of Medieval Europe as they were warriors of unparalleled skill on both sea and land, and they were guilty of unimagined cruelty and mercilessness in their plunder and slaughter.

With their great mobility and swift ships, it did not take long for the Norsemen to discover that the monasteries, particularly of Ireland, England, and along the major rivers in Germany and France, were the repository of Carolingian society's wealth. The Vikings began to occupy the mouth of major rivers in northern Europe as bases from which they might raid every Church and monastery they could find.

The combination of the Norse threat and internal decay of monastic life led to a weakening of monasteries' civilizing influence upon society. Much of their learning, both secular and religious, was forgotten, their discipline fell by the wayside, and some abbots were no better than brigands, who, in order to protect their own monasteries from the Vikings, would lead raids upon other monasteries for food and money.

PART II

Cluny and Monastic Reform

THE FOUNDING

In 909/10 William the Pious, Duke of Aquitaine and a strong supporter of reform, generously and without thought of recompense, donated land in the little town of Cluny in Burgundy, France for the founding of a new monastery.

St. Berno, the first abbot (909/10-927) of the monastery, settled at Cluny with twelve companions. Together they instituted a renewed commitment to the Rule of St. Benedict. The monks imposed demanding austerities on themselves, and put all of their energies into giving glory to God. Soon St. Berno's reputation grew, and Cluny began to be recognized as a center of saintliness in troubled times. Before Berno's death, the Cluniac model was adopted by five or six neighboring monasteries for the purpose of reform; and, even more impressively, over the next two centuries four saints assumed the abbotship of Cluny.

Berno's first successor, St. Odo (927-942), greatly extended the influence of Cluny. Many monasteries in southern France and even some in Italy reformed themselves using the renewed Benedictine rule. One important difference between Cluny and other monastic communities was

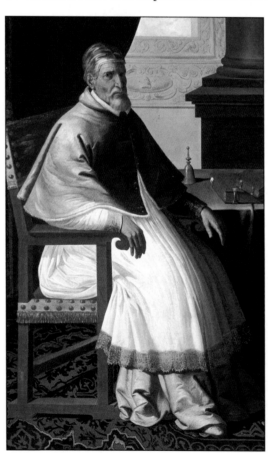

Bl. Urban II consecrated the high altar of the Cluny Church in 1095.

the role played by the abbot. The Cluny monks—in all their various incorporated monasteries—had only one abbot, that of Cluny. Other monasteries followed the tradition of placing an abbot over each individual monastery. Hence the abbot of Cluny was responsible not only for his own monastery at Cluny, but also for all those monasteries that had joined his rule. This helped curb abuse, since it kept wayward abbots from assuming control of monasteries for their own advantage.

The prestige of the monastery spread, and in 1088 Cluny built a new church. Bl. Urban II, a Cluniac monk and one of the period's most upright popes, consecrated the high altar in 1095, and Pope Innocent II consecrated the entire church upon its completion in 1132. At its time of construction the church at Cluny was Europe's largest at 555 feet long.

CLUNIAC SPIRITUALITY

How did the Cluniac monks live out their vocation differently from the regular Benedictine monks? First, as has been noted, the monks at Cluny reinstituted a strict adherence to Benedictine rule. Second, they placed greater emphasis upon the spiritual life of the individual monk. The idea was that a community of holy men was built on the

LIFE AS A MONK AT CLUNY

The daily schedule by which monks at Cluny lived their lives stood in sharp contrast to some other monasteries of the time. The horarium (daily schedule) followed by the monks of Cluny allocated a great portion of time to religious ceremony, and often the observances of Mass and other rites would require that the monks spend almost the entire day in prayer. Psalms and votive offerings were added to the Divine Office, and following the custom introduced into monasteries in France by St. Benedict of Aniane, other devotional exercises were added as well, increasing the hours of the Divine Office. Apart from the increase in the hours of the Divine Office, however, Cluniac observances were similar to that of the Benedictines.

When possible, Cluniac monks would perform as little manual labor as possible to dedicate more time to prayer. Thus, most tasks were delegated to lay servants. In the poorer monasteries further removed from Cluny, however, the monks would have to perform more work in order to survive. While this situation may not have been ideal, it should be noted that every monk was required to spend some years at Cluny itself.

The monks at Cluny placed much emphasis on the observance of the rule of silence in their houses. Conversation was only allowed at certain times and in certain areas. Whenever communication became absolutely necessary, hand gesturing was used. These gestures may have become quite sophisticated over time.

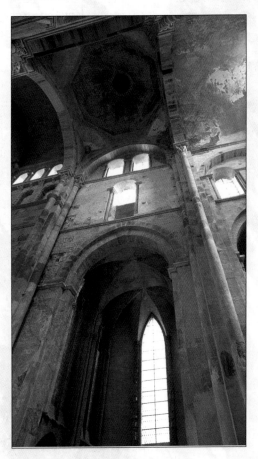

The third church (above) built at the Benedictine Abbey of Cluny was, at the time, the largest church in Christendom.
It was designed by the monk Gunzo. Begun in 1088 and consecrated by Pope Innocent II in 1132, the "great church" or Cluny III was a structure of overwhelming magnificence. The five-aisled nave echoed that of Old St. Peter's in Rome, and unusual for the architectural period, Cluny III had two sets of transepts (the shorter length of the "crossing" of a cruciform church). Only one transept with a bell tower survives today (shown at right). By the time of the French Revolution in 1790 the monks were persecuted by the "enlightened" leaders of the Revolution. As a result, they were suppressed in France, and the Abbey at Cluny was almost completely demolished.

holiness of each member. To this end they reinstated the divine office, which in some monasteries had fallen out of fashion, and decreased manual labor so as to allot more time for spiritual reflection. As an aid to this spiritual reflection, Cluny also lengthened the divine office and the liturgy. The goal was active, continuous, prayer, whether liturgical or meditative, and a close emulation of the life of Christ.

Through asceticism the monk aimed to dwell in the depths of the heart of Christ. Through mastering the body the monks were not only able to free their hearts to love Christ, they were also better equipped to unite themselves to his cross. Through their hidden lives dedicated to prayer and penance, the monks would obtain the grace of conversion of so many individuals alienated from God and the grace to live their faith as well. It was precisely the prayer and self-denial of these monks that revitalized and energized the Church. Such is the efficacy of a life of contemplation, that it bears its fruits across all time and space.

THE INFLUENCE OF THE CLUNIAC MONKS

Within just one hundred years, the monks of Cluny were a force to be reckoned with in the Church. As more and more monasteries signed on to the Cluniac reform, their ranks swelled, and by the year 1100, one thousand four hundred fifty houses inhabited by over ten thousand monks were all under the rule of Cluny.

Neither was Cluny's success confined to monastic communities. As word of the sanctity of Cluny spread, more and more bishops and secular rulers supported their reforms. In 1016 Pope Benedict VIII granted a special privilegium to Cluny: the monastery was to be absolutely free from the authority of kings, bishops, and nobles. Cluny answered directly to the papacy as its final authority. This freed Cluny from the troublesome accompaniments of feudalism already discussed, such as nepotism and simony.

Several of Cluny's monks became the leading churchmen of their day. Abbot Hugh the Great (1049-1109) was the most important churchman of his time and played a pivotal role in the lay investiture controversy. Cardinal Humbert and Frederick of Lorraine, the papal legates to Constantinople, excommunicated the patriarch of Constantinople as part of the Great Schism of 1054. Otto of Lagery became Bl. Urban II, the first pope to preach the Crusades. St. Peter Damian (1007-1072) became the most respected contemporary theologian in Europe.

Cluny exercised considerable influence well into the twelfth century. In the thirteenth century, it reformed itself under the Cistercian model, which by this time had surpassed Cluny in influence and prestige. The later Medieval period saw a precipitous decline in Cluny's influence, which ended in its physical destruction during the French Revolution in 1790.

PART III

The New Temporal Orders

THE OTTONIAN EMPIRE (HOLY ROMAN EMPIRE)

OTTO I, THE GREAT (936-973)

Otto's intention was to secure his own royal power through a mutually beneficial alliance with the Church. He was crowned in Aachen (Germany) by the archbishop of Mainz, which served

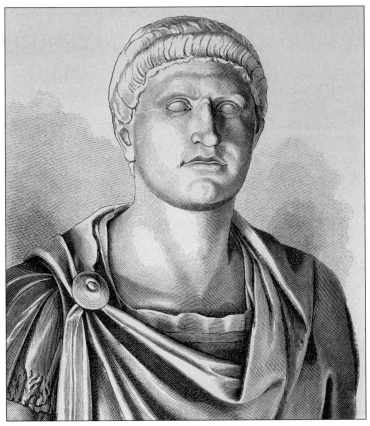

OTTO I, THE GREAT

In 962 Otto the Great traveled to Rome, where Pope John XII crowned him Holy Roman Emperor. The Ottonian Empire provided the Church with the temporal protection that the Carolingian Empire had provided in the previous century, but the Ottonian line ultimately entangled the Church in the lay investiture controversy and similar abuses of authority.

the double purpose of invoking the memory of Charlemagne's authority and wedding the Church to the Ottonian dynasty.

The Ottonian line exercised its influence over the Church in Germany in three different ways: first, through lay investiture, i.e., the appointment of bishops and abbots by secular rulers; second, through the assertion of royal power over proprietary churches, which gave the landowner on which a church stood power to make ecclesiastical appointments; and third, through appropriation of ecclesiastical funds for the royal coffers. In addition, many German ecclesiastical office-holders were vested with secular powers by the royal house in exchange for their allegiance.

By 950 the wealth and power of Germany was unrivaled. And in 955 Otto I decisively defeated the Magyars at the Battle of Lechfeld, winning the support of Western Europe. In 962 Otto I traveled to Rome, where Pope John XII crowned him emperor.

OTTO III AND POPE SYLVESTER II

It was Otto III's Byzantine mother and his grandmother who ruled during his regency. Otto III (983-1002) spent the majority of his reign in Rome with Gerbert of Aurillac, the greatest Latin scholar of his day. Gerbvert had studied in Spain under the Muslims, and this gave him the opportunity to study philosophy and mathematics at Cordoba in an age when the Muslim thinkers were making remarkable headway in both subjects. (Not only had the Muslims preserved ancient Greek writings by conquering Hellenistic cultures, but also they were the sole possessors of most of Aristotle's works.)

Through his power over ecclesiastical affairs, Otto III raised Gerbert to the See of St. Peter as Pope Sylvester II. Together Otto and Sylvester II hoped to build a new empire based in Rome that would incorporate all of Europe. Otto III helped to bring the Poles into the empire in the hopes that a German-Slav contest for eastern hegemony could be averted. Finally, Sylvester II thought that an empire under Otto would eventually secure a lasting peace, which would assist the Church in concentrating on her spiritual mission.

Though Otto III died prematurely in 1002 and Pope Sylvester the following year, their cooperation caused serious difficulties for the Church. Their joint efforts accentuated the problem of temporal interference with ecclesiastical affairs, which gave rise to the lay investiture crisis.

SAINTLY RULERS:
EMPEROR ST. HENRY II AND QUEEN ST. CUNEGOND

St. Henry II (1002-1024), who was cousin to Otto III, succeeded him as emperor. St. Henry II abandoned Otto's grandiose plans of reinstituting a Holy Roman Empire, and was content to maintain his rule over the Italian peninsula. Though a weak and sickly man, St. Henry II traveled throughout his kingdom to maintain peace and ensure that justice was being served.

He was an ardent Catholic and a true reformer and did much to support the Cluny monks. He did, however, involve himself excessively in ecclesiastical governance – and this was true of virtually all leaders of his day–but he did so with grace and humility.

Emperor St. Henry II and Queen St. Cunegond lived a blessed married life. After their deaths, they were both canonized by the Church. Both Sts. Henry II and Cunegond are buried in the cathedral at Bamberg, Germany. In fact, one can view their heads encased in glass with golden crowns.

CAPETIAN FRANCE

In the west, the Carolingian line ended in 987, whereupon Hugh Capet, with the blessing of the Church, became the king of France. The Capetian line would rule France for many centuries, but initially lacked the power to rule the entire area under one centralized government.

NORMANDY: THE VIKINGS,
WILLIAM THE CONQUEROR, AND LANFRANC

One part of France that resisted Capetian rule was Normandy. Normandy first took shape as a duchy in 911 under a band of Norsemen led by the warrior-king Rollo. Rollo planned to establish Normandy as a viable kingdom, and by 980 – chiefly through intermarriage and adaptation–Rollo's band of Vikings transformed this once-backward part of Europe into a formidable power.

The Normans imposed the status of vassalage upon the existing nobility and developed allegiances with the monasteries in the area. Monks, besides providing some amount of credibility to Norman rule, helped raise the cultural bar through their education and writings.

The French Capetian king, Henry I, made the final attempt to bring the Norman duke, William the

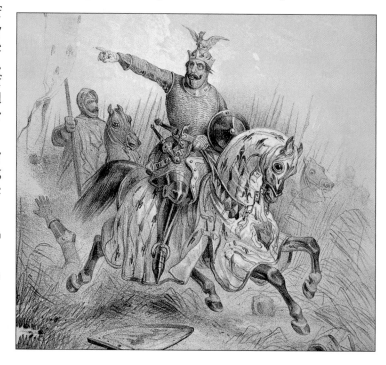

William I (ca. 1027 - September 9, 1087), was King of England from 1066 to 1087. William was the only son of Robert the Magnificent, Duke of Normandy, and Herleva, the daughter of a tanner. Born in Falaise, Normandy, now in France, William succeeded to the throne of England by right of conquest by winning the Battle of Hastings in October of 1066 in what has become known as the Norman Conquest.

William was crowned King of England on December 25, 1066 in Westminster Abbey.

Conqueror (reigned 1035-1087), under his control in the 1040s. William I had the effective support of the nobility and the local church, and Normandy maintained its autonomy in feudal France. Later, in 1066, William headed the last successful invasion of England.

LANFRANC, THE NORMAN ARCHBISHOP OF CANTERBURY

The most important monk brought to Normandy by the Viking dukes was Lanfranc (ca. 1010-1089). He entered the chief monastery founded by the Normans at Bec, located between Rouen and Lisieux, France. At Bec he was a famed educator and prior (his most famous student was St. Anselm) and under William the Conqueror, Lanfranc became the first Archbishop of Canterbury.

Lanfranc was a strong administrator who transformed Bec from an impoverished monastery into one of the leading centers of learning of its day. Equally impressive, he managed to negotiate his allegiance to Church and State in a truly remarkable way. He served at first as counselor to King William I, and later even served as a skilled regent during the king's travels to the continent. But his chief allegiance as Archbishop of Canterbury was to Rome, and though his dual responsibilities seemed at times to be a source of conflict, Lanfranc adroitly walked through the two worlds. Lanfranc supported the reforms of his day, specifically those enforcing clerical celibacy and curbing simony. On the issue of lay investiture, however, he tended to side with secular rulers against the Church. Nonetheless, Lanfranc continually supported the popes even at their weakest moments. Although he supported the secular lords, he refused to recognize any of their anti-popes, even going so far as to send financial aid to the legitimate popes in need.

William I of England likewise remained on good terms with the pope even though he continued to appoint bishops. Because William appointed such good and holy men to these offices, he avoided any direct conflict with Rome.

PART IV

The Lay Investiture Controversies

On the surface, the issue of the lay investiture conflict was relatively clear and could be formulated in a simple question: Who should appoint bishops, secular or religious leaders? But in reality, the depths of this controversy were far more complex. Due to the lack of any clear delineation between the powers of Church and State, those who hoped to rule the State in more than a nominal sense were almost forced to have a hand in ecclesiastical affairs as well. It was common at that time that bishops and abbots of powerful dioceses and monasteries wield considerable political influence. While in principle it was wrong for secular leaders to have any hand in Church matters, given the current state of affairs, it was quite difficult to avoid this secular interference. The crisscrossing of secular and religious authority left little room on either side of the dispute. Moreover, it needs to be pointed out that lay investiture had been going on since the reign of Charlemagne, and in certain cases it worked to the Church's advantage. However, in many instances it proved disastrous. Due to the negative effect lay investiture had on the Church, the reforming popes realized that they needed to retain control over appointments of bishops, thereby reducing the chance of out-and-out political corruption in the episcopacy.

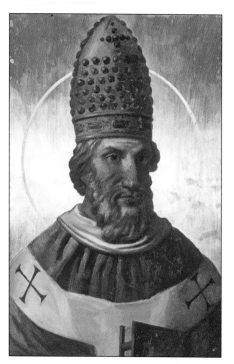

POPE ST. GREGORY VII

Hildebrand, a Cluniac monk and native Roman, was elected Pope Gregory VII in 1073 and served until 1085. Hildebrand entered the Church as a young man, and was for some time an influential leader in the College of Cardinals. In addition, he carried out important tasks for his papal predecessors, particularly for Pope Alexander II (1061-1073). At Alexander II's funeral, the crowd is said to have shouted enthusiastically for Hildebrand as pope. He initially resisted, but understood their call to reflect God's will. And so at fifty-three years of age, Hildebrand took the name Gregory VII. Hildebrand was blessed with a penetrating mind, an iron will, much energy, and relentless perseverance in the face of adversity.

THE DICTATUS PAPÆ

St. Gregory VII wasted little time in making his intentions of reform known. Within a year of becoming pope, he issued a decree called Dictatus Papæ. St. Gregory asserted in his decree that the pope possessed specific powers bestowed by God that rested on him alone. These powers most notably included the power to convene and ratify a council, to define tenets of the faith, and to appoint, transfer, and remove bishops from office. But St. Gregory went further with this, and claimed that the papacy had the power to depose temporal rulers. Furthermore, subjects of any temporal ruler had the right to appeal to the papacy in order to bring charges against their sovereign.

St. Gregory levied stiff penalties for the practice of simony. Anyone who obtained ordination or spiritual benefice through the practice of simony was excluded from the Church hierarchy and lost his authority of governance. In addition, any priest guilty of fornication was barred from saying the Mass, which in effect stripped the priest of his most important function in the Church and the means for his financial support. All church clerics were to avoid and shun any cleric who failed to abide by the pope's decrees.

In addition to St. Gregory's punitive measures, he sought to codify the law of the Church, called canon law, as an effective measure to avoid future abuse. While this project was not completed in his lifetime, he is considered to be the "father of canon law."

"TO GO TO CANOSSA": THE HUMILIATION OF EMPEROR HENRY IV

St. Gregory VII had taken advantage of the papacy's practice of crowning the emperor in order to claim that the papacy held final say on matters of temporal rule. This perceived usurpation of temporal rule placed the Holy Roman Emperor, Henry IV, on a collision course with the pope.

In defiance of the papal decree, Henry on his own appointed the bishop of Milan. St. Gregory VII asked Henry to refrain from carrying out the appointment. Henry declined the pope's request. St. Gregory acted quickly and severely in response, declaring Henry deposed as emperor, and releasing his subjects from his rule. This proved decisive since Henry did not enjoy popular support at home and many of his subjects were opposed to his strong, autocratic rule.

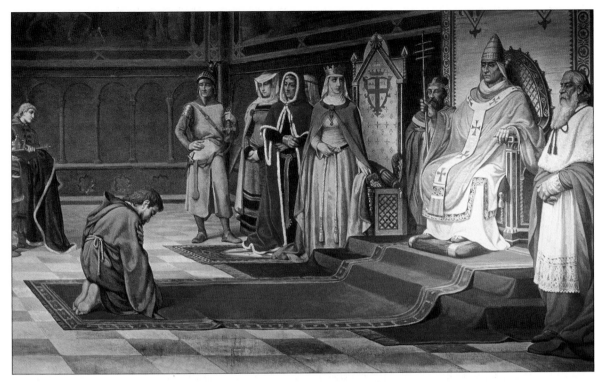

After observing Henry IV's contrition for three days, St. Gregory VII heard Henry's confession, granted him absolution, and restored his royal status.

St. Gregory VII not only deposed Henry IV, but he also excommunicated him. (Excommunication is a censure from a bishop stating a person is cut off from communion with the Church because he is in a persistent state of mortal sin.) The act of excommunication had rarely been used, and caused many of the bishops and important abbots in Germany who had previously supported Henry's cause to withdraw. Since two-thirds of Germany was under the immediate authority of bishops who owned most of the land, it followed that two-thirds of Henry's potential and taxing military power disappeared overnight.

Henry for a time was thus strategically outflanked by the pope. His only recourse was to obtain the pope's forgiveness, thereby being accepted back into the Church, and regaining his office – all before the pope could appoint a new emperor to take his place.

On January 25, 1077, Henry IV set out for Canossa, Italy, with a small party. St. Gregory VII and his entourage were staying there with the Countess Mathilda of Tuscany. Mathilda, who happened to be a relative of Henry, was the first of a group of influential Medieval women who demonstrated great influence at key political and spiritual moments on account of their holiness and wisdom.

Henry arrived at Canossa and stood barefoot in the snow outside the gates of Mathilda's villa for three days. He was dressed in sackcloth. Still, the pope refused to meet with him. St. Gregory doubted Henry's true contrition, and rightfully so. By repenting of his crime, Henry would be reinstituted in the Church and would thereby gain the military support of the bishops he had lost. For some time St. Gregory held back.

Hugh of Cluny, the revered abbot of the famed monastery, appeared on the scene. More than anyone else, he forced St. Gregory's hand. According to long-standing tradition and the rules of the Church, a penitent who requests forgiveness cannot be turned away. St. Gregory knew that he could not dismiss the advice of Hugh, who was the most respected churchman of the day.

Thus after three days St. Gregory relented and agreed to meet with Henry. St. Gregory heard the emperor's confession, granted him absolution, restored his royal status, and admonished him to observe all of the papal decrees.

For a time it appeared that St. Gregory had achieved a tremendous victory: the most important temporal ruler in Christendom had bent to the pope's will. This victory did not last long. Within a year Henry had again rejected St. Gregory's authority and installed Clement III as anti-pope, (i.e., someone who is not–but claims to be–the legitimate successor of St. Peter). St. Gregory and his successors turned to the Normans for protection.

In the end, St. Gregory fled from Henry's army to southern Italy where he died in exile. Henry IV's fate was not much better since he had to fight the nobility and his own son to maintain power.

CONCORDAT OF WORMS

Canossa did not end the struggle between the papacy and the Holy Roman Emperors. Similar, though less dramatic, struggles took place in England and France. After many such battles, the Concordat of Worms (1122) officially ended the investiture matter with a new understanding between the Church and the Holy Roman Empire.

The Concordat of Worms had two parts. First, it left spiritual investiture to the Church alone, and temporal investiture to civil authorities. The emperor renounced all claims to invest churchmen with ring and crosier – symbols of spiritual authority – and had to permit the free election of bishops. The practice of simony was again condemned. The emperor, however, retained veto power over the electoral process since he had the right to invest churchmen with signs of temporal authority. Thus, if an emperor did not like a candidate for the episcopacy, he could withhold the temporal power accompanying the post, and indirectly force the Church to pick another candidate.

INVESTITURE CONFLICT AND THE ENGLISH CHURCH (1154-1189)

Henry II was the most powerful of all Medieval English monarchs. The Church in England had developed its own set of courts and laws independent of the secular administration, but Henry II desired to consolidate the legal structures of England and to place all authority under the crown. Moreover, the English Church, it seemed to him, was growing too powerful and independent. To accomplish this task he chose as Archbishop of Canterbury his trusted friend and advisor St. Thomas à Becket.

St. Thomas à Becket had been Henry II's Chancellor and had worked with him to strengthen the powers of the state. Aware of Henry II's designs for changes within the governance of the English Church – changes that, as archbishop, St. Thomas à Becket knew he could not support or allow – he warned Henry II not to make him archbishop. Henry II and Cardinal Henry of Posa pressured St. Thomas à Becket to accept the position, and he ultimately accepted. With his elevation, he resigned his position as Chancellor and undertook a life of prayer and penance. He resisted the king's effort to overstep his boundaries in violating canon law.

CONSTITUTIONS OF CLARENDON

Henry II asserted his royal authority in the Constitutions of Clarendon in 1164. The king attempted to gain control over the revenues of episcopal sees and abbeys and sought to control the election of all abbots and bishops. All clerics were to be tried in civil courts. Any appeal to Rome first required the consent of the king. The king's court was to be the last resort for ecclesiastical appeals.

St. Thomas à Becket stood almost alone in England in his absolute opposition to the Constitutions of Clarendon, but Pope Alexander III also refused to recognize them. St. Thomas à Becket was forced to flee to France to escape the king's wrath, and he spent time with some Cistercians before Henry II threatened the entire order if they did not give him up. At the same time, fearing excommunication, Henry II feigned reconciliation with St. Thomas à Becket. He returned to England and continued to fight against the king's programs. Out of desperation, Henry II asked if anyone could rid him of this priest. St. Thomas à Becket was murdered in the cathedral by a band of knights in 1170. To what extent Henry II was involved with the murder is unknown. St. Thomas à Becket's martyrdom sparked an almost immediate devotion all across Europe, and it would be the undoing of many of Henry II's programs.

For the remaining 19 years of his rule, Henry II was a haunted man. Betrayed by his wife and children, guilt-ridden by the death of his friend, perhaps a result of a moment of anger, Henry did public penance for his crime—he was violently scourged at the tomb of his old friend, who was canonized only two years after his martyrdom. Disgraced, the king gave up his program of control over the Church.

FREDERICK I, BARBAROSSA (1152-1190)

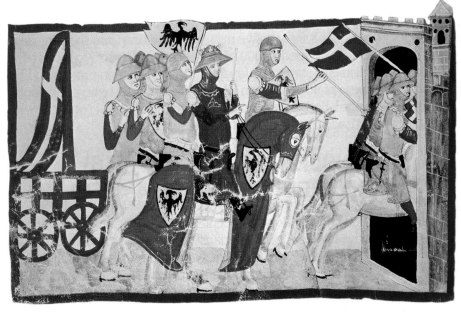

Emperor Frederick I attacks Milan, Italy (1158).

Frederick I, Barbarossa, was the ablest and most powerful ruler of the Holy Roman Empire. He thought his vocation as emperor was to revive the Roman Empire. He believed that absolute power was bestowed upon him directly from God and therefore this power extended over the Church. Since Rome was the first city of the ancient empire, Frederick I believed he should have the authority to appoint the Bishop of Rome.

Pope Adrian IV saw immediately that Frederick I was overstepping his boundaries and threatened him with excommunication if he continued to infringe on the rights of the Church. The Italian city-states also greatly resented the interference of the German emperor. Frederick I, however, continued to appoint bishops in violation of the 1122 Concordat of Worms, and he imprisoned the papal legate sent to stop him.

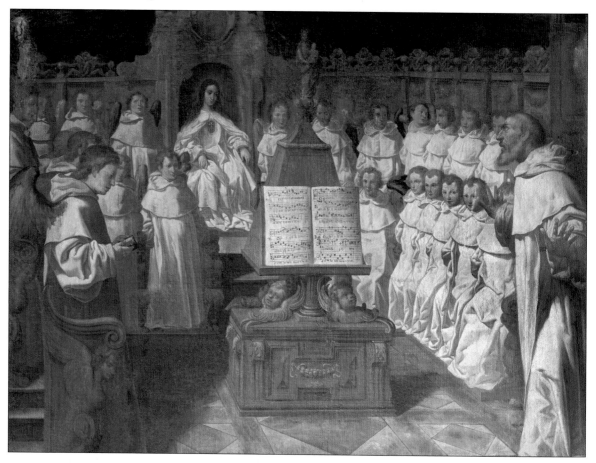

The Carthusians were founded by St. Bruno at Chartreuse, near Grenoble in France.

the Cistercians used the Benedictine rule, though with a special emphasis on austerities, farming, and simplicity of lifestyle. The white habits of the Cistercians were meant to imply their poverty and simplicity; most other monks wore black habits at the time.

The Cistercians were particularly important in the conversion of the Slavic tribes of Poland, Bohemia, and eastern Germany.

ST. BERNARD OF CLAIRVAUX

St. Bernard of Fontaine (1091-1153) joined the Cistercians in 1113 at Citeaux. Known as St. Bernard of Clairvaux, he is often considered the second founder of the order. It was under his leadership that the Cistercians grew dramatically and their influence spread. When he entered the monastery, he brought along thirty friends, four of whom were his brothers. St. Bernard became the first abbot of the new monastery founded at Clairvaux. At Clairvaux the monastery was austere: the walls were barren with small windows, and beds consisting of planks of wood. The monks ate nothing but bread and boiled leaves and roots with some salt and oil.

When he became a monk, St. Bernard focused his studies on the Scriptures and the Fathers of the Church. Profoundly humble, St. Bernard refused all promotions, including the episcopacy and papacy. A major part of his service to the Church was his extraordinary writing to encourage and strengthen others in the Faith. His central theme, in conjunction with extensive quotation of Scriptures, was the divine life communicated to the world in the Person of Jesus Christ.

The middle of the twelfth century was called the "Age of St. Bernard." St. Bernard counseled rulers, bishops, and popes, including Bl. Eugene III, the first pope who was a Cistercian. He carried out a legendary debate with Peter Abelard, the most renowned thinker of the time other than St. Bernard. Abelard had advocated certain theological errors, but St. Bernard, so logically forceful and clear in his condemnation of Abelard's teachings, left the master logician with no response but silence.

THE CARTHUSIANS

The Carthusians were founded by St. Bruno at Chartreuse, near Grenoble in France. Like many churchmen of the day, St. Bruno also served the civil state in France. He was a brilliant scholar and he counted among his pupils Eudes of Châtillon, who would become Bl. Urban II. Despite his prestigious position as chancellor at Rheims, St. Bruno remained a model priest, resisting political pressures. When offered the chance in 1080 to become the bishop of Rheims, he declined.

Instead, inspired by a burning love for God and a desire to live a more spiritually disciplined and simple life, St. Bruno left his position and went off with two friends to live as hermits in the mountains. Like the Egyptian monks centuries before, St. Bruno and his companions lived in isolation, practiced severe mortifications, and observed perpetual silence.

St. Bruno and his two friends settled at Chartreuse in the French Alps where they established a unique monastery for their day. The monks at Chartreuse did not live together like other monks; instead, each had his own cell around the cloister. St. Bruno wanted to bring the ascetic life of the desert hermit into the context of the monastery, establishing an oasis of peace and prayer outside the busy developing cities of the Medieval world.

The Carthusians did not become as numerous as some of the other monastic orders of the day, but their positive example had its own influence. Rumors of their ascetic life spread throughout important centers in Europe, helping to revive Christian devotion to simplicity and prayer.

PART VI

The Crusades

THE FALL OF THE HOLY LAND

Within one hundred years of the death of Muhammad, Islam spread throughout much of the Christian world. As discussed previously, this had as much to do with the success of militant Muslim expansion as it did with authentic religious conversion. Quickly after the birth of the religion, Islamic forces seized most of the Christian world. Palestine, the Holy Land and home of Jesus; Egypt, the birthplace of monasticism; Asia Minor, where St. Paul preached and planted the seeds of early Christian communities; and North Africa had all fallen to Muslim forces. Muslim expansion was finally brought to a halt by Charles Martel's defense of Western Europe in France and the Byzantine Empire's defense in the East. With these new borders established, Muslim and Christian lands remained more or less stable.

After a long period of tolerance, the rise of the Fatimite Muslims in Egypt during the first decades of the eleventh century led to a renewed Christian persecution. In the second half of the century, a new militant Islamic nation, the Seljuk Turks, persecuted

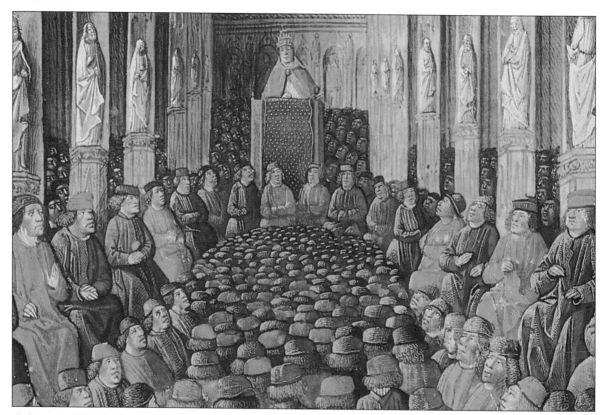

In the summer of 1095, Bl. Urban II preached a momentous sermon in Clermont, France that would launch the First Crusade. "A great commotion arose through all the regions of France, so that if anyone earnestly wished to follow God with pure heart and mind, and wanted to bear the cross faithfully after him, he would hasten to take the road to the Holy Sepulchre" (extract from the *Gesta Francorum*).

Christians, especially in Palestine and Syria, and expanded westwards into lands previously protected by Byzantium. In 1071, in the Battle of Manzikert, the Turks annihilated the Byzantine army and were on the verge of taking Constantinople. By this time, two-thirds of the Christian world had been taken by Muslim forces, and now the last vestiges of the Roman Empire were threatened. The Eastern emperor looked West for assistance, in desperation, asking them to aid their brothers and sisters in the East.

The Western Christians were concerned with their Eastern brethren. Despite the schism of 1054, many (including both Bl. Urban II and the Eastern emperor) hoped that the split could be healed. In 1095, Bl. Urban II held a council in Clermont in central France to try to rouse support from Westerners to aid the Eastern Christians. At Clermont, Bl. Urban II appealed for help.

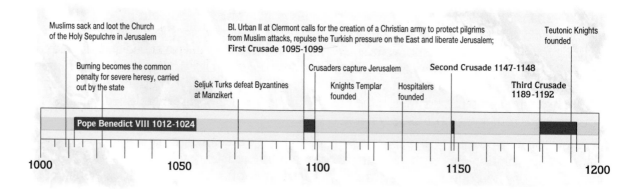

Muslims sack and loot the Church of the Holy Sepulchre in Jerusalem

Bl. Urban II at Clermont calls for the creation of a Christian army to protect pilgrims from Muslim attacks, repulse the Turkish pressure on the East and liberate Jerusalem; **First Crusade 1095-1099**

Teutonic Knights founded

Burning becomes the common penalty for severe heresy, carried out by the state

Seljuk Turks defeat Byzantines at Manzikert

Crusaders capture Jerusalem

Knights Templar founded

Second Crusade 1147-1148

Hospitalers founded

Third Crusade 1189-1192

Pope Benedict VIII 1012-1024

1000   1050   1100   1150   1200

Bl. Urban II began the crusades by proclaiming an organized assault in defense of Christian Europe. Rather than a Christian offensive, the crusades were a desperate attempt to fend off Islamic expansion. Islam was the strongest power of the Medieval world, and it now threatened to overrun the entire West. At some point, Christianity had to defend itself or be taken over by Islam. Islam was born in war and grew the same way. Muslim thought at this time divided the world into two spheres: the abode of Islam and the abode of war. Christianity or any other non-Muslim religion has no abode. Bl. Urban II's crusade was the first of a series of military expeditions meant to ward off the very probable fall of the Christian world to the Muslims.

THE FIRST CRUSADE (1095-1099)

The First Crusade was a popular movement that took place without any direct support or leadership from the kings of Europe, since many of the rulers were either excommunicated or in opposition to the papacy at the time. In northern France and the Rhineland, a number of preachers took Bl. Urban II's message to the people, motivating and organizing armies to set out for the Holy Land. The message was met with enthusiasm throughout all of Europe, and armies from every corner of the continent set out on various routes towards the east. Regretfully with the occasion of the crusades, some crusaders attacked Jewish communities on their way to the Holy Land.

The First Crusade was considered the best organized. The armies were divided into four groups all set to meet in Constantinople. Godfrey of Bouillon, Duke of Lower Lorraine, led the people of Lorraine, the Germans, and the northern French. They followed the valley of the Danube, crossed Hungary, and arrived in Constantinople in late 1096. Hugh of Vermandois, brother of King Philip I of France and Robert Courte-Heuse, the Duke of Normandy and the son of William the Conqueror, led bands of French and Normans across the Alps and set sail from Apulia, on the boot heel of Italy, to Dyrrachium, which is in modern day Albania. From there the army continued overland to Constantinople where they arrived in May of 1097.

The southern French, under the lead of Raymond of Saint-Filles and the bishop of Puy, Adhemar of Moneil, set out overland through the eastern Alps where they met tough resistance from the Slavs, delaying their arrival in Constantinople until the end of April 1097. The fourth army consisted of Normans from Southern Italy led by Bohemund and Tancred, who were both related to the founder of Norman Sicily, Robert Guiscard. On their way across Italy and on through the Byzantine Empire, the army picked up many enthusiastic bands of local crusaders, who joined ranks, and eventually arrived in Constantinople with the Normans in April of 1097. The crusaders came from every corner of Europe, and when they arrived in Constantinople they were a mismatched group and everything but a unified army.

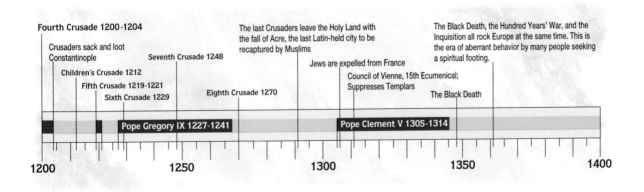

Fourth Crusade 1200-1204

Crusaders sack and loot Constantinople

Children's Crusade 1212

Fifth Crusade 1219-1221

Sixth Crusade 1229

Seventh Crusade 1248

Eighth Crusade 1270

The last Crusaders leave the Holy Land with the fall of Acre, the last Latin-held city to be recaptured by Muslims

Jews are expelled from France

Council of Vienne, 15th Ecumenical; Suppresses Templars

The Black Death, the Hundred Years' War, and the Inquisition all rock Europe at the same time. This is the era of aberrant behavior by many people seeking a spiritual footing.

The Black Death

Pope Gregory IX 1227-1241

Pope Clement V 1305-1314

1200   1250   1300   1350   1400

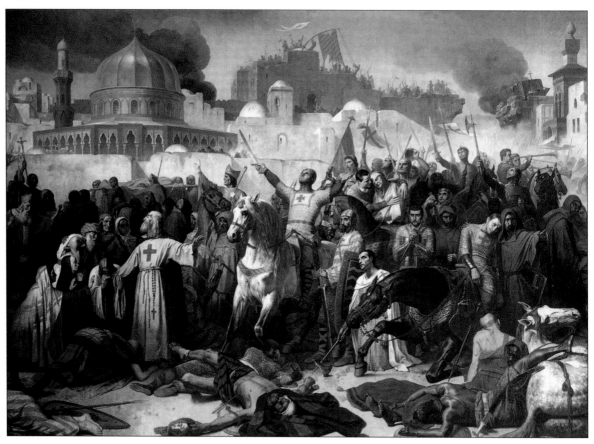

The Taking of Jerusalem by the Crusaders, July 15, 1099

In the spring of 1097 the campaign began, and the four armies proved very successful. First, they staged a successful siege of Nicaea, and after that, moved on to Antioch, which they took in 1098. Jerusalem fell in 1099. Bl. Urban II, whose dream was to recover the Holy Land, died before receiving news of the sacking of Jerusalem. The reconquest of Jerusalem unfortunately resulted in a brutal massacre of the mostly Muslim population.

The First Crusade came at a time when Muslims were politically divided. Seljuk Turks had recently risen to power in the Holy Land and they did not yet have firm control over the area. The crusaders took advantage of their disunity and established authority over Palestine. After the reconquest of Jerusalem, the crusaders organized the lands into a number of counties, fiefs, and principalities based on the Medieval feudal system to build a Christian state in Palestine.

As is still evident today, the organization of a government for a population which included Muslims, Jews, Eastern and Western Christians was no easy task. The job fell to Godfrey of Bouillon, and after his death in 1100, his younger brother Baldwin. Baldwin kept direct control of Jerusalem and its surrounding areas. To the north, three fiefs – the County of Tripoli, the Principality of Antioch, and the County of Edessa were established. Muslims who lived in crusader-won territories were generally allowed to retain their property and livelihood and, as always, their religion.

However, the kingdom of Jerusalem was difficult to maintain, as it shrunk continuously until 1291 when the last acres were overrun. A big problem was that not many Europeans stayed in the Holy Land as settlers, and despite a steady influx of traveling pilgrims and soldiers, the kings found themselves trying to maintain control over a people of largely different faiths, cultures, and sympathies. It is indeed remarkable they were able to maintain control for nearly 200 years.

THE FIRST CRUSADE, 1095-1099

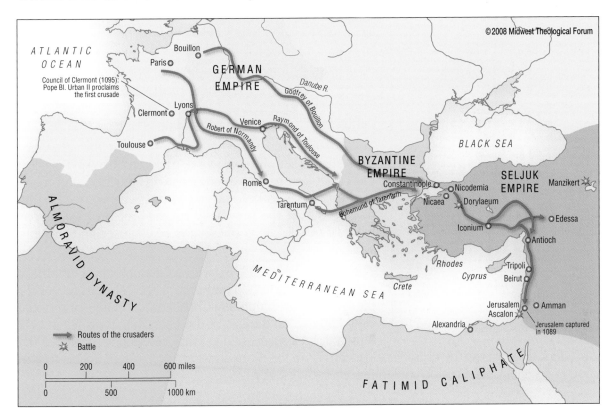

©2008 Midwest Theological Forum

SUCCESSIVE CRUSADES

The popularity and success of the First Crusade inspired a string of crusades that lasted for nearly five centuries. None of these crusades was ever as well organized or effective as the first. In fact, the wars more often resembled a steady stream of people heading east rather than an organized military campaign.

Shortly after the end of the First Crusade, the Christian kingdom in Palestine was under attack. In 1144, the Turks recaptured the city of Edessa in the north. King Louis VII of France and Emperor Conrad II of Germany set out to capture the city of Damascus and establish a defensive front for the Kingdom of Jerusalem. They failed and were forced to retreat. Convinced that God was punishing the West for its sins, lay piety movements arose throughout Europe to purify Christian society in order to be worthy of future victory in the East.

The Third Crusade (1189-1192) is perhaps the most famous due to its role in providing the background of the Robin Hood stories. Richard the Lionheart of England set out with Emperor Frederick I, Barbarossa and King Philip of France to defend the Christian kingdoms against the Turks, who had now unified under their great military leader Saladin. Saladin, the great unifier, had forged the Muslim Near East into a single entity while preaching jihad against the Christians. In 1187 at the Battle of Hattin, his forces wiped out the combined armies of the Christian kingdom of Jerusalem, and they captured the relic of the True Cross. The response was the Third Crusade.

Later crusades failed, abounding with mistakes and accidents. The Fourth Crusade (1201-1204) resulted in the sack of Constantinople, the great Christian city, in 1203. Various conditions led the crusaders to sack the city. The crusaders were significantly in debt to the city of Venice, so

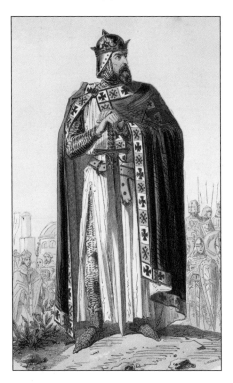

On July 22, 1099, Godfrey of Bouillon was chosen as ruler of Jerusalem with the title "Advocate of the Holy Sepulchre." It was agreed to by the leaders that no one should be called "king" and wear a crown in the land where Christ had worn the crown of thorns. After the majority of pilgrims returned home, Godfrey had only 300 knights and 2,000 foot-soldiers to protect Jerusalem. His one year reign was a struggle to ensure the survival of the infant Christian state.

they favored a Byzantine emperor who would repay the debt for them. The preachers of the crusade thought the Constantinopolitans had sided with Saladin and the Muslims during the Third Crusade and had not assisted in the Second.

In 1212, children, caught up in the popular crusader movements, set off to mount a "Children's Crusade" against the Turks. Before they even arrived in the Holy Land, many of the children either starved to death or were killed by disease during the perilously rugged journey east. Those who did not die along the way were captured and sold into slavery.

These two Crusades, as well as a number of unofficial expeditions, diminished enthusiasm and religious fervor for the Holy Wars. Eventually Christians lost possession of the Holy Land when the last of the Latin Kingdoms fell in 1291. Muslim forces succeeded in killing or ejecting the last of the crusaders, thus erasing the crusader kingdoms from the map. Christian forces were unable to gain another foothold in the region until the nineteenth century.

BYZANTIUM'S RESPONSE

At first, many westerners (especially Pope Innocent III) were optimistic about the positive effect the Crusades might have on the relationship between the western and eastern churches. Politically speaking, the Byzantines needed the help of the western Crusaders to contain the Turks and protect the Byzantine Empire. In addition, the Crusades also allowed for a positive exchange of ideas and culture between the more educated Byzantines and the Western Christians. Many hoped that the constant communication between the west and east would help heal the Great Schism of 1054.

The Eastern Empire, for its part, feared the Crusaders and saw the western armies as a threat against their own territory. Emperor Alexius usually tried to transport the Crusaders as quickly as possible across the Bosporus Straits and out of Byzantine territory given the high intensity of suspicion and hostility many Eastern Christians had for the Latin Church. After the sacking of Constantinople during the fourth Crusade, the relationship between the east and west was ruined.

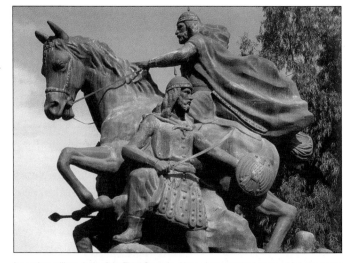

Legendary military rivals of the Third Crusade. *Above*: A monumental statue of Saladin stands in Damascus, the capital of Syria and the site of Saladin's tomb.

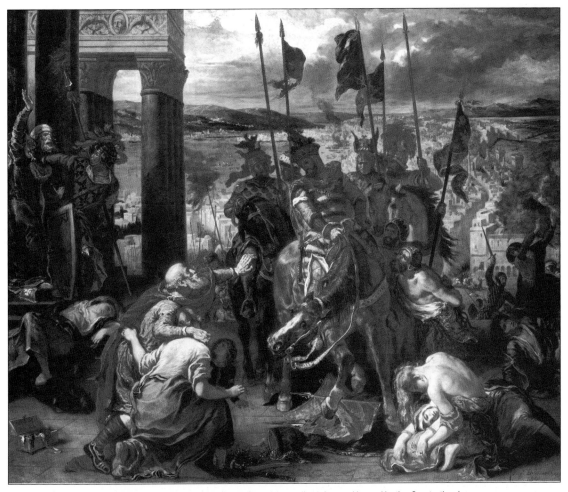

On April 12, 1204 the men of the Fourth Crusade spent three days sacking and looting Constantinople,
a city so filled with treasures and holy relics that it was one of the most destructive and profitable conquests in history.
Many of the looted treasures remain in Venice including the Four Golden Horses of San Marco and a piece of the True Cross.
The feelings of betrayal would create a great rift between the Western and Eastern Churches which still exists today.

The Byzantines regained control over their own capital in 1261, but would be eventually defeated by the Turks in 1453. The Crusades became a turning point in the life of the eastern empire, and the rift created between the Eastern and Western Churches was so great that after eight centuries it still remains open.

OUTCOME OF THE CRUSADES

The main objectives of the Crusades – the deliverance of the Holy Land and the rescue of the Christians in the East – were ultimately frustrated. Nonetheless, the sacrifice of so many lives was not entirely in vain. The Crusades held back Turkish expansion into Europe for four hundred years and gave Christians a

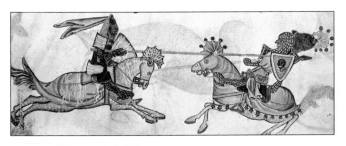

This late medieval illustration depicts Richard the Lionheart and Saladin in a symbolic joust. In a real battle, the crusaders fought with heavy horses and swords wielded with two hands. The Saracens had smaller, quick horses and short, curved scimitars which were slashed at the crusaders from horseback at a full gallop.

more acute consciousness of their Christian unity, which transcended nationality and race. Contact with Eastern Christian culture through the exchange of people, goods, and ideas had an enormous influence on the intellectual life of Europe. The Crusades made pilgrimages to the Holy Land easier, and the Muslims eventually entrusted Christian Holy Places in Palestine to the Franciscans due to St. Francis of Assisi's friendship with Muslim leaders.

The Crusades encouraged travel and fostered a new curiosity for foreign culture among the Latin Christians. Missionaries and merchants set out deep into central Asia, and by the thirteenth century had reached China. The reports from those expeditions (from explorers such as Marco Polo) gave Western Europe abundant information about Asia and fed the desire to explore and evangelize new territories. As a result, the world in many ways became more open for Westerners, and consequently the technological and academic achievements of the Arabic world and the Greek writings on medicine and mathematics facilitated a flowering of Western culture.

PART VII

The Military Orders: The Knights Templar, the Hospitalers, and the Teutonic Knights

With the recovery of the Holy Places in Palestine during the Crusades, Military Orders sprang up out of the necessity to defend the holy sites as well as the pilgrims who traveled there. These orders combined both military and religious life, emphasizing dedication, discipline, and monastic organization. These soldier-monks were bound by vows of poverty, chastity, and obedience and were devoted to the care and defense of pilgrims. Although historians of the military orders have enumerated as many as a hundred different types of orders (stressing the eagerness with which the Middle Ages welcomed an institution so thoroughly corresponding to the two occupations of that period, war and religion), the three oldest and most respected were the Knights Templar, the Knights Hospitalers, and the Teutonic Knights.

The kings and the nobility availed themselves of military orders to strengthen their own position and to protect their kingdoms and fiefdoms. Since this mode of protection, self-defense through warfare, squared so well with Medieval culture, virtually every king and prince had a military order at his disposal.

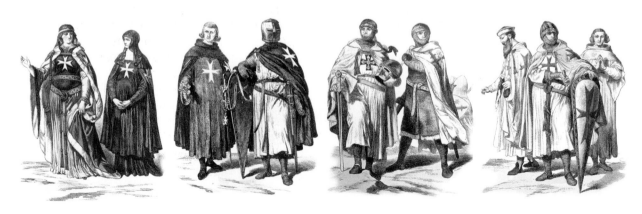

THE KNIGHTS TEMPLAR

In 1118, a group of nine French knights founded the oldest of these three orders, the Knights Templar, specifically to protect pilgrims traveling to Jerusalem. The order derived their name, "The Poor Brothers of the Temple of Jerusalem," or Templars, from the Palace of King Baldwin of Jerusalem, which was built on the site of the ancient Temple of Solomon.

The Pope approved the order at the Council of Troyes in 1128, and St. Bernard of Clairvaux, who was present at the council, wrote a rule for them based on the Cistercian Rule.

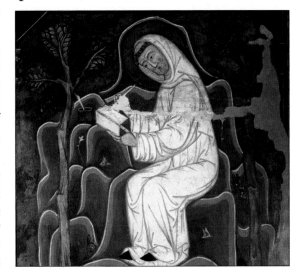
St. Bernard of Clairvaux

St. Bernard saw the military order as an effective way of tempering the knights' bad habits and explicitly tying the mission of the crusading armies to the mission of Christ's Church. These monks made the three traditional vows of poverty, chastity, and obedience and lived lives of monastic warriors.

The Knights Templar were organized in a three rank division with aristocratic soldiers, clergy, and lay brothers from the lower ranks of society who acted as helpers of the aristocratic soldiers. They assumed a major role in the maintenance of safe routes between Europe and the crusader states and the defense of the Kingdom of Jerusalem.

WARRIOR MONKS

The monastic rule drafted by St. Bernard of Clairvaux and followed by the Knights Templar established a strict ascetic way of life that fostered their dedication to physical warfare. According to the rule, the Templars had to wear white monastic garments, distinguishing them on the battlefield where their fierce reputation preceded them. However, off the battlefield the Templars lived the quiet lives of pious monks, exemplifying a seemingly paradoxical existence of war and peace. Their lives of prayer, however, sustained them in war. The prospect of death in battle did not frighten the Templars; they had already given up all worldly pleasures.

Never numerous, at their height there were only four hundred knights in Jerusalem. Nevertheless, these dedicated warrior monks inspired other Christian forces. Never fearing death, if the knights were captured in battle they could not offer a ransom. In addition, those captured would always refuse their freedom if it meant denying their faith. At the siege of Safed in 1264, for example, eighty Templars were taken prisoner. After refusing to yield to their captor's wishes to deny Christ, they all were martyred. Over the course of the first two centuries of their existence, it is estimated that almost twenty thousand Knights Templars were killed.

This often included safeguarding western money that was flowing to the east in support of the western kingdoms there. As a result, the Templars became one of the most important banking institutions of the age.

After the Holy Land fell again to Muslim forces, the Templars returned to their landholdings in Europe, becoming even wealthier and expanding their banking organization even more. Now based out of Paris, the Templars were excellent transferors and loaners of capital. Their clients included the popes and the French kings.

Feeling threatened by their wealth and influence, the French king Philip the Fair maliciously sought to destroy the order. He falsely charged the Templars with heresy and pressured Pope Clement V to suppress it in 1312. These charges, along with other trumped-up accusations of sacrilege, sodomy, and idolatry, made the order increasingly unpopular in France. The French King extracted "confessions" from the members of the Templars through torture, suppressed the order, and seized most of its property. The Templar Grand Master Jacques de Molay was burned at the stake in 1314. He died courageously, publicly condemning the actions of Philip.

THE KNIGHTS HOSPITALERS

Never as numerous or as wealthy as the Templars, The Knights of the Hospital of St. John of Jerusalem, or Hospitalers, founded in about 1130, grew out of an already existing work of charity consisting of the care of sick pilgrims. The knights, typically dressed in a black cloak adorned with

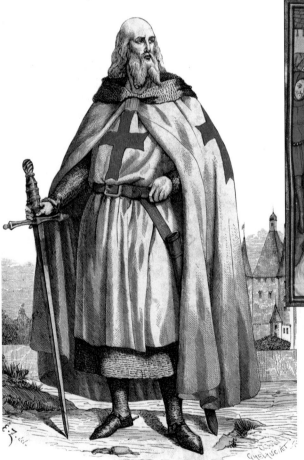

"On Friday 13 October 1307, at precisely the same time, the first glimmer of dawn, all the Templars throughout the kingdom of France were arrested and delivered to various prisons at the command of the king, Philip IV. Among those detained was the master of the whole Order, Jacques of Molay, who was seized at the Templar's Paris house." (from the chronicle of William of Nangis)

Jacques of Molay was burnt at the stake on the Ile-des-Javiaux, an island in the Seine in the center of Paris, on March 18, 1314. He was said to have cursed Philip and Pope Clement V, calling them to join him before God's tribunal. They both died soon after.

a white cloak, made a major contribution in the defense of Jerusalem, and served as a medical corps to the Crusaders. After the fall of the last Christian stronghold in Palestine in 1291, the Hospitalers retreated to the island of Rhodes.

They held Rhodes for two centuries against the Turks. After the capture of Rhodes in 1523 by the Turks, Emperor Charles V bestowed upon them the island of Malta. Although they were expelled from the island in 1798 by Napoleon, the order still exists today. Known as the Knights of Malta, the order has long since put down the sword and exists only as a philanthropic confraternity.

THE TEUTONIC KNIGHTS

Around 1190, a number of crusaders from Bremen and Lübeck in Germany joined with the members of the German Hospital in Jerusalem to form the Order of the Teutonic Knights. Officially known as the Brothers of the Hospital of Saint Mary of Jerusalem, the Teutonic Knights were modeled largely after the Hospitalers and maintained a headquarters in Jerusalem. As early as 1226 they turned their

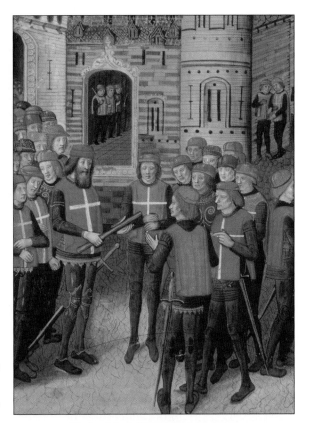

The Hospitalers held Rhodes for two centuries.

attention away from the Holy Land. The King of Prussia and the Bishop Primate of Prussia invited the Teutonic Knights to aid in battles against the heathen Slavs and Tartars. In 1229 the Knights moved their headquarters to Prussia and helped aid the German expansion eastward, conquering lands along the Baltic Sea. The Teutonic Knights took Prussia and other lands of Estonia, Lithuania, and Russia until it finally stopped advancing around 1400. The knights remained a cohesive and efficient group until the sixteenth century, when then grand master, Albert of Hohenzollern, abandoned Catholicism (1525) and became a Lutheran Grand Duke of secularized Prussia.

LEGACY OF THE MILITARY ORDERS

Besides these three orders, there were a great number of lesser military orders. The culture of the Middle Ages offered the right setting for military orders. After the Crusades stopped in the thirteenth century, most of the military orders died out, but their effects on the development of Europe were long lasting.

The Templars were important forerunners in banking, developing an early system of capitalism in Europe. Their immediate successors were the Fugger and Medici families that played important banking roles in the fourteenth and fifteenth centuries. The Teutonic Knights were key in making possible the great German expansion into the East known as the Drang nach Osten (Urge to the East).

Royalty afterwards utilized the model of military orders to form a legion of knights who were ceremoniously invested into the order of knighthood. Some countries today, most notably England, still bestow these titles as a sign of honor or gratitude.

PART VIII

The Inquisition

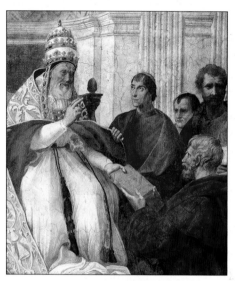

In 1231, Pope Gregory IX established the Inquisition as a means of finding and judging heretics.

The first Christian emperors believed that one of the chief duties of an imperial ruler was to use his political and military power to protect the orthodoxy of the Church. The titles they used, like "Pontifex Maximus" and "Bishop of the Exterior," implied their understanding of their office as a divinely appointed agent of Heaven, a civil authority whose duty was bound up with their service of the Church.

In the Middle Ages, as the Catholic Faith became dominant in Europe, the Church became tied socially, politically, and economically to European life. Christianity provided the moral foundation for law and civil authority. As a major landholder, the Church's well-being had a major economic influence on Europe. Civil authorities, despite their impiety or any dishonest intention, regarded themselves as the political arm of the Church, divinely appointed to assist and preserve the Christian world.

Catholic doctrine and practice was no longer a matter of private belief. Its stability and validity allowed for and protected the stability of Europe. Heretical attacks on the Church were treated as serious threats against the Christian world, and in the thirteenth century, some of these heresies became increasingly more violent.

THE ORIGINS OF THE INQUISITION

The Inquisition began largely in reaction to the Albigensian heresy, which was growing strong and fast during the early part of the thirteenth century in Southern France. Like the Manichean heresy during the time of St. Augustine, Albigensianism appealed to a misunderstood sense of Christian piety and self-sacrifice, as it saw the soul as good and the body evil. Many were attracted to its emphasis on its ostensible fidelity to the Gospel, expressed in austerity regarding poverty and fasting. Their radical asceticism was driven by their belief in the evil of war, physical pleasure, and even matter itself.

The teachings of Albigensianism posed a dangerous threat to the Christian world since their teachings struck at the core of the Catholic Faith. A form of Gnosticism, Albigensianism believed in two gods that governed the universe: one spiritual and good, the other physical and evil. As a result, all things of the temporal world were considered evil and dangerous. The Albigensians were hostile to Christianity, and rejected the Mass, the sacraments, and the ecclesiastical hierarchy and organization. In addition to hating anything that had to do with the world, Albigensians rejected feudal government and refused to abide by oaths or allegiances. They were unaccountable to any authority, religious or civil. Often leaders instructed them to burn down churches and destroy their property. They also forbade marriage and the propagation of the human race, and thus they allowed for homosexual relations as an alternative to heterosexual relations, since producing offspring was considered evil. The Albigensians preached suicide as a way to obtain spiritual purity. By shedding themselves of their bodies through suicide, Albigensians believed they would be pure enough to obtain eternal life.

Both civil and religious authorities in Europe saw this heresy as more than a theological disagreement, but as a destructive illness that would have devastating effects on both the Church and Christian societies.

In 1208, an Albigensian follower killed the Papal Legate Pierre de Castelnau, and Pope Innocent III reacted by calling a crusade to suppress the Albigensians in France and rid the heresy from Christendom.

The purging dragged on for more than twenty years, and although thousands died and Albigensian lands in southern France were seized, many adherents to the heresy were still scattered throughout Europe.

French kings Louis VIII and Louis IX, as well as Emperor Frederick II, took strong measures against the Albigensians by applying capital punishment. Consequently, burning heretics at the stake became a common practice. Civil rulers were becoming increasingly more involved with the prosecution and punishment of heretics to maintain civil order.

In 1231, Pope Gregory IX established the Inquisition as a means of detection and purgation of heresy. He appointed a number of Papal Inquisitors, mostly Dominicans and Franciscans, who could serve as independent judges free from any secular interest and influence.

THE INQUISITORS

The pope did not establish the Inquisition as a distinct tribunal. Rather, he appointed special judges who examined and judged the doctrinal opinions and moral conduct of suspicious individuals. They often worked within the context of the civil system, but with papal authority. The judge, or Inquisitor, had to adhere to the established rules of canonical procedure. Gregory IX also provided that the inquisitional tribunal could only work with the diocesan bishop's cooperation.

The Dominicans and Franciscans were two new orders that enjoyed rigorous and solid theological training and spiritual formation. This education prompted the hierarchy to employ them as inquisitors. Given their spirituality and lifestyle, the Dominicans and Franciscans would be less likely to be swayed by worldly motives or pressure from the secular authorities. It was safe to assume that they were not merely endowed with the requisite knowledge, but that they would also, quite unselfishly fulfill their duty for the good of the Church. In addition, there was reason to hope that, because of their great popularity and moral authority, they would not encounter too much opposition.

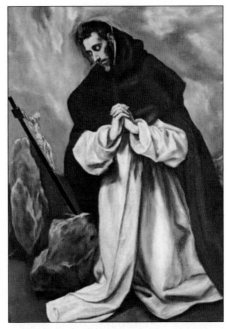

It was a heavy burden of responsibility that fell upon the shoulders of an inquisitor, who was obliged, at least indirectly, to decide between life and death. The Church insisted that he possess the qualities of a good judge expressed in an ardent zeal for protecting and promoting the Faith, the salvation of souls, and the extirpation of heresy. Amid all difficulties, pressures, and dangers of the task, he should never yield to anger or passion. Nevertheless, he should meet hostility fearlessly, but should not encourage it. He should yield to no inducement or threat and yet not be heartless. When circumstances permitted, he should observe mercy in allotting penalties. Finally, he should listen to the counsel of others, and not trust too much in his own opinion or first impressions.

The Spanish friar and papal Inquisitor Dominic Guzman believed in peaceful methods of persuasion such as debating the Albigensians in public.

Inquisitors tried to answer to this ideal. Far from being inhuman, the Church tried to find men with spotless character, and sometimes they were of truly admirable sanctity. A number of them have even been canonized by the Church.

PROCESS FOR INQUISITION

The procedure for inquisition began with a month long "term of grace" proclaimed by the inquisitor when he came into a heresy-ridden district, which allowed the inhabitants to appear before the inquisitor, confess their sins, and perform penance. Of those who confessed heresy of their own accord, a suitable penance (such as a pilgrimage, fasting, or wearing crosses on their clothes) was imposed, but never a severe punishment like incarceration or surrender to the civil power.

If the accused did not confess, the trial began. The accused would be asked to swear his innocence on the four Gospels. If he or she still claimed innocence, there were a number of methods used to extract a confession. First judges would remind the accused the punishment that awaited if he or she were convicted without a confession, hoping that the fear of punishment may convince a guilty

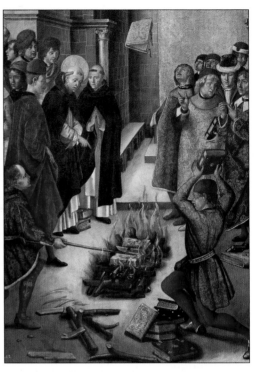

This painting depicts an event that occurred in 1207, in Albi, France, when St. Dominic proved to the Albigensians that their books containing heretic ideas burn in the fire while the Catholic books fly up away from the fire undamaged.

man to admit to the truth, in hopes of a more lenient sentence. If the accused still did not confess, he or she was subject to close confinement (possibly emphasized by curtailment of food), visits of an already tried man (who would attempt to induce free confession through friendly persuasion), and confinement to an inquisition prison for serious offenders. When no voluntary admission was made, evidence was still necessary for conviction. Legally, there had to be at least two witnesses, and conscientious judges often required even more witnesses to convict someone of heresy.

Witnesses for the defense hardly ever appeared, as they would almost inevitably be suspected of being heretics or at least favorable to heresy. For the same reason those impeached rarely secured legal advisers, and therefore made a personal response to the main points of a charge. False witnesses were punished without mercy. If caught, they risked life imprisonment or worse punishment. It must be noted that secret examination of witnesses during the Inquisition was not a peculiarity of the time. This procedure was common to all civil courts as well throughout Europe.

The accused was not given the right to know the names of his accusers. However, the accused was given the right to submit a list of names of his alleged enemies, which often facilitated a just verdict. Furthermore, the accused could appeal to higher authority, including the pope (cf. Shannon, Medieval Inquisition, 1983, pp. 139-140).

In addition to the inquisitor, boni viri (good men) were frequently called upon. Thirty, fifty, eighty, or more persons – laymen and priests; secular and regular – would be summoned, all highly respected and independent men, and sworn to give verdict on the cases before them to the best of their knowledge and belief. They were always called upon to decide two questions: culpability (and the reason for it) and the punishment to be imparted. Although the boni viri were entitled only to an advisory vote, the final ruling was usually in accordance with their views.

The judges were also assisted by a concilium permanens, or standing council, composed of other sworn judges.

THE FINAL VERDICT IN THE INQUISITION

The ultimate decision was usually pronounced with a solemn ceremony. One or two days prior to this ceremony, everyone concerned had the charges read to him again, briefly. The ceremony began very early in the morning. Secular officials were sworn in and made to vow obedience to the inquisitor in all things pertaining to the suppression of heresy. Then the offenses were announced and punishments were assigned to the guilty party. This announcement began with the minor punishments, and went on to the most severe, such as perpetual imprisonment or death. Those found guilty were then turned over to the civil power, whose duty it was to carry out the punishments.

Most of the punishments that were inflicted were largely humane. Most frequently, certain good works were ordered like the building of a church, the visitation to a church, a pilgrimage, the offering of a candle or a chalice, or participation in a crusade. Other stiffer penalties included fines, whose proceeds were devoted to such public purposes as church-building or road-making; whipping with rods during religious service; the pillory; or wearing colored crosses (Livingstone, The Oxford Dictionary of the Christian Church, 1997, p. 836).

The hardest penalties were imprisonment and various degrees of exclusion from the communion of the Church, as well as consequent surrender to the civil power for harsher sentencing.

Imprisonment was not always seen as punishment in the proper sense: it was rather looked on as an opportunity for repentance, a preventive measure against backsliding or infecting others. It was known as immuration (from the Latin murus, a wall), or incarcera-tion, and was inflicted for a definite time or for life. Immuration for life was the lot of those who had perhaps recanted only from fear of death or had once before abjured heresy.

SIMON DE MONTFORT AND THE BATTLE OF MURET

One of the most important battles against the Albigensians took place at Muret, a small town south of Toulouse in southern France, on September 12, 1213. With the support of Pope Innocent III, Simon de Montfort led a small army of Catholics against the Albigensians, led by Count Raymond VI and Peter II of Aragon. The Albigensian army was far larger than that of Simon de Montfort, and so the Catholic general waited for reinforcements to arrive from the North. Help never came.

With about eight hundred cavalry, Simon was facing a heavily reinforced enemy of over two thousand cavalry and fifteen thousand infantry. This massive force marched towards the Catholic position at Muret from Toulouse, intent on crushing the small Catholic resistance. Faced with a seemingly helpless situation, Simon and his army turned to St. Dominic (the founder of Mendicant order that will be studied in the next chapter) for spiritual guidance. At his suggestion the Catholic forces began praying the Rosary, and the night before battle, Simon heard Mass at midnight, and prayed to God for a victory. His enemy Peter II spent the night with his mistress and could barely stand straight the next morning.

That morning Simon's tiny army charged across a mile of open country and attacked the stunned Raymond and Peter. During the course of the battle, St. Dominic knelt before the altar of Saint-Jacque in Muret asking God for a miraculous victory. God answered his prayers, and in a surprisingly short time Peter II was killed and the heretics were defeated. It is believed that Simon erected a chapel dedicated to Our Lady of the Rosary in thanks to St. Dominic and his prayers.

Although it is hard to know exactly how many victims were handed over to civil power, there are some historical approximations. At the height of the Inquisition in southern France in the thirteenth century, three people were burned for heresy per year (Livingstone, The Oxford Dictionary of the Christian Church, 1997, p. 836).

THE INQUISITION IN SPAIN

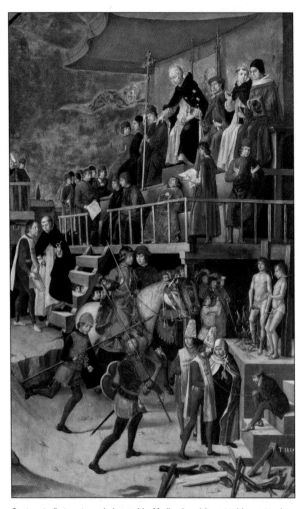

Our twenty-first century minds consider Medieval punishments abhorrent and barbaric, but the punishments inflicted in those times were normal for Medieval cultures.

Religious conditions similar to those in Southern France led to the establishment of the Inquisition in Spain, where it lasted until the eighteenth century. However, motives for the Inquisition developed differently in Spain. The Spanish Inquisition coincided with the *Reconquista*, the reconquering of Spain by the Christians against the Muslims and the Jews. National unification was not completed until 1492, and before and after that date, the Inquisition was used to promote and retain Spanish unity under a common Christian religion.

The Spanish Inquisition formally began after the establishment of the Papal Inquisition around the time of the reign of Ferdinand and Isabella. Beginning in 1480, Spanish civil authorities took over the Inquisition in Spain.

Though the Spanish Inquisition developed into mostly a civil tribunal, theologians never questioned its ecclesiastical nature. The Holy See sanctioned the Spanish Inquisition and granted to the grand inquisitor judicial authority concerning matters of Faith. The grand inquisitor—technically appointed by the pope, though the Spanish Inquisition operated quite independently of the Holy See—could also pass down jurisdiction to subsidiary tribunals under his control. An understanding of Spanish history—uniquely its own—reveals both the perceived and actual threats from Muslim and Jewish militancy against Spain.

The Spanish Inquisition was significantly crueler than the earlier papal inquisition against the Albigensians. Certainly, many reports of the atrocities committed have been the product of fable. Especially with today's much more refined appreciation of human dignity, it is especially clear that many of the methods employed by the Inquisition flagrantly violated the dignity of the person. Nevertheless, disedifying practices of the Medieval churchmen, by modern standards, intended to preserve the purity of Church teaching and protect her children from the corrupting effects of heresy as displayed by the Albigensians. Although some of the disedifying practices of individuals and groups within the Medieval Church have no justification, it is always important to view them in their proper historical context. It bears repeating that heresy was viewed as a serious crime during the Middle Ages, and the usual punishment was excommunication.

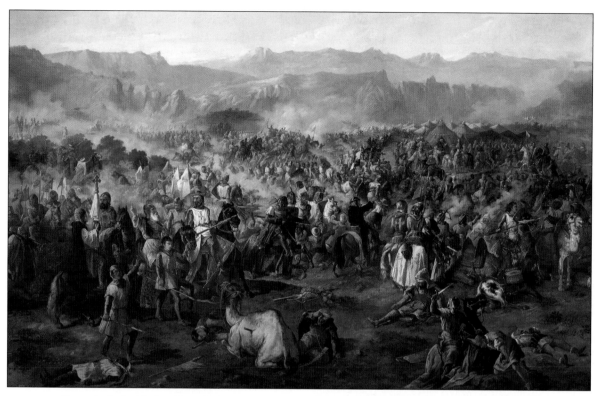

The greatest battle of the *Reconquista* was fought on July 12, 1212 at Las Navas de Tolosa in southern Spain, when the Muslim forces were defeated by a great Christian army which included kings of Aragon, Castile, Navarre, the military orders and 70,000 French crusaders. This battle was decisive, pushing Muslims back to Granada in the far south.

CONCLUSION

The period from Charlemagne's death in the ninth century to the Concordat of Worms in the early twelfth century represents an unstable time in the history of the Church and Europe. The splintering of European political order, external threats of invasion, and conflicts between civil and spiritual authority challenged not only the Church's stability, but its identity as a temporal institution. Regrettably, monastic and diocesan landholdings tied the Church to the developing feudal world in a way that made corruption almost inevitable. Abuses such as simony and nepotism, as well as the weakening of fidelity, celibacy, and piety among the clergy posed a strong threat to the Church. Ironically, at a time when segments of the Church seemed to drift further from the example of the early church, monastic reformers and popes like St. Gregory VII and Innocent III helped transform this period into a time of renewed piety and spiritual devotion. These reformers would begin a rehabilitation that would eventually develop into the golden age of the High Middle Ages.

Like virtually all the periods of the Church's history, the era of the Crusades shows both lights and shadows. Although the guiding light of Divine Providence continually helps the people of God to push the kingdom of God forward, amid the Church's efforts to spread and protect the Faith, sins and shortcomings of her children will always be present. However, without compromising objective moral truth, judgment must take into careful consideration the zeal and uncompromising faith in Christ's Church exemplified by the era of the Crusades. Muslim expansionism "by the sword" posed serious threats to Christian Europe and engulfed and eradicated all the major Christian cities and shrines of the East. Hence, the rigorous response of a people with defects and weaknesses who at the same time see the Catholic tradition as a treasure of inestimable value.

VOCABULARY

AGE OF ST. BERNARD
Refers to the middle of the twelfth century during which St. Bernard of Clairvaux exhibited enormous influence through his counseling of rulers, bishops and popes.

BONI VIRI
Latin meaning "good men," these groups of thirty or more highly respected and independent men, both laymen and priests, were summoned during the Inquisition to give verdict on cases and decide punishment.

CAROLINGIAN
The French dynasty of rulers descended from Charlemagne.

CISTERCIANS
So called "White Monks," after the color of their habits, this order was founded by the Cluniac monk St. Robert of Molesme in 1098. They adopted the Benedictine rule and placed a special emphasis on austerities, farming, simplicity, and strictness in daily life.

CLUNY
City in east-central France which gave birth to monastic reform in 910. The first abbey began with twelve monks committed to renewing the rule of St. Benedict.

CRUSADE
From the Latin word crux (cross) it refers to wars of a religious character, or specifically to a series of eight defensive military expeditions between 1096 and 1270 undertaken by Christians to liberate the Holy Land and stop the expansion of Islam.

FEUDALISM
System that came to organize the politics, economy, and social life of Medieval Europe after the split of the Carolingian empire. Based on the relationship between wealthy, landowning lords and the common villagers, farm-workers, it was a relatively simple arrangement in which the commoners would pay the landowner in labor or services in return for the lord's military protection against foreign or domestic foes.

IMMURATION
Imprisonment for those who recanted their heresy because of fear of punishment or death.

INDULGENCE
A remission before God of temporal punishment due to sins, the guilt of which has already been forgiven through the sacrament of Penance.

INQUISITOR
Special judges appointed by the pope during the Inquisition who examined and judged the doctrinal opinions and moral conduct of suspicious individuals.

LAY INVESTITURE
The appointment of bishops and abbots by secular rulers, often in exchange for temporal protection.

MILITARY ORDER
Arising out of the necessity of defending the Holy Places in Palestine as well as the pilgrims who traveled there, these orders combined both military and religious life, emphasizing dedication, discipline and monastic organization.

NEPOTISM
From the Italian nepote, "nephew" and Latin nepos, "grandson." The appointment of family members to important positions of authority.

SIMONY
The selling of ecclesiastical offices, pardons, or emoluments by either secular or spiritual leaders.

TERM OF GRACE
The procedure for inquisition began with this month long period which allowed for the inhabitants of a heresy-ridden district to appear before the inquisitor, confess their sins, and perform penance.

TREATY OF VERDUN
Signed in 843, the treaty divided the Carolingian empire into three sections, which led to the eventual destruction of Charlemagne's empire.

VOCABULARY Continued

VICAR OF CHRIST
Title used by Pope Innocent III rather than the earlier title, Vicar of St. Peter. "Vicar of Christ" emphasized Innocent III's understanding of the pope as a representative of Christ himself.

STUDY QUESTIONS

1. What three groups coming from which three directions threatened western Europe during the ninth century?

2. Why were monasteries often the targets of the Viking invasions?

3. When and by whom was Cluny founded?

4. What did the monastic reform at Cluny emphasize?

5. What were two things that separated Cluniac monks from other monks?

6. What did Pope Benedict VIII grant to Cluny in 1016? How did this help Cluny not to become involved in the problems of feudalism?

7. Name at least four important Cluniac monks who rose to positions of importance.

8. Otto I's (the Great) coronation at Aachen as Holy Roman emperor served what two purposes?

9. List the three ways in which the Ottonian line exercised influence over the Church.

10. How did Lanfranc negotiate his responsibilities to the Church and his relationship to the state?

11. Why did the Church want to regain control over the ecclesiastical appointments?

12. What act by Henry IV initiated his struggle with St. Gregory VII?

13. What does excommunication mean? Why would Henry IV not ignore the act of excommunication?

14. What was the Concordat of Worms (1122)?

15. What were King Henry II's aims with the Constitutions of Clarendon?

16. How did the contest between St. Thomas à Becket and King Henry II end?

17. What was Pope Innocent III's goal during his papacy?

18. How did Pope Innocent III and his immediate successors view kings? For what kinds of behavior were kings penalized?

19. Which rule do the Cistercians follow and what do they emphasize along with it?

20. What did the color white signify for the Cistercian habit, and what color did most religious orders wear?

21. What were the two areas of focus for St. Bernard's studies, and what was the central theme of his spirituality?

22. Who founded the Carthusians, and how did he live with the earliest Carthusians?

23. What kind of spirituality did the Carthusians create in their order?

24. What were the crusades?

25. What new Muslim people appeared on the scene in the Middle East as a new threat to Byzantium?

STUDY QUESTIONS Continued

26. When was the First Crusade?

27. How was the timing of the First Crusade particularly fortuitous with regard to the Seljuk Turks and other Muslims?

28. How long did the Europeans control Jerusalem?

29. What Seljuk Turkish leader was an excellent military commander and essentially forced the Europeans into a retreat?

30. What was the result of the "Children's Crusade"?

31. How did the Byzantines view the crusaders?

32. What were some of the effects of the crusades?

33. What was a military order?

34. What was the Knights Templar's specific mission?

35. Who wrote the rule for the Knights Templar?

36. How were the Knights Templar organized?

37. How did the Knights Templar become swealthy?

38. When were the Knights Hospitalers founded and what was their vocation?

39. Where did the Knights Hospitalers go after the fall of Palestine?

40. What other island were the Knights Hospitalers given in 1523 by Holy Roman emperor Charles V?

41. The Teutonic Knights did not keep Jerusalem and hospitals for very long before turning their attention to which lands?

42. Who secularized the Teutonic Knights?

43. What was the Inquisition?

44. What two orders were placed in charge of the Inquisition?

45. What group was the initial target of the Inquisition?

46. What were the five methods of extracting a confession from an accused person?

47. Who actually carried out the sentences of the guilty?

48. How was the Spanish Inquisition different from Inquisitions in other parts of Europe?

PRACTICAL EXERCISES

1. Cluny monks lived in isolation. Explain how their isolation did not hinder the beneficial role they served in western European society.

2. One of the criticisms of the Catholic Church is that it was too often involved in a struggle with secular rulers during the Medieval period, and that this involvement led to such corruptions as simony and lay investiture. Is this a fair charge, historically speaking? In what way did the political organization of this era help to ensure justice and moral righteousness on the part of the sovereign? How did it fail to achieve those ends?

3. Explain why the pope was both a temporal ruler and a spiritual ruler. To which aspect of the papacy does infallibility apply? How is the papacy different today than it was in the Middle Ages? How is it the same?

PRACTICAL EXERCISES Continued

4. Many people believe that the Crusades were aggressive excursions with only negative outcomes. Is this true? Cite reasons for your answers.

5. Is there a conflict of interest with the papacy preaching a crusade in a religion that professes peace? Do you think the papacy would call for a crusade today? Do you think the papacy would call for the establishment of a military order today?

6. Why was the Inquisition instituted? What modern ideas make the Inquisition seem absurd by today's standards?

FROM THE CATECHISM

841 The Church's relationship with the Muslims. "The plan of salvation also includes those who acknowledge the Creator, in the first place amongst whom are the Muslims; these profess to hold the faith of Abraham, and together with us they adore the one, merciful God, mankind's judge on the last day" (LG 16; cf. NA 3).

889 In order to preserve the Church in the purity of the faith handed on by the apostles, Christ who is the Truth willed to confer on her a share in his own infallibility. By a "supernatural sense of faith" the People of God, under the guidance of the Church's living Magisterium, "unfailingly adheres to this faith" (LG 12; cf. DV 10).

890 The mission of the Magisterium is linked to the definitive nature of the covenant established by God with his people in Christ. It is this Magisterium's task to preserve God's people from deviations and defections and to guarantee them the objective possibility of professing the true faith without error. Thus, the pastoral duty of the Magisterium is aimed at seeing to it that the People of God abides in the truth that liberates. To fulfill this service, Christ endowed the Church's shepherds with the charism of infallibility in matters of faith and morals. The exercise of this charism takes several forms:

891 "The Roman Pontiff, head of the college of bishops, enjoys this infallibility in virtue of his office, when, as supreme pastor and teacher of all the faithful – who confirms his brethren in the faith – he proclaims by a definitive act a doctrine pertaining to faith or morals….The infallibility promised to the Church is also present in the body of bishops when, together with Peter's successor, they exercise the supreme Magisterium," above all in an Ecumenical Council (LG 25; cf. Vatican Council I: DS 3074). When the Church through its supreme Magisterium proposes a doctrine "for belief as being divinely revealed" (DV 10 § 2), and as the teaching of Christ, the definitions "must be adhered to with the obedience of faith" (LG 25 § 2). This infallibility extends as far as the deposit of divine Revelation itself (cf. LG 25).

2051 The infallibility of the Magisterium of the Pastors extends to all the elements of doctrine, including moral doctrine, without which the saving truths of the faith cannot be preserved, expounded, or observed.

2244 Every institution is inspired, at least implicitly, by a vision of man and his destiny, from which it derives the point of reference for its judgment, its hierarchy of values, its line of conduct. Most societies have formed their institutions in the recognition of a certain preeminence of man over things. Only the divinely revealed religion has clearly recognized man's origin and destiny in God, the Creator and Redeemer. The Church invites political authorities to measure their judgments

FROM THE CATECHISM Continued

and decisions against this inspired truth about God and man:

> Societies not recognizing this vision or rejecting it in the name of their independence from God are brought to seek their criteria and goal in themselves or to borrow them from some ideology. Since they do not admit that one can defend an objective criterion of good and evil, they arrogate to themselves an explicit or implicit totalitarian power over man and his destiny, as history shows (cf. CA 45; 46).

2245 The Church, because of her commission and competence, is not to be confused in any way with the political community. She is both the sign and the safeguard of the transcendent character of the human person. "The Church respects and encourages the political freedom and responsibility of the citizen" (GS 76 § 3).

2266 The efforts of the state to curb the spread of behavior harmful to people's rights and to the basic rules of civil society correspond to the requirement of safeguarding the common good. Legitimate public authority has the right and the duty to inflict punishment proportionate to the gravity of the offense. Punishment has the primary aim of redressing the disorder introduced by the offense. When it is willingly accepted by the guilty party, it assumes the value of expiation. Punishment then, in addition to defending public order and protecting people's safety, has a medicinal purpose: as far as possible, it must contribute to the correction of the guilty party (cf. Lk 23: 4-43).

2297 Kidnapping and hostage taking bring on a reign of terror; by means of threats they subject their victims to intolerable pressures. They are morally wrong. Terrorism threatens, wounds, and kills indiscriminately is gravely against justice and charity. Torture which uses physical or moral violence to extract confessions, punish the guilty, frighten opponents, or satisfy hatred is contrary to respect for the person and for human dignity. Except when performed for strictly therapeutic medical reasons, directly intended amputations, mutilations, and sterilizations performed on innocent persons are against the moral law (cf. DS 3722).

2298 In times past, cruel practices were commonly used by legitimate governments to maintain law and order, often without protest from the Pastors of the Church, who themselves adopted in their own tribunals the prescriptions of Roman law concerning torture. Regrettable as these facts are, the Church always taught the duty of clemency and mercy. She forbade clerics to shed blood. In recent times it has become evident that these cruel practices were neither necessary for public order, nor in conformity with the legitimate rights of the human person. On the contrary, these practices led to ones even more degrading. It is necessary to work for their abolition. We must pray for the victims and their tormentors.

2309 The strict conditions for legitimate defense by military force require rigorous consideration. The gravity of such a decision makes it subject to rigorous conditions of moral legitimacy. At one and the same time:

– the damage inflicted by the aggressor on the nation or community of nations must be lasting, grave, and certain;

– all other means of putting an end to it must have been shown to be impractical or ineffective;

– there must be serious prospects of success;

– the use of arms must not produce evils and disorders graver than the evil to be eliminated. The power of modern means of destruction weighs very heavily in evaluating this condition.

These are the traditional elements enumerated in what is called the "just war" doctrine.

The evaluation of these conditions for moral legitimacy belongs to the prudential judgment of those who have responsibility for the common good.

CHAPTER 5

The Renaissance

Christian philosophy, piety, and art boldly ventured into new depths, and the saints of the period showed how sanctity can pervade all of our human endeavors.

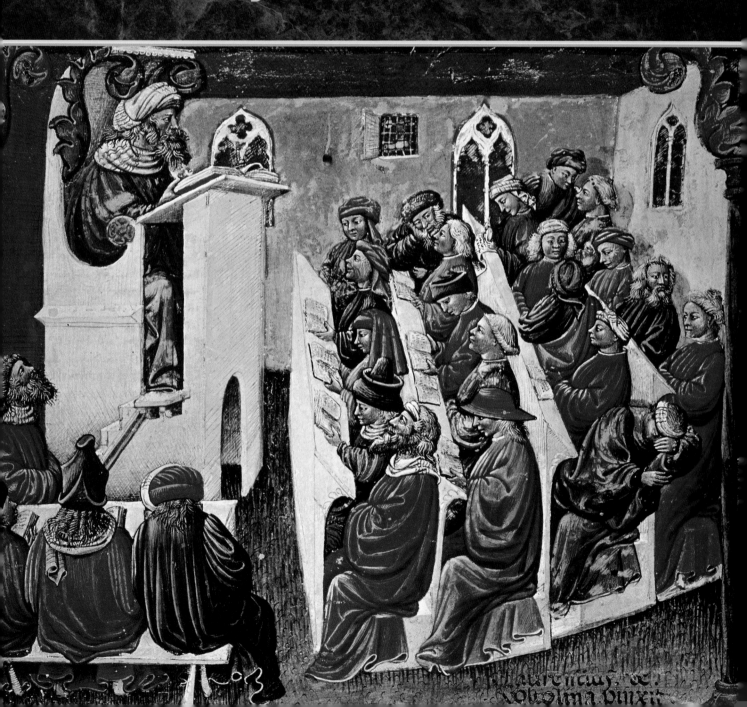

CHAPTER 5

The Renaissance

Before the twelfth and thirteenth centuries, most educational activity in Europe took place in monasteries and cathedral schools. Over time, as the demand for education among monks and nobles increased, these schools began to develop expanded areas of study for their student bodies. The schools added philosophy, astronomy, civil and canon law, and medicine to their curricula and reorganized to meet administrative demands. Modeling themselves after feudal trade guilds, schools began to develop into university systems that provided the proper environment for unprecedented educational and intellectual advancement.

One result of the Medieval university system was Scholasticism. Led by thinkers like St. Thomas Aquinas, St. Bonaventure, and the English Franciscan Bl. John Duns Scotus, Scholasticism grew out of the style of Medieval teaching, combining theological and philosophical methods in their efforts to understand the highest truths of philosophy and theology and man's relationship to God and his Church. These Scholastics produced some of the most lasting and valuable works in the Western Tradition.

In the midst of this flourishing of Medieval thought there came another movement led by two extraordinary saints. St. Francis of Assisi and St. Dominic founded the first two mendicant orders whose devotion to simple piety and poverty helped rejuvenate religious zeal in the late Medieval age.

With the pontificates of Innocent III, Gregory IX, and Boniface VIII, Church authority together with a united Western Christendom reached its zenith. During the thirteenth century, the Church established the legal foundation of the Medieval state, combated heresy and contested with emperors and kings for its legitimate role in regulating society. During this period, the Church finally achieved a balance between its temporal responsibilities and its spiritual authority.

The fourteenth century, however, would witness a dramatic change sweep across the face of Europe, and the accomplishments of the thirteenth century would begin to unravel. The rising kingdoms of France, Germany, and England would no longer be willing to submit themselves to the leadership of the pope. Furthermore Church authority would be almost fatally eroded by its long tenure under the influence of the French Kings at Avignon and by forty years of schism.

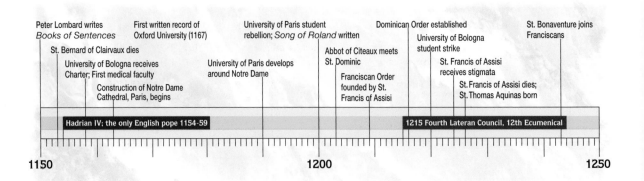

Peter Lombard writes *Books of Sentences*

First written record of Oxford University (1167)

University of Paris student rebellion; *Song of Roland* written

Dominican Order established

St. Bonaventure joins Franciscans

St. Bernard of Clairvaux dies

University of Bologna receives Charter; First medical faculty

Construction of Notre Dame Cathedral, Paris, begins

University of Paris develops around Notre Dame

Abbot of Citeaux meets St. Dominic

Franciscan Order founded by St. Francis of Assisi

University of Bologna student strike

St. Francis of Assisi receives stigmata

St. Francis of Assisi dies; St. Thomas Aquinas born

Hadrian IV; the only English pope 1154-59

1215 Fourth Lateran Council, 12th Ecumenical

1150   1200   1250

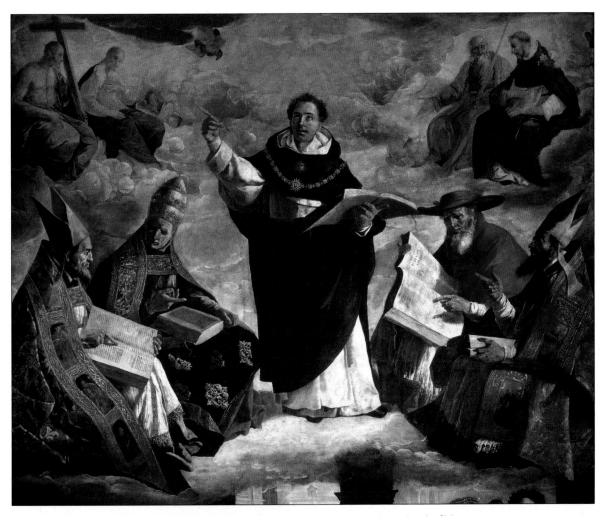

It is training and spiritual life, faith and love of God that leads us closer to knowing Christ.

The survival of Europe would be threatened by both internal and external forces. Plague and famine would shake Medieval society to its very foundations; war within Christendom (between England and France) would destroy the flower of feudal aristocracy; and the Turks would ravage Constantinople and threaten further expansion into Christendom.

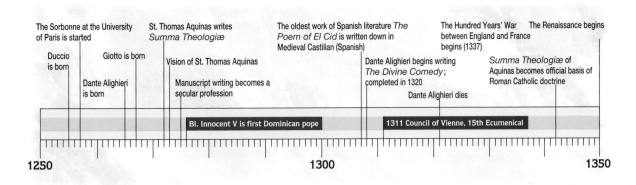

The Sorbonne at the University of Paris is started

St. Thomas Aquinas writes *Summa Theologiæ*

The oldest work of Spanish literature *The Poem of El Cid* is written down in Medieval Castilian (Spanish)

The Hundred Years' War between England and France begins (1337)

The Renaissance begins

Duccio is born

Giotto is born

Vision of St. Thomas Aquinas

Dante Alighieri begins writing *The Divine Comedy*; completed in 1320

Summa Theologiæ of Aquinas becomes official basis of Roman Catholic doctrine

Dante Alighieri is born

Manuscript writing becomes a secular profession

Dante Alighieri dies

Bl. Innocent V is first Dominican pope

1311 Council of Vienne, 15th Ecumenical

1250

1300

1350

As the fourteenth century ended, the Church and Europe were changing. In the wake of war, plague, and schism, feudalism was crumbling as new political and social entities were emerging. All the achievements of the Middle Ages – the creation of the Western monarchies, the development of English law and Parliament, the foundation of universities, the beginning of great vernacular works of literature, and the revival of commerce – pushed Western civilization in a new direction. The nation-state began to rise from the collections of kingdoms and fiefs, and universal access to commerce and capital began to erode the feudal system's vassal-lord relationship.

Along with these social-political changes, there were changes in people's intellectual pursuits. As education became more widely available, people looked away from the theological Scholasticism that flourished in the days of St. Thomas Aquinas and instead turned to the ancient Latin and Greek classics. Familiarity with these texts gave rise to a popular desire to return to the civilization of the Greco-Roman world, to re-awaken a sense of human beauty and appreciate man's achievements. The name given to this movement by its contemporaries was the "Renaissance," a French word meaning "rebirth," and it was a period of rebirth in almost every area of study. With this phenomenon came new challenges for the Church, but in many ways, it also opened the door for much needed humanistic growth and reform.

PART I

The Universities

Beginning in the mid-eleventh century, the demand for education among both clergy and nobles increased dramatically. More and more students flocked to schools, and as the student bodies began to outgrow the cathedral and monastic schools, teachers and students alike recognized the need to reorganize the established educational systems. Following Feudal organizations, schools began to restructure into guilds. Rather than training as a knight or a craftsman, many people began to study at the universities, apprenticing to expert teachers and eventually mastering their disciplines. Degrees awarded to students reflected the same type of recognition bestowed upon members of other trades.

In the North, masters united to form a *universitas*, a type of corporation that protected the educational and administrative interests of its members. In Southern Europe, students formed similar organizations that helped ensure their safety and the quality of their education. As it were, the students at those universities held authority over their teachers, hiring and firing them as they saw fit. In the North, teachers determined the curriculum and the nature of the student body.

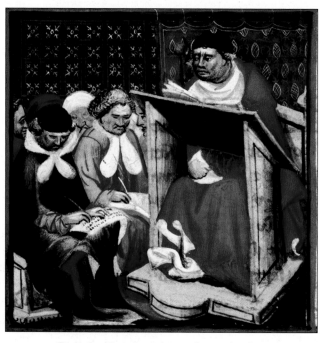

This Medieval illustration depicts a professor and students at the University of Paris.

ORIGIN OF UNIVERSITIES

The development of the University of Paris in 1175 typified the growth of most northern universities. In Paris, there existed three cathedral schools that became especially famous during the early part of the Medieval period: the Palatine or palace school, the school of Notre-Dame, and Sainte-Geneviève. Over time these schools began producing renowned professors, and as their reputations grew, more pupils enrolled in schools where these celebrated lecturers taught. As schools expanded, more lodging was provided, and the numbers of courses increased. Eventually the three schools formed a corporation that protected the professors and combined each individual school's discipline. Although each school continued to teach its specialty, students could now receive a broader education from the unified schools that made up the University of Paris.

In the South, the Italian city of Bologna succeeded Ravenna as the home of jurisprudence in Europe. As the Lombard cities grew together with the demand for legal instruction, the school at Bologna in 1088 became a center for legal study. The University of Bologna began teaching the *Dictamen*, or Art of Composition, which included rules for drawing up briefs and other legal documents. This specialized training attracted many students, and there soon developed another intense program specializing in grammar and rhetoric, which were both closely connected with the study of law. As the number of disciplines increased, students organized to help ensure their educational security. Bologna became the undisputed center of legal training in Europe, and almost all of the important scholars of canon and Roman law studied, at least for some time, at that school.

The school at Salerno had more singular origins. The Benedictine monastery of Salerno, established in 794, devoted much of its work to the study of ancient works on botanical and medical sciences. The fame of the monastery's expertise in these areas grew after Constantino Africano, a Christian who studied in the Arabic schools in Babylon, Baghdad, and in Egypt, took up residence at the monastery around the year 1070. Under the influence of Africano, the monastery school added philosophical and Arabic works to the medical studies, helping the school advance its reputation as an institution with a superior understanding of medicine. As the school grew, it became the first university in Europe to offer degrees and licenses for its studies.

ORGANIZATION OF THE UNIVERSITY

Although the organization of Northern and Southern European universities differed, normally both were collections of different schools that taught their respective disciplines. It was not until 1230 that several branches of learning were taught at one university.

At Bologna, Italy, which became the template for most of the Southern European universities, students from all over Europe came to the city to study. For protection and housing, foreign students formed groups called "nations." They elected a rector who led the nation and helped administer the affairs of the university.

Paris is the center that typified the structure of the northern European universities; the chancellor had full authority over issuing licenses to teach and awarding degrees. Naturally, this led to friction between teachers and the chancellor. To protect their own interests and authority, teachers bound together to form a guild, or *universitates*. The students also organized into nations, but they never had the same authority as those in Southern Europe. By the middle of the thirteenth century, the teachers' guilds had separated into faculties according to the corresponding discipline that was being taught. A dean headed each faculty, and those same deans voted for a rector who was the head of all the faculties and the university (similar to the modern-day president).

The guild organizations allowed these universities to remain independent, and they were theoretically exempt from arrest or punishment by the secular authorities. Each university eventually secured independence from both lay and local ecclesiastical authorities. This fostered an environment of free inquiry and unobstructed explorations into all aspects of learning.

ACADEMIC COURSEWORK

By unifying various schools and disciplines, the universities were able to offer a program called *studium generale,* which included the study of theology (including philosophy), law (both civil and canon law), medicine, which was called physics, and the arts. The arts were also divided into two main sections: the *trivium* (Latin for "three ways"), in which Latin grammar, rhetoric, and logic were studied, and the *quadrivium* (four ways), which included arithmetic, geometry, astronomy, and music.

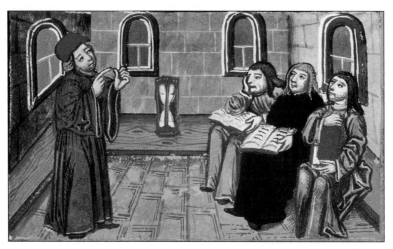

A student needed to be able to read and write in Latin before being admitted into the university.

A student needed to be able to read and write in Latin before being admitted into the university. Once admitted, he began his studies with the *trivium,* mastering writing and reading and studying Classical and Christian works on the subjects. The teacher, or master, would read the text of a work on a topic along with his predecessors' comments on the text before adding his own ideas. This method of teaching was called "hearing" a book, i.e., lecture (from the Latin *lectio,* the act of reading). After completing the *trivium,* the student became a "bachelor of arts," and was considered qualified to instruct others in those subjects. He then moved on to study the *quadrivium,* during which he spent five or six years studying before earning a "master of arts" degree. All students who finished university studies received both degrees, and they could then leave the school or continue on to study more intensively for a doctorate degree in law, medicine, or theology. To earn these higher degrees, students not only "heard" books, but also debated their professors on the subjects and prepared formal responses to tough questions posed by their superiors.

THE EFFECTS OF THE UNIVERSITY

The cultural exchange brought about by the Crusades ushered in a flood of previously unknown books and ideas into Western Europe. The universities were able to maintain significant academic liveliness through the continued introduction of these new books to their curriculum. As works in mathematics, philosophy, and theology were discovered or written, they would be adopted into various university studies. Legal studies at Bologna advanced the understanding of canon law and produced skilled and scholarly clergy who became experts in both Roman and Church law. These hubs of expert academic learning helped lead Europe into a period of exceptional intellectual growth.

PART II

Scholasticism

New philosophical texts entered into Europe as the crusaders returned, and scholars set about the task of reconciling these "new" ideas with over a thousand years of Christian belief and doctrine. Previously, European scholars only had access to neo-Platonic philosophy and Aristotle's logic to use as a tool for their theology. Until the latter part of the twelfth century and the beginning of the thirteenth, most of Aristotle's words were unknown in the West. By contrast, in the East there existed both Arab and Jewish commentaries on Aristotle's works, espeially his *Metaphysics*. This new discovery of Aristotle's thought would revolutionize theology and subsequently elicit debate and controversy.

With access to Aristotle's works, universities fostered a new style of inquiry in philosophy, known as Scholasticism, or "science of the schools." This method led to a rebirth of interest in Classical philosophy and the relationship between Faith and reason.

METHODS AND MYSTERY

The methods of Scholasticism came largely out of a teaching technique that developed in the universities. When a scholar read an ancient or authoritative text, he drew up lists of contradictory statements. Then, by means of logical reasoning, the scholar tried to reveal the underlying agreement between these points of contradiction, hoping to attain the central and underlying truths of the work. Over time this system of philosophical and theological inquiry developed in the Medieval schools of Christian Europe, creating its own technical language and methodology. This method became known as Scholasticism.

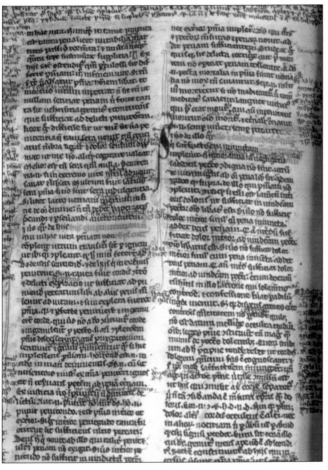

A 13th century manuscript of Peter Lombard's *Books of Sentences*, IV. Written ca. 1150, this work became a standard university textbook.

Anselm of Laon was a student of St. Anselm, who is known as the "father of Scholasticism" because he first studied and analyzed the beliefs of Christian Faith resorting to logic and discursive reasoning while lecturing on Scripture at Paris. He achieved it mainly by following the methods of Boethius, Charlemagne, and Alcuin that were available to him, Anselm collected authoritative statements from the Church Fathers and attached them to matching texts in the Bible. When two Fathers differed in their interpretation, their contradictory statements were compared in Anselm's classroom. Students would argue, debate, and hope to find the underlying truths behind the contradictions.

Peter Lombard further refined this method of questioning. He set forth two requirements for the Scholastic method. First he proposed that questioning is the key to perceiving truth. Scholasticism, in this way, did not grow as an independent school of thought, but rather out of a continual questioning of the contradictions that arose in already formulated schools of thought. Secondly, he proposed that the differences that will arise in questioning could usually be resolved by determining the meaning of terms used by different authors in varying ways. Thus, out of comparatively studying the works and the language of the great thinkers, truth and clarity can be drawn between them. In his four *Books of Sentences,* Peter Lombard collected and discussed the opinions of the Church Fathers and earlier theologians on all questions pertaining to Revelation. His thorough and comprehensive work on the rational understanding of God's revealed truth; this opus became the handbook of theologians and part of every professor's curriculum.

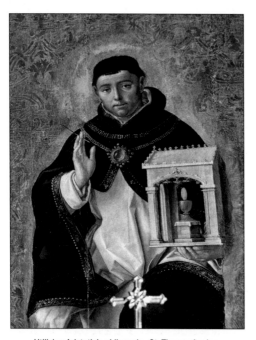

Utilizing Aristotle's philosophy, St. Thomas Aquinas was able to discuss in a cogent way Christ's dual nature as God and man and his presence in the Eucharist.

ST. THOMAS AQUINAS

Many insightful commentaries came out of this approach to learning, but perhaps none can match the work of the Dominican friar St. Thomas Aquinas during the thirteenth century. St. Thomas Aquinas studied theology at the University of Paris and then returned to hold a chair of theology at the university. St. Thomas systematically approached virtually all the questions that confronted Christianity, eventually creating his encyclopedic work, the *Summa Theologiæ.* The *Summa* sets about understanding the most fundamental tenets of Christianity, including, among other things, the existence of God, the divinity of Christ, and Christian morality.

Much of St. Thomas's work was directed toward rectifying a philosophical problem that arose from the rediscovery of the Greek philosopher Aristotle. Many feared that Aristotle's works would undermine the truth of Christianity. St. Thomas showed by his integration of Aristotelian philosophy with Christian belief that Aristotle's thought was an added tool for Catholic theology.

During the Middle Ages, some of Aristotle's work was known in the West through Boethius, but many of Aristotle's books, most notably the *Metaphysics,* were not. In the East, both Muslims and Jews had a tradition of thought included Aristotelian philosophy. During the time of the Crusades, both Aristotle's works and the commentaries began circulating in Europe.

Until Aristotle's works were made known again to the West, most Christian thinkers since the time of the Church Fathers looked to Plato and Plotinus for a philosophical tool to explain the theological truths of Christianity. Neo-Platonism appeared as the ideal philosophy for a deeper understanding of Christian teaching. Plato's ideas about God and contemplation appeared to reinforce Christian teaching. Plato deduced a world of ideas, or "forms" emanating from the highest form, called the *Logos*. Some Christian thinkers equated the *Logos* with the Second Person of the Trinity. Aristotle broke ranks with his former teacher and contended that the universe was infinite and that the individual soul was mortal. This directly contradicted Christian teachings of creation and the immortality of the soul. Aristotle and Plato disagreed with each other concerning the reality of material existence. Whereas Plato held that matter was a pale shadow of the eternal form (idea) of a material object, Aristotle argued that the reality of each material being pertains to both its form and

its material component. For example, all trees are not simply shadows of a greater perfect form of a tree, the philosopher would contend. Rather, each tree is a unity of form and matter, which makes it an individual tree.

While most Christians held to the Platonic camp, St. Thomas Aquinas was convinced of Aristotle's superior logic and sought to reconcile the compatibility between reason and revelation. He set out to systematically employ the philosophy of Aristotle to expound on the Christian Faith. Rather than dismiss the problems that arose between Aristotle's logic and Christian doctrine, the dutiful Scholastic thinker set out to ask questions and arrive at a fundamental conclusion in their mutual applicability. Faith and reason, St. Thomas contended, did not need to be opposed to one another.

St. Thomas Aquinas was able to use this reasoned approach with respect to Faith and reason in updating Catholic theology. For instance, utilizing Aristotle's philosophy, he was able to discuss in a cogent way Christ's dual nature as God and man and his presence in the Eucharist. St. Thomas used philosophy to shed light

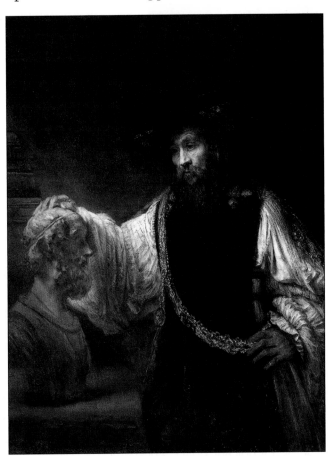

Rembrandt's portrait of Aristotle.
St. Thomas Aquinas was convinced of Aristotle's superior logic and sought to reconcile Aristotelian logic and Christian Faith.

on the mysteries of Christian doctrine, explaining theology in a philosophical context. The saint never subjugated reason to revelation. He said that even some truths that are available to man through reason would be very hard, if not nearly impossible to understand were it not for God's revelation. This wise thinker, together with his brilliant mind, retained a childlike faith throughout his life. Towards the end of his life, he had a mystical vision while offering Mass in Naples in 1273. After that vision, he stopped his philosophical work, saying that "Everything I have written seems like straw by comparison to what I have seen and what has been revealed to me" (quoted in Livingstone, *The Oxford Dictionary of the Christian Church*, 1997, pp. 1614-15.). Despite his incredible philosophical output, the Angelic Doctor saw himself as a teacher of theology in service of the Church. St. Thomas Aquinas's books and treatises remain unsurpassed in offering a comprehensive and thorough theological and philosophical understanding of God, his works, and his laws.

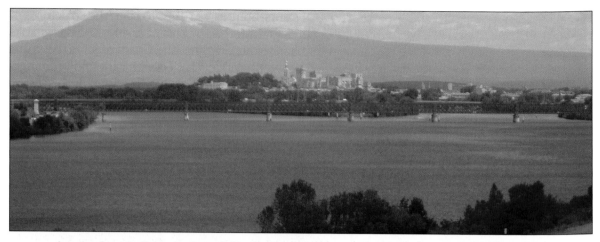

In southern France, the *Palais des Papes* (Palace of the Popes), now a museum, towers over the city of Avignon and the Rhône River. Beginning with Clement V, seven popes resided in Avignon from 1309-1377. It remained a papal possession until the French Revolution incorporated Avignon into France in 1791. Avignon is 400 miles southeast of Paris.

PART V

The Road to Avignon

POPE ST. CELESTINE V

After Pope Nicolas IV died in 1294, the papal throne remained vacant for more than two years while rival Italian parties vied for their own papal candidate. In order to break the deadlock, three cardinals sought a compromise candidate. In the hills of Abruzzi there lived an 80-year-old saintly hermit by the name of Peter Murrone. He spent much of his life in a small cave, living a rigorously ascetic existence of prayer, labor, and fasting. In 1294, the three dignitaries, accompanied by a huge gathering of monks, priests, and laymen, begged Peter to accept the papacy. Though he did not wish to leave his simple life of prayer and solitude, Peter accepted, choosing the name Celestine V. As pope, this simple, holy, old man was beloved by the people, but before the year was out, the immense task of shepherding the Church proved too much for him. Without training or experience, especially in dealing with the various political machinations of certain cardinals, nobles, and emperors, the task of directing all of Christendom was humanly overwhelming and certainly beyond this hermit's abilities. After making many imprudent and ill-informed political decisions,

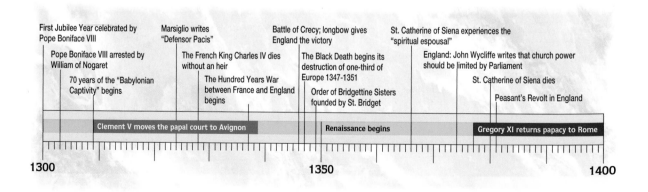

First Jubilee Year celebrated by Pope Boniface VIII

Pope Boniface VIII arrested by William of Nogaret

70 years of the "Babylonian Captivity" begins

Marsiglio writes "Defensor Pacis"

The French King Charles IV dies without an heir

The Hundred Years War between France and England begins

Battle of Crecy; longbow gives England the victory

The Black Death begins its destruction of one-third of Europe 1347-1351

Order of Bridgettine Sisters founded by St. Bridget

St. Catherine of Siena experiences the "spiritual espousal"

England: John Wycliffe writes that church power should be limited by Parliament

St. Catherine of Siena dies

Peasant's Revolt in England

Clement V moves the papal court to Avignon

Renaissance begins

Gregory XI returns papacy to Rome

1300   1350   1400

he, without precedent and in the face of much opposition, chose to resign his office and return to his private life of prayer and penance. Most of his decisions and official acts not affecting Faith and morals were annulled by the succeeding pope, Boniface VIII (Benedetto Gaetani). While pope, St. Celestine split the College of Cardinals, appointing twelve new cardinals in his short, five month pontificate – seven of them French, the rest, Neapolitan.

Free of the burden of the papacy, St. Celestine sought to return to his beloved eremitic life. Boniface VIII feared that the previous pope might be used by certain oppositional groups who wished to advance schism in the Church. The new pope attempted to apprehend St. Celestine in order to keep him in confinement. St. Celestine avoided capture for some time, but was eventually imprisoned quite uncomfortably for the remaining ten months of his life. While prudence dictated to Boniface VIII to protect St. Celestine, and with him the integrity of the Church, the unfortunate treatment of this simple, saintly man remains a regrettable chapter in Boniface's pontificate.

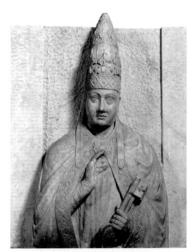

Pope Boniface VIII (1294-1303) was in certain ways like a Renaissance pope. He was a patron of artists, Giotto in particular, and of sculptors; he founded the University of Rome; he reorganized the Vatican archives and had the Vatican library catalogued.

BONIFACE VIII AND PHILIP IV

Though a courageous man of action, with political experience and knowledge of the current situation of the Church, Boniface VIII also lacked the necessary diplomacy required to deal with the difficult and changing political landscape. Tension would soon mount between pope and king over the temporal authority of the Church, and Pope Boniface VIII found that wielding these two swords would be nearly impossible in the changing European political climate.

The grandson of the late King St. Louis IX of France shared none of his predecessor's saintly admiration for the Church. Philip, called the Fair, assumed the throne in 1285, and, intent on extending the boundaries of France, he undertook a series of wars, particularly against England. These wars depleted Philip's funds, and he turned to Church lands to supplement his royal treasury. Except in times of a crusade, the Church had always been exempt from the taxation policies of the royal government, but the king ignored this precedent, collecting revenue from Church estates and confiscating properties to suit his desires.

In 1296, to chastise Philip, Boniface wrote *Clericis laicos* in which he asserted that kings did not have the right to tax clergy without the permission of the pope. Philip responded by cutting off

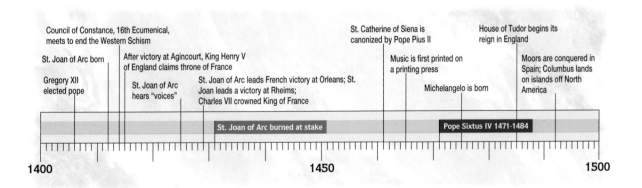

Council of Constance, 16th Ecumenical, meets to end the Western Schism

St. Catherine of Siena is canonized by Pope Pius II

House of Tudor begins its reign in England

St. Joan of Arc born

After victory at Agincourt, King Henry V of England claims throne of France

Music is first printed on a printing press

Moors are conquered in Spain; Columbus lands on islands off North America

Gregory XII elected pope

St. Joan of Arc hears "voices"

St. Joan of Arc leads French victory at Orleans; St. Joan leads a victory at Rheims; Charles VII crowned King of France

Michelangelo is born

St. Joan of Arc burned at stake

Pope Sixtus IV 1471-1484

1400   1450   1500

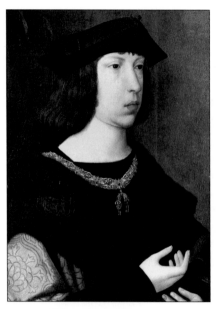

Philip the Fair was King of France from 1285 until his death in 1314.

all French shipments of gold, silver, and jewels to Italy. The loss of Church revenue from this action forced Boniface to compromise on this issue.

In 1301, a more serious dispute broke out between Philip and Pope Boniface. Philip, in order to assert his authority over the Church in France, arrested Pope Boniface's papal legate on a series of secular charges. Pope Boniface condemned Philip's actions and ordered the prelate released. In the letter *Unam Sanctam*, Boniface declared that in order to save his or her soul, every human being – including the king – must be subject to the pope. Philip responded by calling his own national council, the Estates General, to condemn and depose the pope. Boniface was falsely charged with a ridiculous list of crimes ranging from idolatry and magic, to the death of St. Celestine V and the loss of the Holy Land. In 1303 with some six hundred men, William of Nogaret, advisor to King Philip, and Sciarra Colonna, head of a powerful Roman family, marched through Italy to the small town of Anagni. There they stormed the papal palace to find Boniface dressed in full papal regalia, waiting calmly and righteously, resolute in the authority and integrity of his exalted position as the Vicar of Christ. He was captured, slapped, and held prisoner at Anagni for three days. Though he was soon released, the affair and the abuse he suffered during his short captivity ruined his health. He soon died of a raging fever.

THE AVIGNON PAPACY

In the aftermath of the death of Pope Boniface VIII, Italy fell into a state of turmoil. Rome was subjected to the semi-anarchy of the masses and powerful Italian families, and the Italian peninsula began breaking up into a series of independent city-states. Pope Boniface VIII was succeeded by Bl. Benedict XI, who attempted to work out some sort of peace with King Philip. The king clamored for the formal condemnation of Boniface VIII, but Bl. Benedict XI resisted, taking steps to redress the scandalous events surrounding the last days of Boniface's pontificate by excommunicating William of Nogaret, Sciarra Colonna, and their accomplices. The pope's bold move was not met lightly, and within eight months of ascending the papal throne, Bl. Benedict XI was found dead. Though the cause of his death is listed as acute dysentery, many suspect the cause of his death to be a fatal combination of an angry William of Nogaret and poison.

For nearly a year, the chair of St. Peter remained vacant. Under pressure from King Philip IV, the eleven-month conclave finally appointed Bertrand de Got, the Archbishop of Bordeaux and personal friend of the French king, who took the name Clement V. In order to avoid the political chaos of Rome, Clement chose to establish his papal court elsewhere, eventually settling in the town of Avignon (at that time beholden to Naples), near the French border. In Avignon, the pope surrounded himself with French cardinals, a move that exposed Pope Clement, and the Church, to the pressures and whims of the French crown. A far cry from Pope Boniface VIII's exposé of symbolic temporal power, Pope Clement V never left French soil, and for the next 70 years (1305-1377), the popes (all French) would reside in Avignon under the watchful eye of the French king in what would be called "The Babylonian Captivity."

Pope Clement and King Philip were boyhood friends. The king hoped that this new pope would vindicate his recent actions by declaring Pope Boniface VIII a heretic and revoking all of Boniface's anti-regal acts. Pope Clement V refused to give in to this demand. Wishing to placate the powerful

French king, nonetheless, Pope Clement allowed the inquisition in France to investigate the military order of the Knights Templar; this affair would end in a terrible disaster. The inquisition spun away from papal control as Clement was too weak and indecisive to keep it under his charge. Though accused of heresy and worldliness, the Templars' real "crime" was possessing property and wealth coveted by the king. Those knights captured by King Philip were brutally tortured until they admitted to all of the various crimes with which they were falsely charged. Many knights were eventually burned as heretics, and when the order was permanently dissolved, King Philip seized half of their possessions.

The Church at Avignon tried to stem the threats posed by the rising tide of secular governments by strengthening its own administrative system. Though not completely under the influence of the French king, the papacy at Avignon seemed to have lost its independent position in Christendom. The Medieval popes had fought German Imperial designs on Italy to secure the independence of the Church, but by staying at Avignon, they lost this same independence to the French King. The growth of nationalism at this time made it imperative that the pope remain above particular national interests. Since this was not the case with the Avignon popes, the prestige and authority of the papacy quickly declined. England and Germany began to view the pope more as a puppet of the French king than the supreme pastor of the universal Church.

To make matters more difficult for the popes, the idea that the kings' power extended into ecclesiastical affairs favored the nationalization of the Church in each European kingdom. This phenomenon became especially more widespread as the papacy took up residence at Avignon. Gallicanism (the idea that the French Roman Catholic clergy favored the restriction of papal control and the achievement by each nation of individual autonomy) has its origins in this period of history, emerging in France when King Philip IV called for his Estates General to move against Pope Boniface VIII. English laws of 1351-1393 helped to establish the foundations for an Anglican Church years before the Reformation and King Henry VIII. The German Emperor Louis IV of Bavaria, fearing French influence over the pope at Avignon, harbored a large number of anti-papal agitators at his court, including the Englishman William of Ockham who strongly supported the democratization of Church government. Pope Clement V only exacerbated the situation when, in order to please King Philip IV, he retracted Pope Boniface VIII's *Clericis laicos* and reinterpreted *Unam Sanctam*, stripping the document of any claims to temporal authority.

In 1324, the most damaging attack from the proponents of Gallicanism came from a former rector of the University of Paris by the name of Marsiglio of Padua. In the book *Defensor Pacis* (Defender of Peace), Marsiglio made the first clear assertion of the supremacy of secular rulers over the Church. He declared that the faithful were the true authority of the Church. This book held that the pope derived his authority not from Christ, but from the General Council, a body made up of clergymen and laymen and directed by the state. It further maintained that the emperor, as the representative of the people, had the right to depose and punish Church officials and dispose of ecclesiastical property as he saw fit.

As long as the pope remained in Avignon, the independence of the papacy was severely compromised. Writers such as William of Ockham and Marsiglio of Padua paved the way for anti-clerical attacks on the authority of the pope and sowed the seeds of religious rebellion. As if the situation was not grim enough, in the midst of these troubles came a series of events that would by themselves shake the very foundation of Medieval society.

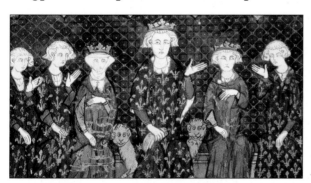

King Philip IV and his children. Three of Philip's sons became kings of France: Louis X, Philip V and Charles IV. His daughter Isabella became Queen Consort of England.

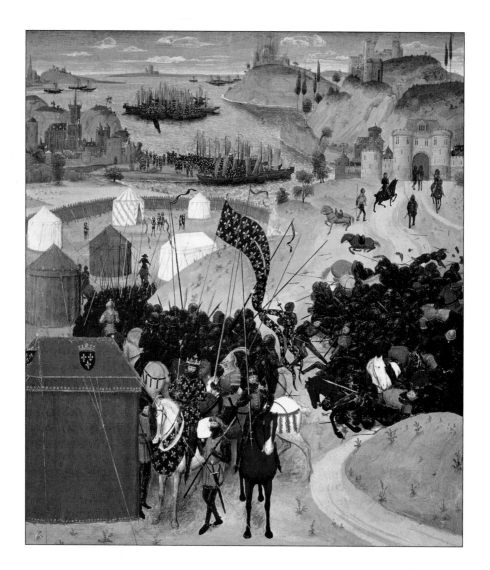

PART VI

The Hundred Years War (1337-1453)

Another major crisis struck Medieval Europe while the popes took up residence in Avignon. For much of the Middle Ages, the Church had managed to prevent and avoid major confrontations between the various kings of Christendom through what was known as the Peace and Truce of God. According to this principle, European kings recognized a common unity of Faith, keeping peace between European peoples who otherwise did not share nationality or custom. Those religious bonds were no longer held sacred, and the problems of inheritance and conflicting economic interest that arose out of the feudal system put many kings at odds against each other. Ultimately, the conflict that arose between England and France during the fourteenth century would change the nature of knightly warfare and transform not only the kingdoms of England and France, but also the entire political makeup of Europe. Out of the ashes of more than one hundred years of warring rose a new sense of national identity – the first steps towards the formation of the European nation-states.

THE ENGLISH IN FRANCE

Since the time of William the Conqueror in the eleventh century, the English and French thrones were linked through a number of matrimonial alliances. Through those marriages, England had inherited large portions of French land. The largest portion came from Henry II's marriage to Eleanor of Aquitaine, through which the king acquired the huge Duchy of Aquitaine in south-western France. Although officially Henry held this land as a vassal of the French king, the English kings never really considered their possessions subject to the foreign ruler. Hostile to the foreign occupiers, the French kings long aspired to drive the English from their feudal estates in France.

All these hostilities exploded when the French king Charles IV (Charles the Fair), the last son of the French king Philip IV, died without an heir in 1328. The Capetian line was broken and no one was left with a clear claim on the throne of France. Both King Philip IV's nephew (the grandson of King Philip III) and King Edward III of England (whose mother was the sister of King Charles IV of France) claimed the right of succession. This dispute began the long series of armed conflicts between England and France, known as the Hundred Years War.

THE HUNDRED YEARS WAR

The Hundred Years War was in fact a series of short battles interrupted by long periods of relative peace. The English gained the upper hand early in the conflict. Though outnumbered, English forces destroyed the French knights at Crecy in 1346, thanks in part to the introduction of the long bow. This new weapon could shoot a yard-long arrow as far as 400 yards at the rate of five to six arrows a minute. It was one of the many deadly military innovations that would change the style of combat during the Hundred Years War.

In 1356, King Edward III's eldest son Edward (the Black Prince) led an English offensive at Poitiers. Both sides exhausted each other through a long battle of attrition, and eventually a truce was signed. However, peace lasted only four years before war broke out again in 1360. Learning from Crecy and Poitiers, the French knights avoided meeting the English in full-scale battles; instead, they skirmished with the English, scattering the troops. This style of warfare proved slow and deadly, never allowing either side to gain a clear upper hand. Twenty years of grueling fighting passed.

By 1380 both King Edward III and the Black Prince were dead, and England held only the coastal towns of Bordeaux, Bayonne, and Calais. England was on her heels, and an end to the war was in sight. But a civil war between the major noble houses of France broke out, helping to prolong the military conflict. The new French king, Charles VI, took the throne at the age of twelve, and besides being too young to rule in his own right, he was exceedingly mad. (Among his many fits and eccentricities, he believed himself to be made of glass and about to break.) The Dukes of Burgundy and Orléans took advantage

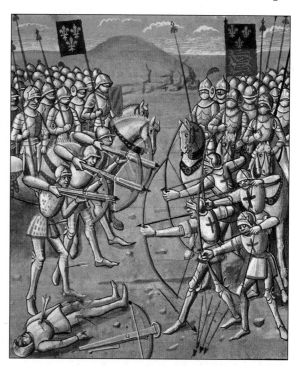

The English defeated the French at Crecy in 1346 with the help of the deadly long bow which could shoot an arrow 400 yards.

of Charles's handicap and fought for control of France. The infighting left France vulnerable to an invasion, and England's King Henry V did not miss his opportunity.

King Henry V destroyed the elite of the French aristocracy and overwhelmed the king of France at Agincourt in 1415. The aftermath of Henry's victory at Agincourt demonstrated the failing legacy of the Medieval feudal system. French cavalry butchered young pages waiting at the wagons off the field of battle and French prisoners were executed rather than ransomed, as was the custom. Henry V claimed the throne of France and married the French king's daughter, Catherine. Henry only ruled for two years before his death, after which he left his infant son Henry VI on the throne.

A succession of young, incompetent, and partially mad kings left France demoralized and subject to the English crown. As the Hundred Years War dragged on, the future of France looked bleak. The ominous fate of the kingdom was radically changed by the appearance of a young peasant girl named Joan.

ST. JOAN OF ARC

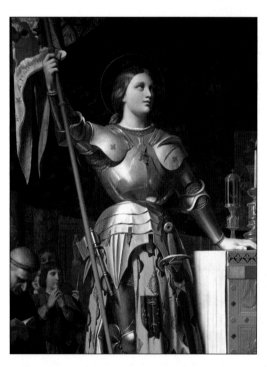

St. Joan was born at Domremy in Champagne, probably on January 6, 1412. At the age of 13, she began to hear voices and had a vision of light in which St. Michael the Archangel, St. Margaret, and St. Catherine of Alexandria appeared to her. These guiding councilors elected her as liberator of France and, in particular, the city of Orléans. St. Joan was instructed by the saints to inform Charles VII that she would make possible his coronation.

Dressed in men's clothes, St. Joan succeeded in convincing the king of the sincerity of her mission, and in May 1429, she led a small army against the captured city of Orléans. Under her leadership, French soldiers overwhelmed English fortifications and drove them from the city, liberating the regions of Loire, Troyes, and Châlons. During the battle, St. Joan was wounded by an arrow, but desired to move on to Rheims. Rheims was finally captured in July 1429, and there Charles was formally crowned king Charles VII.

With the crowning of King Charles VII, St. Joan's principal aim was complete, and after a failed attack on Paris, she did not lead any assaults until the following year. During the winter, Charles and his advisors grew increasingly apathetic to her mission. The following May, St. Joan led a small army of five hundred soldiers against a far stronger force. During the attack she was captured by the English.

Charles dvid not attempt to bargain for St. Joan's life, and with no support from the French, St. Joan was put on trial for heresy and witchcraft by Pierre Cauchon, the Bishop of Beauvais. The Bishop was an unscrupulous, ambitious man and a puppet of the English rulers in Burgundy. St. Joan was convicted of heresy, largely because she was allowed no defense of her supernatural premonitions. Before leading her first strike with French forces, King Charles had St. Joan examined by a number of doctors and bishops. They found nothing sick or heretical in St. Joan's message, but neither those officials nor their documents proving St. Joan's innocence were allowed to be used in St. Joan's defense during her English trial. St. Joan was burned at the stake on May 30, 1431.

ST. JOAN OF ARC'S IMPOSSIBLE MISSION

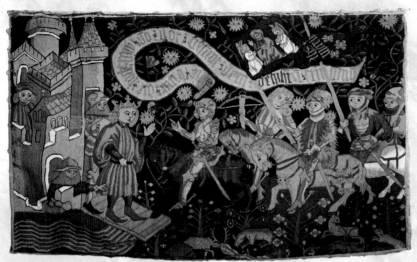

This tapestry depicts the meeting of St. Joan of Arc and King Charles VII at Chinon in March 1429.

God made it clear to St. Joan that she was to lead an army against the English. Despite the certainty of God's will for her life, her mission was no easy task. Nevertheless, through St. Joan's strong faith and committed persistence, God enabled her to carry out this nearly impossible mission.

The first obstacle to St. Joan's mission was the king. Securing an audience with the French monarch was difficult enough, let alone persuading him to let a poor peasant girl lead one of the French armies in battle. Initially, she could not get into the king's court. St. Joan continued to hear mystical voices that instructed her on how to proceed. In May 1428, these voices told her to seek out Robert Baudricourt, a commander of the king's army in the nearby town of Vaucouleurs.

Accompanied by her cousin, St. Joan traveled to Vaucouleurs and spoke with Baudricourt about her instructions to lead an army. The commander remained skeptical, to the say the least, and rather then helping St. Joan, he told St. Joan's cousin to bring the girl home and have her whipped. Despite Baudricourt's indignation, the voices persisted in urging St. Joan to seek the commander's help. St. Joan returned to Vaucouleurs, this time with a prophetic message. Although it was too soon for anyone in Vaucouleurs to have known about a recent French defeat at the Battle of Herrings, she told Baudricourt about the details of the battle. Baudricourt, struck by St. Joan's prophetic insight, sent the young girl to see the king at Chinon in March 1429.

St. Joan finally had her chance to speak with the king, but convincing the king to allow her to lead an army still did not seem likely. St. Joan would be aided, ironically, by the king's own trickery. Seeking to test her, the king disguised an aid as king. Upon entering the court, however, St. Joan saluted the real king, who disguised himself as a simple attendant. She then revealed to the king a secret sign that the Lord disclosed to St. Joan before her arrival. While no one knows what the secret was, many believe it had to do with the king's doubts about the legitimacy of his birth. After these revelations, the king was convinced and proceeded to help St. Joan carry out her mission.

Twenty-five years later, in 1456, the sentence was lifted after a re-examination by Pope Callistus III. St. Joan was eventually beatified in 1909 and canonized by Pope Benedict XV in 1920.

Through the services of St. Joan of Arc, the tide of battle turned against the English. Although St. Joan was captured and killed, her efforts enabled the French army to begin a counter-offensive against the English. Now fighting a divided enemy, the French retook Paris in 1436. One by one, English posts fell rapidly, and by 1453 the English only controlled Calais. The memory of St. Joan was vindicated, and popular devotion to her grew. The people of France rallied around St. Joan of Arc, and by the end of the Hundred Years War, St. Joan became a symbol of French unity and national spirit.

PART VII

Return to Rome and Schism

Plague and war had devastating effects on the institutions and leadership of Medieval Europe, and the continuing presence of the popes at Avignon undermined the ability of the Holy See to reform itself and restore order to Christendom. The long-awaited return of the pope to Rome finally came in 1377 during the pontificate of Gregory XI. Avignon itself was no longer safe as French and English armies fought for domination of the French mainland. Ongoing civil war in Italy, including war between Florence and the papacy (1375), made it clear to Pope Gregory XI that the Holy See needed to return to the City of St. Peter in order to recover its absent leadership. Gregory hesitated to take the fateful step. Nevertheless, the pope would receive the strength and confidence to return to Rome through the work of another extraordinary woman of the fourteenth century, the Dominican Tertiary mystic St. Catherine of Siena.

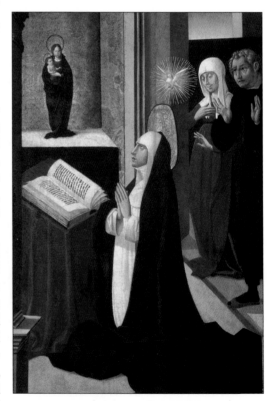

St. Catherine underwent a mystical experience common to many saints known as the "spiritual espousal."

ST. CATHERINE OF SIENA

St. Catherine (1347-1380) was the youngest of twenty-five children. As a young girl, St. Catherine had a precocious understanding of her own vocation and by age seven had consecrated her virginity to Christ. St. Catherine began to receive visions and wasted no time in committing herself to God's mission for her. At sixteen years of age, she joined the Dominican Tertiaries.

For a time she lived a secluded and demanding ascetical life during which she had visions and strong mystical experiences, including conversations with Christ. In 1366, St. Catherine underwent a mystical experience common to a number of saints known as a "spiritual espousal." In this "mystical marriage," Christ tells a soul that he takes it for his bride. The apparition is accompanied by a ceremony in which the Blessed Virgin, saints, and angels are present, after which the soul receives a sudden surge of charity and an increased familiarity with God.

After her spiritual espousal and years of seclusion, St. Catherine returned to the world to dedicate herself to the service of the poor and the sick – especially those suffering from the plague.

St. Catherine lived extreme poverty amongst the sick and constantly suffered physical pain. She went for long periods with practically no food, save Holy Communion. Despite these physical deprivations, she was radiantly happy and full of practical wisdom and spiritual insight. Even members of her own order who saw her extraordinary personal charm, despite her physical sufferings, teased and tormented her. Nonetheless, her spiritual purity and charisma drew followers, both men and women, who flocked to her, united by the bonds of mystical love. She continued to experience all types of visions, including a series of special manifestations of the Divine mysteries and a prolonged ecstasy in which she had a vision of Hell, Purgatory, and Heaven. During that vision, St. Catherine heard God ask her to enter public life and help "heal the wounds of the Church."

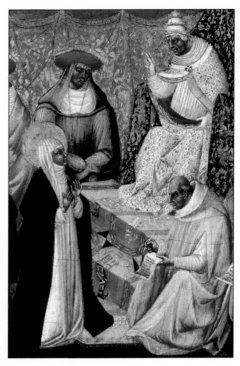

Upon meeting with Pope Gregory XI, St. Catherine reminded him of a personal vow he had made to himself.

St. Catherine began to send letters to men and women of every walk of life. She entered into correspondence with many princes and leaders of Italy and began imploring Pope Gregory XI to return to Rome. Upon meeting with Pope Gregory, God miraculously revealed to St. Catherine Gregory's secret desire to return the papacy to Rome, a personal vow he had never disclosed to any human being. "Fulfill what you have promised," she told him, and the pope knew that she was indeed sent from God (quoted in "Saint Catherine of Siena, Virgin," taken from Crawley, *Lives of the Saints*, 1954).

Amid storms and frightening intrigues, Pope Gregory XI returned to Rome on January 17, 1377, with the hope of bringing reform and peace to the Church in Italy. He sent St. Catherine to Florence hoping that she could negotiate peace between some of the Italian princes, but her efforts proved fruitless against the chaotic politics of the Italian city-states. She narrowly escaped an attempt on her life. St. Catherine went from Florence to Siena where she rested for some time and dictated her *Dialogue*, the book containing her meditations and revelations.

In November 1378, St. Catherine was summoned back to Rome by Pope Urban VI. In her absence, the Great Western Schism had broken out, and the pope sought St. Catherine's help. In Rome, she spent the remainder of her life working to reform the Church, serving the destitute and afflicted, and writing eloquent letters in support of Pope Urban's legitimacy. She continued to suffer immense physical pain, and in her prayers, asked Christ to allow her to bear the punishment for all the sins of the world and to sacrifice her body for the unity of the Church. She received the stigmata, but prayed that it would not show on the surface of her skin. The marks only became visible after her death.

After a prolonged and mysterious agony, which she bore with happiness for three months, St. Catherine of Siena died on the Sunday before the Ascension in 1380 at the age of thirty-three. The Stigmata was revealed, and in 1430 her body was discovered incorruptible. St. Catherine was canonized in 1461, and her relics are the object of pilgrimages and venerated to this day. Her feast day is celebrated on April 29. She is a Doctor of the Church.

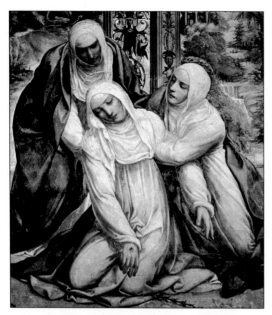

In her prayers, St. Catherine asked Christ to allow her to bear the punishment for all the sins of the world and to sacrifice her body for the unity of the Church. During her intense ecstasies, St. Catherine received the wounds of Christ, the stigmata.

THE WESTERN SCHISM

The jubilation over the pope's return to Rome did not last after the death of Pope Gregory XI. After seventy years of French domination, the people of Italy desired an Italian pope. A mob of Romans, tired of the Avignon papacy, had invaded the conclave, violently demanding an Italian pope. The cardinals elected the Italian archbishop of Bari, Bartolomeo Prignano, who chose the name Urban VI. After the crowd had calmed, these same cardinals confirmed their choice, gave a sign of obedience to Urban, sent letters throughout Christendom announcing the election of the new pope. They reported to their colleagues at Avignon that they had voted "freely and unanimously."

The Avignon cardinals had thought they had found a docile and malleable candidate for the papacy, but Urban VI turned out to be an inflexible and aggressive reformer. Urban clearly stated that there would be no return to Avignon; he declared war on every moral abuse, harshly criticizing the materialistic lifestyle of the worldly cardinals. His overzealous and violent character soured the previously favorable opinions of many of his electors. Even St. Catherine, who supported the new pope for the remainder of her life, attempted to intervene. She pleaded with Urban: "For the love of Christ, moderate a little the violent actions to which your nature drives you!" (St. Catherine, *Letter to Urban VI*, January 29, 1380). Six months after his election, the French cardinals returned to Avignon and declared that they had invalidly elected Urban out of fear and under duress. The French Cardinals then voted for the antipope Clement VII in place of Urban VI. The Western Schism, which would open gaping wounds in the Church, had begun.

Each country of Europe rallied around its own choice for pope. Western Christendom was split into two camps. Even many saints were confused as to who was the real pope. At a time when the Church needed to bring together the faithful, division and chaos became the order of the day. Bishops and abbots contested for the same benefices and monasteries. Church authorities conceded large control of ecclesiastical affairs to secular rulers to gain political support. The absence of strong papal leadership allowed new antipapal heresies, which especially included Conciliarism, Gallicanism, Wycliffeism and Hussitism to gain followers. This schism, which lasted for forty years, would result in untold confusion and a weaker Church and would pave the way for mass defections in the sixteenth century.

RESOLUTION OF THE SCHISM: COUNCIL OF CONSTANCE

By 1400, the situation of the Church seemed hopeless. The schism had lasted twenty-two years and no end was in sight; efforts to resolve the schism had failed. Many within the Church began to believe that only a general church council could solve the dilemma. This belief resulted in the Conciliar Movement and its attendant heresy, Conciliarism. Taking its authority from such works as *Defensor Pacis*, the Conciliarists tried to maintain that a Council could depose the rival claimants to the papacy and choose a compromise candidate. The first attempt to end the schism in this way occurred at Pisa, Italy, in 1409. However, neither Gregory XII, the legitimate pope, nor Benedict XIII, the antipope, would abdicate, so the Pisan Council deposed them both and chose a second antipope,

Alexander V, to replace both of them. The authority of Pisa was rejected by Gregory, Benedict, and key European kings, and rather than having solved the problem, the predicament was merely compounded. There were now three claimants to the papacy.

It would take another five years to find a more lasting solution. The Holy Roman emperor Sigismund, then in the imperial city of Constance, dedicated great efforts to achieve Church unity. He forced the Pisan antipope John XXIII to call a council at Constance and to resign his position. Peace between France and England as well as the protection of Sigismund were key to the success of the Council of Constance. Pope Gregory XII sent a representative to the Council of Constance (1414-1418) with the offer that he would recognize the authority of Constance and would abdicate if the Council would recognize him as pope. Benedict XIII refused to cooperate with the council, and as a result, he lost most of his support. Gregory's abdication cleared the way for the election of Pope Martin V and an end to the Western Schism.

Conciliarism would continue in the aftermath of Constance, and regular councils were held to direct the leadership of the Church. The Council of Constance had only succeeded due to the support of Pope Gregory XII, and many of the later councils failed through lack of participation or quarrels between rival groups. Finally, in 1439 at Ferrara-Florence, the pope's superiority over a general council was established. It was decided that three essential characteristics must be maintained for a council to be valid. First, it must be called by the pope; second, it must be presided over by the pope or his legate; finally, its dogmatic decrees are considered valid only if they are accepted and approved by the pope.

PART VIII

Decline of Scholastic Philosophy and Theology and the Rise of Heresy

WILLIAM OF OCKHAM

Intellectual life of the fourteenth century was undergoing subtle changes. Scholastic theology and its handmaiden, philosophy, which had reached their pinnacle in the works of St. Thomas Aquinas and Bl. John Duns Scotus, were now in decline. Scholasticism became increasingly technical, to the point of quibbling over insignificancies, and it had lost the rich content and understanding of purpose it once held. Challenges to Scholastic thought arose, and a new debate began over the relationship of reason to revelation. The Franciscan friar William of Ockham was one of the early critics of the old Scholastic tradition. He attempted to "simplify" the excessive formalism of the Scholastic method by separating what he claimed could truly be known by reason and what must be accepted only on faith. Ockham was an intensely religious individual, but he made the mistake of confusing philosophy and theology. His guiding philosophical principle was a theological tenet: "I believe in God, the Father Almighty."

With this statement of faith as his philosophical foundation, Ockham concluded that God, if he is almighty, must be the only and direct reason why things are true or false. Ockham's "nominalism" taught that the human mind can only know individual, sensible objects, such as "this textbook right here." Universal concepts (such as "what it means to be a textbook in general") are not concepts but merely general names – in Latin, *nomina*. Only God guarantees that knowledge of particular things consistently correspond to the *nomina*, which people have falsely assumed to be self-generated concepts. From this way of thinking, it follows that moral and religious truths are inaccessible through mere human reason, and can only be known through revelation. This is problematic since actions can no longer be said to be good or bad by nature. Instead, it is only because God determines an action to be good or bad that it is morally right or wrong. Religion, he argued, is a mystery of faith with no room for philosophical discourse. Ockham's philosophy is one of the roots of the skeptical crisis in metaphysics that finally erupted in the seventeenth century with René Descartes and has continued for hundreds of years in modern philosophy.

Ockham was an early critic of Church authority and, with his companion Marsiglio of Padua, advocated the supreme authority of the state. Since the Church deals with mysteries of Faith and the state works with empirical and therefore sure facts, according to Ockham, the Church should be subordinate to the authority of the state. As the unity of Christendom faded and nationalistic movements spread, similar heretical ideas began to appear throughout Europe. Writers such as the Englishman John Wycliffe and the Bohemian Jan Hus began to attack the authority of the Holy See and traditional beliefs of the Catholic Church.

JOHN WYCLIFFE

John Wycliffe's popularity in England arose in conjunction with some of the difficulties posed by the Hundred Years War. The Avignon popes were seen as allies of the enemies of England, and the need for new revenues directed the English crown's attention to the wealth of Church lands. John Wycliffe, a professor at the University of Oxford, had long been a critic of the temporal practices and material possessions of the Church. He had advocated that the Church should rid itself of all political power and practice strict poverty. "Dominion is founded in grace" he claimed, believing that no monks or clergy, not even the righteous, could hold temporal possessions without sin. Through this principle he advocated that it was lawful for the king to seize Church lands.

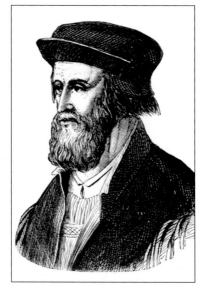

Wycliffe was one of the first pre-Protestant thinkers. In addition to attacking the authority of the pope, he rejected Scholastic theology and claimed that religious knowledge was derived from the Bible only, and not from Tradition. He advocated predestination and concluded that the Church did not need the clergy or the Sacraments. Together with the renunciation of the priesthood, he attacked the validity of indulgences, and denied man's free will, claiming that man was completely subjected to the will of God. Like many critics of the twelfth and thirteenth centuries, Wycliffe began with an attack on clerical wealth; but he then went on to dispute the authority of the Church and, finally, he attacked its sacramental system.

Popular support among the upper classes for Wycliffe's ideas began to wane after the Peasants' Revolt of 1381. Many nobles feared that Wycliffe's attack on the authority of the Church would find a parallel in the relationship between the peasants and the aristocracy or king. The Lollards, those who embraced Wycliffe's ideas in the late fourteenth and fifteenth centuries, helped pave the way for Protestantism in England during the sixteenth century.

JAN HUS

Like Wycliffe, Hus attacked the abuses of the clergy and the authority of the Church. He proclaimed the supremacy of private judgment over Church pronouncements and advocated the free interpretation of the Bible. He denied the authority of tradition, attacked the veneration of relics and

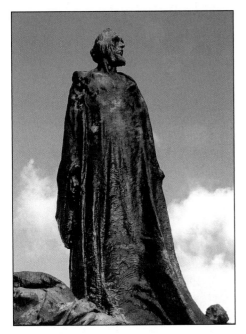

This monument to Jan Hus stands in the city of Prague, Czechoslovakia.

rejected the existence of Purgatory. While rejecting many of the Sacraments, he advocated Communion under both species, but denied Transubstantiation. He was the spiritual precursor to Martin Luther, arguing that Faith alone, apart from good works, is the means of salvation.

Holy Roman Emperor Sigismund had pushed the Council of Constance to resolve the crisis of the Western Schism. Hus, being excommunicated, was granted a pass of safe conduct by Sigismund to plead his case in Constance. There Hus was imprisoned and brought to trial for heresy. The council was not anxious to execute Hus, and they encouraged him to admit his errors and recant. With full knowledge of the consequences, Hus refused to accept the judgment of the Council and was tragically burned at the stake on July 6, 1415. National strife continued in Bohemia after the death of Hus, who came to be revered as a martyr for the Czech national cause. Churches were burned and priests killed during the Husite wars, and the conflict would not be resolved until the Thirty Years War of the seventeenth century.

PART IX

The Fall of Constantinople and the Rise of the Italian Free Cities

The economic growth of the Italian cities was a key contribution to the Renaissance. Throughout the thirteenth and fourteenth centuries, as the rest of Europe warred with each other, the Italian cities became centers of commerce – trading ports of diverse peoples who exchanged goods and ideas. Cities like Florence, Venice, and Genoa were ruled by noble families whose interest in trade, wealth, and power helped form a society based on merchants and commerce. These merchants enjoyed the freedom to buy and sell as they pleased. The economic growth of these Italian "free cities" was also aided by the seventy-year papal absence from Rome. As Italy decentralized, noble families set up their own means of governing. This rise in independence among the nobility occasioned petty wars as these ruling families expanded their sphere of influence into new lands.

As the Byzantine Empire declined in the East, the center of trade shifted to the Italian cities, bringing a burgeoning business economy with a dramatic increase of goods and merchants. Along with the growth in trade, there was a significant increase of scholarship due to the influx of Greek intellectuals. Fleeing the instability of Constantinople and the surrounding lands, Greek scholars sought after safer employment in the Italian cities. This greatly enhanced a rich exchange of ideas already enjoyed by the Italian cities.

THE COUNCIL OF BASEL-FERRARA-FLORENCE (1431-1445) AND THE END OF THE BYZANTINE EMPIRE

The Byzantine Empire never really recovered from the aftermath of the Fourth Crusade, which involved the sacking of Constantinople together with the establishment of a Latin empire on Byzantine soil. During the fourteenth century there arose a new threat to the Byzantine Empire and the whole of Europe: the Ottoman Turks. The Turks, an Islamic people with ties to the nomadic central Asians, were emigrating into the Baltic Peninsula. They conquered Gallipoli (northwest Turkey) in 1354, and moved as far west as Kosovo, Serbia, by 1389, and then north to Bucharest, Hungary, in 1393. The weakened Byzantine Empire was no match for the Turkish armies who, in addition to massive numbers, used cannons to breach city walls. In 1391, the Turks put Constantinople under siege, but due to Mongol attacks on the eastern Ottoman Empire, the siege was abandoned.

At first, the serious threat posed by the Turks on the Byzantine Empire seemed to strengthen relations between the Latin and Greek churches. Recognizing a common enemy and a mutual danger to their safety, Greeks and Latins were drawn together in a common cause, which helped heal some of the wounds that divided the Church. Venetians, fearful that any further Turkish advance would severely threaten their trade and territory, were particularly concerned with reestablishing favorable relations with the Greeks. Taking advantage of his Venetian background, Eugene IV, who became pope in 1431, sought reunification of the East and West and dreamed of launching a unified crusade against the Turks.

The Council of Basel-Ferrara-Florence was convoked just before Pope Martin V's death in 1431, and it initially dealt with problems of heresy arising in central Europe; however, Pope Eugene IV later decided to use the council as an opportunity to reunite the Western and Eastern Churches. He worked busily, sending delegates to every corner of the Christian world for support. Finally, in 1437, Greek churchmen sailed from Constantinople to Ferrara, where the council resumed. The council had a rocky start. Since the Eastern Emperor John VIII sought a firm military alliance against the Turks, he tried to avoid theological debates that might cause friction between the East and West. The Latin Bishops carefully steered the discussions towards the objections the Greek bishops had with the Latin Church.

There were four major points of disagreement between the two churches that were anything but easy to resolve. First, the Greeks objected to the Latin Church's teaching about the relation of the Holy Spirit to the other two Persons of the Blessed Trinity. They rejected the *Filioque* clause, which stated that the Holy Spirit proceeded from both the Father and the Son, whereas the Greeks professed that the Holy Spirit proceeded from the Father *through* the Son. The Greeks also used

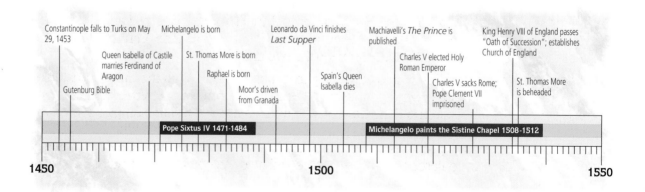

Constantinople falls to Turks on May 29, 1453

Michelangelo is born

Leonardo da Vinci finishes *Last Supper*

Machiavelli's *The Prince* is published

King Henry VIII of England passes "Oath of Succession"; establishes Church of England

Queen Isabella of Castile marries Ferdinand of Aragon

St. Thomas More is born

Charles V elected Holy Roman Emperor

Raphael is born

Spain's Queen Isabella dies

Charles V sacks Rome; Pope Clement VII imprisoned

St. Thomas More is beheaded

Gutenburg Bible

Moor's driven from Granada

Pope Sixtus IV 1471-1484

Michelangelo paints the Sistine Chapel 1508-1512

1450   1500   1550

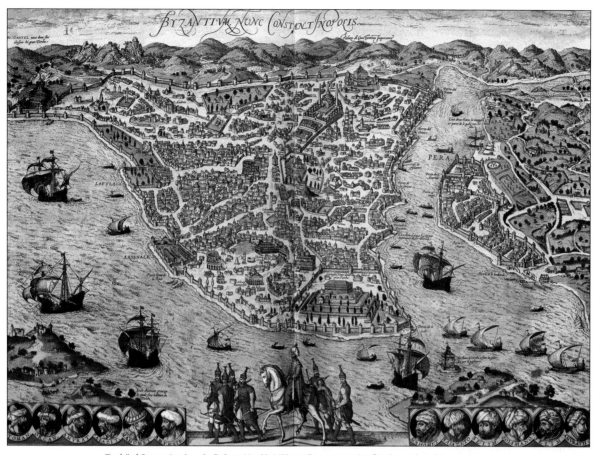

The fall of Constantinople to the Turks on May 29, 1453 was disastrous. In spite of its thousand-year history in the city,
Christianity would be immediately replaced by the Muslim culture of the Ottoman Turks. The magnificent Hagia Sophia's mosaics
would be plastered over, the High Altar destroyed and what was once the center of Byzantine Christianity would become a mosque.

leavened bread for the celebration of the Eucharist and disagreed with the Latin insistence on using only unleavened bread. Two old disagreements with the Latin Church – the existence of Purgatory and the primacy of the Roman See over the whole Church of Christ – were also debated during the council. In order to discuss these issues, the pope formed commissions consisting of both Greeks and Latins that could argue out and draft clear conclusions to these theological questions.

Much to the disappointment of the Eastern Emperor, these theological discussions, which lasted for more than a year, totally absorbed the attention of the Council Fathers to the detriment of addressing the issue of military defense. In any case, the emperor did manage to pressure the bishops to come to an agreement, which was finally reached in 1439 and recorded in Pope Eugene IV's bull *Lætentur cœli* (Let the Heavens Rejoice). Much to the joy of the Latin Church, the Greeks accepted the question of *Filioque*, the existence of Purgatory, and the primacy of the pope, and there was a temporary reunification between the two churches.

Unfortunately, the reunification existed more on paper than in reality. With the Turks threatening Constantinople, popular Greek sentiment against the Latin Church was extremely acute. Many Greeks blamed the Latin Church and the Crusades for weakening the Byzantine Empire. Moreover, once they were away from the pressures of the council, many Greek bishops who accepted the agreements reversed their positions and campaigned against the Latin Church. Indeed, popular hatred of the West was so fierce that the emperors withheld the documents of reunification for fifteen years.

Emperor John VIII was dissatisfied with the council since it was limited to theological matters and that none of the Western princes attended. His hopes for an effective military alliance were dashed since it was already too late. Furthermore, much of the fear and negative sentiment that preceded the city's fall was directed towards the West. A popular line was heard in the city: "Better the turban of the Prophet than the Pope's tiara" (quoted in Hughes, *A History of the Church to the Eve of the Reformation*, 1976, p. 351). In December 1452, the reunion of the two Churches was finally proclaimed by the bishops in a ceremony at Hagia Sophia. The people vehemently refused to accept the proclamation and it only fueled their deep resentment toward the West.

Five months later, papal ships arrived to aid the city in the ensuing battle with the Turks, but it was too late. The population of Constantinople watched as 160,000 Turkish troops surrounded the city. After two months of siege, on May 29, 1453, Constantinople fell to Turkish Muslim forces, bringing down a thousand-year-old Christian empire.

The fall of Constantinople solidified the split between the Western and Eastern Churches and created an animosity and historical sense of injustice that has yet to be overcome. It seems probable that if the Latin kingdoms had defeated the Ottomans, it would only have meant years of occupation by Western princes. It can only be speculated that this hypothetical scenario would have further inflamed hatred of the West by the Greeks. Nonetheless, the fall of Constantinople was disastrous. In spite of its thousand-year history and tradition in the city, Christianity would be immediately replaced by the Muslim culture of the Ottoman Turks, subjugating the Greeks to foreign rule. After the siege, the Ottomans pillaged Constantinople for three days and three nights. They stripped Hagia Sophia, turning it into a mosque.

Despite their efforts in defending Constantinople, the Italian city-states benefited greatly from its fall because trade shifted from the "Golden Horn" of Constantinople to Venice, Genoa, and Florence. Italian ports became even greater centers of ideas from areas outside of Christendom with their cosmopolitan bazaars bustling with people from all over the world. Christians, Jews, and Muslims bought and sold side by side, experiencing a level of toleration unseen elsewhere in Europe.

PART X

The Birth of Humanism and the Flourishing of Arts and Letters

HUMANISM

Like the word "Renaissance," "humanism" also carries with it a certain ambiguity. Humanism denotes a certain general mood and intellectual climate which focuses on the richness of the human spirit over the almost exclusive theological focus of the Medieval era. Nevertheless, the writers and thinkers who fall under its broad umbrella are often so diverse in their aims and beliefs that the term loses much precision without the clarifying prefixes of "theistic," "atheistic," "secular," "aesthetic," "Christian," "pagan," and the like. Humanism was a literary genre that would elaborate on different facets of human life. This fascination with humanity spilled over into the fine arts as well, beginning in the Italian city-states during the late fourteenth century. Medieval Scholastic education was a very specialized, practical aim; for example, one studied medicine to become a doctor; logic, philosophy, and theology to become a theologian; law to become a lawyer. The humanists reacted against this functional specialization of education since it did not include the exciting subject matter of the human condition. Education not only should offer training, but must have the moral purpose of making the individual wiser and more virtuous.

The humanists revived the study of the many texts of the great authors of ancient Rome: Virgil, Cicero, Ovid, Seneca, Tacitus, and Catullus. Eventually, as knowledge of Greek culture was acquired in the West, mostly through Byzantine refugees after 1453, they retrieved the works of ancient Greek thinkers: Homer, Aristotle, Plato, and Thucydides. The humanists called their works the *bonae litterae* (good letters) or *litterae humaniores* (more humane letters), as these texts focused on man's relation to the world rather than man's relation to God and eternal salvation.

Certainly this opened the door to a worldly outlook devoid of a true Catholic sentiment as many humanists displayed an inordinate reverence for pagan thinkers and writers. The Catholic Church developed a Christian humanism to the already rich storehouse of theological and philosophical thought. The Renaissance, from a Christian perspective, underscored the revealed truth that the human person is made in the image and likeness of God.

Fourteenth and fifteenth century humanism walked a fine line between fascination with the grandeur of the human person and the fact that every person is a fruit of God's creative power.

DANTE ALIGHIERI (1265-1321)

Dante Alighieri had been the premier Florentine writer at the close of the Medieval Era. He had suffered amid the political turmoil of the Italian citystates and had been a victim of the many power struggles and political intrigues. His writings struck a balance between the person's earthly condition and life after death. His epic poem, *The Divine Comedy*, is a poetic reflection in many ways reflective of the Scholastic tradition. At the same time, he had a great admiration for the classical writers in their dedication to the pursuit of natural truth. In *The Divine Comedy*, the poet assigns the souls of pagan writers and thinkers to limbo, a place where they are not condemned by God, but do not share the Beatific Vision since they are not baptized in the Catholic Church and therefore do not have the fullness of truth. Christian revelation provides the necessary divine light that would have guided them to knowledge of God.

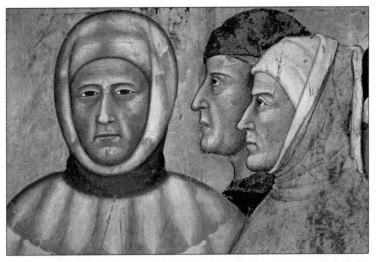

Petrarch, Boccaccio and Dante — Petrarch succeeded Dante as the great sage of Florence. He was crowned "poet laureate" by a Roman senator when he was only thirty.

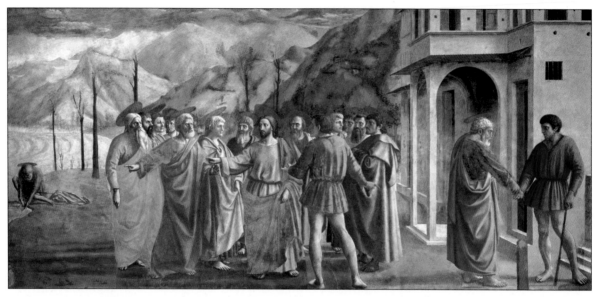

Tribute Money by **Masaccio** (1401-1427?), the first great Italian Renaissance painter. Masaccio's innovations in the use of scientific perspective (knowledge of mathematical proportion acquired from Brunelleschi) inaugurated the modern era in painting. Masaccio's work exerted a strong influence on later Florentine art and particularly on the work of Michelangelo. This painting depicts the arrival in Capernaum of Jesus and the Apostles, based on Matthew 17: 24-27. Masaccio has included the three different moments of the story: the tax collector's request, with Jesus indicating to Peter how to find the money, in the center; Peter catching the fish in Lake Genezaret and extracting the coin, on the left; and Peter handing the tribute money to the tax collector in front of his house, on the right.

HUMANISM IN PAINTING AND SCULPTURE

The rebirth of art in Italy during the fifteenth century expressed similar cultural changes, as was the case regarding philosophy and literature. Increased interest in classical literature and art prompted a new resolve for observation of the individual and study of the natural world. Subjects from Greek and Roman mythology found their way into the art of the day in response to the renewed interest in the classical era. The study of ancient architecture also inspired new techniques in building involving spatial perspective, elegance of form, and symmetry.

The first generation of Renaissance artists (most notably Donatello, Brunelleschi and Masaccio) applied rational inquiry to discover laws of proportion, formal balance, and symmetry. They remained keenly observant of natural phenomena, but also sought to render spiritual ideals through their art forms of painting and architecture.

The late fifteenth century, the period known as the High Renaissance, produced some of the most magnificent works of art ever seen. Commissioned by wealthy families, kings, and popes alike, artists such as Leonardo da Vinci, Michelangelo, and Raphael filled Italian churches and palaces with breathtaking paintings and sculptures which alternated between religious and secular themes. More than just thematic content, these artists presented unified balance and color composition with a talent that combined the dramatic force of a physical representation with sublime harmonic and lyric beauty.

MICHELANGELO

Michelangelo Buonarroti, born in 1475, played an unparalleled role in the development of Western art. He embodies the Renaissance man who excels in many disciplines in a way that is larger than

MICHELANGELO AND THE POPES

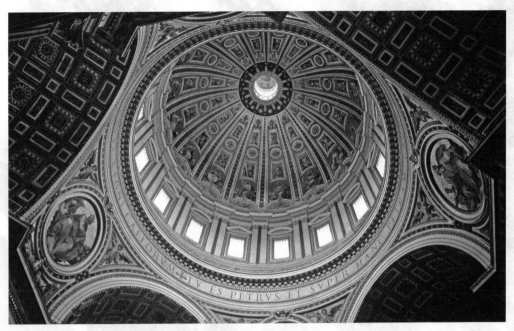

Interior of the dome of St. Peter's Basilica designed by Michelangelo. The shape is a parabola which gives it more strength. The dome was completed by the architect Giacomo della Porta after Michelangelo's death.

The sculptor and painter Michelangelo lived for ninety years and received commissions from four different popes. Unfortunately, as he lived during a time when corruption and intrigue dominated the papacy, relations with these popes were often strained.

Born in Florence, Michelangelo was thirty years old when he was first called to Rome by Pope Julius II. Michelangelo was commissioned by Pope Julius II to design and erect a stately tomb for himself, a four-sided marble structure decorated with forty massive figures. The planning went on for a year, but Julius suddenly changed his mind and began to focus exclusively on the rebuilding of St. Peter's Basilica. Losing his commission and abandoning the mausoleum, Michelangelo left Rome for Florence in despair and even considered moving to Constantinople. At Julius' insistence, Michelangelo eventually returned to Rome in order to paint the ceiling of the Sistine Chapel. When Julius II died in 1513, Michelangelo labored for two years on a scaled-down version of the original mausoleum, adorning it with the famous "Moses" found today in the church of St. Peter in Chains, located in Rome.

Before he could complete the mausoleum, the sculptor was again interrupted by the new pope, Leo X, who asked Michelangelo to construct a new facade for a church at San Lorenzo. After four years, that contract was rescinded, and this project was also left incomplete. In 1523 a new pope, Clement VII, was elected after the short reign of Adrian VI. Pope Clement commissioned Michelangelo to build a mortuary chapel for the Medici family. Surprisingly, this commission was not revoked, and Michelangelo completed the chapel in 1524. After Clement VII died, Pope Paul III appointed Michelangelo as chief architect for the reconstruction of St. Peter's Basilica in 1546. Before he died, Michelangelo almost completed the dome of the church and four columns for its base.

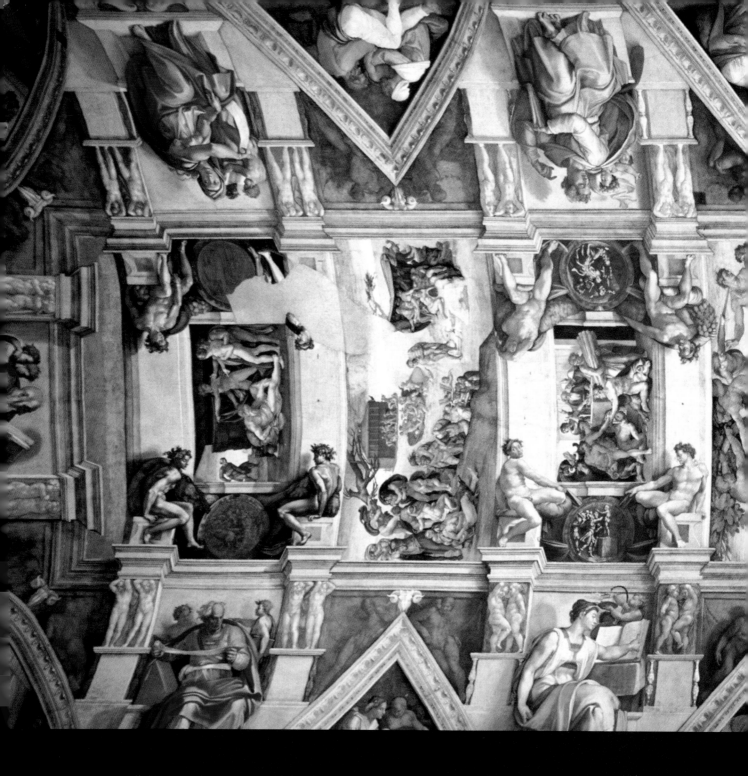

"From here can be heard the voice of Michelangelo who in the Sistine Chapel has presented the drama and mystery of the world from the Creation to the Last Judgement, giving a face to God the Father, to Christ the Judge, and to man on his arduous journey from the dawn to the consummation of history." –St. John Paul II, Letter to Artists, 1999

life. Michelangelo was a sculptor, painter, and architect of almost superhuman capacity, whose works hold the viewer of every age in utter amazement.

An unmistakable quality of Michelangelo's art was his depiction of the contours of the human body in such a manner that the grandeur of man comes out with overwhelming force. His sculpture "David" typifies the artist's use of scale and exaggeration along with detailed studies of the human anatomy to create this massive figure that exudes power and strength.

Like many artists of the time, Michelangelo was supported financially by the popes. His relationship with these men was not always cordial. Commissioned to paint the Sistine Chapel as well as to design the dome of St. Peter's Basilica, the popes needed to coerce Michelangelo to complete the task. Painted from 1508 until 1512, the ceiling of the Sistine

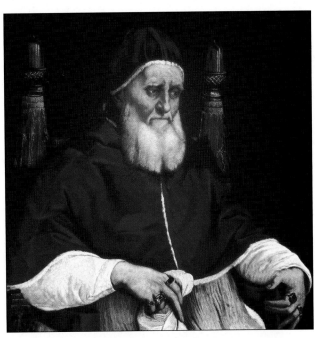

Portrait of Pope Julius II by Raphael. Julius II was a great patron of the arts. Michelangelo, Bramante and Raphael all benefited from his commissions.

Chapel was a painstaking and torturous endeavor for the artist who was left nearly blind by the time of its completion. The chapel ceiling remains an incredible achievement in Renaissance art that perfectly displays dazzling beauty through an idealized human form.

RAPHAEL

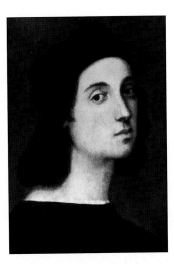

Self-Portrait by Raphael

Another painter commissioned by the pope and a contemporary of Michelangelo was Raphael Sanzio (1483-1520), admired for his clarity of form and ease of composition. Whereas Michelangelo preferred sculpture, Raphael was primarily a painter best known for his Madonnas (Italian for "my Lady"; paintings of the Blessed Virgin Mary) as well as his large paintings in the Vatican apartments.

Like most artists of the day, Raphael spent much of his life in Florence. There he immersed himself in the artistic milieu of the day which helped shape his own ideas and methods. In Florence, Raphael's principal teachers were Leonardo da Vinci and Michelangelo. During his early years in Florence, Raphael worked to perfect his painting of the Madonna, concentrating on creating intimate and simple paintings that masterfully balanced the use of light, composition, and a sense of depth.

During the last twelve years of his life, Raphael worked in Rome and was commissioned by popes and wealthy families alike. Pope Julius II hired this artist to paint a series of rooms in the papal apartments, and these murals are still considered some of Raphael's greatest works. Demonstrating the humanistic trends of his period, these paintings also deal with philosophical themes.

Like many of the artists of the Renaissance, Raphael was well known and admired during his life. The artist died on his thirty-seventh birthday and was given a funeral in St. Peter's in Rome. Since many held him in very high esteem, Pope Leo X had him buried in the Pantheon in Rome.

HUMANISM IN THE NORTH

The Renaissance in the North was more of a blend between the Christian-centered Medieval world and the new mindset exhibited by the Renaissance. Rather than wholeheartedly embracing the traditions of antiquity, they integrated and elaborated on the human person in relation to Christianity. It would take longer for a Christian orientation to be lost in the humanistic literature of the North. Moreover, that region would see some of the greatest Christian humanists.

ST. THOMAS MORE (1478-1535)

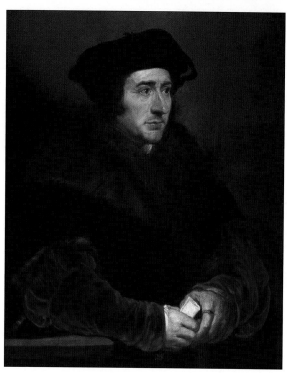

St. Thomas More by Peter Paul Rubens

On the opposite end of the political spectrum from Machiavelli, there appears another renowned humanist, a certain lawyer, knight, Lord Chancellor, saint, martyr, and one of the greatest minds of the Renaissance: St. Thomas More (1478-1535). He mastered Greek, French, and Latin; studied mathematics, history, music, law, and philosophy; and wrote numerous works, among them his famous *Utopia*. The word "utopia," first coined by St. Thomas More himself, is Greek meaning "no place." In this modern parallel to Plato's *Republic*, More described a religious society, heavily influenced by divine revelation, in which goods were held in common and the state regulated business. More meant exactly what the etymology implied by the name of his island—Utopia is no place, and can never be, but it offers a remarkable humanist critique of the socio-political state of sixteenth century England.

Besides his work *Utopia*, St. Thomas More is best remembered for his heroic Christian witness during the tumultuous events surrounding Henry VIII's defection from the Catholic Church. More served as Lord Chancellor for Henry VIII until 1532. When Henry, whom the pope once named *Defensor Fidei* (Defender of the Faith) because of his work against Lutheran heresies, passed the *Act of Succession and Oath of Supremacy* in 1534, thereby establishing the Church of England. St. Thomas More refused to swear allegiance to these schismatic decrees. He was accused of high treason and imprisoned in the Tower of London, where he remained until his beheading on July 6, 1535. Pope Pius XI canonized St. Thomas More in 1935. His feast day is celebrated on June 22.

ERASMUS OF ROTTERDAM (ca. 1466-1536)

Perhaps the most renowned of all Renaissance humanists is Desiderius Erasmus of Rotterdam (ca. 1466-1536), who was a close friend and correspondent of St. Thomas More. This father of Northern humanism was recognized throughout Europe—by King Henry VIII, Holy Roman Emperor Charles V, various popes, St. Thomas More, and Martin Luther—for his brilliance and intellect. A master of Greek and Latin, Erasmus traveled all over Europe, lecturing, counseling, and writing. He epitomized the intellectual character of humanism. He saw the Middle Ages and Scholasticism as unenlightened and stagnant while holding the classical thinkers in highest esteem. He extolled the primacy of human virtues such as prudence, intellectual honesty, zeal for truth, and consideration for others. He had deep desires for reform and progress through education and tolerance. Although he never spoke against its divine origin and fundamental beliefs, Erasmus was highly critical of the way many societies within the Church functioned. His biting and sarcastic critiques of ecclesiastical and monastic life brought out the need for a profound spiritual renewal of the sixteenth-century Church.

In his *Handbook of a Christian Knight*, Erasmus confronted the difficult question Petrarch and many Christian humanists raised: How does one remain a good Christian while taking part in world affairs? Unhappy with the contemporary structure and practices of the Church from the popes to Christian rulers to everyday people, Erasmus suggested a more personal and subjective spirituality and understanding of the Faith. He called for study and meditation on the writings of the Church Fathers and the Scriptures. He strongly encouraged research into the classical thinkers together with continuous practice of rational virtue and adherence to the "philosophy of Christ." His most famous work, however, is *Moriae encomium* (Praise of Folly), written for his friend St. Thomas More. In this short work, Folly speaks on the state of human society. From ruler to peasant, she says, all favor Folly over Reason, though they are dishonest about their preference and give her disparaging names. The work, a satirical exposition of the Renaissance world, is at once a celebration and a critique that harshly criticizes members of the Church. Erasmus remained a Christian throughout his life, and he never balked at criticizing the Church's many members who did not uphold the dignity and respect of the Church. Because his faith and love of the Church was devoted and deep, Erasmus continually expressed zeal for necessary reform.

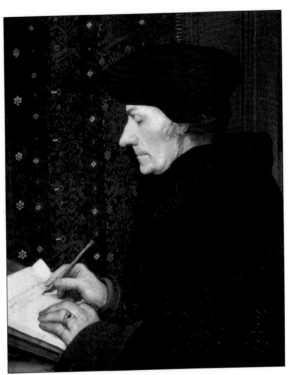

Erasmus of Rotterdam by Hans Holbein

PART XI

Popes and Politics

THE RENAISSANCE POPES

Much has been said of the worldly lives of the Renaissance popes. Unfortunately, these popes lived more like worldly princes than men called to reflect the holiness of Christ's vicar and successor of St. Peter. It is worth mentioning that the popes of the Renaissance acted as temporal princes who were trying to strengthen the temporal authority of the Church after the long period of schism and establish a stronger security for the Papal States. Some of the popes were men of letters who helped sponsor the artistic works of the Renaissance, whereas others acted more as princes interested in increasing their power.

NICHOLAS V (1447-1455)

Born Tommaso Parentucelli, Pope Nicholas V ascended to the papacy in 1447 and remains one of the greatest of the Renaissance popes. From an early age he took up the burgeoning humanism of that period, serving for some twenty years under the patronage of Nicolò Albergati, the bishop of Bologna. During that time he began his lifelong hobby of collecting and caring for rare books and at the same time demonstrated a deep capacity for learning and scholarship. At the Council of Basel-Ferrara-Florence (1431-45), Parentucelli's familiarity with Scholastic philosophy and the Church Fathers gave him prominence during the discussions with the Greek bishops who had come to reconcile with Rome. He became a cardinal in 1446 and was elected to the papacy the following year upon the death of Eugene IV. In thankful remembrance of his longtime patron Nicolò, he took the name Nicholas.

As pope, Nicholas V undertook three major tasks: to make Rome once again a city of grand monuments; to make Rome a center of art and literature; and to strengthen, both spiritually and temporally, the capital of Christendom. He set about restoring churches, repairing the Roman infrastructure, cleaning the city, and repairing the ancient aqueducts. He also made many grandiose plans and laid the foundation for the future St. Peter's Basilica. Nicholas, driven by his love of literature and beautiful books, vigorously searched the monasteries and palaces of Europe, and saved thousands of ancient and precious texts from being swallowed by neglect. Perhaps the greatest achievement of his pontificate was founding the Vatican Library, which, by the end of his life, had accumulated more than five thousand works. Nicholas also generously sponsored many humanist writers as well as the translation of Greek classics, thus reintroducing to the West the great works of Thucydides, Herodotus, and Xenophon.

Nicholas V continued to work at restoring the authority of the Church by finalizing the condemnation of the Conciliarist heresy and winning the submission of the antipope Felix V. He sent Cardinal Nicholas of Cusa, one of the greatest theological and philosophical minds of the age, to England and Northern Germany, and sent the Franciscan St. John of Capistrano to southern Germany in the hope of stemming the growing religious dissension among both the clergy and laity. He also made valiant attempts at achieving greater political unity in Europe as a way of counteracting the growing Turkish threat. Unfortunately, the ongoing division among the Italian states and the lack of cooperation among the competing European states made it impossible for Nicholas to organize sufficient resistance to the Turkish threat to Constantinople. The Byzantine Empire fell to the Turks in 1453.

CALLISTUS III (1455-58)

The Spanish-born Alfonso Borgia became Pope Callistus III in 1455. Callistus was preoccupied with the looming Turkish threat. He sent missionaries throughout the West to preach a crusade and to recruit volunteers and money. Bells were rung at midday to remind the faithful to pray for the welfare of the Crusades. Unfortunately, the temporal rulers of the West, still embittered and embattled against each other, were slow to respond to the pope's call. France and England were still engaged in the Hundred Years War and the German Empire was at odds with Polish and Hungarian princes who were fighting the Turks. Even though the crusaders won a major victory in July 1456 at Belgrade, the absence of leadership among the Western states, the continuing Hussite conflict in Bohemia, and the general lack of cohesion among European states all prevented any chance of completely driving out the Turks after this victory. Put simply, Christendom was in no condition to wage war in the hopes of a resounding victory.

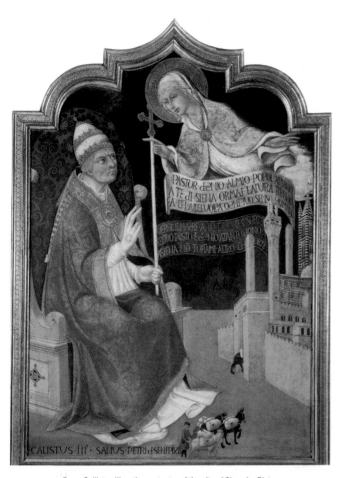

Pope Callistus III as the protector of the city of Siena by Pietro.
Pope Callistus III reversed Joan of Arc's sentence and proclaimed her innocent.

Though nearly all of his energies throughout his pontificate were focused upon stemming the Turkish threat, Callistus enjoyed a number of accomplishments. He oversaw the reversal of the sentence against St. Joan of Arc and formally proclaimed her innocence. Though he was not a great literary patron, Callistus did spend a good amount of time, money, and effort in securing artistic treasures for the Vatican. Furthermore, Callistus began to realize, through his futile attempts to unite Europe against the Turks, that responsibility for the military security of the West lay outside the capacity and duty of the papacy. Unfortunately, this understanding would be forgotten by succeeding popes. Nevertheless, the distraction of a Turkish invasion remained an obstacle to Church reform as it would occupy the mind of the popes for years.

PIUS II (1458-64)

Pope Pius II, born Enea Silvio de'Piccolomini, was a man of multiple facets and in his youth was marked by moral laxity. He possessed an extraordinary intellectual acumen and, as a young man before his ordination, had become passionately involved in the humanist movement. Unfortunately, his fervent embrace of the pagan culture of the past led him to indulge in many worldly pursuits, and for a time he lived a dissolute life, though he was known to have inflicted great penances upon himself. He had been politically involved with various Italian and German princes and at one time supported the Conciliar movement against the pope, serving as secretary for the antipope Felix V. In 1445, however, he reconciled with Pope Eugene IV and underwent a spiritual conversion.

Like his predecessor, the central focus of Pius's pontificate was overcoming the Turkish threat. Again like Callistus, Pius could not win the support of the many feuding princes constantly at war with each other. In addition to his abortive attempts at launching a successful crusade, Pius seriously endeavored to restore monastic discipline and canonized St. Catherine of Siena. He continued giving papal support for humanist writing and penned a number of literary works.

SIXTUS IV (1471-84)

Francesco della Rovere was a virtuous Franciscan monk and professor of philosophy and theology at a number of Italian universities before being called to Rome as a cardinal in 1467. As a scholar, he devoted his time to writing a number of theological and philosophical works, taking special interest in the greatest and most notable of Scholastic philosophers, St. Thomas Aquinas and Bl. John Duns Scotus. He was elected Pope in 1471 and took the name Sixtus IV.

Like his predecessors, Sixtus IV continued to fight the advance of the Turks, but with little success. He commenced dialogue with the Russian Orthodox Church in the hopes of reunion, but failed at this as well.

Most of Sixtus IV's efforts as pope were devoted to maintaining Church strength and independence amid continual growth of nationalism in Europe. The Gallican movement continued to erode papal authority in France. Internal fighting among the Italian states also drew Sixtus into the political fray. Sixtus compounded these political difficulties through rampant nepotism, as he mistakenly tried to build up Church unity by filling its administration with friends and relatives. To his credit, other than his political shortcomings, Sixtus IV lived the rest of his days in blamelessness and virtue. He took steps to suppress abuses in the Inquisition and continued the fight against heresy. He was a patron of the arts and letters, improved the sanitary conditions of Rome, and built the famous Sistine (Sixtine) Chapel.

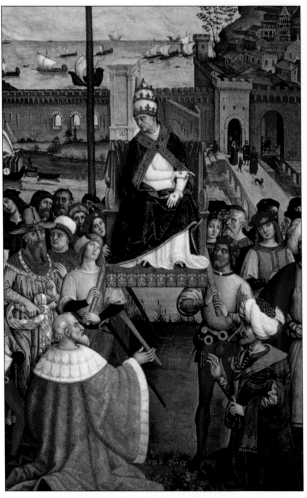

Pope Pius II in Ancona trying to raise a crusade against the Turks threatening Constantinople.

After the papacy of Sixtus IV to the time of the Reformation, secular interests dominated the policies of the popes. The need to maintain and protect papal independence against rival Italian city-states together with an inordinate interest in worldly matters made the leaders of the Church appear more like princes than Vicars of Christ. Nevertheless, it is important to remember that even though the papacy has not been at all immune to weakness, the teaching of the popes on Faith and morals has never changed. Moreover, the Lord's words, "the powers of death shall not prevail against it" (Mt 16:18), assures the Church of her perseverance in spite of the frailty of her children or officeholders. It bears repeating that the Church is not a mere human institution; rather, it is the Mystical Body of Christ guided and enlivened by the Holy Spirit.

INNOCENT VIII, ALEXANDER VI, AND JULIUS II

The end of the fifteenth and beginning of the sixteenth centuries brought the Church three popes who demonstrated poor moral leadership and worldly attitudes unfit for the Vicar of Christ. The first of these, Innocent VIII, the son of a Roman noble, rose to the papal throne in 1484. He lived a worldly life and primarily tried to restore order to the chaotic Italian political scene. Though earnestly interested in unifying Europe against the possible onslaught of Islam, he failed to take any significant action. While he was pope, the Moors and Jews were expelled from Spain in 1492 during the *Reconquista*.

The most notorious of the Renaissance popes was Alexander VI, born Rodrigo Borgia. This ambitious man attempted to unify Italy under his control by placing family members as the heads of various states and by embroiling himself in a variety of political intrigues. Despite his moral shortcomings and religious insincerity, Alexander was a gifted leader and an able administrator. He dispensed justice in an admirable way and put an end to the lawlessness in Rome. He also was able to negotiate a peace settlement between Spain and Portugal, dividing their colonial possessions with the famous Line of Demarcation. Alexander also sent the first missionaries to the New World.

Like most Renaissance popes, Alexander was a generous patron of the arts, particularly embellishing the art and architecture of Rome. Among other improvements he made to the city, Alexander decorated the ceiling of Santa Maria Maggiore with a shipment of gold from Columbus's voyage to America.

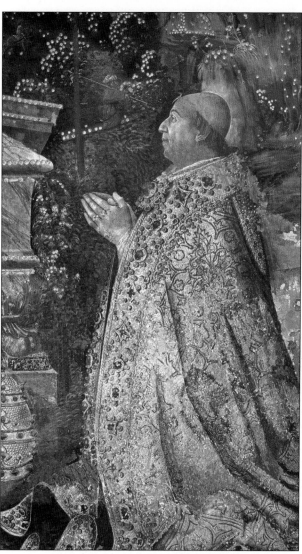

Alexander VI's political skill made him a strong secular leader, but his political involvement and his scandalous personal life (fathering nine illegitimate children) tarnished the moral authority of the Church and made many political enemies. Alexander divided the papal lands for his sons and formed many political marriages with his children. Much to the pope's historical shame, Alexander's son Cesare was the model ruler for Machiavelli's famous treatise on political intrigue, *The Prince.*

The successor to Alexander was his powerful rival in the College of Cardinals, Giuliano della Rovere, who took the name Julius II. Julius continued Alexander's attempt to pacify the Italian peninsula and devoted his pontificate to military endeavors and the artistic glorification of Rome. He was a great patron of the arts and sponsored the great works of Michelangelo and Raphael as well as a host of other builders and artists whose works have beautified the Eternal City. Julius, like Alexander, was a strong military and secular leader who firmly established the temporal

The most notorious Renaissance pope, Alexander VI.

authority of the Church over the Papal States. Despite his secular interests, Julius did help bring about some minor reforms in the Church. He abolished simony in the papacy, established the first bishoprics in the New World, and authorized Henry VIII to marry Catherine of Aragon.

Although the private lives of the Renaissance popes were quite unbecoming for the successor of St. Peter, remarkably, they still fulfilled their religious duties as popes. In a time of confusion and secularization, they upheld the teachings of the Church. Still, they failed to live good, moral lives and missed opportunities for much-needed reform.

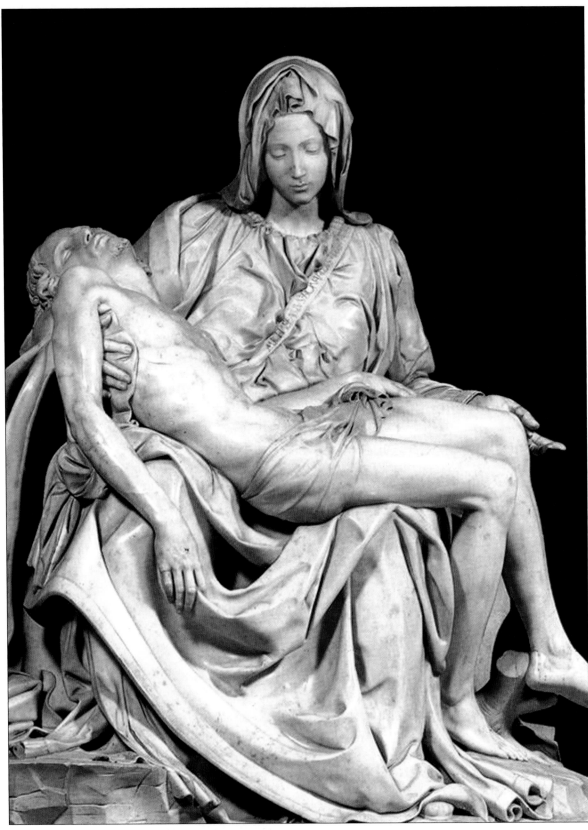

Michelangelo's *Pieta*. The Renaissance offered the social climate perfect for the rise of Christian humanism, a rebirth in Classical principles, and magnificent developments in the fine arts.

CONCLUSION

The High Middle Ages saw a significant flourishing in Christ's Church, and in many ways, this period of time was a golden age in the history of the Church. Christian philosophy, piety, and art boldly ventured into new heights, and the saints of the period showed how holiness redounds to the benefit of all of society. This does not mean, of course, that the Medieval period was bereft of dark shadows in its reflection of Christ's Gospel. Nonetheless, Medieval culture, expressed in its breakthroughs in philosophy, theology, architecture, art, and literature, offers a glimmer of the magnificent ramifications of the Christian ideal.

Though often heralded as one of the pinnacle moments in human history, the Renaissance did not pass without its high and low points. At its best the Renaissance offered the social climate perfect for the rise of Christian humanism, a rebirth in classical principles, and magnificent developments in the fine arts. However, the Renaissance in its excesses exaggerated the understanding of human capacity and encouraged a false sense of self-sufficiency. This period represents a significant crossroads in the history of the West, a time when thinkers and artists grew confident enough to explore human understanding and beauty outside the realm of religion. New developments in art, politics, and economics showed the people of the Renaissance that society could function, and function effectively, outside the traditional restraints of religion and morality. This confidence helped advance the material quality of life, but in many ways it also led to the indulgence and extravagance of the baroque and rococo periods.

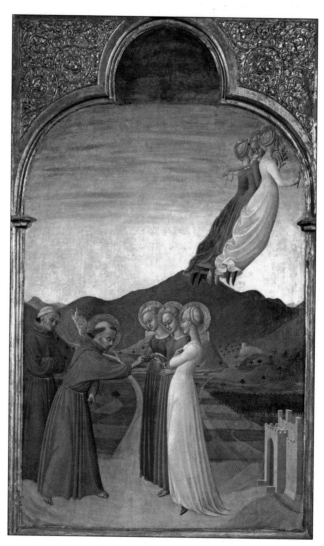

St. Francis's Mystical Marriage with Poverty

The contradictions of the Renaissance are no better exemplified than in the lives of the popes of that period. Certainly much has been said about the gross excesses and hypocritical immorality of these men. At the same time, their artistic and intellectual heritage survives to this day. These men did much to advance the quality of life both in Rome and in the rest of Italy, and they helped to reestablish the papacy as a patron of intellectual and spiritual exploration. It bears mentioning that some of the most pious popes have not always been effective in governing the Church from a political, social, artistic, and economic viewpoint, whereas these "princes of men" helped protect and strengthen the Church according to the ways and means of their time. They represent the ironic reality familiar to the hierarchical Church: often in history, less than worthy men are chosen to carry and sustain the Mystical Body of Christ.

VOCABULARY

BABYLONIAN CAPTIVITY
The seventy years (1305-1377) the papacy spent in Avignon under the watchful eye of the French kings.

BONÆ LITTERÆ OR LITTERÆ HUMANIORES
Latin for "good letters" or "more humane letters," these terms were used by humanists to describe works which focused on man's relation to the world rather than man's relation to God and eternal salvation.

CLERICIS LAICOS
Written by Pope Boniface VIII to King Philip the Fair in 1296, this letter asserted that kings did not have the right to tax clergy without permission from the pope. Philip responded by cutting off all French shipments of gold, silver, and jewels to Italy. The loss of Church revenues from this action forced Boniface to back down.

CONCILIARISM
Movement which supported the power of a council to appoint a candidate for the papacy, thus placing a council's authority over that of the pope.

DEFENSOR PACIS (DEFENDER OF PEACE)
Written by Marsiglio of Padua, a former rector of the University of Paris, this book made the first clear assertion of the supremacy of secular powers over the Church. He declared that the faithful were the true authority of the Church.

DICTAMEN
The "Art of Composition" taught at Bologna, which included rules for drawing up briefs and other legal documents. This training attracted many students and soon developed into another intense program specializing in grammar and rhetoric.

FREE CITIES
Italian cities ruled by noble families whose interest in trade, wealth, and power helped form a society based on commerce in which merchants were free to trade with whomever they pleased.

GALLICANISM
The idea that the French Roman Catholic clergy favored the restriction of papal control and the achievement by each nation of individual administrative autonomy.

GOTHIC
Style of Medieval building that flourished from 1200-1500. By using pointed arches, ribbed vaulting and flying buttresses, this style created an airy and well-lit space and gave masons, artists, and architects the freedom to adorn buildings with works of art.

HIGH RENAISSANCE
Period beginning in the late fifteenth century, it produced some of the most well-known religious and secular artwork of the period from such figures as Leonardo, Raphael and Michelangelo.

HUMANISM
An intellectual and literary movement that began in the city-states of Italy during the late fourteenth century. Moving away from the Scholastic education of the Medieval era, the humanists thought that education had a moral purpose, the end of which was to make the individual a better, wiser, and more virtuous human being. To achieve this, they aimed to base every branch of learning on classical Greek and Roman culture.

HUSITISM
Movement started by Jan Hus which denied the authority of tradition, the existence of Purgatory, transubstantiation, and the necessity of good works in salvation. It was especially popular in Bohemia.

MENDICANT FRIARS
From the Latin word mendicare, meaning "to beg," this new type of religious order was not bound to a place or community and subsisted entirely on alms. The Franciscans and Dominicans are the largest orders of mendicant friars.

VOCABULARY

NOMINALISM
Put forth by William of Ockham, this theory taught that the human mind can only know individual, sensible objects, and that universal ideas, like truth, goodness, and humanity are only names – *nomina*. Only God guarantees that individual experiences properly and consistently correspond to the *nomina*, which people have falsely assumed to be self-generated concepts. From this way of thinking it follows that moral and religious truths are inaccessible through mere human reason, and can only be known through revelation.

NORTHERN HUMANISM
Humanism had a different effect in Northern Europe where there were not the same economic and social changes as there were in Italy. Life was much like it was during the Medieval age, and rather than redirecting study to classical, pagan culture, those in the North sought to reconcile humanism with Christianity.

PEACE AND TRUCE OF GOD
Principle which, for much of the Middle Ages, kept European kings at peace by recognizing a common unity in Faith between European peoples who otherwise did not share common nationalities or customs.

PLATONIC FORMS
Philosophical construct developed by the fifth century Greek philosopher Plato that held that all things that exist emanate from the primal unity of the unseen idea, at the very core of which is the Form of the Good.

QUADRIVIUM
Latin for "four ways." More advanced program in the Medieval liberal arts program, it included the study of arithmetic, geometry, astronomy, and music.

RENAISSANCE
French for "re-birth," this period is characterized by the popular desire to return to the civilization of the Greco-Roman world and re-awaken a sense of human beauty and personal achievement.

SCHOLASTICISM
The system of philosophical and theological inquiry first developed in the Medieval schools of Christian Europe, creating its own technical language and methodology.

SPIRITUAL ESPOUSAL
These "Mystical Marriages" were experienced by a number of great saints, most notably St. Catherine of Siena. They occur when Christ takes a soul as his bride, leading it to an increase of charity and familiarity with Christ.

STIGMATA
Phenomenon in which a person bears all or some of the wounds of Christ in his or her own body.

STUDIUM GENERALE
Unified program of study offered by Medieval universities which included theology, law, medicine and the arts.

STUDIUM HUMANITAS
Study of the humanities which placed a great emphasis on Classical texts and literature, as well as revival of the study of Greek and Latin.

TRIVIUM
Latin for "three ways," this was one of two sections into which the arts were divided in Medieval universities. It referred to the three primary branches of Medieval education: grammar, rhetoric and dialectic.

UNAM SANCTAM
Letter written by Pope Boniface claiming that in order to save his or her soul, every human being – including the king – must be subject to the pope. King Philip responded by calling his own national council, the Estates General, to condemn and depose the pope.

UNIVERSITAS
A type of corporation that protected the educational and administrative needs of masters and students in schools of the mid-eleventh century.

VOCABULARY

UTOPIA

Meaning "no place," this term was coined by St. Thomas More who, in his book by that name, describes a religious society, heavily influenced by divine revelation, in which goods were held in common and the state regulated business.

WYCLIFFEISM

Heretical movement founded by John Wycliffe which held that authority to rule depends on moral virtue; the Bible alone contains all divine revelation, preaching is more important than the sacraments or the Mass, and the pope has no primacy of jurisdiction.

STUDY QUESTIONS

1. What is Scholasticism?

2. Which university became the most famous during the Medieval period because of the talent that it attracted?

3. Which university became known for its study of jurisprudence?

4. Which university became an important center for the sciences and later added philosophy and Arabic related texts to its curriculum?

5. What did the guild system and the independence from lay and ecclesiastical authorities create on the university campus that is still highly regarded on today's college campus?

6. What was the *studium generale* at the universities?

7. What was St. Thomas Aquinas's largest work, and what are two of the topics that this work addresses?

8. Until St. Thomas Aquinas, what ancient Greek philosopher had given the philosophical framework within which Christianity usually operated?

9. Why did Aristotle need to be "re-discovered"?

10. What was the main task of St. Thomas Aquinas?

11. What is St. Thomas Aquinas reported to have said after his mystical experience in Naples?

12. Why is St. Thomas's work so valuable to the Christian tradition?

13. How did Bl. John Duns Scotus negotiate St. Augustine's neo-Platonism and St. Thomas Aquinas's Scholasticism?

14. What are the two mendicant orders and who founded them?

15. How were the mendicants different than the monks of previous centuries?

16. What was St. Francis's dream as a young man? How did he live?

17. How did St. Francis organize the common life of his followers?

18. Pope Innocent III and the Vatican were initially suspect of St. Francis. What reportedly happened that changed Pope Innocent's mind?

19. What order oversees many of the holy shrines in the Holy Land?

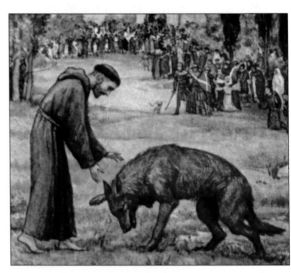

St. Francis Talks to Brother Wolf; Friends of St. Francis of Assisi

STUDY QUESTIONS

20. What rule of life did St. Dominic take for his order?

21. What color habit did the Dominicans take?

22. What heresy did the Dominicans set out to correct?

23. What devotion did the Dominicans advocate as a means of evangelization?

24. What was the legacy of the mendicant friars?

25. What architectural innovations were developed for gothic churches?

26. What was the purpose of Medieval Church art?

27. How did St. Celestine V contribute to the problems of the Avignon papacy and the Western Schism?

28. What did Philip the Fair want that instigated a struggle with the papacy?

29. What did *Clericis laicos* by Pope Boniface VIII state?

30. What did Pope Boniface assert in *Unam Sanctam?*

31. How did the Babylonian Captivity compromise the papacy and the Church?

32. Define Gallicanism.

33. How did the English king come to govern a large section of western France?

34. What were the three main battles of the Hundred Years War?

35. How did St. Joan of Arc give new hope to the French?

36. Describe St. Catherine's spirituality.

37. What is the Western Schism?

38. How did the co-existence of three "popes" prove to be a scandal to the faithful?

39. How did the Council of Constance handle the situation of three popes?

40. When was conciliarism definitively defeated?

41. Of what was William of Ockham critical?

42. What was John Wycliffe's profession?

43. What did Wycliffe criticize?

44. What English movement used Wycliffe as a basis for their criticism of the Church?

45. In what empire did John Hus live?

46. What did Hus criticize?

47. What does the French word Renaissance mean in English?

48. Name three important cities involved in trade and commerce in Italy other than Rome.

49. When did Constantinople fall?

50. What was the main topic handled by the Council of Basel-Ferrara-Florence (1431-45)?

51. Was the council's aim successful?

52. To what did the Italian city-states aspire to return in the fifteenth century?

53. What was another over-arching theme of the Renaissance that stood out in contrast not only to the Medieval period, but also the classical age?

54. What discipline was considered the pinnacle of human achievement during the Renaissance?

55. Who authored Utopia?

56. Name two works written by Erasmus.

57. What qualities led to Erasmus's recognition as a humanist?

58. Who was St. Thomas More?

59. Characterize the holiness of the Renaissance popes.

PRACTICAL EXERCISES

1. The Scholastic method answered questions by first stating objections to a statement, then giving an answer, and finally offering replies to each of the initial objections. Following the method of inquiry used in St. Thomas Aquinas's Summa Theologiæ, answer the following questions by using the Scholastic method:

    a) Is the Scholastic method an effective way of reaching philosophic conclusions?

    b) Were the Mendicant Orders really following the words of Christ?

    c) Did the High Middle Ages experience a true flowering of culture?

2. St. Joan of Arc and St. Catherine of Siena are too very different saints. Explain how the lives of these two great women reflect the multifaceted role of women in fourteenth century society. What were each saint's great accomplishments? How did they serve God? How did they serve society?

3. How did both the Avignon papacy and the Hundred Years War reflect a changing sense of social identity in western Europeans?

4. Throughout the history of the Church, many heresies have threatened the Faith. Why were the writings of the three heretics described in this chapter so influential?

5. What distinguished the Renaissance from the High Middle Ages? Compare and contrast an artist or writer from each period to explain your answer.

6. The Renaissance held art in very high esteem. How does the way that the Renaissance culture understood art help explain the motives for the Renaissance popes? Choose two popes and explain how they might defend their decisions to a contemporary audience.

FROM THE CATECHISM Continued

35 Man's faculties make him capable of coming to a knowledge of the existence of a personal God. But for man to be able to enter into real intimacy with him, God willed both to reveal himself to man, and to give him the grace of being able to welcome this revelation in faith. The proofs of God's existence, however, can predispose one to faith and help one to see that faith is not opposed to reason.

36 "Our holy mother, the Church, holds and teaches that God, the first principle and last end of all things, can be known with certainty from the created world by the natural light of human reason" (Vatican Council I, Dei Filius 2: DS 3004 cf. 3026; Vatican Council II, Dei Verbum 6). Without this capacity, man would not be able to welcome God's revelation. Man has this capacity because he is created "in the image of God" (cf. Gen 1:27).

159 Faith and science: "Though faith is above reason, there can never be any real discrepancy between faith and reason. Since the same God who reveals mysteries and infuses faith has bestowed the light of reason on the human mind, God cannot deny himself, nor can truth ever contradict truth" (Dei Filius 4: DS 3017). "Consequently, methodical research in all branches of knowledge, provided it is carried out in a truly scientific manner and does not override moral laws, can never conflict with the faith, because the things of the world and the things of faith derive from the same God. The humble and persevering investigator of the secrets of nature is being led, as it were,

FROM THE CATECHISM Continued

by the hand of God in spite of himself, for it is God, the conserver of all things, who made them what they are" (GS 36 § 1).

815 What are these bonds of unity? Above all, charity "binds everything together in perfect harmony" (Col 3:14). But the unity of the pilgrim Church is also assured by visible bonds of communion:
– profession of one faith received from the Apostles;
– common celebration of divine worship, especially of the sacraments;
– apostolic succession through the sacrament of Holy Orders, maintaining the fraternal concord of God's family (cf. UR 2; LG 14; CIC, can. 205).

817 In fact, "in this one and only Church of God from its very beginnings there arose certain rifts, which the Apostle strongly censures as damnable. But in subsequent centuries much more serious dissensions appeared and large communities became separated from full communion with the Catholic Church – for which, often enough, men of both sides were to blame" (UR 3 § 1). The ruptures that wound the unity of Christ's Body – here we must distinguish heresy, apostasy, and schism (cf. CIC, can. 751) – do not occur without human sin:

> Where there are sins, there are also divisions, schisms, heresies, and disputes. Where there is virtue, however, there also are harmony and unity, from which arise the one heart and one soul of all believers (Origen, *Hom. in Ezech.* 9, 1: PG 13, 732).

820 "Christ bestowed unity on his Church from the beginning. This unity, we believe, subsists in the Catholic Church as something she can never lose, and we hope that it will continue to increase until the end of time" (UR 4 § 3). Christ always gives his Church the gift of unity, but the Church must always pray and work to maintain, reinforce, and perfect the unity that Christ wills for her. This is

why Jesus himself prayed at the hour of his Passion, and does not cease praying to his Father, for the unity of his disciples: "That they may all be one. As you, Father, are in me and I am in you, may they also be one in us,... so that the world may know that you have sent me" (Jn 17:21; cf. Heb 7:25). The desire to recover the unity of all Christians is a gift of Christ and a call of the Holy Spirit (cf. UR 1).

822 Concern for achieving unity "involves the whole Church, faithful and clergy alike" (UR 5). But we must realize "that this holy objective – the reconciliation of all Christians in the unity of the one and only Church of Christ – transcends human powers and gifts." That is why we place all our hope "in the prayer of Christ for the Church, in the love of the Father for us, and in the power of the Holy Spirit" (UR 24 § 2).

1915 As far as possible citizens should take an active part *in public life*. The manner of this participation may vary from one country or culture to another. "One must pay tribute to those nations whose systems permit the largest possible number of the citizens to take part in public life in a climate of genuine freedom" (GS 31 § 3).

2089 *Incredulity* is the neglect of revealed truth or the willful refusal to assent to it. "*Heresy* is the obstinate post-baptismal denial of some truth which must be believed with divine and catholic faith, or it is likewise an obstinate doubt concerning the same; *apostasy* is the total repudiation of the Christian faith; *schism* is the refusal of submission to the Roman Pontiff or of communion with the members of the Church subject to him" (CIC, can. 751: emphasis added).

2245 The Church, because of her commission and competence, is not to be confused in any way with the political community. She is both the sign and the safeguard of the transcendent character of the human person.

"The Church respects and encourages the political freedom and responsibility of the citizen" (GS 76 § 3).

2293 Basic scientific research, as well as applied research, is a significant expression of man's dominion over creation. Science and technology are precious resources when placed at the service of man and promote his integral development for the benefit of all. By themselves however they cannot disclose the meaning of existence and of human progress. Science and technology are ordered to man, from whom they take their origin and development; hence they find in the person and in his moral values both evidence of their purpose and awareness of their limits.

2462 Giving alms to the poor is a witness to fraternal charity: it is also a work of justice pleasing to God.

2502 Sacred art is true and beautiful when its form corresponds to its particular vocation: evoking and glorifying, in faith and adoration, the transcendent mystery of God – the surpassing invisible beauty of truth and love visible in Christ, who "reflects the glory of God and bears the very stamp of his nature," in whom "the whole fullness of deity dwells bodily" (Heb 1: 3; Col 2: 9). This spiritual beauty of God is reflected in the most holy Virgin Mother of God, the angels, and saints. Genuine sacred art draws man to adoration, to prayer, and to the love of God, Creator and Savior, the Holy One and Sanctifier.

2544 Jesus enjoins his disciples to prefer him to everything and everyone, and bids them "renounce all that [they have]" for his sake and that of the Gospel (Lk 14: 33; cf. Mk 8: 35). Shortly before his passion he gave them the example of the poor widow of Jerusalem who, out of her poverty, gave all that she had to live on (cf. Lk 21: 4). The precept of detachment from riches is obligatory for entrance into the Kingdom of heaven.

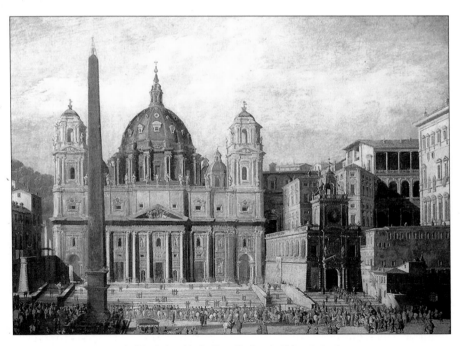

A 1630 painting of the Basilica of St. Peter by Viviano Codazzi.

The Reformation: Protestant And Catholic

The political chaos resulting from the Hundred Years War, the breakdown of feudal loyalties, and the tarnished moral authority of the papacy created an environment ripe for rebellion.

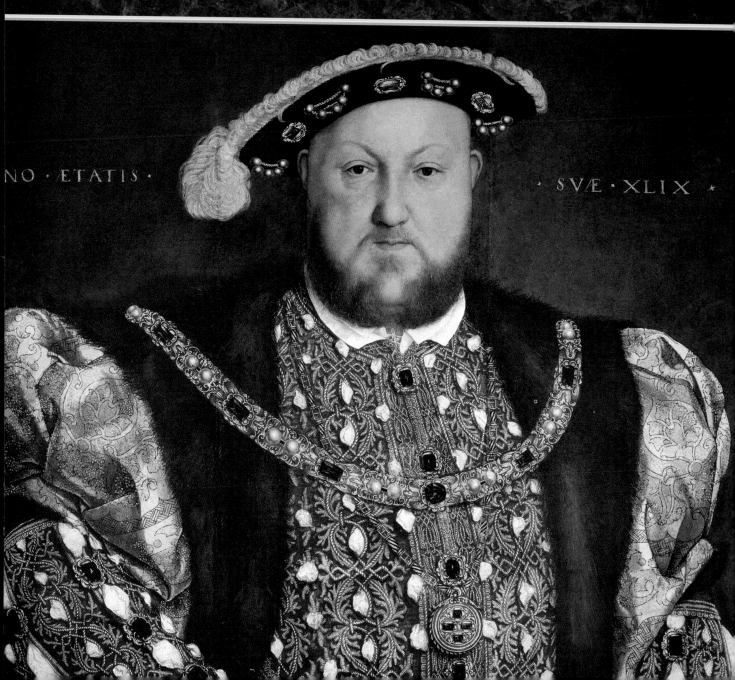

NO · ÆTATIS ·   · SVÆ · XLIX ·

CHAPTER 6

The Reformation: Protestant And Catholic

In the middle of the sixteenth century, a series of reformers began to question the teaching of the Church, shaking the very foundations of Christendom. Many of these reformers' ideas can be traced to the earlier heresies of Jan Hus and John Wycliffe. With this new movement, heretical ideas took hold in Europe in an unprecedented way. The political chaos caused by the Hundred Years War, the breakdown of feudal loyalties resulting from the plague, and the tarnished moral authority of the papacy after years of schism and political preoccupations, created a situation ripe for rebellion. Worldliness in the hierarchy, clerical abuses, rising nationalism, and unsupervised individual preaching contributed to what would be known as the Protestant Reformation.

PART I

The Protestant Revolt

Reform was needed in the Church. Simony, nepotism, and the abuse of indulgences and improper veneration of relics had spread throughout Western Europe. Many clerics collected benefices for personal gain, some failed to keep their promises of celibacy and obedience, and others had been corrupted by the lure of wealth and worldliness. Along with moral character, the level of learning among parish priests had also declined. Many could neither read nor write in Latin, and superstition grew in many rural areas where ignorant peasants often resorted to witchcraft or astrology to determine the fate of their lives. Leo X (1425-1521), the reigning pope who excommunicated Luther, typified the worldly lifestyle of Renaissance Rome.

MARTIN LUTHER'S EARLY LIFE

Martin Luther was born in Eisleben, Saxony, in 1483. He was the second of eight children, and he received the customary education of his time. Luther's father had risen slightly in society, starting

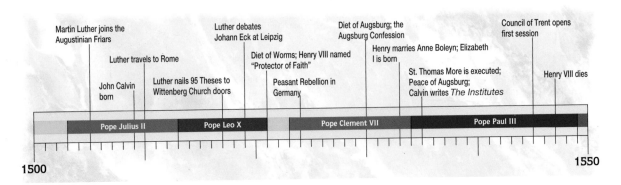

Martin Luther joins the Augustinian Friars

Luther travels to Rome

John Calvin born

Luther nails 95 Theses to Wittenberg Church doors

Luther debates Johann Eck at Leipzig

Diet of Worms; Henry VIII named "Protector of Faith"

Peasant Rebellion in Germany

Diet of Augsburg; the Augsburg Confession

Henry marries Anne Boleyn; Elizabeth I is born

St. Thomas More is executed; Peace of Augsburg; Calvin writes The Institutes

Council of Trent opens first session

Henry VIII dies

Pope Julius II   Pope Leo X   Pope Clement VII   Pope Paul III

1500   1550

as a poor peasant and then a copper miner, eventually gaining some wealth and obtaining a minor elected position in his village. As a father, he was a strict disciplinarian, and he had hoped that his son would enter the field of law. However, Martin Luther would choose a very different path.

Rather than study law, Luther joined the Augustinian Friars in 1505. Legend has it that he made the decision to enter the monastery after surviving a violent thunderstorm. After a bolt of lightning crashed near the young Luther, he made a vow, promising that if he survived the storm he would dedicate his life to God. As a monk, Luther believed he could better seek perfection and forgiveness from a God who seemed indifferent to the life and death of his people.

IN THE MONASTERY

Luther took his vows and was ordained after only nine months in the monastery. He showed to be a promising scholar and lived an exemplary life as far as his piety and ascetical struggle were concerned. Luther was promoted rapidly as a professor, and after only a year and a half of formal theological studies, he was appointed to lecture at the university. But despite his success, Luther's life in the monastery was far from happy.

It was during his early years in monastic life that he had a problem with scrupulosity, the habit of imagining sin when none exists or grave sin when the matter is not serious. More and more, Luther began to see God exclusively as a righteous lawgiver and administrator of justice. Much of Luther's understanding of God's judgment and his misconception of his love and mercy–through grace–was a consequence of the severe image of God stirred up by the culture of the day, particularly in Germany. The heavy emphasis on damnation, divine justice, and the absolute necessity of contrite repentance fostered the notion of a god who would deal out abundant punishment and whose wrath towards sinners was difficult to appease. Luther wondered how much penance a sinner could possibly do before finally obtaining God's mercy.

Martin Luther (1483-1546) painted by his friend Lucas Cranach the Elder in 1529.

Luther's objections to the Church developed over time, and in some sense, they were all rooted in the spiritual struggles of his own soul, and not the politics of ecclesiastical life. Luther's exaggerated understanding of God as judge began to influence his conception of God's love and mercy. His own

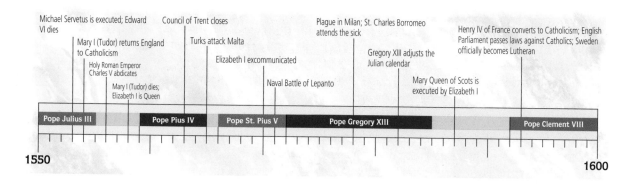

Michael Servetus is executed; Edward VI dies

Mary I (Tudor) returns England to Catholicism

Holy Roman Emperor Charles V abdicates

Mary I (Tudor) dies; Elizabeth I is Queen

Council of Trent closes

Turks attack Malta

Elizabeth I excommunicated

Naval Battle of Lepanto

Plague in Milan; St. Charles Borromeo attends the sick

Gregory XIII adjusts the Julian calendar

Mary Queen of Scots is executed by Elizabeth I

Henry IV of France converts to Catholicism; English Parliament passes laws against Catholics; Sweden officially becomes Lutheran

Pope Julius III | Pope Pius IV | Pope St. Pius V | Pope Gregory XIII | Pope Clement VIII

1550

1600

theological inclinations found a counterpart in a popular, though heretical, theologian that Luther encountered in his studies: William of Ockham. For someone like Luther, the teachings of William of Ockham offered little comfort. Ockham taught that man could not overcome sin alone, and that all meritorious human action must be willed by God. This reduced man's ability to perform good deeds. The teachings of Ockham appealed to Luther, and he began to speculate about similar theological tendencies in the writings of St. Paul and St. Augustine. These misreadings and miscomprehensions of the nature of Divine justice and man's sinfulness laid the foundation for Luther's future heresy, and in 1517, they helped fuel his distaste for the practice of selling indulgences. Outraged with the Church's teaching that indulgences, when obtained within the context of the Sacrament of Penance, could help lessen or remit one's temporal punishment due to sin. His inner tensions over personal salvation and the practice of selling indulgences prompted him to write and nail the Ninety-five Theses to the door of the Church at Wittenberg.

THE NINETY-FIVE THESES

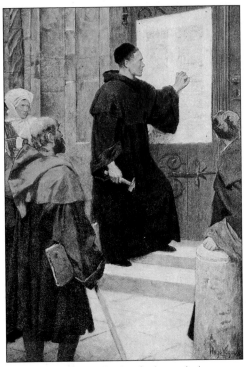

Martin Luther nailed his ninety-five theses to the door of the Church of All Saints in Wittenberg (the University's customary notice board) as an open invitation to debate his objections.

None of Luther's theses was explicitly heretical, but implicitly because they directly undermine the teaching authority of the Church. In them, Luther criticizes the use of indulgences for distracting sinners from true repentance. Luther argued that indulgences imply the forgiveness of sin through human as opposed to divine authority, and he saw this as a grave deviation. Luther questioned the validity of indulgences since the Church seemed to be usurping the authority of Christ in his role as mediator of grace and reconciliation with God the Father. Moreover, Luther started to place personal interpretation of Scripture over the teaching authority of the Church. These arguments reveal trends in Luther's thought that, in hindsight, point towards his future break with the Catholic Church.

FROM DEBATE TO DISSENSION

Luther's posting of the Ninety-five Theses to the door of the church at Wittenberg was not, in and of itself, an action provoking scandal. It was the academic custom of the age to offer an argument in this manner and invite public debate on an issue. At first, no one came forward to argue with Luther on the subject of indulgences. In earlier years, this kind of dissent would not have spread, but due to the advent of the printing press, copies of Luther's theses were able to be printed and circulated, finding their way to the doorsteps of most of the prominent clerics and scholars in Germany. His ideas met a mixed response. The theses, which now sound unmistakably Protestant, were not immediately condemned. In fact, many students began to rally behind Luther and praise the monk's bold criticism of the abuses that detracted from the Church's spiritual mission.

Luther's criticism did, however, upset the Archbishop of Mainz who forwarded Luther's theses to Rome. At first Pope Leo X considered the critique a minor incident. Luther was summoned before the Dominican Cardinal Cajetan at Augsburg who asked the theologian Sylvester Prierias to study Luther's theses and issue a rebuttal. Applying Prierias's findings, Cajetan objected to Luther's attack on the notion of merit and his questioning of the Church's infallibility. He sent a response to Luther that the pope himself hoped would settle the matter and allow the monk to fade back into obscurity.

Luther did not recant. Instead, while retaining a certain tone of respect and subordination towards the pope, he issued his Resolution on the Virtue of Indulgences, which restated his position on the matter. Surprised by Luther's bold reply, the Holy See responded more authoritatively. Pope Leo had the head of the Dominican order draw up an indictment that summoned Luther to Rome in order to explain his position before Cardinal Cajetan. In his efforts to drive home his theological position, the Dominican's letter, which was a strong reprimand of Luther, gave much importance to some of the points of disagreement, including the scope of papal authority. The change in tone

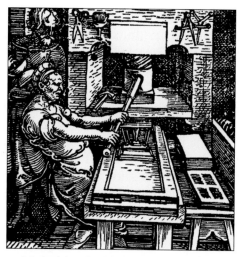

Gutenberg's invention of the printing press allowed mass circulation of Luther's ideas and criticism of Rome.

and severity on the part of the papal representative angered Luther, who still believed that his arguments were sound. He also reacted to the harsh letter from Rome by becoming firmer in his sense of righteousness.

Rather than having Luther travel to Rome, Duke Frederick of Saxony intervened on behalf of Luther and arranged for a public debate between Cajetan and Luther in Augsburg (Germany). When Luther arrived, Cajetan instructed Luther, scolding him like a father and urging him to return to the teachings of the Church. However correct Cajetan's theology was, his fatherly method did not take into account that Luther, more than a simple wayward monk, was a celebrated theologian and considered an expert in his field. Tired of dismissals and still desiring a debate, Luther felt very much offended and did not recant.

At this point Luther still did not wish to break with the Church. He wrote a letter to Leo X, subordinating himself to the authority of the supreme pontiff and showing his desire for the problem to be resolved. Theologically, Luther was still unconvinced, and the longer his points remained unresolved, the more justified he felt in his position.

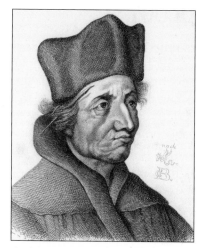

In a Leipzig debate, Professor Johann Eck forced Luther to reveal the heretical content of his ideas.

Luther was finally invited to debate beginning on June 27, 1519, at Leipzig. There, many of the foremost Catholic theologians of the day met with Luther, hoping to put the matter to rest for good. Among them was Johann Eck, the well-known professor at Ingoldstagt. Eck, a master rhetorician, required Luther to expound on his positions more extensively and concretely than ever before, perhaps in much more depth than Luther had actually considered up until that time. Then Johann Eck revealed the true philosophy behind Martin Luther's thought, which led him to voice direct opposition to the Church. Luther dismissed papal supremacy, the authority of the councils, and at one point, the Epistle of St. James because that portion of Scripture disagreed with Luther's own ideas about the effectiveness of good works. Backed into a corner, Luther further committed himself to the idea of justification by faith alone and the limitations of free will.

By the end of the debate, Luther's ideas were clearly heretical. Even those scholars who had at one time sympathized with Luther's criticisms, such as the renowned humanist Erasmus, began to withdraw their support. Germany was divided into two camps: those who supported Luther and those who recognized his heresy and stood firmly with the Church. Pope Leo X issued a bull, which gave Luther two months to formally retract his opinions under threat of excommunication. He was now forced with the decision to save or split the Church.

Despite Luther's mixed emotions over the matter, he responded to the bull in a proud and aggressive manner, burning it in a bonfire along with the code of canon law. During his lecture on the following day, Luther said that the act was symbolic since it was the pope who should have been burned. Luther then wrote the pamphlet Against the Bull of the Antichrist, which called for an all-out rebellion against the Church. His words did not fall on passive ears, and shortly after there were disorders at Leipzig, Erfurt, and Magdeburg.

The matter now fell into the hands of the new Holy Roman Emperor, Charles V, who had risen to the throne in October 1520 at the age of nineteen. Threatened with revolts throughout his realm, Charles called the Diet (Assembly) of Worms in January 1521. There Luther was again questioned on his position, and when asked to retract his writings, the

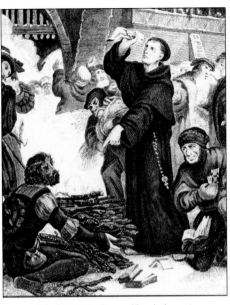

If the Reformation began with a single event, it's possible that it was not the posting of the ninety-five theses, but the burning of the papal bull *Exsurge Domine* and the canon law by Martin Luther in 1520.

reformer famously retorted, "I cannot submit my faith either to the Pope or the Councils, because it is clear as day that they have frequently erred and contradicted each other. Unless I am convinced by the testimony of Scripture or on plain and clear grounds of reason, so that conscience shall bind me to make acknowledgement of error, I cannot and will not retract, for it is neither safe nor wise to do anything contrary to conscience. Here I stand, I can do no other. May God help me. Amen" (quoted in Oberman, Luther, 1992, pp. 39-40). Judgment was passed, and Luther was granted twenty-four hours of safe passage before being subject to execution. Under fear of death, Luther fled to Wittenberg. Along the journey, he was escorted by a band of knights who brought the monk to the Castle of Wartburg where he was kept in hiding under the protection of Duke Frederick of Saxony.

LUTHER DEVELOPS HIS THEOLOGY

Luther remained at the castle in Wartburg for one year. During this time he translated the New Testament into German and continued to develop his theories, writing his three most famous

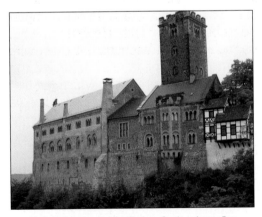

Martin Luther stayed at the Wartburg Castle under an alias: the Knight George. Duke Frederick had little personal contact with him and remained a Catholic.

works: Address to the Christian Nobility of the German Nation, On the Babylonian Captivity of the Church, and On the Freedom of a Christian. In these works, Luther worked out the theological principles that would become the cornerstone of Protestantism.

Many of Luther's ideas were inspired by the writings of John Wycliffe, William of Ockham, and Jan Hus. These writers, who criticized the Church and downplayed man's capacity for theological knowledge and the merit of good works, appealed to Luther's pessimistic view of human nature. Luther believed that sinfulness was impossible to overcome and that man could never fully escape the deceptive attraction to sin. Since any act was essentially sinful, for Luther, good works could

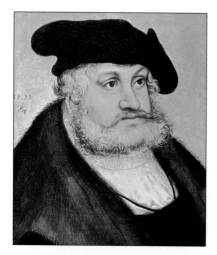

The protection of Duke Frederick of Saxony at the Castle of Wartburg provided Luther with safeharbor to translate the Bible into German and to develop his theological principles.

not play a role in perfecting the human person or obtaining God's forgiveness. Incapacitated by sin, an individual can simply have faith in God, and it is through this faith that God will grant salvation. For Luther, salvation is not a matter of perfecting oneself for God by taking advantage of his grace, but simply believing that God's mercy will ultimately grant salvation. He thought the soul will always remain corrupt, but through faith, the grace of Jesus Christ covers over sin so that one may be saved.

Luther referred to this idea of justification through faith alone as his major theological "discovery." Taking a passage from the letter of St. Paul to the Romans which reads, "For in it the righteous-ness of God is revealed through faith for faith; as it is written, 'He who through faith is righteous shall live'" (Rom 1:17), Luther began to believe that it is only "through faith" that one becomes righteous. In this passage, Luther thought that he finally found the answer to his scrupulosity and spiritual anguish. Righteousness, that lofty goal towards which Luther's thought rendered man incapable, was now possible through faith. Good deeds, penance, and works of charity do not contribute to righteousness. Faith alone saves a person, he concluded.

From this idea of justification through faith, Luther developed four major theological principles: sola Scriptura, sola fide, sola gratia, and solo Christo (Scripture alone, faith alone, grace alone, and Christ alone). Each of Luther's four main theological principles was conceived in reaction to what he believed were false teachings of the Church. Scripture alone (which held Sacred Scripture as the sole authority on Faith and doctrine) rejected tradition's role in its close link with the Scriptures, the authority of the councils and the pope, and the idea that the Holy Spirit continues to dwell and teach through the Church. Faith alone dismissed the value of corporal and spiritual works of mercy as a means to attaining righteousness. His teaching, "grace alone," held that every good action is a direct result of God's saving grace since it is beyond human capacity to do good. Along with this principle of sola gratia, Luther abandoned the idea that people can freely choose to do good (although he would certainly hold that they can choose evil freely and that they sin by their own will). At the center of these three principles was solo Christo. Martin Luther held that Christ must be the sole content of the Scriptures, the mediator of grace, and the subject of faith. Luther objected to some books of Scripture, including the Epistle of St. James, which he considered insufficiently centered on the Person of Christ.

Luther's theology brought into question the entirety of Christian worship and practice. He attacked the sacraments, arguing that God did not need material means through which he could impart grace, so one is normally saved not through the sacraments but only by faith. He denied all but the two sacraments explicitly instituted in the Gospels, Eucharist and Baptism, but even with those, he gradually replaced the Church's teaching with his own interpretation. He maintained that after the consecration, both the substance of bread and wine together with Christ's Body and Blood are present. He used the term consubstantiation, explaining that Christ is present in the Eucharist in the same way heat is present in a red-hot iron. His

Martin Luther's German Bible was the first mass produced book on the Gutenberg press. It had great impact on unifying German culture. Its language became the people's language. Regions which previously had multiple dialects now could communicate with each other.

THE EPISTLE OF ST. JAMES

The only place where the expression "faith alone" appears in the Bible is in the Epistle of St. James. Therein he offers a strong argument against Martin Luther's theology of sola fide (faith alone):

> What does it profit, my bretheren, if a man says he has faith but has not works? Can his faith save him?... So faith by itself, if it has no works is dead.... Do you want to be shown, you foolish fellow, that faith apart from works is barren? Was not Abraham our father justified by works, when he offered his son Isaac upon the altar? You see that faith was active along with his works, and faith was completed by works, and the scripture was fulfilled which says, "Abraham believed God and it was reckoned to him as righteousness"; and he was called the friend of God. You see that a man is justified by works and not by faith alone.... For as the body apart from the spirit is dead, so faith apart from works is dead. (Jas 2:14, 17-18, 20-24, 26)

This passage contradicts Martin Luther's position on the effectiveness of good works. Needless to say, it was not one of his favorites. In fact, Luther once referred to this letter as "an epistle of straw" and, comparing the work to other parts of the New Testament, Luther considered "throwing Jimmy into the fire." Luther

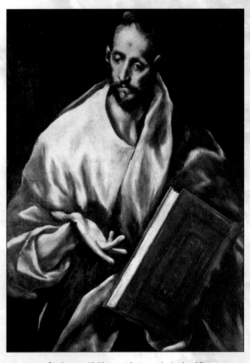

St. James: "faith apart from works is dead."

also had problems with the Book of Revelation, Hebrews, Jude, and 2 Peter. In addition to these New Testament books, Martin Luther attacked the Old Testament deuterocanonical texts, although he did not take them out of his translation of the Bible, where they remained as an appendix (cf. The Canon of Scripture in chapter four).

ideas about consubstantiation contradict the Church's teaching that the substance of the bread and wine completely change into the Body and Blood of Christ, called transubstantiation, with only the accidents (or properties) remaining.

In addition to his translation of the Bible and major theological works, Luther wrote On Monastic Vows and The Abolition of Private Masses while at Wartburg. In these works, Luther virulently attacks celibacy and the monastic life. He claimed that living celibacy was an impossible burden and called for all religious to break their vows and marry. In 1525, Luther himself married an ex-nun, Katherine von Bora.

While Luther was hiding in Wartburg, the Reformation began to gain momentum. In Wittenberg, two friends and followers of Luther, Carlstadt and Melanchthon, brought extreme reforms to the university town. The Augustinian monastery saw forty members leave their order and a Franciscan monastery was attacked, its altars demolished and its windows smashed. In answer to Luther's call to marriage, Carlstadt married, and on Christmas Day 1521, Carlstadt proceeded to say Mass in German without vestments, publicly denying the real presence of Christ in the Eucharist. Luther would condemn Carlstadt and try to bring about more moderate reforms. Carlstadt, and later his successor Zwingli, would continue to push his ideas further, contributing to the eventual growth of Calvinism, as will be explained later.

PART II

The Peasant Rebellion and the Splintering of Protestantism

THE GERMAN PRINCES

Frederick of Saxony and other princes of the realm became concerned with some of Carlstadt's tendencies and called upon Luther to moderate affairs in Wittenberg. The princes of Germany had little in common with Luther's religious sentiments. They did, however, share in his rebelliousness toward the papacy. They saw in Luther's new movement a way to free themselves from the pope and the Catholic emperor and to enrich themselves with expropriated Church lands.

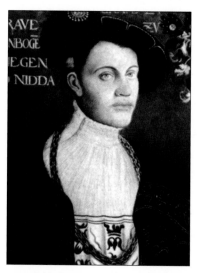

Prince Philip I of Hesse. When Luther was asked to condone the bigamy of Prince Philip I of Hesse, he granted him a dispensation to keep his two wives.

After 1524 other German princes joined Frederick of Saxony in support of Luther. Knights of the Empire, such as Franz von Sickingen and Ulrich von Hutten, used their private armies to press for Lutheran reforms. In 1522, von Sickingen laid siege to Trier whose bishop was a strong opponent of Luther. Albert of Brandenburg, the cousin of the Bishop of Mainz and head of the Teutonic Knights, used the Lutheran cause to declare himself Duke of Prussia. The Teutonic Order was disbanded and Albert, a priest, broke his vows in order to marry. The future kings of Germany would now descend from the House of Brandenburg.

Other relations between Luther and the princes proved embarrassing. Philip of Hesse demanded that Luther support his bigamous marriage, a measure he was hesitant to condone.

A compromise was made with Philip. There would be no general law permitting dual marriage, but Philip would be granted a dispensation and he would thus continue to live with both wives. In defending his position, Luther argued that all things are proper for the sake of the Church. Luther said, "What harm would there be, if a man to accomplish better things and for the sake of the Christian Church, does tell a good thumping lie" (Lenz, Briefwechsel, I, p. 382; Kolde, Analecta, p. 356).

THE PEASANT REBELLION

Luther became a pawn of the German princes. The greatest example of this was his reaction to the great peasant uprising in 1524. Luther's attack on the authority of the Church had wide-ranging consequences. Denying the authority of the Church was a kind of model for denying secular authority. This radical democratization of the Church, which gave everyone the same authority to preach and interpret the Gospel, led to an attempt to overthrow the feudal system of rule by the nobility. Peasants throughout Germany rebelled in social revolution.

Luther was called upon to condemn the uprising. He urged the princes to "Strike, slay front and rear; nothing is more devilish than sedition. There must be no sleep, no patience, no mercy; they are the children of the devil" (quoted in Harney, The Catholic Church Through the Ages, 1974, p. 239). Over 100,000 men, women, and children were slain; hundreds of villages were burned and crops destroyed. The civil authorities were willing to usurp the authority of the Church in Germany, but not share that same power with common people below them.

THE AUGSBURG CONFESSION

In 1530 a diet (legislative assembly) was to be held in Augsburg to attempt to resolve the conflict between Lutherans and Catholics in the hopes of forming an alliance against Turkish aggression. Melanchthon was sent to draft a list of principles from which a compromise could be made. The draft of these principles became known as the Augsburg Confession, establishing the basic tenets of Lutheranism for the future. The principles understated the basic theological differences between Lutheran theology and the teachings of the Catholic Church. Cardinal Campeggio, the papal legate at Augsburg, noted these divergent views and admitted the need for studying a reform of some of these abuses in the Catholic Church. The diet ended with a call for reform and for the princes of the north to return to the Church.

In response to the Diet of Augsburg, the northern princes met in Schmalkalden, Thuringia (Germany). The Northern princes formed a pact among themselves that insisted on their rights as independent monarchs, refusing to accept the terms of Augsburg in order to increase their control. With the need to gain their support in his wars against the Turks, Charles V authorized a temporary truce with the League of Schmalkalden in 1532, a turning point in the history of the conflict. The truce allowed the rebellious nobles equal rights and was a latent recognition of the existence of a permanent Protestant state. Though future conflict would erupt between Charles V and the League of Schmalkalden, a precedent was created and would be formalized thirty years later at the Peace of Augsburg in 1555. There it would be decided that the religion of the prince would be the religion of the people within his realm.

THE DEATH OF LUTHER

Luther was eventually pushed to the side in the newly constituted Protestant Germany. His marriage to Katherine von Bora gave him six children. In his later life, he would continue to write, but his style became increasingly coarse and crude. He continued attacking the papacy and added anti-Semitic attacks as well. Slowly his irascible nature caused by physical impairments and unchecked disease, along with a vicious temper, would drive his friends and colleagues away. "Hardly one of us," lamented one of his followers, "can escape Luther's anger and his public scourging" (Corp. Ref., V, 314).

Luther died in his sleep on February 18, 1546, without having reconciled with the Church.

JOHN CALVIN

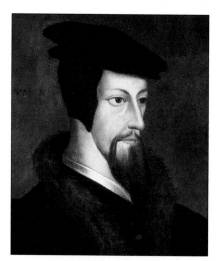

John Calvin held that human nature
is totally corrupted, rotten, and vicious.

The second major figure of the Protestant reformation was John Calvin. Born in 1509 in Noyon, France, Calvin was the son of a middle-class attorney. In many ways Calvin was a great contrast to Luther. Where Luther was born of peasant stock, uncouth in language and mystical in his religious zeal, Calvin was born into a middle-class family and in his growing years was in contact with intellectuals. His strong intellectual inclinations are especially seen in his rational treatises and humorless sermons. Luther was a monk who had forsaken his vows and left his Church to lead his religious crusade; Calvin was a layman who never took vows, who structured and codified the reform movement and turned it into a militant crusade.

Early in his life, Calvin studied for an ecclesiastical career at the University of Paris. Because of disagreements between his father and his family's local bishop, Calvin's father had his son study law. For three years Calvin studied philosophy and law and afterwards he became familiar with humanistic writings at the University of Orléans (France). Much of the structure and spirit of his celebrated work Institutes of the Christian Religion can be attributed to his study of Roman law and the Codex Justinianus. After his father's death, Calvin returned to Paris where he finished his theological studies. While at university, Calvin discovered the teachings of Luther. Shortly after his return to Paris, Calvin was implicated in the "Affair of the Placards," which consisted of scurrilous literature appearing all over Paris attacking the Catholic Church in a degrading way. Because of this, Calvin was forced to flee the city to avoid arrest and punishment. He reached Basel, Switzerland, in January 1535 where he undertook the first draft of his major work, Institutes of the Christian Religion. The book began as an apology of Protestantism written to the king of France, Francis I, whom Calvin hoped to convert to the cause.

THE INSTITUTES OF THE CHRISTIAN RELIGION

The Institutes contained four books with a complete presentation by Calvin of his view concerning Protestant theology and church organization. It was a law manual codifying the principles first taught by Luther. After numerous revisions and editions, it became the most widely read book of the sixteenth century.

Ultimate authority, according to Calvin, is contained in the Scriptures. Following the tradition of Wycliffe and Luther, he stated that the Bible is the only source of revelation. Calvin was a great Scripture scholar and used his knowledge of Sacred Scripture to present rationally the teachings of Protestant theology. Like Hus and Luther, Calvin rejected the power of human freedom to elicit good actions and the ability of man to merit through good works. For Calvin, human nature is totally corrupted, rotten and vicious; man is no more than a savage beast. Like Luther, Calvin maintained that man's sinfulness is so great that he can never overcome it. However, Calvin went even further than Luther regarding the Sacraments. Whereas Luther maintained some sacramental elements of Baptism and Eucharist, Calvin denied all sacramental grace. Baptism and the Eucharist became merely memorials, and he rejected all Catholic practices that were not explicitly based in Scripture. He directed iconoclastic actions against all crucifixes, statues, sacred paintings, vestments, altars, confessionals, and stained-glass windows depicting saints. His followers would move through towns leveling destruction against Catholic churches throughout Europe.

PREDESTINATION

Since salvation depended solely on God's free decision, Calvin maintained that some were predestined to Heaven and most others to Hell. Those who were chosen by God – through no effort of their own – were known as the elect. These few elect had some inclination of their salvation by their good moral behavior and their earthly success. This principle was eagerly accepted by the middle classes who began to favor Calvinist doctrine. Just as some were chosen for Heaven, others were chosen by God for damnation. This damnation, according to Calvin, was necessary to show God's great justice. It would follow, therefore, that the sorry lot of the underprivileged and those considered reprobated would be the just chastisement for those doomed to the fires of Hell.

THEOCRACY IN GENEVA

Calvin first came to Geneva in 1536 when he was passing through on his way to Strasbourg. At the time, Geneva was in the midst of religious turmoil. Guillaume Farel, a Lutheran, sought Calvin's aid in persuading the town council to accept the Lutheran position. At first, the town fathers accepted Calvin's reforms, but by 1538 the implementation seemed too severe, and Calvin was forced into exile for four years. He traveled to Strasbourg where he married Idelette de Bure, the widow of an Anabaptist whom he had converted. Idelette gave birth to Calvin's only son who died in infancy. She also died not too long after in 1541. In that same year, Calvin was summoned back to Geneva.

In Geneva, Calvin transformed the city's government into a theocracy dominated by Calvin himself. Although the city council never elected him, through his influence, Calvin would make the state subservient to the Church.

In Geneva no expression of religious freedom was tolerated. The old, Catholic creed was forbidden, no prayer could be said in Latin, and no words of sympathy for or recognition of the pope could ever be uttered. Disagreement with Calvin, or even criticizing his preaching, could easily result in punishment. One unfortunate individual, Jacques Gouet, was imprisoned on charges of impiety in June 1547, and after severe torture, was beheaded in July. It was said that coughing during a sermon or making other such rude noises could bring a prison sentence. Under Calvin, one citizen of Geneva remarked:

> No tyrant of our own times was more terribly the master of men's lives than this long gray beard, old long before his time, whose eyes flashed so terribly when justly angered – and of course when angered it was always justly. (quoted in Hughes, A History of the Church to the Eve of the Reformation, 1976, p. 230)

The most famous episode of religious intolerance was with the execution of Michael Servetus in 1553. Servetus, a Spanish Unitarian, had met with Calvin and debated against him in Paris in 1534. (A Unitarian believes in individual freedom of belief from any authority.) In a series of letters, Servetus had criticized Calvin's Institutes. Calvin railed against Servetus and was reported to have said, "If he comes here and I have any authority, I will never let him leave the place alive." Calvin's prediction came true when Servetus was passing through Geneva in 1553. The Spaniard was arrested and burned at the stake. Adultery, pregnancy outside of marriage, heresy, striking a parent, and blasphemy all incurred the death penalty. During a five-year period, fifty-five people were executed and another seventy-six were driven into exile.

Calvin's church was organized with pastors, doctors, elders, and deacons with the supreme power given to the magistrate. Divine worship was reduced to prayers, sermons, and singing psalms. Each congregation elected its own pastor, and the congregations were overseen by a local synod. Moral behavior was strictly regulated, and church attendance and conduct were carefully monitored. There were punishments for dancing, card playing, drinking, braiding hair, or falling asleep during sermons. Twice a year a commission of inquisitors inspected every home to ensure orthodoxy. Any new book or manuscript was censored and had to include the author's initials and the censor's initials on every page. All findings of the commission were listed in a book where each person's name would be followed with the notation of "pious," "lukewarm," or "corrupt."

Calvin justified and maintained this severe environment by his appeal for an impeccable moral life and habitual practice of prayer. The example of his personal virtue and mastery of Scripture called upon everyone to forsake any disposition toward materialism and seek the holiness of the

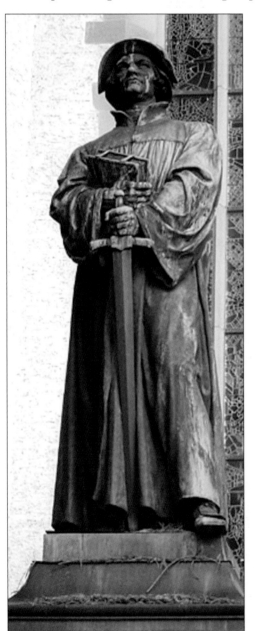

elect. His teachings rapidly spread throughout Europe as other reform movements adapted his teachings. John Knox would create the Presbyterian Church according to Calvinist teachings, as would the Huguenots in France and the Puritans in England. Thus John Calvin can be credited with the explosive diffusion of Protestantism throughout Europe.

ULRICH ZWINGLI

Ulrich Zwingli (1484-1531) was the third major reformer and founder of the Reformation in Switzerland. His humanistic studies, beginning in the university where he studied for the priesthood, led him to study Greek and read the classics and the Fathers of the Church. He became acquainted with and entered into friendly discussions with the leading humanists of his day: Heinrich Loriti (Glareanus), Erasmus, and Vadian. While serving as a priest in Zurich, he fell into sins against priestly celibacy (like many Renaissance-era clerics), and before long converted many of the faithful to his increasingly anti-Catholic views on Church-state relations, the veneration of the saints, the removal of images, good works, and the Sacraments. With much political power behind him, he used the state to seize Church property, suppress the Mass and Sacraments such as Penance and Anointing of the Sick, destroy images, statues, relics, altars, and organs (regardless of even their artistic value), and melt down chalices and monstrances into coins. As the head of both government and church in Zurich, Zwingli was able to establish and stabilize the Reformation during his lifetime.

Ulrich Zwingli's reformation spread from the Zürich canton (Swiss state) to five other cantons of the Swiss Confederation. The remaining five cantons firmly held onto the Catholic Faith.

Ulrich Zwingli was killed in a military battle between the Zürich canton and the Catholic cantons at Kappel am Albis.

PART III
The English Reformation

The last of the movements to bring about a Protestant revolution occurred in England. The spread of Protestantism in England did not originate from theological or dogmatic issues, but over the issue of papal authority, specifically regarding the issue of the king's marriage and, later, with the English monarch as head of the Church in England.

The Catholic Church in England at the beginning of the sixteenth century was in better condition than in any country in Europe save Spain. Relations between the clergy and the laity were very good; there were relatively few clerical scandals and there was popular support for the religious and the Church in general. A visitor to the British island at the time could admire the universal observation of Catholic practices and the general manifestation of English piety. The king himself had been named "Protector of the Faith" by the pope in 1520 for defending the Church against Lutheran attacks in the work entitled Defense of the Seven Sacraments (Livingstone, The Oxford Dictionary of the Christian Church, 1997, p. 752).

HENRY VIII

The Tudors had come to the throne at the end of the English civil war (War of the Roses). This forty-year struggle wrought havoc on the island nation and brought it to the brink of destruction. Henry VII ended the conflict and restored calm and prosperity to England. He managed to increase his treasury by avoiding war and allying himself with Spain, the strongest European state. (His eldest son Arthur was betrothed to Catherine of Aragon, the daughter of the king and queen of Spain.) Henry's second son, only seventeen at the time, was never supposed to be king. He was a handsome, popular youth

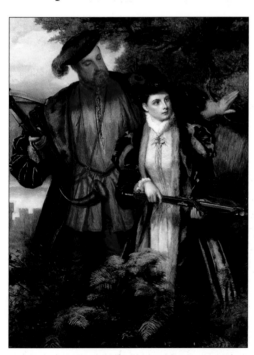

Henry VIII and Anne Boleyn.
Henry was a hunter, a dancer and a womanizer. He wanted Anne and would turn the world upside-down to have her.

who was a renowned wrestler, hunter, dancer, and womanizer. The life of this young man, however, would be forever changed by the death of his older brother. In order to save the Spanish alliance, young Henry was given to the older Catherine in marriage. Legally, a dispensation was needed since, technically, Catherine was Henry's sister through marriage. Pope Julius II granted the dispensation, and the Spanish alliance was preserved through Catherine and Henry's marriage.

The marriage at first was a happy one. Catherine gave Henry a daughter whom they named Mary. Other children soon came, including a number of sons, but all died before their first year. As Catherine grew older, the 35-year-old Henry realized that he would not have a male heir. To complicate the problem, Henry's affections were drawn toward one of his Queen's attendants, Anne Boleyn. Henry began to seek a way to end his marriage with Catherine. Quoting Leviticus, King Henry asserted that Julius II had wrongfully granted a dispensation; God was punishing Henry by refusing him an heir for having taken his brother's wife. Henry sent his legates to Rome and asked Pope Clement VII for an annulment.

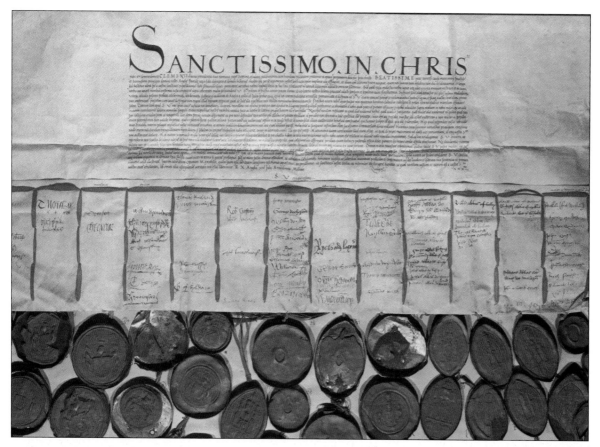

A letter from King Henry VIII to Pope Clement, July 13, 1530. The letter is composed on behalf of the Peers of the realm requesting that the Pope annul the first marriage of their king to Catherine of Aragon. The document bears the personal signatures of the petitioners and 85 red wax seals.

CARDINAL WOLSEY

The legate in charge of the annulment was Cardinal Wolsey, Chancellor and the most powerful churchman in England. He had accumulated large benefices throughout England and at one time strove for the papacy itself. Wolsey was not a scholar trained in law or theology, but a skillful and pragmatic chancellor. A few years before, he tried to gain Henry the title "Holy Roman Emperor," and although he had failed, Wolsey's efforts clearly showed him to be the most capable advocate for Henry's cause.

Wolsey obtained permission from Rome to begin the trial for the annulment case in England, where he would be able to control the outcome. At first, he was given assurances from Rome that the decision would not be questioned regardless of the outcome. Since Pope Clement VII was a cautious man and realized that England might fall into schism over the issue of the annulment, he insisted on a legitimate trial for Catherine. Clement also had to contend with Catherine's powerful nephew, Emperor Charles V of Spain, and so before judgment was reached, Clement ordered the case to be brought to Rome.

Henry VIII derided the pope's decision and declared Wolsey a traitor to England, claiming that he was attempting to enforce the laws of a foreign ruler. Wolsey was stripped of his power and ordered back to London to answer the charges. On this journey the cardinal died in a monastery at Leicester. When Wolsey's body was prepared for burial, caretakers discovered that he was wearing a hair shirt for penance under his splendid robes.

THE ACT OF SUPREMACY

After Wolsey's death, relations between England and Rome became even more strained. Henry wanted desperately to resolve his problem. He had turned to his friend St. Thomas More in the hopes that the scholar's good reputation would sway the mind of the pope. More became Chancellor and helped Henry reform the Church in England, but he refused to touch the matter of the annulment. Henry would find an answer to his problem in Thomas Cranmer and Thomas Cromwell.

When Archbishop William Warham of Canterbury died, Henry named Thomas Cranmer, the personal confessor of Anne Boleyn and a secret Lutheran, as the new archbishop. Cranmer had officiated over the illicit marriage of Henry and the now pregnant Anne in a secret ceremony on January 25, 1533. In May of that year, Archbishop Cranmer nullified Henry's first marriage to Catherine and recognized the validity of Henry's new marriage to Anne and the legitimacy of her unborn child. On September 7, 1533, Anne gave birth to a girl, Elizabeth.

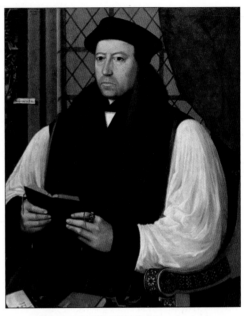

Archbishop Cranmer nullified Henry's first marriage and recognized Henry's new marriage to Anne Boleyn.

Henry turned to parliament for an acknowledgement of his supremacy. With the "Act of Supremacy" law, the king was proclaimed the supreme head of the Church in England, and Anne Boleyn was recognized as Queen. Their daughter Elizabeth would become heir to the throne of England. The pope was no longer recognized as having even any religious authority within England, so all matters of faith, ecclesiastical appointment, and maintenance of ecclesiastical properties were in the hands of the king. All subjects of the crown were required to take an oath of allegiance to the king under penalty of imprisonment, and anyone who spoke against the Act of Supremacy would be punished by death.

BISHOP STS. JOHN FISHER AND THOMAS MORE

Henry was determined to enforce his will upon England. A young Benedictine nun, Elizabeth Barton, known as the Holy Maid of Kent, and four parish priests were executed after they had called upon the king to return to the Faith and send Anne away. Only one of England's Bishops refused to go along with Henry's actions: St. John Fisher, the Bishop of Rochester. St. John Fisher refused to sign the allegiance to the royal supremacy, and was imprisoned. With the idea of saving his life, Pope Paul III made St. John Fisher a cardinal while he was imprisoned. This elevation backfired and so enraged Henry that the king had the cardinal beheaded in 1535, less than one month later.

St. Thomas More, Chancellor of England, a renowned humanist writer and lifelong friend of Henry, also refused to take the oath of supremacy. His high standing in England threatened Henry's plans, so St. Thomas More was arrested and sent to the Tower of London. He was a gifted lawyer and writer who struggled heroically to make his Catholic Faith an absolute priority. He had a jovial and cheerful nature and a great sense of humor. He would frequently have the poor and destitute join him and his family for meals. Though a layman, he habitually wore a hair shirt and regularly engaged in other penitential practices. He was a family man, devoted to his wife and daughters. A leading humanist writer of his time, he undertook the education of his daughters in Latin and classical literature.

ST. JOHN HOUGHTON AND THE BLESSED MARTYRS OF THE CARTHUSIAN ORDER

Some of the earliest martyrs of the English Reformation were members of the Carthusian Charterhouse of London. The Carthusian order, founded by St. Bruno in France during the eleventh century, is unique among western monastic orders for its nearly eremitical life and emphasis on strict austerity. According to the Carthusian rule, each monk lives alone in a cell with a small garden, and the monks come together only for communal worship.

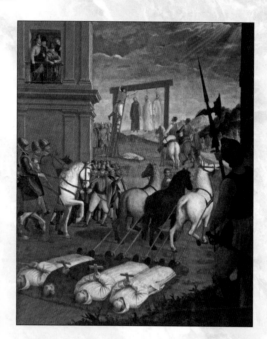

In sixteenth-century England, the Carthusians were held in such high regard that Henry VIII was set on winning them over to Anglicanism or destroying the order. The Prior of the Carthusian Charterhouse in London, St. John Houghton, was the first man who refused Henry VIII's Oath of Supremacy. On May 4, 1535, just weeks before the deaths of Sts. Thomas More and John Fisher, three Carthusians, including St. John Houghton, were hanged, drawn, and quartered at Tyburn for their fidelity to the Church of Rome. During the subsequent five years, fifteen more Carthusians were martyred for the Faith. The eighteen Carthusian martyrs were beatified by Pope Leo XIII in 1886. Pope Paul VI canonized St. John Houghton in 1970, including him among the Forty Martyrs of England and Wales, a group representative of the English and Welsh martyrs of the Reformation who died at various dates between 1535 and 1679.

St. Thomas More was learned in the law and knew he could be imprisoned but not executed for refusing to sign the Oath of Supremacy. For more than one year, St. Thomas More was kept in the Tower where he refused to speak for or against the Oath. When asked, his only response was:

> I am (quoth I) the king's true faithful subject and daily bedesman, and pray for His Highness, and all his, and all the realm. I do nobody harm, I say none harm, I think none harm, but wish everybody good. And if this be not enough to keep a man alive, in good faith I long not to live. (quoted in Hughes, A History of the Church to the Eve of the Reformation, 1976, p. 182)

Henry turned this case over to his new Chancellor, Thomas Cromwell. Using perjured testimony, Cromwell gained a conviction. Originally sentenced to be hanged, drawn, and quartered, St. Thomas More was beheaded on July 6, 1535, two weeks after St. John Fisher. On the scaffold he said, "I die the King's good servant, but God's first" (quoted in Hughes, A History of the Church to the Eve of the Reformation, 1976, p. 183). Both Sts. John Fisher and Thomas More were canonized in 1935, 400 years after they were martyred; they share a feast day celebrated on June 22.

CONFISCATION OF CHURCH PROPERTIES

Thomas Cromwell became the major advocate for Henry's new regime. As an administrator under Cardinal Wolsey, it had been Cromwell's task to administer the confiscation of monastic properties that were declared vacated. Cromwell oversaw the seizure of monastic lands now that the king was the new head of the church. Nearly a third of English property was held by the Church, a gross income of nearly £300,000 a year. The first move by Cromwell was to take over the small monastic lands. In the Act for the Dissolution of the Lesser Monasteries, some 318 houses were closed, displacing nearly 1500 religious. The larger monasteries met the same fate shortly after. Lead was stripped from the roofs of the monasteries and melted down; jewels and plate were confiscated and sent to Henry's treasury. This greatest land redistribution in England since the time of William the Conqueror occurred between 1533 and 1536, vastly enriching the nobility loyal to Henry and his new church.

Not all were pleased with Henry's new policies. Many peasants suffered tremendously as towns were ruined by the wholesale redistribution of land. An insurrection broke out in October 1536, known as the Pilgrimage of Grace. Lincolnshire and Yorkshire exploded in open rebellion with over 40,000 well-armed men. The Duke of Norfolk was called upon to quell the uprising. He met with the leaders and agreed to take their terms of reform to the king. The leaders of the uprising believed they could impress the king with their demands by a show of force, but Norfolk undermined the resistance by appeasing the leaders of the uprising. After the mobs subsided, the leadership was arrested and executed.

AFTERMATH OF HENRY VIII: ENGLAND BECOMES PROTESTANT

In spite of his break from Rome, Henry still considered himself a Catholic, and he continued to fight against the introduction of Lutheran ideas into his realm. In 1539 Henry compelled Parliament to adopt his Six Articles that determined the main teachings of the English Church. These articles included maintaining the doctrine of transubstantiation, Communion under one species, Masses for the dead, the Sacrament of Penance, vows, and celibacy of the clergy. Tyndale's English translation of the Bible was condemned and heretics were still to be burned at the stake.

Henry soon grew tired of Anne Boleyn. He was angry that she had born him a daughter instead of a son and blamed her for the presence of Lutheranism in England. He had also fallen in love with one of Anne's attendants, Jane Seymour. With Catherine of Aragon's death in January 1536 the way was clear for Henry to rid himself of Anne and marry Jane. Thomas Cromwell brought charges of adultery against Anne who was beheaded in 1536. Henry married Jane who gave birth to Henry's heir, Edward VI.

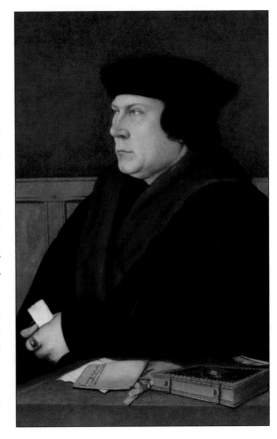

Henry fought any introduction of Lutheran ideas into his realm. Thomas Cromwell tried to unite England with Protestant Germany through Henry's marriage to Anne of Cleves. He paid for this final manipulation with his life.

Thomas Cromwell would also lose favor with Henry by trying to unite England with Protestant Germany. After Jane Seymour died during childbirth, Cromwell arranged a marriage between Henry and a German princess, Anne of Cleves. Henry was angered at being drawn into a conflict with Spain because of the union, and he executed Cromwell for treason.

Henry married two more times before his own death. Aged before his time, obese and racked with gout, Henry died on January 28, 1547, at age 55. He left an infant son to deal with the growing Protestant movement in England.

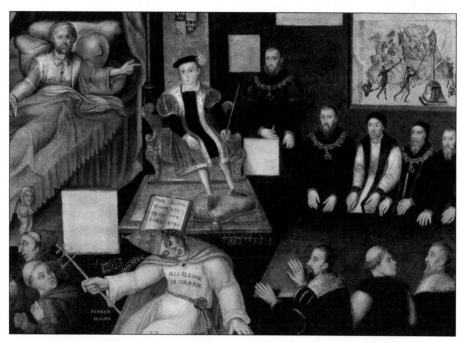

This allegorical painting from 1548 shows the dying Henry VIII pointing to the new order of Edward VI. Edward is surrounded by his council, the Duke of Sommerset and Thomas Cranmer. The pope and monks are deposed, while through the window Calvinist iconoclasts are destroying religious images. Under the boy king, there was a dramatic shift to a Swiss-style theology. The Reformation was given free rein, the Mass was essentially abolished, and Cranmer wrote two prayerbooks which introduced English into the church liturgy.

EDWARD VI

The Protestant cause seemed triumphant with the death of Henry VIII. The Six Articles of Henry were quickly repealed and the seat of government fell into the hands of Edward VI's two major ministers: the Duke of Sommerset (Edward's uncle) and Thomas Cranmer, the Archbishop of Canterbury. The two would attempt to turn Anglican England into a Lutheran-Calvinist country.

England was flooded with translations of Lutheran writings. Cranmer published a Lutheran catechism and The Book of Common Prayer. Altars were destroyed and replaced by simple tables as the essential parts of the Mass were swept away. Bishops who protested the changes were imprisoned, and political opportunists took control of the government. Public outcry to the changes led to a series of local rebellions, but the regency did not last. In 1553, Edward, who had always been sickly, died at age 15. The Duke of Northumberland tried unsuccessfully to place a distant cousin, Lady Jane Grey, on the throne in order to maintain Protestant succession. Support, however, turned to Henry's eldest daughter, Mary Tudor.

MARY I

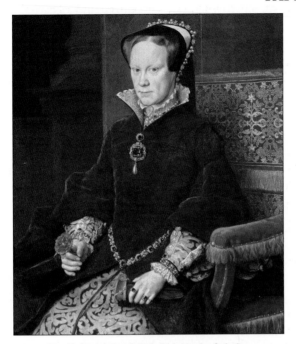

Mary Tudor, an ardent Catholic like her mother Catherine, repealed all of Edward VI's Protestant changes and executed Cranmer and other Reformation proponents.

Mary was the daughter of Catherine of Aragon and an ardent Catholic. She acted quickly to restore the Church of England to the old Faith. All of the Edwardian enactments were repealed, and England was reunited with Rome in 1554. She accepted the advice of her cousin Charles V not to press for the return of Church lands confiscated by her father. Mary attempted to strengthen her reforms by marrying Charles's son, Philip II, King of Spain.

Later English writers have vilified Mary's short-lived reign. However, one must keep in mind that Mary's reign was a hard and volatile time. Many of the leaders of Edward VI's reign attempted to keep Mary from the throne and further the Lutheran cause. They continuously fought Mary's Catholic reforms. In response, Mary had Cranmer and other leading opponents tried for heresy and burned at the stake. In all, 277 were executed under Mary's rule, hence, her legendary nickname, Bloody Mary.

Mary had only ruled England for five years upon her death in 1558. These troubled years were too short to bring about permanent reform. After Mary's death, her half sister Elizabeth would undo the positive effects of Mary's reign, and push England even further away from th;e Catholic Faith.

ELIZABETH I

Elizabeth's reign began with many questions of succession. She was the daughter of Anne Boleyn whose marriage to Henry VIII had been annulled, calling into question Elizabeth's legitimacy. Without Elizabeth, the throne would have fallen to the young Mary Stuart of Scotland. Unfortunately for Mary, she was recently married to the King of France and the English Parliament was wary of an alliance between the two countries. Henry's confiscation of Church lands had made Parliament very wealthy, and it was now concerned with retaining the power that resulted from that expropriation. Enmity with Catholic France

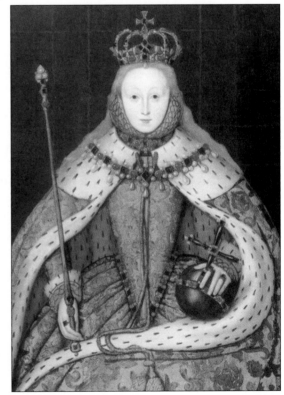

Elizabeth I was crowned on January 15, 1559. There was no Archbishop of Canterbury at the time. The last Roman Catholic Archbishop had died shortly after Mary I. Senior bishops declined to participate in the coronation since Elizabeth was illegitimate under both canon law and statute and because she was a Protestant. The Communion was celebrated by the Queen's personal chaplain, to avoid the use of the Roman Catholic rites. Elizabeth I's coronation was the last coronation to use a Latin service.

encouraged Parliament to support Elizabeth's claim to the throne. In short, Elizabeth's forty-year reign reflected the desire of Parliament to hold on to their wealth and property and Elizabeth's uncanny capacity to maintain her royal power. The result of her alliance with Parliament cemented the Protestant cause in England.

Elizabeth surrounded herself with strong advisors, the most important being William Cecil, the Lord Burghley who helped her complete the Protestant revolution in England. Maintaining all the outward appearances of Catholicism, Elizabeth incorporated Protestant doctrine into the Church of England. The majority of England was still Catholic in practice and custom, and so Elizabeth worked on the Anglican Compromise to help make the transition to Protestantism smoother for the English. She issued the Thirty-Nine Articles. In those articles, Elizabeth kept the old organization of the Church with its ceremonies and vestments, but rigorously re-imposed the Oath of Royal Supremacy and decreed a uniformity of prayer following Protestant lines.

In 1563, The Council of Trent closed after accomplishing a monumental effort to reform the Catholic Church. Legates of the pope attempted to meet with Elizabeth and reconcile the differences between the Anglican and Roman Churches, but Elizabeth refused to meet with the Papal representatives. Instead, the Queen threatened to execute any papal representative who set foot in England. In 1569, Elizabeth ruthlessly put down a series of uprisings against her rule. Elizabeth began a campaign of legislation that tore away Catholicism from the English countryside. She forbade any public celebration of Catholic rites and imprisoned her Catholic cousin, Mary of Scotland. After St. Pius V excommunicated the queen in 1570, persecution followed in 1571. Parliament made it treasonable for any papal document to be published in England or any English subject to be reconciled with Rome. Fines and imprisonment were imposed for celebrating or attending Mass; fines were imposed for failing to show up for Anglican services. Elizabeth would eventually execute 189 Catholic priests and imprison hundreds of English gentry and thousands among the lower classes on account of their practice of the Catholic Faith.

PART IV

The Catholic Revival

In the midst of the religious revolution of the sixteenth century, the Catholic Church had its own spiritual revival. Opposition to the Catholic Church during the sixteenth century was both so strong and damaging that its steady progress of reform is an indication that the Church was indeed guided by the Holy Spirit and not merely a human institution. Unfortunately, reform was delayed by war between the major Christian kings and the interference of secular rulers. Many Protestant reformers were afraid that a successful council might undermine their doctrinal changes, and they used their political and military influence to try to thwart Catholic revival. In spite of these difficulties, the Council of Trent would meet the challenge of the Protestant reformers and bring about a renewed spirit of Catholicism.

ADRIAN VI AND CLEMENT VII

The forerunner to the Catholic Reformation was Pope Adrian VI. The Dutch-born Adrian was the last non-Italian to be Pope before St. John Paul II. As bishop of Tortosa in Spain, Adrian became an associate of Cardinal Ximenes de Cisneros in the Spanish reform. He was a man of impeccable morals with deep piety and a strong penitential asceticism. As pope he attempted to bring the Spanish revival to Rome. He wanted to win back the Lutherans by force of good example and dialogue. He worked tirelessly to reform the Church but tragically died only one year after his election. Though little progress was made towards reform during his short pontificate, Adrian identified the major areas that needed a change for the better, and many of his recommendations would eventually be put into practice.

Adrian's successor was Clement VII, a man of strong intellectual ability, but indecisive in action. Clement wanted to reform the clergy and religious orders, while the Christian kingdoms were looking for a response to Lutheran challenges to Catholic doctrine. In his attempt to call a council for renewal of the Church, Clement found himself stuck between political infighting of Emperor Charles V and Francis I of France. These rulers wanted to dominate any council of the Church and refused to allow bishops to attend in areas out of their control. Wars between Charles and Francis continuously delayed attempts to call an ecumenical council. In addition to the Lutheran challenge, Clement also had to deal with Henry VIII's marital situation.

PAUL III AND CALLING OF THE COUNCIL OF TRENT

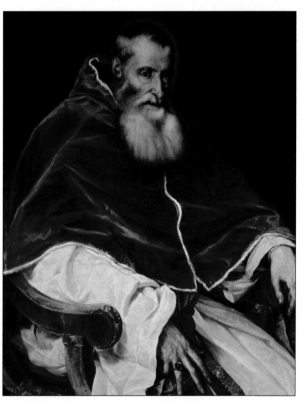

Many credit Pope Paul III with the official start of the Catholic revival.

Alessandro Farnese became Pope Paul III in 1534. Before his election he had been a Renaissance Cardinal who loved the arts and raucous parties. Farnese underwent a late spiritual conversion and was ordained to the priesthood at age 51. He immediately began to dedicate his life to reforming the Church. For this reason, many credit Paul III with the official start of the Catholic revival. Paul III appointed exemplary cardinals and bishops to study the problems needing to be addressed, approved the Jesuit order, and launched the Council of Trent.

Paul III took strong action to begin revitalizing the Church. He excommunicated Henry VIII in 1538 for his rebellious actions and placed England under interdict. He urged the Catholic princes of Germany to unite against their Lutheran counterparts and managed to convince Charles V and Francis I to call a ten-year truce. Capitalizing on the truce as an opportunity for a council, in 1537 he appointed Consilium de emendanda Ecclesia, a commission to study and report on needed Church reform. He chose for this commission Cardinals Gasparo Contarini as president, Gian Pietro Caraffa (the future Pope Paul IV), Jacopo Sadoleto, and Reginald Pole (almost elected pope in 1549); Archbishops Federigo Fregoso and Jerome Aleander; Bishop Gian Matteo Giberti; Abbot Gregorio Cortese; and Friar Tommaso Badia. (cf. Olin, Catholic Reform from Cardinal Ximenes to the Council of Trent, 1495-1563, 1994, p. 79) This commission established a blueprint for the upcoming Council of Trent.

There were many obstacles for Paul III in the calling of a general council. Many of his closest advisers were against a council, fearing an end to patronage and financial benefits of their positions that reform might bring. Lutheran reformers wanted acceptance of their theological positions in

POPULAR RELIGIONS IN 1560

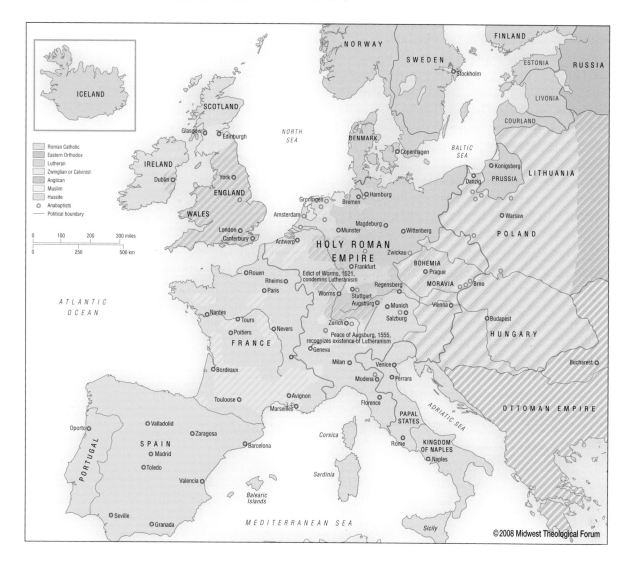

advance of a council. They wanted to be on equal footing with the bishops present and demanded that only the gospels be used in the deliberations and pronouncements. When it was clear they would not get their way, the Protestant League of Schmalkalden attempted to disrupt the council.

Secular rulers were also opposed to a council: Henry VIII had started his own church, Francis I did not want the French Church to lose its independence, and Charles V was afraid his subjects would react badly to a condemnation of Lutheranism. The secular princes wanted no dogmatic decrees discussed at the council and argued that only matters of discipline should be addressed. A compromise was established which agreed to have each session of the council deal with both doctrine and reform. Paul III summoned a council to meet in Mantua in 1537, but Francis I refused to allow any French Bishops to attend, and Charles V did not want the location in an Italian city outside his control. Consequently, when the Duke of Mantua could not guarantee the safety of the members, the council disbanded. It was finally agreed that the Italian city of Trent, a city under Charles V's jurisdiction, should host the council. However, war broke out again between Charles V and Francis I, and the council was delayed for another three years. Finally, on December 13, 1545, the Council of Trent opened its first session.

CHURCH'S TEACHING

Luther's theology broke away from the Church's teaching mainly in its deflated view of humanity. The Church teaches that no one can merit the initial grace of forgiveness and justification, this grace is granted by God at Baptism and the other sacraments. However, Catholics believe that "moved by the Holy Spirit and by charity, we can then merit for ourselves and others the graces needed for our sanctification, for the increase of grace and charity, and for the attainment of eternal life" (CCC 2010). Works are more than mere indicators of one's faith, but free actions inspired by faith through which grace is obtained, flowing from Christ's redemptive sacrifice.

Original sin does not leave man totally corrupt, as Luther believed, but rather wounds his nature. Human freedom, aided by grace, makes it possible for man to cooperate with God and to unite his personal good works to the merits of Christ, thereby meriting further grace. By Baptism Christians are incorporated into the Mystical Body of Christ whereby they become children of God the Father. Through this divine filiation, obtained through the goodness and mercy of God, they gain grace through good works, whereby they grow in sanctity and win graces for others as well.

The contents of the Bible is considered divine revelation and therefore the word of God. Nevertheless, it is the work of man in its composition and expression of the divinely inspired teaching. "'God chose certain men who, all the while he employed them in this task, made full use of their own faculties and powers so that, though he acted in them and by them, it was as true authors that they consigned to writing whatever he wanted written, and no more' (DV 11)" (CCC 106). Luther denied the role played by human cooperation in the transmission of divine revelation; this erroneous opinion lines up with his view of fallen humanity. The approval and explanation of Sacred Scripture is also intimately bound up with the early tradition of the Church: without the clarification of Sacred Tradition and the guiding light of the Church there would be confusion and uncertainty regarding the identification of inspired texts and its right interpretation. In summary, the traditions of the Church ultimately come from Christ through his Apostles and their successors (bishops) under the authority of the pope.

The Seven Sacraments were instituted over time by Christ as a means of salvation. Christ, who perfectly knew human nature, instituted the Sacraments to impart all the necessary graces for forgiveness, healing, conversion, and ultimately salvation. Due to Luther's attack on the Sacraments, the Council of Trent would elucidate on each Sacrament with a thorough theological explanation which would cogently and logically counteract all the erroneous ideas in circulation at the time.

Luther's original and chief criticism of the Church regarded the sale of indulgences. Indulgences concern the forgiveness of temporal punishment in Purgatory due to sins. Even after Penance, which forgives the guilt associated with sin, the penitent still needs to make reparation and undergo purification for sins committed. This can take the

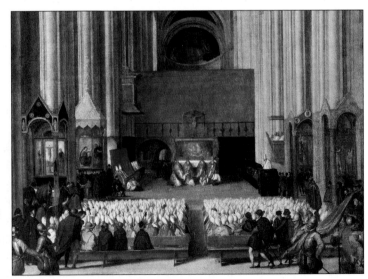

The Council of Trent turned out to be a detailed response to all the Protestant theological positions. Council sessions were held in the Trent's Romanesque cathedral and in the Church of Santa Maria Maggiore. Many of the reforms and doctrinal formulations worked out over twenty-five sessions remained the framework of Catholicism until the 1960s.

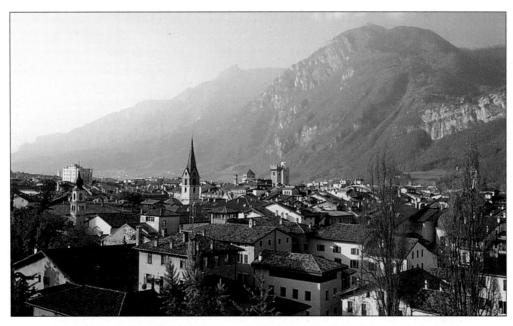

A view of Trento (Trent) from Castello del Buonconsiglio. In the background is the Monte Bondone. Trent, in English, Italian *Trento*, German *Trient*, Latin *Tridentum* (the Latin form is the source of the adjective *Tridentine*) is located in the Adige river valley in the Italian region of Trentino-Alto Adige. It is the capital of the region and of the autonomous province of Trento. Originally a Celtic city, Trent was later conquered by the Romans in the first Century BC In 1027, the Holy Roman Emperor Conrad II created the Prince, Bishop of Trent, who wielded both temporal and religious powers.

form of prayer, almsgiving, or corporal works of mercy. Indulgences are granted for certain good acts of piety or charitable actions. The Church teaches that through Christ's merits an individual can make reparation for sin and thereby cooperate with that grace through his willing efforts to please God. Therefore, the efficacy of indulgences comes from Christ's redemption applied to an individual who appeals to God's mercy expressed in devotions and good actions. The abuse of indulgences, which was prevalent during Luther's time, was to preach that a monetary sum could gain such release from temporal punishment without the proper interior dispositions of sorrow for sin and efforts to follow Christ. This abuse was corrected and condemned by the Church.

THE COUNCIL OF TRENT (1545-47): SESSIONS 1-10

The Council of Trent was in session at irregular intervals for eighteen years throughout three pontificates. When the first session of Trent convened, three papal cardinal legates directed the affairs of the council: Gian Maria del Monte, Marcello Cervinni, and Reginald Pole. Over sixty bishops and fifty other theologians met to discuss the reform agenda put forward by Paul III's Consilium of 1537. The secretary of the council, Angelo Massarelli, later Bishop of Telese, compiled a detailed diary of the events of the council. The council met in Particular Congregations where theologians and laymen discussed the topic of each session. Decisions of these Congregations would be sent to the General Congregation of Bishops for their review. Final promulgation of each topic occurred at the end of each session. All decisions were then sent to the pope for his final approval.

The first seven sessions of Trent addressed a number of doctrinal issues. The first topic dealt with the question of Sacred Scripture. Two decrees came out of the fourth session, which declared that in matters of Faith and morals, the Tradition of the Church together with the Bible is the source of Catholic belief. This session also indicated that the Latin Vulgate (originally translated into Latin by St. Jerome) was the authoritative text for Sacred Scripture and the books contained therein was the complete canonical list, though nothing was decided concerning translation of the Bible into vernacular languages.

Original sin was the second topic discussed at Trent: its nature, consequences, and its remission through Baptism. The council discredited the notion that original sin destroyed human freedom and man's ability to cooperate with grace. This led the council to begin the discussion brought up by Luther on the topic of justification. Perhaps the most divisive topic among the Germanic princes of the North, the council nevertheless took up this stormy debate with sessions of sixty-one general congregations and forty-four particular congregations. Though it is true that Christ justifies and restores each person's relationship to God the Father by his death on the Cross, the council declared that Baptism makes people "sons of God" who can freely choose to cooperate with God's salvific mission. Although Faith is a gratuitous gift, good works guided by faith are necessary for salvation.

During these sessions the council also took up the topic of the Sacraments in general and identified those seven which were instituted by Christ. They then proceeded to examine each of the Sacraments in turn. Baptism and Confirmation were the first discussed in detail by the council.

In matters of reform, the council candidly addressed abuses of clerical benefices and the need to provide better training for the clergy. Pluralism, i.e., having charge over more than one diocese, was strictly forbidden, and strict laws were devised for the appointment of bishops and the awarding of benefices.

Before the seventh session was complete, war broke out between the Emperor and the Protestant League of Schmalkalden. Plague also killed many in Trent, including the general of the Franciscan order. The cardinal legates proposed in the eighth session of Trent to move the council to Bologna for protection from war and disease. Though Paul III had not ordered the move, both Francis I and Charles V were outraged by the relocation. Due to the political interference of the secular princes, nothing further was accomplished during the ninth and tenth sessions. The council itself was temporarily closed with the death of Paul III on November 10, 1549.

THE COUNCIL OF TRENT (1551-1553): SESSIONS 11-16 UNDER JULIUS III

Paul III's successor was the first cardinal legate of the council, Giovanni del Monte, who took the name Julius III. Though fearful of the growing power of the Emperor Charles V, Julius pushed for the re-opening of the council in Trent in May 1551. The council continued to undertake a detailed discussion of each of the Seven Sacraments. During sessions thirteen and fourteen, the congregations outlined the doctrines of the Eucharist, Penance, and Anointing of the Sick. In addition to these doctrinal issues, the council continued its reform with further discussion on discipline of clergy regarding benefices and jurisdictional questions and supervision of bishops.

A delegation of Protestant theologians arrived in Trent demanding participation in the council. The first demand of this party was to throw out the work of the preceding sessions of the council and begin anew. They again set before the council the demand that their theological arguments be accepted as the starting point of discussion and that the subordination of the pope to the council be defined. The fifteenth session of the council began to honor the requests of the Protestants by postponing the consideration of any further issues. The appearance of the League of Schmalkalden, however, placed Trent and the members of the council in danger. Subsequently, the council was again forced to close temporarily.

PAUL IV

After the death of Julius III in 1555 and the short-lived pontificate of Marcellus II, the papacy fell to the austere reformer Cardinal Carafa who took the name Paul IV. This 80-year-old pope had been a co-founder of the Theatine order and sought to bring about internal reform throughout the Roman Curia rather than continue with the council. Paul IV was an ascetical and pious man who zealously sought to free the Church from imperial control. He recreated the inquisition in Rome to root out heresy and demanded that members of the Roman Curia give up their materialistic lifestyle. Those who refused to give up pluralistic benefices were severely disciplined. He ended the practice of collecting payment for many clerical appointments, cutting papal revenues and making it less financially lucrative to seek such appointment. He tried to stop Spanish political influence in Rome, but was soundly defeated by the armies of the new Spanish king Philip II. Paul IV also refused to recognize the elevation of Elizabeth I as Queen of England due to her illegitimacy. Although many historians have criticized Paul IV's rigid reform, his actions helped to restore the Papacy to its spiritual mission.

THE COUNCIL OF TRENT (1562-1563): SESSIONS 17-25 UNDER PIUS IV

The final stage of the Council of Trent took place with the elevation of Pius IV in 1559. The major adversaries of the council were gone: Charles V had abdicated his throne in 1557, dividing his empire between his son Philip II of Spain and his brother Ferdinand of Germany. Charles then entered a monastery to live out the last years of his life. Francis I of France had died. The council re-convened in 1562, and there were nine sessions in three months. These sessions finished the discussion of the remaining sacraments with declarations on the Sacrifice of the Mass, Holy Orders, and Matrimony. The council also covered the topics of veneration of saints and relics and more clearly defined the true nature of indulgences. Probably the greatest reform was accomplished during these sessions. The council established the seminary system for the education of the clergy, directly attacking the problem of ignorance among parish priests. The seminaries established liturgical guidelines insuring

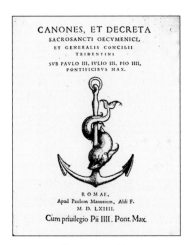

The title page of the
Council of Trent Canons.

adequate priestly guidance and uniform practice of the Faith among the Christian faithful. A list of forbidden books was established as well as the authorization to publish a new catechism for the faithful. To help curb episcopal abuses, bishops were not permitted to be away from their diocese for more than three months, and they were urged to visit all their Churches and care for the clergy and people.

The Council of Trent turned out to be a detailed response to all the Protestant theological positions. Each dogmatic decree included a canon anathematizing (denouncing as accursed) those who deny the doctrine in question. The contents filled fourteen volumes addressing the major concerns brought by the Protestants regarding justification, grace, Sacred Scripture, original sin, and the Seven Sacraments. The reform that began in Rome would work its way down to the laity. All bishops were required to faithfully bind themselves to uphold the conciliar decrees.

APPLICATION OF THE TRIDENTINE REFORM

The conclusion of the Council of Trent did not bring about immediate reforms. Many secular princes refused to accept the council's statements and would not allow the publication of its decrees. It was only through the personal example and dedicated holiness of a number of particular individuals that the fruits of Trent were bought forth.

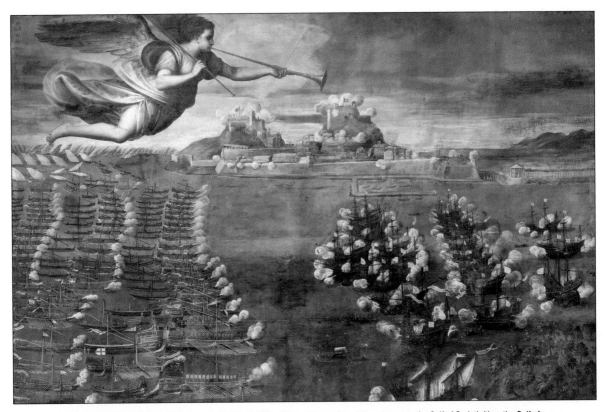

The naval Battle of Lepanto took place on October 7, 1571, at the northern edge of the entrance to the Gulf of Corinth (then the Gulf of Lepanto), off western Greece. A galley fleet of the Holy League, a coalition of St. Pius V, Spain, Venice, Genoa, Savoy, Naples, the Knights of Malta and others, defeated a force of 230 Ottoman galleys and 60 galliots. The Holy League fleet consisted of 206 galleys and 6 galleasses, and was ably commanded by Don Juan of Austria. The League suffered 9,000 casualties and lost 12 ships; the Ottomans suffered 30,000 casualties and lost 240 ships. The famous Spanish author Cervantes was wounded in this battle and lost the use of his left hand.

ST. PIUS V

Michele Ghislieri was elected Pope Pius V in January 1566. A Dominican monk, St. Pius spread the religious reform of Trent throughout Christendom by living in a monastic cell as pope. He fasted, did penance, and passed long hours of the night in meditation and prayer. Despite the heavy labors and anxieties of his office, his piety did not diminish. He abolished lavish feasts and the use of fancy carriages by cardinals. He visited churches barefoot and cared for the poor and sick of Rome. An English nobleman was converted to the Faith upon seeing this holy man kiss the feet of a beggar who was covered in ulcerous sores. In his bull, In cœna Domini, St. Pius V strove for the independence of the Church and of churchmen everywhere against dominance by secular powers. He fought German Emperor Maximilian II's attempt to abolish celibacy among the clergy, excommunicated Elizabeth I for her imprisonment of Mary Stuart and her attacks upon the Catholic faithful in England, and helped stem the tide of the Turkish threat from the East.

THE TURKISH THREAT AND THE BATTLE OF LEPANTO

By the late 1560s, the Turks were reaching the height of their power. Under the leadership of Suleiman the Magnificent, the Turkish fleet controlled the Mediterranean. In 1521 Belgrade fell, and the following year the Knights Hospitalers were driven from the Island of Rhodes. Hungary fell to Turkish forces in 1526, and Vienna itself was placed under siege in 1529. At sea, Tripoli became the harbor of Corsair raiding ships that struck at Sicily and Southern Italy.

St. Pius V had concerns that Turkish armies could overwhelm the Austrians in Vienna or that a Turkish fleet amassing in Greece could invade any part of Europe. He worked tirelessly to form a league of Christian princes to stop the Turkish menace. In 1565 this threat seemed about to be realized when the Island of Malta, a very strategic center of the Mediterranean, was attacked by 30,000 Turkish soldiers. The Knights Hospitalers with only 600 knights and 8000 men outlasted a summer-long siege and nearly total annihilation before the Turkish force withdrew. St. Pius feared that the Turkish fleet in the Gulf of Patros near Greece would bring Europe to its knees within the year. To offset this imminent danger St. Pius financed a Christian fleet to be led by Don Juan of Austria, the illegitimate son of Charles V, the former Holy Roman emperor.

The Christian League was beset by internal rivalry. The largest fleets of Europe were held by Venice and Spain, but Venice attempted diplomacy with the Turks in the hope of maintaining its large trading empire in the East. They were loath to aid in a war that could bring them financial ruin. The Spanish fleet was expensive to maintain, and Philip II was not eager to risk his entire fleet in a single engagement.

The turning point came when Turkish forces attacked Famagusta on Cyprus where the Venetians had established a diplomatic enclave. The Turks had previously guaranteed security for the Venetians, but during the attack, the entire Venetian delegation was murdered. This drove the Venetians into the Christian League against the Turks, and the Spanish fleet agreed to join the coalition if the young Spaniard Don Juan of Austria would lead it.

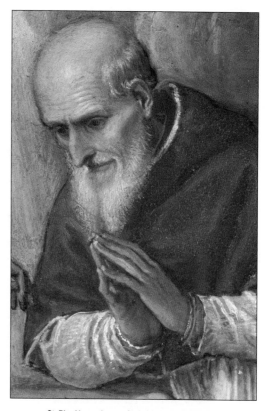

St. Pius V urged every Christian to prepare for the naval battle at Lepanto by reciting the Rosary.

St. Pius V was dedicated to implementing the decisions of the Council of Trent. He was canonized in 1712 by Clement XI.

With the alliance strengthened and the attack approaching, St. Pius V urged every Christian to prepare for the naval offensive by praying the Rosary. On October 7, 1571, the Christian fleet met the Turkish fleet at Lepanto. Owing to superiority in gun power and a sudden shift in the wind, the Christian fleet defeated the larger Turkish force. The Turkish fleet was broken, and the Christian powers were freed from the fear of the Mediterranean becoming a "Muslim lake." In thanksgiving for this victory in the crucial Battle of Lepanto, St. Pius V added "Help of Christians," to the Litany of Loreto. Mary's assistance is remembered on every October 7, the Feast of Our Lady of the Rosary.

ST. CHARLES BORROMEO

St. Charles Borromeo was named a cardinal and made secretary of state under his uncle, Pope Pius IV, where he oversaw the final sessions of the Council of Trent. It was through his efforts that the successful completion of the Council of Trent was accomplished. St. Charles was one of those remarkably able men whose personal example managed to bring about effective reform. After the council, St. Charles was made Archbishop of Milan, one of the most important archdioceses outside of Rome and one that did not have a resident bishop for over eighty years. Milan was beset with all the problems of the contemporary age. Many of its clergy were ignorant or ill-equipped to fulfill

ST. PETER CANISIUS

For his work in successfully implementing the reforms of the Council of Trent in Germany and defending the Church against the spread of Protestantism, St. Peter Canisius is often called the "Second Apostle of Germany" (St. Boniface being the first—cf. chapter five). Born in 1521, St. Peter began his studies at the University of Cologne at the age of fifteen. In 1543, still only twenty-two, he went on a retreat directed by St. Peter Faber, a Jesuit and companion of St. Ignatius of Loyola, where he decided to enter the Society of Jesus. St. Peter founded the first Jesuit house in Germany, and for fourteen years served as the first Jesuit provincial to that country.

Attending a session of the Council of Trent in 1547, St. Peter Canisius became deeply involved in the debates and issues surrounding the reform of the Church. In 1549, at the request of the Pope, he was entrusted with the nearly impossible task of stopping defections of Catholics in Germany and bringing back into the Church those who had already left. Realizing that one way to prevent the spread of Protestantism was through the teaching of proper Catholic doctrine, he helped develop or establish colleges at Ingolstadt, Vienna, Prague, Munich, Innsbruck, Dillingen, Tyrnau, Hall-in-Tyrol, and other places in the Protestant North of Germany.

In 1555 St. Peter Canisius introduced what is considered his most lasting contribution. In response to the Reformation, many German Catholics left the faith out of ignorance of the teachings of their own Church. To respond to the problem, Canisius was asked to write a Catholic Catechism that offered a clear and readable exposition of Catholic doctrine. St. Peter Canisius ended up writing three Catechisms: one for children, one for students, and one for adults. The impact of his work was immediate. These immensely popular Catechisms were translated into fifteen languages and used for centuries.

In 1925 Pope Pius XI canonized St. Peter Canisius and named him a Doctor of the Church. His feast day is celebrated on December 21.

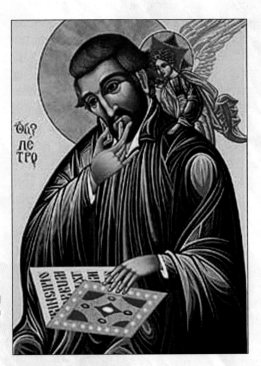

In 1925 Pope Pius XI canonized St. Peter Canisius and named him a Doctor of the Church.

their pastoral duties. It naturally followed that due to a weak clergy, the laity were deprived of the guidance and direction to lead good Christian lives. This weakened faith among both priests and laity created an ideal situation for heresy and immorality.

To accomplish this great reform, St. Charles set about reorganizing his archdiocese. During his tenure as archbishop, he held a series of provincial councils and diocesan synods to implement the terms of Trent. He established three seminaries for training clergy and required annual retreats for all clerics. His reforms were published in Acts of the Church of Milan, which became a pattern for reform throughout Europe. St. Charles Borromeo regularly made visits to his parishes and brought to his aid the services of other reforming orders such as the Barnabites and Jesuits. St. Charles founded the Confraternity of Christian Doctrine with 2,000 teachers to instruct the children of Milan in over 740 schools.

Resistance to reform in Milan was strong. Agents of the secular powers sought to block his authority, and some religious communities attempted to block his entry. Someone even attempted to assassinate this zealous reformer. In the summer of 1578, plague raged throughout Milan and most of the important dignitaries left the city. Throughout the epidemic, St. Charles

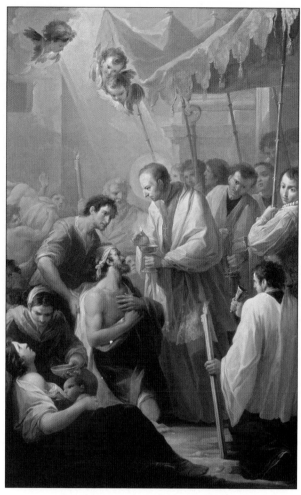

St. Charles Borromeo personally attended to plague victims in Milan in 1578.

continued his work in the city and personally helped to provide food for the poor and care for the sick and dying. Personal example and strong determination helped bring about an exemplary archdiocese in Milan, showing that the Tridentine reforms could be put into practice.

REFORMING THE ORDERS: STS. PHILIP NERI AND TERESA OF AVILA

Equally important to post-Tridentine reform was the need to revive the old religious orders. The renewed spiritual example of monks and friars would help influence the reform of diocesan clergy and lay faithful. This reform especially prompted monastic orders to return to their original spirit expressed in a serious practice of prayer and penance and a strict observation of the evangelical counsels through vows of poverty, chastity, and obedience. The Council of Trent provided invaluable support for the renewal of the older orders and the establishment of new "regular" orders created to serve the Church in its task of reform.

Sometimes referred to as the "Reformer of Rome," St. Philip of Neri helped to bring back a spirit of piety to the Eternal City. St. Philip founded the Oratorians, a congregation of secular priests who dedicated themselves to the spiritual formation and support of the clergy. For forty years St. Philip helped restore Rome as the central city of Catholicism. In 1559 one of the first Protestant works on

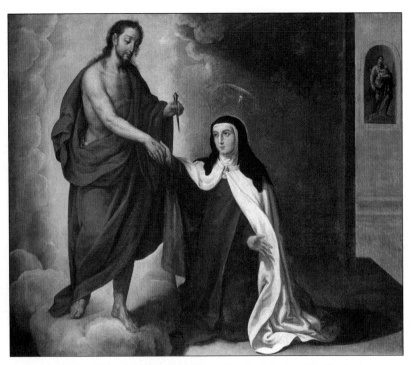

The Spanish mystic St. Teresa of Avila is one of four female Doctors of the Church.

the history of the Church appeared. Entitled The Centuries, this book attempted to discredit the Church hierarchy and attack the authority of the pope. St. Philip appointed the Venerable Cardinal Baronius to write a suitable response, and Baronius published his Annales Ecclesiastici in twelve volumes in response to The Centuries. His work became a pioneer in historical criticism and easily eclipsed its Protestant counterpart. His feast day is celebrated on May 26.

A spiritual resurgence took place in the wake of the Tridentine reforms. In place of the pessimistic outlook toward the unworthiness of man, the denial of free will, and the futility of good deeds, there came about an optimistic spirit that placed trust in the goodness of human nature and in the beauty of the human soul. One of the great representatives of this movement was the Spanish mystic St. Teresa of Avila. As a young Carmelite nun, St. Teresa's early life was wracked with serious illnesses and suffered from failed medical treatment that reduced her health to a pitiful state. Through her sufferings, St. Teresa began the practice of mental prayer (meditation) and became immersed in God. She was granted a series of ecstasies from God and gained a great reputation among those around her. Believing God wanted her to found a convent of perpetual prayer, she established the Discalced Carmelites. Within her lifetime she founded sixteen houses for her new order. St. Teresa wrote magnificent treatises on the interior life that have become part of the patrimony of the Church's spirituality, including *The Way of Perfection*, *Foundations*, and *Life* (her autobiography). Pope Paul VI proclaimed her a Doctor of the Church in 1970; St. Teresa of Avila – along with Sts. Catherine of Siena, Therese of Lisieux, and Hildegard of Bingen – is one of four female Doctors of the Church. St. Teresa of Avila's feast day is celebrated on October 15.

ST. IGNATIUS OF LOYOLA AND THE SOCIETY OF JESUS

Probably the most significant of the new orders brought about to help realize Tridentine reform involved the Society of Jesus founded by St. Ignatius of Loyola. In 1491, St. Ignatius was born in a castle in Loyola, Spain, and he trained from boyhood to be a knight. He served at court where he lived the worldly life of a typical young nobleman. In 1517 he was transferred to Pamplona. When war broke out between Charles V and Francis I in 1521, St. Ignatius led the defense of the fortress at Pamplona where he was seriously injured in both legs. His captors, much impressed by his courage, attempted to dress his wounds and set his bones. During his return to his castle in Loyola, it was apparent that a second operation would be necessary. In order to save his leg, the surgeons attempted to saw off part of the bone that protruded. This operation left St. Ignatius permanently crippled and it ended his military career.

During his convalescence, St. Ignatius read all the romantic books and books of chivalry he could find. After finishing all those, he grudgingly read the remaining two books: one on the life of Christ and the other on the lives of the saints. These last two books had a profound effect on St. Ignatius and led to his conversion. His injuries left him unable to be a soldier for the king, so he sought to be a soldier for Christ.

After spending the night dressed in military regalia praying before an image of Mary, St. Ignatius set out to the shrine of Our Lady of Montserrat. At the shrine he made a general confession, laid his sword and dagger at the feet of Mary, and exchanged clothes with a poor beggar. He proceeded to spend a year in the seclusion of a cave called Manresa, near the town of Cataluña. For an entire year, he knelt everyday for seven hours at a time, completely absorbed in prayer. He hardly ate and eventually became very sick. Despite his physical discomfort, during his year in seclusion, St. Ignatius realized that God had called him for a special task. He was inspired to write *Spiritual Exercises*, a guide for spiritual perfection meant to help the believer learn to emulate Christ.

St. Ignatius left his sanctuary to study at the University of Alcala in Barcelona and eventually went to study at Paris. Already forty, St. Ignatius was unimpressive in appearance. He had a severe limp, was a poor speaker, and was not especially brilliant. He did, however, have a high capacity for work and a serene and self-controlled temperament. His spiritual example alone began to attract a number of followers. On August 15, 1524, St. Ignatius gathered seven companions from the Sorbonne to climb a mountain, on top of which, in a small Benedictine chapel, they made a vow of poverty and selfless service to others. St. Ignatius of Loyola's feast day is celebrated on July 31.

Pope Paul III approved this new order founded by St. Ignatius – known as the Society of Jesus or Jesuits – with the bull Regimini militantis Ecclesiae. St. Ignatius of Loyola's Spiritual Exercises was written for the Jesuits, who were growing in number, as a response to the rising militancy of Protestantism and Calvin's Institutes. The new Jesuit order added a vow of obedience to the pope himself to the traditional vows of poverty, chastity, and obedience. The order became characterized by militaristic discipline and total availability to the service of the Church and the poor. Wherever the pope sent them, they would go.

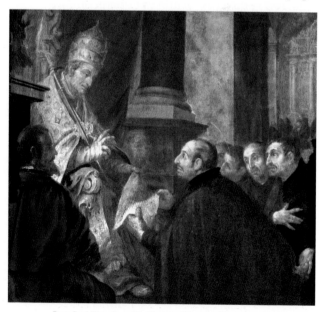

Jesuits soon became involved in every facet of the Church's ministry. They served as nuncios, theologians, professors, and missionaries. They were sent all over the globe – especially to the wilderness of the Americas and Asia – to spread the Gospel. The Jesuits also suffered persecution in England and other Protestant countries. For the next four centuries, Jesuits stood out as exceptional servants to Christ, the Church, and the pope, leading the world as saints, martyrs, intellectuals, advisors and confessors.

Pope Paul III confirmed the Society of Jesus on September 27, 1540.

PART V
Spain and the Empire of Philip II
THE CRUSADE OF CATHOLIC SPAIN

Philip II was an ardent Catholic, and the Catholic Faith permeated every facet of Philip's life. He was a grave and somber man known for working tirelessly for 12 hours at a time. He spent hours in prayer, frequently confessed his sins, had the Blessed Sacrament close to his room, and only read works on spirituality. His palace, the cold and austere El Escorial, was built as a reflection of his personality. His private room in the massive palace complex, for example, was as simple as a monk's cell.

Philip II sought to root out heresy and rebellion throughout his realm and provide a good centralized government to all his provinces. Absolutism seemed to work in Spain, and Philip attempted to impose this same rigorous form of rule in all the territories under his control. Spanish governors were sent out to enforce the will of the king, who issued thousands of orders throughout the world from his small cell.

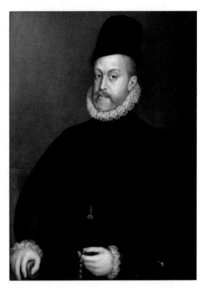

An ardent Catholic, Philip II worked tirelessly for twelve hours at a time. He spent hours in prayer and frequently confessed his sins. His private room in his palace, El Escorial, was as simple as a monk's cell.

Early in Philip's reign, the *Moriscos*, descendants of the Islamic conquerors of the Spanish kingdom of Granada, rebelled against his rule. The *Moriscos* were in close communication with Turkish agents who were trying to prepare for a Turkish assault on Spain. The Austrian Don Juan, the half brother of Philip, was sent to remove this danger and transplant all of the *Moriscos* to the interior of Spain where communication with the Turks was near impossible. The Turks would continue to threaten Spain until they were defeated at the great Battle of Lepanto in 1571.

THE REVOLT OF THE LOW COUNTRIES

The seventeen provinces making up the Low Countries included some of the richest and most populous regions in Europe. It was a cosmopolitan area made up of Dutch in the north, Flemish in the center, and Walloons (Francophones) in the south. An industrious people, they had a thriving

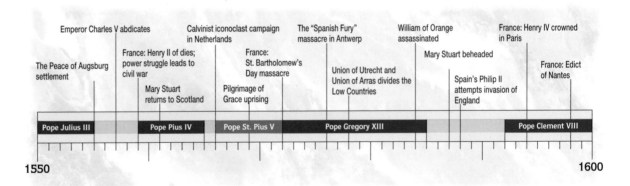

Emperor Charles V abdicates

Calvinist iconoclast campaign in Netherlands

The "Spanish Fury" massacre in Antwerp

William of Orange assassinated

France: Henry IV crowned in Paris

The Peace of Augsburg settlement

France: Henry II of dies; power struggle leads to civil war

France: St. Bartholomew's Day massacre

Mary Stuart beheaded

France: Edict of Nantes

Mary Stuart returns to Scotland

Pilgrimage of Grace uprising

Union of Utrecht and Union of Arras divides the Low Countries

Spain's Philip II attempts invasion of England

Pope Julius III | Pope Pius IV | Pope St. Pius V | Pope Gregory XIII | Pope Clement VIII

1550 — 1600

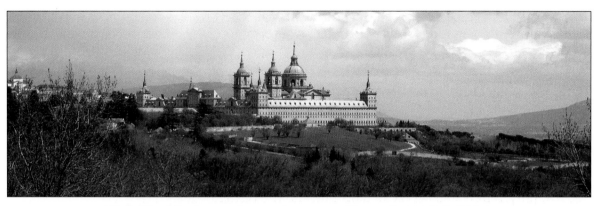

Philip II's El Escorial is an immense palace, monastery, museum, and library complex located in Madrid, Spain.

agricultural and commercial economy and were ruggedly independent. Few countries, it was said, were so well governed, and none was richer. The city of Antwerp was a commercial metropolis; everyday a fleet of 500 seafaring vessels would enter and leave its port.

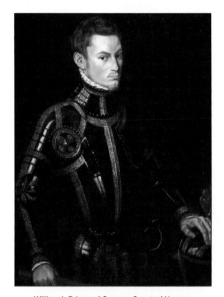

William I, Prince of Orange, Count of Nassau (1533-1584), was the main leader of the Dutch revolt against the Spanish. In the Netherlands, he is also known as the *Vader des vaderlands*, "Father of the Fatherland." The Dutch national anthem, the *Wilhelmus*, was written in his honor.

Each province in the Low Countries was a state unto itself, and each had its own legislature and local customs. A central government, or Estates General, was located in Brussels and was led by the traditional local prince known as the "Stadtholder" who led the provinces in times of trouble. Otherwise, business and politics were carried out locally and independently.

The House of Burgundy reigned over the territory of the Netherlands since the preceding century, and with Charles V's ascent, it became part of his greater empire. Charles V was, in fact, born in the Low Countries and spoke Flemish from birth. As a ruler, he respected the unwritten constitution of the provinces (known as the Joyeuse Entrée), and gave lucrative government positions to the local nobles. Because of his fair and evenhanded treatment of the Low Countries, Charles and Catholic Spain were popular. When Protestantism crept into the area, it took hold of only a minority of the population. But as the region's weaving industry opened itself to trade with England and Bohemia, Calvinism and Anabaptism began to appear. French Calvinists also arrived in the Low Countries

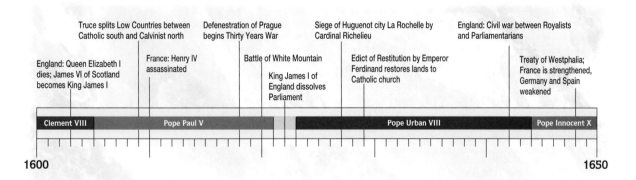

Truce splits Low Countries between Catholic south and Calvinist north

Defenestration of Prague begins Thirty Years War

Siege of Huguenot city La Rochelle by Cardinal Richelieu

England: Civil war between Royalists and Parliamentarians

England: Queen Elizabeth I dies; James VI of Scotland becomes King James I

France: Henry IV assassinated

Battle of White Mountain

King James I of England dissolves Parliament

Edict of Restitution by Emperor Ferdinand restores lands to Catholic church

Treaty of Westphalia; France is strengthened, Germany and Spain weakened

| Clement VIII | Pope Paul V | Pope Urban VIII | Pope Innocent X |

1600

1650

fleeing violence in France. Although Charles V had passed certain laws against heresy, he did not largely enforce them, still respecting the tradition of toleration. When Philip ascended the throne, that policy changed. He quickly sent Spanish governors to enforce his own jurisdiction over the Low Countries – a move that pushed the local rulers to revolt.

The revolt against Philip II in the Low Countries had both political and religious dimensions. Politically the nobility of the Low Countries became resentful that Spanish governors were sent to rule their land. At first, when Philip's regent, Margaret of Parma, was sent to the region, she tried to rule with a moderate hand. But her efforts were frustrated by the presence of 3000 Spanish troops sent by the king to protect the southern frontier with France. The arrival of the Spanish dashed the local nobility's hopes for gaining privileged and lucrative positions in Philip's government. Furthermore, the high cost of maintaining these foreigners' lavish lifestyles intensely embittered the Dutch.

Philip also tried to implement religious reforms that were spelled out by the Council of Trent. Prior to Philip's rule, the heavily populated Low Countries had only three dioceses, which were governed by foreign bishops. Pope Paul IV attempted to apply the Tridentine Reforms by restructuring the current dioceses and adding fourteen more. This redistribution of authority from the older system took power away from local nobles and abbots. Adding to the discontent, rumors began to spread that the inquisition was going to be brought into the Low Countries.

Two local princes, William of Orange and the Count of Egmont, protested the presence of Spanish troops in the region and asked Philip to moderate his program for religious reform. At their request, Philip did remove some Spanish soldiers, but the king refused to alter his position on doctrinal uniformity.

Conflict between Spain and the Low Countries erupted when small Calvinist groups launched an iconoclastic campaign across the countryside in late August 1566. Over 1000 churches and monasteries, including the cathedral of Antwerp, were plundered over a two-week period. Manuscripts, paintings, and statues were destroyed; gold chalices were stolen and tabernacles desecrated. At first, public opinion condemned the outrage and sided with the government. Philip mishandled the situation and lost any good will he might have gained. Rather than skillfully capitalizing on this turn of events to win back those who were shocked by the violence of the Calvinists, he looked upon all his subjects in the Low Countries as equally guilty. His regent, Margaret of Parma, was beginning to win favor among the people, but instead of supporting her efforts to handle the rebellion locally, Philip swore by his father's soul to make an example of the rebels. He condemned the people of the Low Countries for the atrocities, and against the advice of the regent and in spite of the pope's exhortation to clemency, he sent a Spanish army led by the Duke of Alba to restore order.

THE COUNCIL OF TROUBLES AND WILLIAM OF ORANGE

Alba was a superior general, but not a gifted statesman. Under his governance, Spanish soldiers began a system of merciless repression; blood flowed freely, and all the traditional rights of the people were discarded. The dissident Stadtholder William of Orange fled into exile

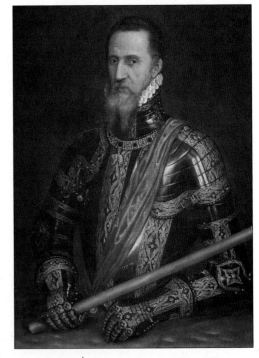

Fernando Álvarez de Toledo, the third Duke of Alba (or Alva) (1508-1583), was nicknamed "the Iron Duke" by Protestants of the Low Countries because of his harshness. His cruelty united the Dutch against the Spanish.

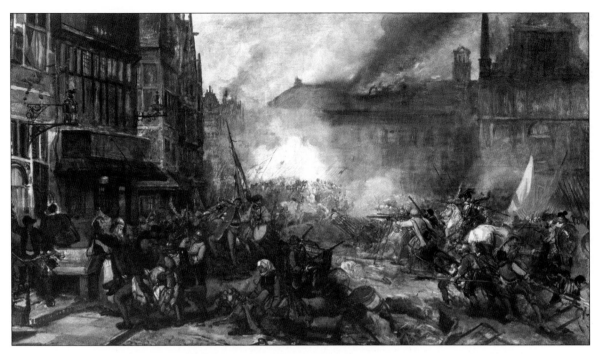

The Spanish Fury. On November 4,1576, Spanish troops began the sack of Antwerp, three days of horror among the Flemish population. The Spanish soldiers, tired of fighting the Dutch without rest and without payment from Philip II, decided to take their "salary" from the population of Antwerp. The mutinous troops destroyed six hundred houses and killed over six thousand people.

while the Catholic nobleman, Count of Egmont, remained to deal with the Spanish assault. Without trial, the Duke of Alba executed the Count of Egmont, and sentenced thousands to death. The land of the aristocracy was confiscated, and the Duke of Alba levied heavy taxes to finance his military campaign. His policies consequently brought trade to a virtual standstill throughout the Low Countries, and general public outrage united peasants and nobles alike against the Spanish.

In exile, William of Orange tried to use his position as Stadtholder to gain support and muster a military force against the Spanish invasion. To generate strong opposition to Spain, William wielded religion as a political mechanism. He was a Catholic in the court of Philip II, but a Lutheran when dealing with the German princes whom he hoped would aid him against the Spanish. When Calvinism emerged as the prominent religious denomination among the Dutch, he in turn adopted their creed.

Encouraged by local support, William and his brother invaded the Low Countries with an army of German mercenaries, but was quickly driven back by the Spanish soldiers. The Duke of Alba pompously thought he secured victory, and he had a statue of himself erected in the city of Antwerp. News soon reached the general of a rebel fleet attacking the port of Den Briel and rebel forces advancing against a number of other cities. The war was far from over.

DIVISION OF THE LOW COUNTRIES

William of Orange strove to unite the Low Countries against the Spanish, and Protestant minorities flocked to him. Because of the Spanish repression, leading Catholic lords also joined William's camp. By 1576, whatever Catholic support remained in the Low Countries was destroyed after the Spanish army mutinied. The army had not received pay, and they rebelled against their commanders and unleashed terrible violence. Known as the "Spanish Fury," soldiers pillaged the country and killed over six thousand people. Any resistance to William dissolved. The Estates General signed the

THE REVOLT OF THE LOW COUNTRIES AGAINST SPAIN, 1559-1592

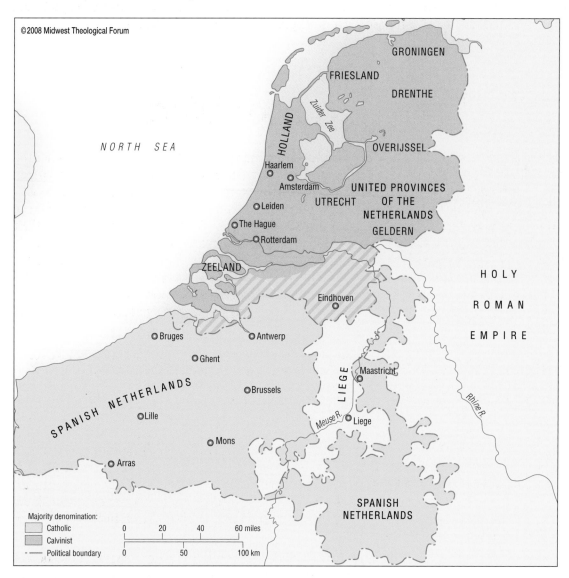

©2008 Midwest Theological Forum

Majority denomination:
Catholic
Calvinist
--- Political boundary

0   20   40   60 miles
0   50   100 km

Pacification of Ghent in November of that year, granting toleration of worship and placing authority of the provinces under the Calvinist regions of Holland and Zeeland. Practicing the Catholic religion was no longer allowed in the North, and the southern provinces were becoming Protestant.

Philip II, realizing that the Duke of Alba had failed to subdue the Low Countries, recalled the governor to Spain. In his place, Philip sent the victor of Lepanto, Don Juan of Austria. Don Juan realized that William of Orange was playing upon the fear of the provinces, and so he accepted the Pacification of Ghent and sought to win back the Low Countries to Spain. After a series of military victories, it appeared that Don Juan was on the verge of defeating the Protestant forces and re-uniting the provinces. However, an illness took his life in 1578. Another great general and diplomat replaced Don Juan: the son of Margaret of Parma, Alessandro Farnese. This Prince of Parma broke up the unity of the seventeen provinces by promising a return to their original liberties enjoyed before the fighting. Catholics who had become fearful of William of Orange's growing power were drawn back to the Spanish throne. William, whose ambitions were thwarted by this reversal of Dutch sentiment, united the seven Northern provinces in an alliance called the Union of Utrecht. This union declared their independence from Spain, and re-organized as the United Provinces of the Netherlands or the Dutch Republic. In 1578, the ten southern provinces that remained loyal to the Spanish crown formed the Union of Arras or the Spanish Netherlands (Belgium).

PART VI

The Huguenot Wars

France was the most populous and powerful of all the European kingdoms. It was three times the size of England and five times as populated. Like Germany, the kingdom of France was made up of some three hundred areas with their own legal systems and specific liberties. Traditionally the nobles of these regions wielded strong influence. As the public began to seek relief from these powerful lords, they supported the rising tide of the French kings. Seeking to defend their power, more than a third, and possibly half of the nobility in France turned to Protestantism in the 1560s and 1570s. Many regions defied the local bishop and adopted Protestant services. Unlike Anglicanism in England and Lutheranism in Germany, Calvinism was a pretext used by the nobles against the monarchy in France, and thus both Francis I and Henry II opposed its spread. After the death of Henry II in 1559, the stage was set for a confrontation among the various nobles over the control of France.

THREE FACTIONS: GUISE, HUGUENOT, AND *POLITIQUE*

After the death of Henry II, France was split between three major groups. The House of Guise was an ardent Catholic faction that was led by the Dukes and Cardinals of Lorraine. The Guise family had aided Francis I in his many wars against Charles V and had become very influential in directing the affairs of France. As descendants of Charlemagne, the Guise family also had a distant claim to the French throne. Adding to their power and prestige, Mary of Guise was Queen of Scotland, and her daughter Mary Stuart was once Queen of France and heir to the English Throne. The Guise family made an aggressive bid for the throne and pressed their political and hereditary advantage during the ensuing conflicts to such an extent that it tarnished their prior reputation as Catholic reformers.

The Huguenot faction was led by the Prince of Conde and the Admiral de Coligny. These nobles sought to undermine the authority of the Guise family and fought for local liberties in religious worship. They were opposed to Spanish influence in France and hoped to convince the kings of France to support the Protestants in the Low Countries against Philip II. Being part of the professional warrior class, the Huguenot nobles aggressively waged war to press their demands. No less than nine civil wars were fought in the concluding four decades of the sixteenth century.

Between the Catholic and Huguenot sectors were the politiques. This group had no strong religious ties, but used the political situation to further their own ambitions. The most famous of these politiques was the Queen mother of France, Catherine de Medici. Her three young sons, the future Francis II, Charles IX and Henry III, would be little more than puppets of the queen mother. Lacking any real religious conviction, Catherine de Medici tried to play the Catholics and Protestants off each other to maintain her own power. Eventually her intrigues would backfire and the throne would fall to the French Huguenot House of Navarre.

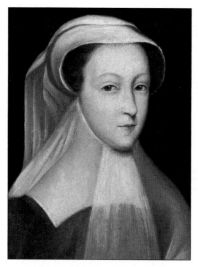

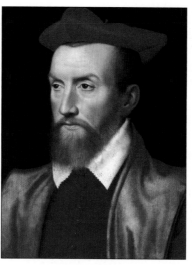

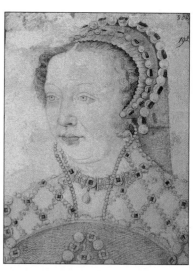

Mary Stuart, daughter of Mary of Guise, Queen of Scotland; widow of King Francis II of France; heir to the throne of England.

Huguenot leader Admiral Gaspard de Coligny of France was murdered during the St. Bartholomew's Day massacre.

Catherine de Medici, the Queen mother of France, an influential *politique*, the instigator of the St. Bartholomew's Day massacre.

FRANCIS II AND CHARLES IX

Francis II came to the throne at age fifteen after his father Henry II was killed in an accident during a tournament in 1559. Francis's uncles, Francis, Duke of Lorraine, and Charles, Cardinal of Lorraine, dominated the young king's reign, and their policies improved religious unity in France. This effort to maintain Catholicism as the only licit religion in France led to an ongoing persecution of various Huguenot factions, which helped sharply define the divisions between the Huguenot, Guise, and politique factions. Catherine de Medici remained powerless against the rise of the Guise family, who continued to strengthen their position in France. After an unsuccessful war against Spain, Catherine sent her daughter Elizabeth to wed the young king of Spain, Francis II, giving France a greater Catholic influence. Francis died of an ear infection after only two short years in power, leaving his ten-year-old brother Charles IX on the throne.

Now Catherine was able to use her regency of Charles to offset the influence of the Guise family over France. She supported further toleration of the Huguenots and named the Protestant Anthony of Bourbon lieutenant general of the kingdom. Catherine also blocked Mary Stuart's attempted marriage to Philip II's son, which she regarded as an excessive consolidation of Catholic power. Instead, Catherine tried to arrange a marriage between her son Charles and Elizabeth I of England. Catherine also worked to arrange another marriage, this one successfully, between her daughter Margaret and the Huguenot prince Henry of Navarre. Strengthening her ties with French Protestants seemed the best way to offset the power of the Catholic Guise Family. But just as she seemed to reach the pinnacle of her power, Catherine's scheming fell apart. In February 1563, Francis, Duke of Guise, was assassinated, and civil war broke out between the Catholics and the Huguenots, thrusting Catherine, Charles, and the crown in the middle of the "French Wars of Religion," a bloody power struggle that would last eighteen years.

THE ST. BARTHOLOMEW'S DAY MASSACRE

During the eighteen years of civil war, many attacks and brutalities were meted out by both Protestants and Catholics. Perhaps the worst atrocity was schemed by Catherine herself. The Huguenot Admiral Coligny was a very close advisor and friend of Catherine's son, King Charles. Fearing the influence

Admiral Coligny could have over her son, Catherine looked for a way to assassinate the admiral. At the time, many of the leading Huguenots were in Paris attending the marriage of Henry of Navarre to Catherine's daughter, Margaret. Seizing the opportunity, the queen mother spread rumors of a Protestant insurrection being planned in Paris during the wedding. Catholic supporters were outraged and they responded to the rumors by planning a preemptive counterattack.

On the night of St. Bartholomew's Feast Day (August 24) 1572, Catholics took to the streets, butchering Protestants. Catherine's menacing scheme was successful, as the Admiral Coligny was indeed killed. The admiral was first stabbed to death in his apartment, and then thrown out of the window into the garden, where he was beheaded and his body was burned. The admiral was not the only victim, as the same violent and brutal end met much of the Huguenot nobility that night. The estimated number of victims in Paris exceeded 2000, but violence spread to the surrounding regions, and victims from mob attacks over the next few weeks throughout all of France have been estimated between 2000 and 100,000 people. Huguenots, furious over the attacks, renewed the civil war, and both parties hired companies of mercenary soldiers that slaughtered each other and terrorized civilians. In the wake of the war, more than 20,000 Catholic churches in France were sacked, looted, and destroyed by Huguenot mobs. Thousands of priests and religious were also massacred.

THE WAR OF THE THREE HENRYS

Catherine's third son Henry became king after Charles died from tuberculosis in May 1574. King Henry III attempted to end the religious conflict by agreeing to concessions of toleration. This move led Henry of Guise to form the Catholic League, which demanded an end to toleration of Protestants. When Catherine's youngest son Francis died, thus making the Protestant Henry of Navarre heir to

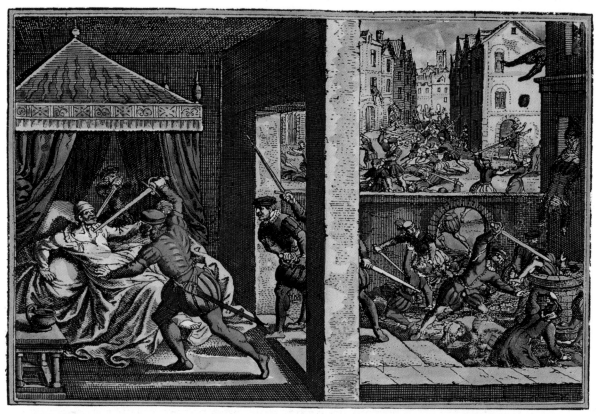

Admiral Coligny was murdered in his apartment on a bloody St. Bartholomew's Feast Day, August 24, 1572. The mob violence against the Protestants lasted for several months. This massacre stiffened Huguenot resistance and was a turning point in the French Wars of Religion.

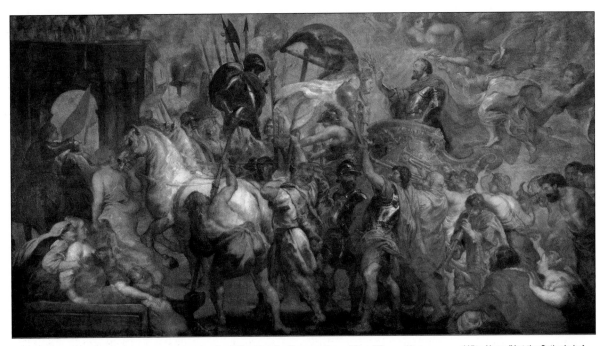

The reconverted Catholic Henry of Navarre rides triumphantly into Paris for his coronation as King of France. He was crowned King Henry IV at the Cathedral of Chartres on February 27, 1594. He was a popular king showing great care for the welfare of his subjects, as well as displaying an unusual religious tolerance for the time. He was murdered by a disturbed man, Ravaillac, on May 14, 1610. Henry IV is informally nicknamed *le bon roi Henri* ("good king Henry"). He had six children with Marie de Medici.

the French throne, the Catholic League forced Henry III to issue an edict suppressing Protestantism and excluding Henry of Navarre from the throne. Henry of Navarre resisted the measure, and civil war once again erupted between Henry III, Henry of Guise, and Henry of Navarre. Henry III allied himself with Henry of Navarre against the Catholic League and orchestrated the assassination of the head of the Guise family in 1589. Afterwards, Henry III was himself assassinated, which left only Henry of Navarre alive, and therefore victorious and king by default.

At first, the Catholics refused to recognize Henry of Navarre and sought Spanish aid to resist the Protestant king. This pressure, in addition to Henry of Navarre's fear that Philip II might use disunity in France to claim the throne for himself, convinced Henry that it was unwise to place his hopes in the Huguenot minority. Henry, therefore, reconverted to the Catholic Faith, justifying his conversion by saying infamously: "Paris is well worth a Mass." The phrase adequately reflected the less than pious attitude that was typical of the majority of rulers of Europe at that time. The new Catholic king was welcomed into Paris where he was crowned King Henry IV.

THE EDICT OF NANTES

After years of civil war, Henry understood well that religious tensions could destroy his tenuous hold on the throne. The Huguenots demanded positive guarantees protecting their religious liberties, and Henry responded by issuing the Edict of Nantes in 1598. The Edict allowed every noble who was also a landholder the right to hold Protestant services in the privacy of his own household. It also allowed legal practice of Protestantism in towns where the majority of the population was Protestant, excluding diocesan sees and towns in and around Paris. About a hundred towns were also granted the right to fortify themselves with Protestant garrisons under Protestant commanders. The Edict promised Protestants the same civil rights as Catholics and the same chances for public office and admittance into Catholic universities. By granting toleration to the Huguenots, Henry removed the main cause of conflict in France and helped the country recover from the long era of civil war.

CARDINAL RICHELIEU

In 1610, Henry IV was assassinated, leaving the throne to his very young son, Louis XIII. Too young to wield full power over France, the affairs of state fell into the hands of his secretary of state, Cardinal Richelieu. Richelieu worked tirelessly to centralize the government and advance the power of the monarchy by fostering religious unity and promoting anti-Hapsburg policies. He helped France recover financially from the civil wars by encouraging a mercantile economic system that included oversees exploration. In an effort to increase

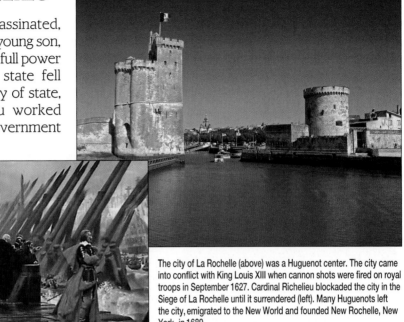

The city of La Rochelle (above) was a Huguenot center. The city came into conflict with King Louis XIII when cannon shots were fired on royal troops in September 1627. Cardinal Richelieu blockaded the city in the Siege of La Rochelle until it surrendered (left). Many Huguenots left the city, emigrated to the New World and founded New Rochelle, New York, in 1689.

the power of the French monarchy, Richelieu ordered the destruction of all fortified castles that were not manned by the king's forces. The Huguenot towns created by the Edict of Nantes acted like virtual states within a state and were hostile to monarchical centralization. Richelieu responded by suppressing these towns and the Protestant nobility that led them.

Backed by the English, a Huguenot rebellion broke out in La Rochelle in 1627, which Richelieu quickly put down. Richelieu used the opportunity to modify the Edict of Nantes. Through the king, he issued "The Peace of Alais" which retracted the right of Huguenots to fortify and garrison towns and forbade Protestants from actively participating in the functions of government. Huguenots were still allowed to practice religion in their own private homes, but Richelieu made Protestantism an obstacle to political advancement in France. He kept Protestants out of government, thus protecting the country against more civil unrest by strengthening and centralizing authority around the king.

PART VII

The British Isles

THE FIRST COVENANT

The Protestant preacher John Knox founded the Presbyterian Church of Scotland. Knox encouraged violence against Catholics, and his preaching and writing inspired a wave of iconoclastic attacks in Scotland that saw the destruction of many churches and monasteries. Driven by both political and religious motives, Scottish lords resolved to do everything in their power to renounce and destroy the Catholic Church. They signed a document known as the "First Covenant" that adopted a Calvinistic profession of faith and rejected the jurisdiction of the pope. Though Mary, Queen of Scots, tried for more than seven years to save the Church in Scotland, Catholic priests were forced to flee as church lands were confiscated and the practice of the Catholic Faith was suppressed.

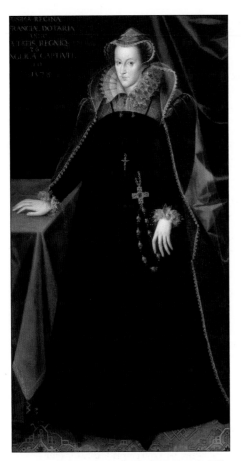

When Mary Stuart returned to Scotland from France in 1561, she found herself alone in her Catholic beliefs.

Mary's position in England was continually entangled in controversy. The possibility for her to become heir to the English crown made her a threat to Elizabeth. Even though Mary herself never voiced any desire for the English crown, others wanted her to be queen of England to further their own ends. Rumors of her involvement in plots against Elizabeth circulated, and eventually the queen reacted by leveling false charges against Mary, including marital infidelity and murder. These charges forced Mary to abdicate her claim to the crown in favor of her one-year-old son, James. Furthermore, Scottish unrest forced Mary to hand over rule of Scotland to her half brother (also named James). In addition, her son, the future James I of England, was raised a Protestant. Mary finally fled Scotland seeking sanctuary in England. Elizabeth answered Mary's pleas for protection by placing her under house arrest for nineteen years.

CONTINUING PERSECUTION IN ENGLAND

With the rise of the Presbyterian Church in Scotland and the dominance of the Church of England, Catholics were quickly losing their place in British society. Many saw Catholics as traitors disloyal to the English Crown. In 1559, Elizabeth took discrimination against Catholics to an extreme by prohibiting the practice of the Catholic Faith. The queen hoped that most Catholics would convert to the Church of England, and those who did not would simply die out quietly. Many Catholics refused to give up their Faith and continued to practice in secret. At first, they were tolerated, but it soon became clear that Catholics in England were not fading out of the population as quickly or as quietly as Elizabeth had hoped. Catholics continued to call for a return to union with Rome, and Elizabeth, angered by the failure to stop allegiance to the Catholic Faith, increased the severity of the penal laws against the Church. Finally, she made the practice of the Catholic Faith or adherence to Rome a treasonable offense.

Now with their religion publicly abolished, a major problem that faced English Catholics was the shortage of priests. Without a seminary to train new priests, the English clergy was in danger of dying out. In 1568, Cardinal William Allen helped found a seminary for the English at Douay in the Spanish Netherlands. This seminary would for

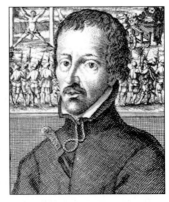

St. Edmund Campion (1540-1581) was an English Jesuit and martyr.

generations help keep the Catholic Faith alive in England by sending missionary priests to administer the sacraments and uphold the teachings of the Catholic Church in the British Isles.

During the reign of Elizabeth, there were many martyrs accused of treason on account of their Catholic Faith. One of the greatest examples of the English martyrs under Elizabeth I was St. Edmund Campion. Campion was a young Oxford scholar who, in 1568, became a celebrated leader of the Anglican Church. Wooed by the success and advancement that membership in the Church of England promised for him, St. Edmund Campion took the Oath of Supremacy.

Soon after having taken the oath, St. Edmund Campion had a personal conversion, left his promising teaching position, and fled England in order to study at the seminary at Douay. There he joined the Society of Jesus in 1573 and was ordained in 1578. Upon his return to England in 1581, St. Edmund Campion was arrested and charged with treason. Once convicted, he suffered a cruel and public punishment. Amid violent excitement, he was paraded through the streets of London, bound hand and foot, riding backwards, with a paper stuck in his hat to denote him as a Jesuit. On the scaffold, St. Edmund Campion was taunted by the crowd concerning the bull of St. Pius V excommunicating Queen Elizabeth. Reminiscent of St. Thomas More, St. Edmund Campion simply prayed for her, proclaiming loudly: "your Queen and my Queen." His feast day is celebrated on December 1.

St. Edmund Campion's death encouraged some growth of Catholicism in England. Among those who returned to the Faith was St. Henry Walpole. The young St. Henry was at St. Edmund's execution, and the incident had a powerful effect on him. St. Henry's shirt was splattered with St. Edmund's blood as he was being drawn and quartered. Afterward St. Henry Walpole converted and lived to become a Jesuit martyr as well.

THE EXECUTION OF MARY, QUEEN OF SCOTS

Mary Stuart was executed at Fotheringhay Castle on February 8, 1587, on suspicion of having been involved in a plot to murder Elizabeth I. She chose to wear red, thereby declaring herself a Catholic martyr.

Below: Mary Stuart was initially buried at Peterborough Cathedral, but her body was exhumed in 1612 when her son, King James I of England, ordered she be reinterred in Westminster Abbey.
It remains there, only thirty feet from the grave of her cousin Elizabeth I.

The growth of Catholic resistance within England and the imminent threat of foreign invasion made Mary Stuart, Queen of Scots, potentially dangerous to Elizabeth's rule. In 1569, an uprising took place in the north of the country where the Catholic Faith remained strong. The uprising, known as the second "Pilgrimage of Grace," tried to restore the Catholic religion, drive Protestant leadership out of London, and acknowledge Mary Stuart as heir and successor to the English throne because Elizabeth I was illegitimate. This rebellion was crushed, and in turn Elizabeth's vengeance was terrible. The queen declared martial law throughout the North, and English troops conducted house-to-house searches to find and execute Catholic priests. The Duke of Norfolk, who sought to marry Mary Stuart and gain the throne of England, was executed in 1572 after he was caught negotiating with the Spanish. Her crown threatened on so many fronts, Elizabeth looked for a way to rid herself of Mary Stuart.

Elizabeth held Mary under house arrest for 19 years while the queen's chief secretary, Francis Walsingham, tried to find evidence that could lead to Mary's execution. Lacking data of any credible crimes, Walsingham sent a spy named Gilbert Gifford to encourage a young admirer of Mary named Babington to plot an escape. The young accomplice wrote letters to Mary discussing his escape plans and desire to assassinate Elizabeth. Mary never received the letters. Instead, Gifford intercepted the letters and forged responses from Mary that urged Babington to reveal his accomplices. This forgery allowed Walsingham to put together a case accusing Mary Stuart of conspiracy to commit treason. Consequently, Babington and his companions were executed in 1586, and Mary was tried for treason. Mary freely confessed to her attempts at escaping Elizabeth's confinement but insisted on her innocence regarding any designs on Elizabeth's life. Nonetheless, Mary was convicted based on the forged documents and beheaded on February 8, 1587.

THE SPANISH ARMADA

The beheading of Mary and the continuing persecution of Catholics in Britain enraged Philip II of Spain, and he planned to lead a crusade against the heretical queen of England. Philip had a claim to the English throne through his marriage to Mary Tudor, and Elizabeth's continuing support of the Protestant cause in Europe further prompted the Spanish king to take up arms against the island nation. Elizabeth aided the Dutch revolution of Utrecht and supported the Huguenot cause in France. Her "Sea-Dogs" led by Francis Drake attacked Spanish treasure ships in the New World and pirated Spanish gold for England. To add to the insult, rather than punish Drake's piracy, Elizabeth knighted him and granted him a new fleet of ships. As a consequence, Philip II set out to invade England and remove Elizabeth from the throne. In 1588 he launched an invasion using his "invincible armada."

The planned invasion was unsuccessful. The Spanish admiral was delayed by poor organization, and Spanish troops waiting to invade from the Netherlands were not prepared in time. The smaller and better-equipped English fleet harried the bigger and clumsy Spanish ships for two weeks without sustaining significant damage. An unexpected storm eventually drove the Spanish fleet to the north where many ships were lost while attempting to return to Spain. The defeat of the Spanish Armada shattered the image of an invincible Spain, establishing an English naval supremacy that continued to support the Protestant cause.

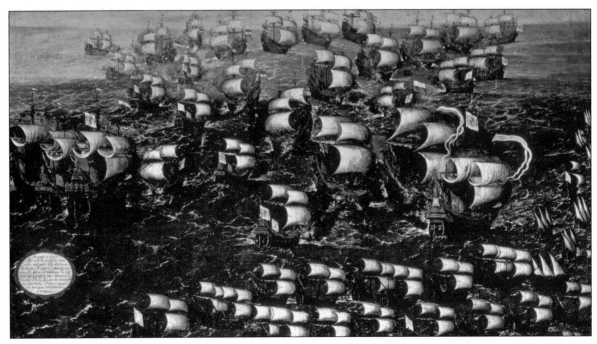

The Spanish fleet was scattered by an English fire ship attack sent in by Francis Drake in the Battle of Gravelines.

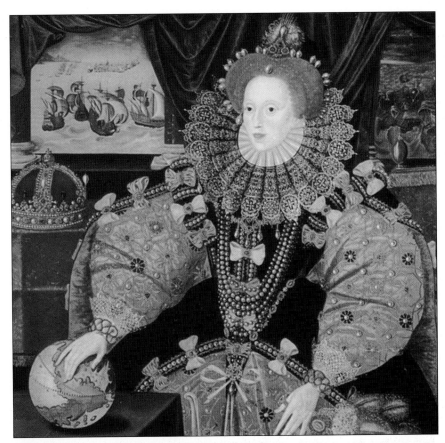

The *Queen Elizabeth Armada Portrait.* The battle between the English fleet and the Spanish Armada lasted from June 19 to August 12, 1588. On August 8, Elizabeth went to Tilbury to encourage her forces. The next day she gave to them what is considered her most famous speech: "…I am come amongst you as you see, at this time…in the midst and heat of the battle to live or die amongst you all, to lay down for my God and for my kingdom, and for my people, my honour and my blood, even in the dust. I know I have the body of a weak and feeble woman, but I have the heart and stomach of a king."

WAR IN IRELAND

Ireland did not fare well during the reign of Elizabeth. Elizabeth inherited Ireland from her father Henry VIII, and after declaring the kingdom Protestant, she waged a war of extermination against the Emerald Isle. English troops butchered men, women, and children. The decimated and demoralized Irish fought back, staging three revolts in an effort to hold on to their religion and culture. All three rebellions failed, and Elizabeth responded to the revolts by launching a complete military conquest and legal suppression of the island. The Gaelic language was abolished, and Protestant overlords were sent to control the agricultural estates. Soldiers destroyed all the crops and livestock in areas of rebellion and implemented systematic starvation. The Annals of the Four Masters describes the plight of the provinces: "neither the lowing of a cow nor the voices of a ploughman was heard from Cashel to the farthermost parts of Kerry" (Vidmar, The Catholic Church through the Ages, 2005, p. 352). According to an English official in the year 1582, over a six-month period more than 30,000 people starved to death. By the end of that ordeal, Elizabeth had little to rule except ashes and carcasses.

Ireland would continue its fight against English Protestantism, while the Faith of the Irish deepened in the face of persecution. Irish seminaries were established in Spain, Portugal, the Low Countries, France, and Rome, where Irish boys were smuggled out of Ireland to be trained for the priesthood. These renegade Irish priests would return to their island to administer the sacraments and preach the word of God to their persecuted flock.

ST. JOHN OGILVIE

The most prominent Scottish martyr of the Reformation was St. John Ogilvie, a Jesuit priest and convert to Catholicism. St. John was born to Calvinist parents in Banfshire, Scotland, around the year 1579. When he was thirteen, St. John was sent abroad by his parents in order to receive a French Calvinist education at Louvain, France. In France it was common for Catholic and Calvinist scholars to debate religion, and while at school, St. John came to know the teachings of the Catholic Church. St. John was deeply impressed by how the Roman Catholic Church was comprised of all types of people. Kings, princes, peasants, and beggars could all renounce the world and devote their lives wholly to God. Furthermore, many of these people had given their lives as martyrs, a reality that had a tremendous influence on St. John Ogilvie.

In 1600 at the age of seventeen, St. John converted to Catholicism at Louvain. Four years later, he joined the Jesuit novitiate at Brünn, and for ten years worked in Austria, mostly at Graz and Vienna, before being sent to the French province. Finally ordained in 1610, St. John expressed a desire to return to his Scottish homeland and minister to the persecuted Catholics who remained there. He received per-mission, and in 1613, St. John disguised himself as a soldier returning to Scotland

from the wars in Europe. Upon his return, he ministered to many Catholics and even won back some converts to the Church. Unfortunately, St. John was betrayed by someone pretending to be interested in the Faith. St. John was eventually imprisoned and tortured by the authorities for refusing to give the names of other Catholics he knew. On March 10, 1615, St. John Ogilvie, who so admired the martyrs of the Church, was himself martyred for his faith by being hanged for high treason. He was canonized by Pope Paul VI in 1976. His feast day is celebrated on March 10.

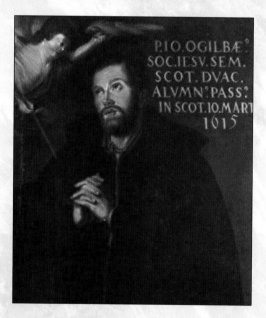

PART VIII

The Thirty Years War (1618-1648)

The final great war of religion took place within the Holy Roman Empire between 1618 and 1648. This last religious conflict would permanently divide Germany between Protestant and Catholic camps and undermine the political development of a unified Germany. Whereas the rest of Europe, in the aftermath of the seventeenth-century wars, developed into powerful nation-states, the Thirty Years War crippled the German states and insured that they would remain a collection of small, disunited kingdoms.

Many different factors brought about the war within Germany. A religious war pitted Protestants and Catholics against each other, each vying for domination of the region. The Thirty Years War was waged by independent German princes, both Catholic and Protestant, who resisted the growing imperial designs of the Austrian Hapsburgs. In the end, with the aid of Richelieu's France, the Hapsburgs would be defeated, and as a result, Christendom would be permanently divided.

The Peace of Augsburg (1555) divided Germany roughly between Lutheran Princes in the North and Catholics in the South. The Peace's famous line "cuius regio huius religio" (whose region, his the religion), provided that each prince determine the faith of his region. The Peace of Augsburg succeeded in pacifying each individual region from infighting, and the Ecclesiastical Reservation Clause protected Catholic regions from further territorial expansion by Protestant princes. But as weak emperors succeeded Charles V, they proved incapable of protecting Catholic interests, and consequently allowed several violations of the Ecclesiastical Reservation Clause to occur. Quarrels also broke out in Protestant areas between Lutheran princes and the members of the newly-emerging Calvinist faith. Not included in the Augsburg settlement, Calvinist princes made efforts to gain ecclesiastical properties from both Catholics and Lutherans.

These scuffles took on new severity as they soon affected religious change in the seats of the imperial electors. Two out of seven total imperial electorships (the Palatinate and Brandenburg) transferred from Lutheranism to Calvinism. With the loss of these seats, Lutheran princes began to fear a loss of influence in the empire. To add to Lutherans' dismay, one of the new electors,

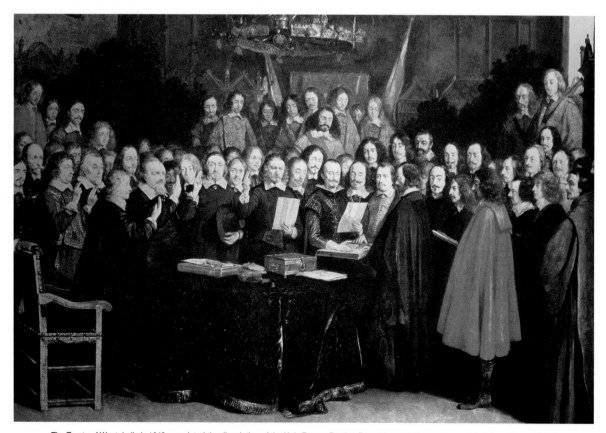

The Treaty of Westphalia in 1648 completed the dissolution of the Holy Roman Empire. France became the most powerful state on the continent.

AFTER THE WARS...THE CATHOLIC RECOVERY, 1650

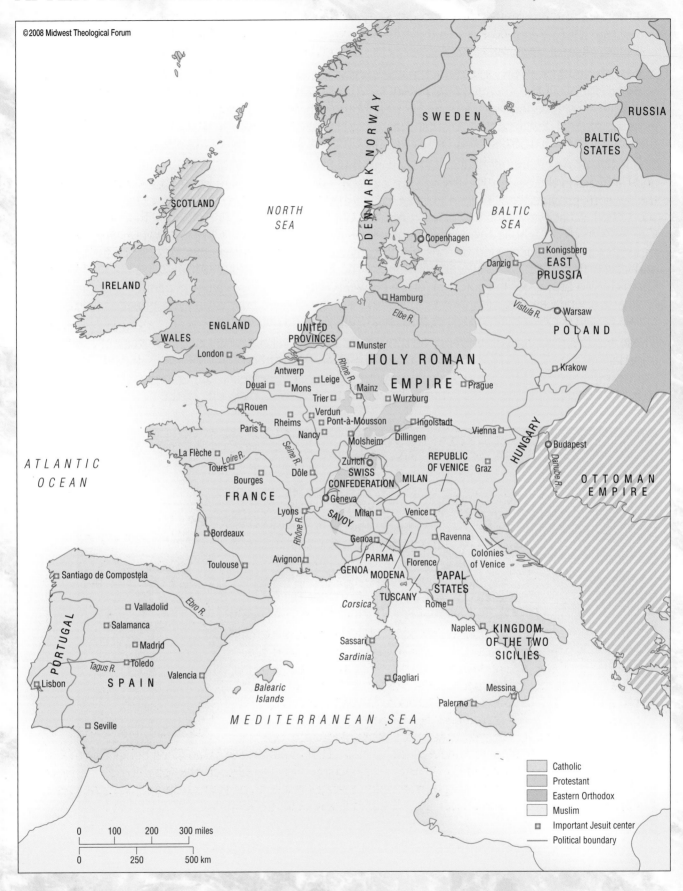

©2008 Midwest Theological Forum

NORWAY

SWEDEN

RUSSIA

BALTIC
STATES

SCOTLAND

NORTH
SEA

DENMARK

BALTIC
SEA

Copenhagen

Konigsberg

EAST
PRUSSIA

Danzig

IRELAND

Hamburg

Elbe R.

Vistula R.

Warsaw

POLAND

ENGLAND

UNITED
PROVINCES

Munster

HOLY ROMAN

Krakow

WALES

London

Antwerp

Rhine R.

Leige

Mainz

EMPIRE

Prague

Douai

Mons

Trier

Wurzburg

Rouen

Verdun

Rheims

Pont-à-Mousson

Ingolstadt

Vienna

HUNGARY

Paris

Nancy

Molsheim

Dillingen

La Flèche

Loire R.

Seine R.

Budapest

Danube R.

OTTOMAN
EMPIRE

ATLANTIC
OCEAN

Tours

Dôle

Zurich

SWISS
CONFEDERATION

REPUBLIC
OF VENICE

Graz

Bourges

MILAN

FRANCE

Geneva

Lyons

Rhône R.

SAVOY

Milan

Venice

Ravenna

Bordeaux

Genoa

Colonies
of Venice

Toulouse

Avignon

PARMA

Florence

GENOA

MODENA

PAPAL
STATES

Santiago de Compostela

TUSCANY

Rome

Corsica

Valladolid

Naples

KINGDOM
OF THE TWO
SICILIES

Salamanca

Madrid

Ebro R.

Sassari

PORTUGAL

Toledo

Tagus R.

SPAIN

Valencia

Sardinia

Cagliari

Lisbon

Seville

Balearic
Islands

Messina

Palermo

MEDITERRANEAN SEA

0 100 200 300 miles	
0 250 500 km	

	Catholic
	Protestant
	Eastern Orthodox
	Muslim
◻	Important Jesuit center
——	Political boundary

Frederick of the Palatinate, was supported by the Dutch Republic and his father-in-law, James I of England, and he formed a Calvinist league known as the Evangelical Union. The Union backed up Frederick's Calvinist policies with militarily might, and their aggression disrupted peace in Germany.

Catholic reform also changed the political landscape in southern Germany. Since the Augsburg settlement, St. Peter Canisius's Catechism of Trent and the preaching of Capuchin friars and Jesuits helped energize the Catholic reform movement. Thousands returned to the Catholic Faith, and with the aid of the king of Spain and the pope, the Bavarian Duke Maximilian formed the Catholic League in 1620 to oppose Frederick's Evangelical Union. The Austrian Ferdinand of Styria (the future Ferdinand II) restored Catholic unity in Austria and the Hapsburg domains.

In 1621, the twelve-year truce that ended the Dutch conflict lapsed, and the Spanish saw an opportunity to renew the struggle and re-establish a Catholic presence in Europe. Philip II launched a campaign from Spanish-controlled Burgundy, through the Calvinist Palatinate and into the Netherlands. Through this campaign, the Spanish hoped to deliver a resounding defeat to rising Calvinist power with one blow. However, the military campaign did not prove easy, and it eventually sparked the long and arduous Thirty Years War, which played out in four phases: the Bohemian (1618-1625), Danish (1625-1629), Swedish (1630-1635), and French (1635-1648).

The Thirty Years War concluded, the wars of religion essentially divided Europe into two camps: Protestant and Catholic. What had begun as a war to restore religious unity became a war that ended in political compromise. Although the papal nuncio at Westphalia protested the compromise, the secular leaders in attendance ignored his concerns, and the pope refused to sign the terms of the treaty.

PART IX

Missionary Apostolate

While Europe was divided along religious and political lines in the sixteenth century, the Church embarked upon the greatest missionary expansion of her history, reaching out to millions of new faithful around the world. This remarkable period of evangelization came about through the efforts of a relatively small number of holy missionaries who truly believed that "God desires the salvation of everyone." Through their courageous travels, the good news of Christ was being preached in Asia, Africa, and the New World.

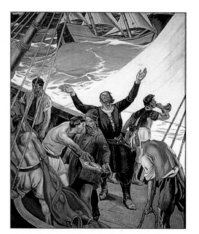

Dias rounded the tip of Africa in 1487.

These missionary expeditions followed in the wake of new explorations throughout the world. The curiosity for discovery so characteristic of the Renaissance together with new navigational advancements helped to open trade routes to the Orient and lead to monumental achievements in exploration. In 1487, the Portuguese sailor Bartholomew Dias rounded the southern tip of Africa opening a new way to India. Five years later another ambitious explorer set off westwards to find an alternative route to India. That explorer, the Italian Christopher Columbus, discovered a New World in the Western hemisphere. For the Church, the "opening of the New World" would provide a new opportunity for evangelization, a chance to help people from every corner of the globe find, as St. John Paul II said, "fullness of life in God."

Settlement into the New World opened new apostolic opportunities just as the Church was undergoing a renewal. The Catholic Reformation helped enthuse dedicated missionaries who ardently desired to spread the Good News of Christ into these newly-founded territories. Older orders were refilled with zealous and disciplined monks and friars, and newer religious orders, such as the Jesuits, Capuchins, and Vincentians, turned out many priests eager to evangelize the indigenous peoples of the New World. The popes encouraged these missions and often helped finance these apostolic ventures. In 1622, Pope Gregory XV founded the congregation De propaganda Fide to promote and establish apostolic missions, and in 1627, the Urbanian University was established in Rome to help educate missionary priests.

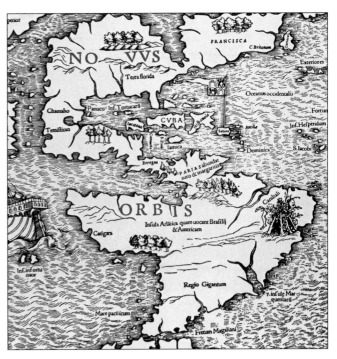

A 1540 map of the New World, the Americas

ST. FRANCIS XAVIER

In 1500, missionary friars arrived at the small trading port of Goa in India established by the Portuguese. As they began preaching to the Indians, they discovered a group of Christians who claimed descent from the original missionary activity of the Apostle St. Thomas. Encouraged by these "St. Thomas Christians," as they were called, a diocese was established in 1533 in Goa with a seminary for training native priests. Unfortunately, many difficulties limited the success of these first missionary friars. The vast Indian subcontinent, with its densely packed populations, the highly structured caste system of the Hindu culture, and the abysmal example of the many recently arrived colonists made progress for conversion slow and difficult.

In 1542, one of the greatest missionary apostles of the age, St. Francis Xavier, arrived in India to help the struggling mission. St. Francis Xavier was one of the founding members of the Society of Jesus; he helped form the order after he met St. Ignatius Loyola at the University of Paris. After his ordination, St. Francis's exceptional zeal for the Gospel was recognized by Pope Paul III, and the pontiff designated him a special emissary for the evangelization of the Indian people.

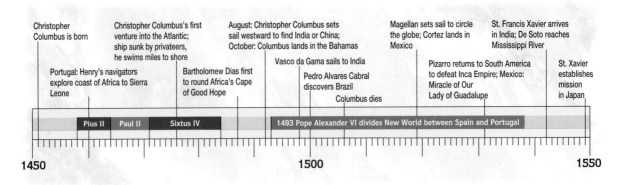

Over the next ten years, St. Francis traveled across the subcontinent, helped strengthen the faith of the nominal St. Thomas Christians, and baptized thousands of local people. He later continued on to the city of Malacca in modern day Sri Lanka, the second most important trading post of the Portuguese empire, where St. Francis established his headquarters. From Malacca, he made many journeys further eastward to the Molucca (Spice Islands), and some accounts say he traveled as far as the Philippines. St. Francis's simple charity and straightforward approach (he always tried to learn the native tongue of the regions he visited) helped convert many people wherever he traveled. St. Francis's missionary work was further strengthened by the strong administrative systems he established for the missions he founded. After St. Francis left a region, he instructed well-trained successors to continue ministering to the newly evangelized peoples.

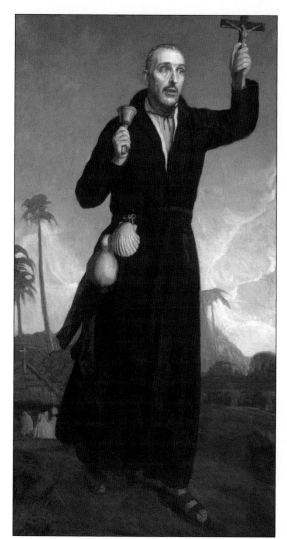

In 1549, St. Francis traveled to Japan along with Jesuit Father de Torres and three Japanese converts to set up a mission on the island farthest east. He spent his first year in Japan familiarizing himself with the culture, learning the language, and translating the principal articles of the Faith into Japanese. Unfortunately for St. Francis, the political situation in Japan was unlike the countries he had already visited. At the time, Japan had an established feudal structure, and as in Medieval Europe, Japanese

Pope Paul III sent St. Francis Xavier to Goa, India, as a special emissary to evangelize the Indian people. For five months Francis worked to remedy the appalling behavior of the Portuguese against the Indians. He worked in the city's three prisons, in the hospital and among the lepers. Moving around the country with only an umbrella and a piece of leather to mend his shoes, he found the language barrier his greatest problem. He had the *Creed, Ten Commandments, Lord's Prayer, Hail Mary, Salve Regina* and the *Rite of Confession* translated into pidgin Tamil and memorized them. He gathered flocks of children by walking with a handbell and taught them to chant the prayers. In one month he had baptized 10,000 people.

(Excerpted from *Cultural Atlas of the Christian World*, Graham Speake, Editor, 1987, p.122)

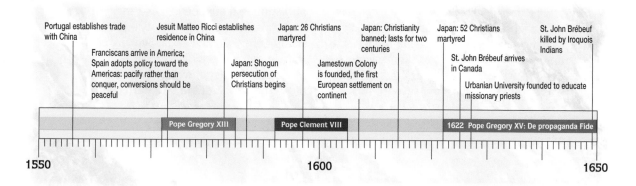

Portugal establishes trade with China

Franciscans arrive in America; Spain adopts policy toward the Americas: pacify rather than conquer, conversions should be peaceful

Jesuit Matteo Ricci establishes residence in China

Japan: Shogun persecution of Christians begins

Japan: 26 Christians martyred

Jamestown Colony is founded, the first European settlement on continent

Japan: Christianity banned; lasts for two centuries

Japan: 52 Christians martyred

St. John Brébeuf arrives in Canada

Urbanian University founded to educate missionary priests

St. John Brébeuf killed by Iroquois Indians

Pope Gregory XIII

Pope Clement VIII

1622 Pope Gregory XV: De propaganda Fide

1550   1600   1650

ST. THOMAS CHRISTIANS

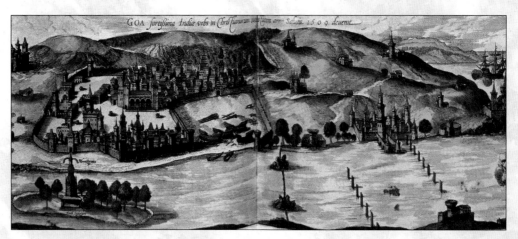

The city of Goa, India in the sixteenth century. Encouraged by the presence of the group called "St. Thomas Christians," a diocese was established in 1533 in Goa with a seminary for training native priests. St. Francis Xavier was sent to Goa to help the struggling mission in 1542.

St. Thomas Christians are Christians from the Malabar Coast (west coast) in southern India whose customs date back to the evangelization of St. Thomas the Apostle. According to their tradition, St. Thomas traveled from the Holy Land to India in AD 52 and established seven Churches in Maliankara, Palayur, Kottakavu, Quilon, Niranom, Nilakkal, and Chayal. He was killed in AD 72 and buried in Mylapore on the East coast of India (although his relics were later relocated to Edessa). This tradition has been consistently agreed to by many scholars from the third century onwards and seems to be supported by modern developments and advances in archaeology, geography, anthropology and other disciplines.

In the fourth century, a group of Jewish Christians led by Thomas Cana settled in Kerala at the request of the Assyrian Church of the East. Thomas Cana was said to have collected seventy-two Christian families and settled on the southern shore of the Perigar. In the fifth century, the Christians of Malabar were exposed to the Nestorian churches of Iraq, whose theology and doctrine influenced the St. Thomas Christians until the arrival of the Portuguese in the sixteenth century.

Before the arrival of the Portuguese, St. Thomas Christians were able to obtain high social status and were granted privileges within the complex caste system of southern India. The head of the Church was the archdeacon, and "Palliyogams"—Parish Councils—were given charge of temporal matters. The lives of the St. Thomas Christians were centered on a liturgy that included days of fasting and abstinence, and their churches were of a similar style to Hindu Temples and Jewish Synagogues. Unfortunately, no written records of the St. Thomas Christians exist from the time of St. Thomas until the sixteenth century.

priests (bonzes) were tied to the political system. They saw St. Francis and his missionaries as a danger to their traditional authority and worked to oust him. Evangelizing in Japan became even more difficult for St. Francis when he petitioned the emperor for protection from the bonzes and, to his dismay, found that the ruler was simply a puppet dominated by strong feudal lords. St. Francis understood that the rigid society in Japan would make long-term growth of Christianity difficult. St. Francis left Japan in 1552 after converting two thousand Japanese. He now set his sights on the nearby kingdom of China.

In Japan, St. Francis had heard stories and myths about the "Celestial Empire," as China was known at the time. Hearing of a magnificent culture across the sea in China, St. Francis was eager to bring the Faith to the legendary empire. Just before he set off, the Viceroy of India appointed St. Francis ambassador and the Holy See made him a Papal Nuncio, giving the missionary diplomatic prestige to bolster his efforts in China.

At the time, China was closed to foreigners, and anyone who tried to enter the country was subject to immediate execution. To avoid this peril, St. Francis appealed to some Chinese smugglers who promised to help him enter the mainland. Tragically, on his way to China, St. Francis caught a serious fever. The smugglers abandoned him in a small hut on the island of Sancian, and he died five days later. St. Francis Xavier was only forty-six years of age when he died in 1552, and he was canonized just seventy years later. His feast day is celebrated on December 3.

INDIA

When missionaries landed in a new area of India, they would encounter a complex multiplicity of cultures. Missionaries had to work at winning acceptance from tightly closed communities and adapt the practice of Christianity to the particular cultural traditions of the people. To achieve this, missionaries dedicated a huge part of their efforts to assimilating local customs, learning dialects, and earning the trust of the locals by integrating themselves into the community. By understanding the culture thoroughly, missionaries could tailor the teachings of Christ in a more effective and convincing way.

In India, the missionary Robert de Nobili exemplified the effectiveness of this "inculturation." Catholic missionaries had difficulties reaching India's intellectual class, the Brahmins. The Portuguese missionaries who preceded de Nobili won over many converts among the lower classes. However, the Brahmins rejected Christianity since it was perceived as unfit for the upper class. De Nobili realized that in Indian society divisions were so strong that Christianity had to be presented differently to each caste. He took a year to master Hindi, Sanskrit, and the local dialects. He studied the Brahmin caste and learned about what they held sacred and worthy of reverence. De Nobili then asked permission from his archbishop to present himself as a Christian Brahmin holy man as a way of showing Christian virtue in a form understandable to the Indian Brahmin. He followed the Brahmins' rigorous traditions of fasting and abstaining from foods considered unclean. The leaders of the Brahmin class were also impressed by de Nobili's goodness and kindness. Gradually, de Nobili showed how Christianity could be adapted to their philosophical and religious ideas. Some estimate that around 150,000 Brahmin converted through de Nobili's work.

Maintaining a vibrant and active church in India proved difficult in subsequent centuries. The strong divisions between upper- and lower-class Christians in India was criticized by many Westerners. In 1742, Pope Benedict XIV, insisting that missions publicly admit members of the lower classes into full communion with the Church, condemned some Indian Christian rites. These changes were not welcomed by local Indians, and after the suppression of the Jesuit order during the eighteenth century, the Christian population in India shrank.

CHINA

St. Francis Xavier was not the only missionary who could not penetrate China's closed borders. Despite the flourishing missions in the surrounding lands, China resisted Christian and European visitors for years. In 1583 (thirty years after St. Francis Xavier's death), an Italian Jesuit named Matteo Ricci was finally able to set up a permanent residence in China. Like de Nobili in India, Ricci understood that the best way to reach the Chinese people was to adopt their local customs and traditions. However, China posed particular problems for Catholic missionaries. The Chinese culture prided themselves on adherence to traditions of family worship and philosophical principles of truth and justice. These traditions were old and deep-rooted, and they had produced many centuries of sophisticated and refined civilization. The Chinese were satisfied with their ways and proud of their culture, with no inclination to embrace a new one.

Ricci understood this and recognized the beauty and richness of the Chinese culture. Rather than preach in opposition to these traditions, Ricci blended the Eastern and Western worlds in an attractive and compatible way. He dressed as a Mandarin scholar but filled his residence in Canton with western works of art and scientific instruments. Ricci lived as a public witness to the Christian Faith, and he offered a moving example of charity and patience that won the admiration of the Chinese. Through his exemplary virtue, as well as exposing them to the fruits of Western civilization, he won the respect of the local people. Eventually, the emperor summoned Ricci to his court, and the two developed a friendship. While in the emperor's court, Ricci gave lectures on science and astronomy, translated Christian principles into Chinese, and developed a Chinese liturgical rite that used the Chinese language, not Latin, in the Mass. Ricci wrote a treatise on the Catholic Faith in Chinese called The True Doctrine of God, in which he was able to express the complex theological dogmas and concepts of Catholicism in a language that had never before conveyed Christian ideas. By his death in 1610, Ricci had established five residences in China and brought two thousand converts to the Faith.

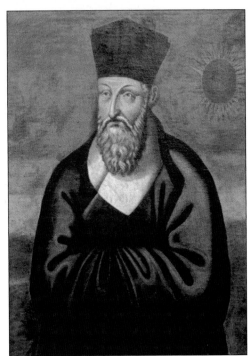

Matteo Ricci (1552-1610) was an Italian Jesuit priest whose missionary activity in China during the Ming Dynasty marked the beginning of modern Chinese Christianity. The church he built remains the largest Catholic church to survive the Cultural Revolution.

Father Johann Adam Schall succeeded Ricci in China, and the number of converted Chinese Christians rose to over 237,000 by 1664. Father Schall continued to expose the Chinese to Western culture. He held the presidency of the Mathematical Tribunal in the Imperial City and was made a first class citizen by the emperor. In many ways, the success of his missionary activity depended upon the support and good graces of the emperor. In 1692, the emperor issued an edict giving complete toleration to the Church, and by 1724, the number of Chinese Catholics rose to 800,000.

Nonetheless, the Church did not remain in good graces with the emperors of China for long. As western nations expanded their trading empires in the East, the Chinese became wary of Western domination, and Western Christian missionaries began to lose favor. In 1724 persecutions of Christians in China resumed and missionary activity quickly declined. The suppression of the Society of Jesus in 1773 also diminished the number of available missionary priests. By the end of the eighteenth century, China's faithful numbered around 300,000, less than half the number at the beginning the the century.

JAPAN

Persecution posed a difficult obstacle for Christian missionaries in Japan as well. Within thirty years of St. Francis Xavier's work in Japan, Japanese converts numbered over 200,000. However, the success of the Church in Japan was at the mercy of the whims of the strong feudal warlords that dominated Japanese society. As long as the leading warlord, the Shogun, permitted missionary activity, Christianity thrived. In 1587 power shifted, and the Shogun Hideyoshi began a new era of persecution.

This persecution was largely the result of paranoia affecting many Asian countries at that time. Western expansion made many ancient civilizations fearful of invasion and suppression. In Japan, a ship captain suggested that the missionaries were preparing for a larger European invasion, and Japanese authorities responded by arresting the missionaries. Twenty-six of them were martyred by crucifixion in Nagasaki on February 5, 1597 (canonized by Bl. Pius IX in 1862). Persecution intensified in 1614 after the Shogun officially outlawed the practice of Christianity in Japan. In 1622, fifty-two Christians were killed, and the faithful were driven underground.

Japanese martyrs came from all classes of society. Clergy and laity, Europeans and Japanese, men and women, elderly and children were all subject to persecution, and the punishments were especially cruel.

Years later, in 1865, Japan was reopened to the West, and French missionaries returned to the Islands. To their surprise, the French discovered over 50,000 Japanese Christians in hiding. Despite persecutions, these Christians had kept the Faith alive, passing it down from generation to generation for nearly three centuries. Remarkably, these Japanese Christians retained their orthodoxy, finding solidarity with the French missionaries in their mutual obedience to the pope in Rome, veneration of the Blessed Virgin, and practice of celibacy by the clergy.

THE CHURCH IN CHINA TODAY

Christianity in China appeared to be on the rise during the early part of the twentieth century. However, when the communists came to power in 1949, Christian Churches were seized, missionaries forced to leave, and Christians were pressured to follow the strict requirements of the communist party. In 1957 the situation worsened as the Roman Catholics who remained in China were forced to sever relations with Rome, driving those who pledged allegiance to the Holy Pontiff underground. This has resulted in the existence of two Churches in China: the official or government-sanctioned church ("Patriotic Church"), which does not recognize the supremacy of the pope, and the unofficial or "underground" Church, which is still united with Rome.

The underground Church today continues to suffer fierce persecution. Both clergy and laity are regularly detained and beaten, and Churches and shrines destroyed. Nevertheless, as occurred in Eastern Europe, the underground Church is also growing in popularity as those disillusioned with communist ideology join the fold. The underground Church continually asks all Catholics to pray that their government stop persecution and grant the freedom to practice Catholicism.

THE PHILIPPINES AND AFRICA

By far the most successful missionary effort in the East occurred in the Philippines. Various religious, including the Augustinians, Dominicans, and Franciscans, flocked to the Spanish colony, teaching the natives, among other skills, new farming techniques and textile manufacturing. These missionaries also helped build roads and bridges throughout the islands, and in 1611, the University of Santo Tomas was established.

The missionary efforts gave rise to an improved capacity to work efficiently and a higher standard of living. These advances had a positive impact on the general moral character of the people. These long-lasting effects of these missionary achievements in the Philippines is still strongly reflected in the deep faith of the Filipino people.

During this period of great missionary activity, Africa showed the least results. Disease proved to be the harshest opponent to opening the vast interior of the African Continent to the Christian Faith. Nearly every missionary who entered the Dark Continent before the middle of the nineteenth century would succumb to a variety of lethal tropical diseases. In addition, hostile Muslims, reprisals over the slave trade, and jealous pagan priests took a great toll on the missionaries. During this time, many lost their lives to persecution, and since it was nearly impossible to maintain a steady missionary presence, only a few would convert to the Catholic Faith. But the late nineteenth and twentieth centuries saw new and effective inroads in the evangelization of Africa where now the Church in a number of countries is thriving.

PART X

The New World

Although at first many explorers thought that they had discovered a new route to the Orient, they soon realized that they had come across a new continent. Anything but a disappointment, this New World provided a wealth of opportunity. Land-starved Spanish nobles carved out feudal estates, while others looked for easy access to new sources of gold, silver, and other goods. To achieve these ends, the Conquistadors let nothing stand in their way. They conquered the large Aztec and Inca empires as well as countless other native cultures in order to establish a strong and affluent hold on Central and South America.

For the Catholic kings Charles V and Philip II, the propagation of Christianity was a primary goal in the New World. Since the very first explorations, priests accompanied the various expeditions, seeking to bring native peoples to Christ. The Spanish crown generously supported the missionary clerics and passed legislation that protected the basic human rights of the Indians.

Missionaries did not simply introduce the Christian religion. As in other parts of the world, they learned native traditions and dialects and helped teach and train the Indians in agriculture and technical crafts. Thanks to work of the missionaries, Spanish culture intermingled with the culture of America and eventually the natives intermarried with Spanish settlers. These efforts brought millions to the Church and helped bring a Christian culture to the Latin world.

OUR LADY OF GUADALUPE

The early missionaries had a difficult time eradicating the superstition of the Indian people. Initially the cessation of human sacrifices and the destruction of the pagan temples by the Spanish hindered

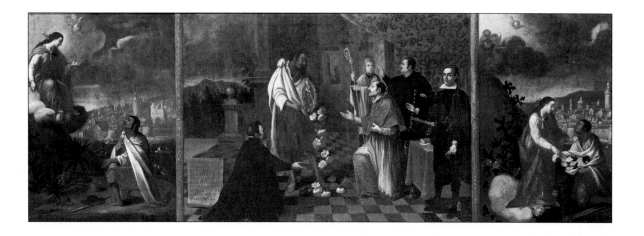

the missionaries' efforts to win converts to Christ. However, a spectacular intervention of Mary would help remedy this lackluster interest in Christianity by occasioning a staggering number of converts to the Church. Within ten years, nine million Indians would receive Baptism.

On December 9, 1531, ten years after the conquest of Mexico, a new convert to the Faith, St. Juan Diego, was walking his usual six miles to attend Holy Mass, when he heard angelic voices and saw a rainbow of dazzling colors. Mary appeared to St. Juan Diego and asked him to go to the Bishop to ask that a temple be erected in her name. St. Juan Diego obeyed and informed the bishop of the apparition. Bishop Juan de Zumarraga listened patiently to St. Juan Diego's account, but was skeptical. He told St. Juan Diego to return another day.

St. Juan Diego returned to his home feeling he had failed Mary. As the sun set, she appeared again to St. Juan Diego and encouraged him to return the next day to the bishop to again make her request. Upon his return the next day, the bishop asked that she give a sign to prove the veracity of her visitation. St. Juan Diego returned home, once again disappointed.

On December 12, St. Juan Diego's uncle became very ill, and fearing that his uncle might die, he summoned a priest to give his uncle the last rites. Because of the urgency to attend to his uncle, he tried to detour away from the hill where Mary had first appeared to him, but it made no difference. She appeared to St. Juan Diego again, and asked him about her request for the church. When St. Juan Diego spoke about his sick uncle, she reassured him that she had already seen to his uncle's recovery. As for the bishop's request for a sign, she directed St. Juan Diego to a nearby hill to collect the roses he found there and deliver them to the bishop. It was not the season for roses; nonetheless, St. Juan Diego discovered a large patch of roses in full bloom. He filled his tilma (cloak) with the flowers and rushed to the bishop's residence. When Bishop Zumarraga received St. Juan Diego, he asked about the sign. He opened his cloak and dozens of red roses fell to the floor. The bishop immediately fell to his knees, and St. Juan Diego eventually realized that Mary's image was imprinted on his tilma (cloak made of cactus fibers). This miracle prompted Bishop Zumarraga to build her church.

The image of Our Lady of Guadalupe was a message to all the people of America. In the image, Mary appeared greater than the sun, moon, stars, and all the pagan deities. Yet Mary was bowing in submission. She herself was not a god, the image seemed to say, but she prayed to the one God. The cross around her neck was the same that flew on Cortes's flag, and through this image, Indians began to embrace the Catholic Faith. For over four hundred thirty years, the image that first appeared on St. Juan Diego's cloak has expressed the protection of Our Lady for all the Americas. She is the patroness of the Americas. Her feast day is celebrated on December 12 in the universal Church.

SPANISH MISSIONS

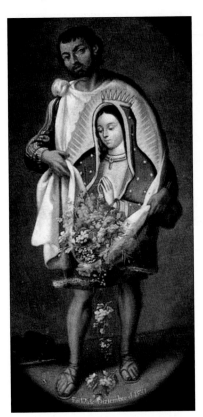

St. Juan Diego opened his cloak, and dozens of red roses fell to the floor. Appearing on his *tilma* was the image of Mary, a message to all the people of America.

Spanish missionaries wanted to create Indian communities away from the influence of the white settlers so that their efforts at evangelization would be untouched by the bad example and meddling of outsiders. They received permission from the king to found mission settlements. These missions gave Indians complete control over their own affairs. The Indians chose their own civic authorities and judges and were protected by their own warriors. Only the missionaries were able to visit these settlements. Two priests and up to four laymen were assigned to each community. They taught the Faith, established schools, and transcribed the spoken native language into a written language. They also taught natives reading and writing, modern farming techniques, and industrial crafts.

Between 1610 and 1767, thirty-two mission settlements were established within newly-acquired Spanish territories, ministering to over 700,000 neophyte Catholics. Father Bl. Junipero Serra began similar settlements along the coast of California. Bl. Junipero Serra founded nine missions, and his collaborators twelve more after his death, for a total of twenty-one California missions.

SLAVERY AND ST. PETER CLAVER

The Portuguese, like the Arabs in the Middle East and Africa, introduced slavery to Europe in the sixteenth century in an effort to solve its labor shortages. During their expeditions along the coast of Africa, Portuguese sailors enslaved many Africans and helped create a market for slave labor. As their trading empires grew, the Dutch and English would eventually dominate the traffic in African slaves in the West, bringing thousands of Africans to their colonies in North America. This dark period of European and American history lasted through the end of the nineteenth century.

The horrors of the slave trade were numerous and well-documented. Travel was extremely hazardous, and many of the Africans taken from Africa died during the long, disease-ridden voyages to the New World. Families suffered as children were separated from their parents and husbands from their wives.

In the Spanish missions, one missionary in particular did much to alleviate the suffering of the African slaves. In 1610, St. Peter Claver landed in Cartagena (Colombia), the chief slave market in the New World. He was appalled by the harsh, inhumane treatment of the African slaves, and decided to devote himself to their care. Although St. Peter Claver could not single-handedly stop the slave trade, for forty years he attempted to temper its evils. When ships arrived from Africa, St. Peter Claver would meet them on a pilot boat bringing food for the slaves. He helped care for the sick, tended their sores, and offered kind words and support to the wounded victims of the trade. After they arrived, while the slaves were waiting to be traded, St. Peter Claver instructed them in the Catholic Faith. During his tenure in Cartagena, he baptized over 300,000 slaves. He declared himself "the slave of the Negroes forever." St. Peter Claver's feast day is celebrated on September 9.

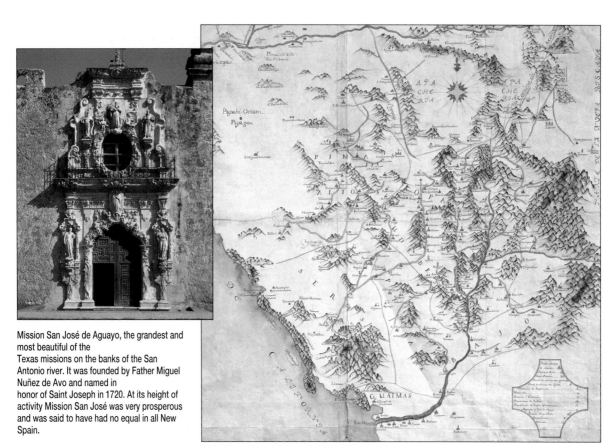

Mission San José de Aguayo, the grandest and most beautiful of the
Texas missions on the banks of the San Antonio river. It was founded by Father Miguel Nuñez de Avo and named in
honor of Saint Joseph in 1720. At its height of activity Mission San José was very prosperous and was said to have had no equal in all New Spain.

A map of Missions in Mexico.

MISSIONARY ACTIVITY IN NORTH AMERICA

The French first colonized North America in the seventeenth century while searching for fur skins to sell in Europe. French trappers lived among the Indians and established trading posts along the St. Lawrence River Valley and down the Mississippi River to New Orleans. Jesuit missionaries accompanied the French settlers and made heroic efforts to convert the scattered Indian tribes that dominated the interior of the continent. Although their success was limited, the Jesuit missionaries persevered in faith and sanctity, even to the point of martyrdom.

Among these missionaries were the Jesuits St. John de Brébeuf and St. Isaac Jogues. St. John de Brébeuf arrived in Canada in 1625 and established a mission among the Huron Indians. For sixteen years St. John de Brébeuf endured grueling poverty as he worked to evangelize the Indian tribes. In 1647, war broke out among the Huron and Iroquois tribes, and although St. John de Brébeuf and his missionaries had the opportunity to leave the area, they chose to stay with their mission. In March 1649, St. John de Brébeuf was seized by Iroquois Indians and tortured mercilessly before being killed in a disgusting and blasphemous fashion. Boiling water was poured over his head in a mockery of Baptism and a red-hot iron was thrust down his throat. Throughout the entire ordeal, St. John de Brébeuf never cried out in pain, suffering his torment in silence.

St. Isaac Jogues also suffered at the hands of the Iroquois tribes. While working on a mission near the Great Lakes, he was taken prisoner in August 1642 and forced into slavery for thirteen months. When St. Isaac Jogues was rescued, he was near death and the fingers of his hands were mutilated from being bitten off. St. Isaac Jogues returned to France, but soon insisted upon returning to Canada to negotiate a peace settlement to the Indian wars. St. Isaac Jogues returned to Canada and was successful with the negotiations at first. Unfortunately, blight struck the crops in the region, and some Indians accused him of sorcery, insisting that the priest had caused the famine. In 1646 Iroquois warriors seized St. Isaac Jogues and beat him to death with a tomahawk. Sts. John de Brébeuf, Isaac Jogues, and their companions, known as the North American martyrs, share a feast day celebrated on October 19.

FOUNDING THE CATHOLIC COLONY OF MARYLAND

Unlike the Spanish and French missionaries, English Catholics came to the New World in order to seek refuge from fierce persecution in their native country and practice the Faith. In 1632, the Lord of Baltimore, George Calvert, used his influence with King Charles I to gain a charter for colonization. The king granted the charter, and Calvert and a group of Catholics left England to establish the colony of Maryland.

At first, Catholics and Protestants coexisted peacefully in Maryland thanks to the Act of Toleration (1649). The act was originally passed to pacify conflict between English Protestants and French Canadians, but some Protestants in Maryland soon felt that it did not protect the English Catholic settlers. As Protestant numbers grew in Maryland, Catholics began to suffer restrictions on their religious freedom. In order to protect the Catholic minority in the colony, the colonial representative legislature was split into two parts. This precedent would eventually influence the establishment of a bicameral (two-house) legislature specified by the U.S. Constitution.

Maryland was not the only safe haven for Catholics in America. Pennsylvania also granted religious toleration to Catholics. Set up as a Quaker colony, Pennsylvania allowed the free expression of any Christian religion. The American Revolution solidified freedom for the Catholic faithful in all the colonies by creating a republic which endorsed and promoted religious toleration. Non-establishment of religion would be legally enshrined in the first amendment to the Constitution. After the revolution, the Holy See appointed John Carroll of Baltimore, the brother of one of the signers of the Declaration of Independence, as the first Catholic bishop in the United States.

CONCLUSION

The unfailing light and strength of the Holy Spirit explains not only the Church's survival amid one of the greatest crises She has ever faced, but also her vigorous renewal. It is indeed remarkable that in the face of the Church's greatest upheaval, renewal and revitalization within the Church reflected in a special way the power of the Holy Spirit to protect and renew the Church. The many and varied examples of saints is a marvelous testimony to the perennial truth that the Church is always young and vibrant in spite of the constant need of purification of her children. The political and religious upheavals of the sixteenth century would challenge the Church's part to play as leaven for society but would never manage to stop her work in extending Christ's kingdom.

By the end of the seventeenth century, the pope would no longer play a significant role in the political development of Europe, and religion would no longer be the chief motivating factor in political affairs. Instead, politics and economics would drive the leaders of Europe as they sought to transform their realms into powerful and self-sufficient nations. Exploration in the New World turned the interests of many leaders towards the economic possibilities which overseas expansion offered. Through these wars of religion, the Christian world was reshaped and reorganized as new values and interests began to overshadow their Christian heritage.

In light of the Wars of Religion, the need for dialogue and mutual Christian charity becomes quite obvious. This period of history is a powerful reminder that the heart of the Christian message to love as Christ loved must always be an absolute priority for all Christians, both rulers and citizens. The

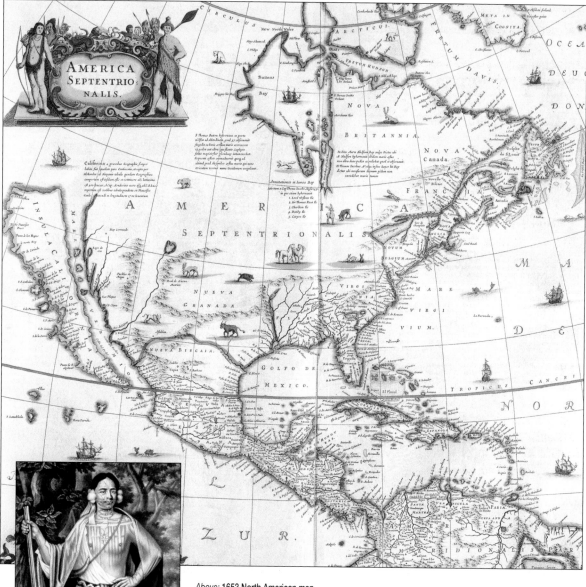

Above: 1653 North American map.
Left: Engraving of an Iroquois Chief from 1710. His linen shirt, wool blanket, beaded moccasins, and musket are the result of contact with European traders.

alternative to Christ's new law of love is tragedy expressed in terrible violations of human dignity.

In spite of the tragic divisions between the Protestants and Catholics in sixteenth century Europe, divine providence was at work in the newly-discovered lands. As millions of Christians separated from the Church of Rome, millions of indigenous peoples of the New World of Central and South America embraced the Catholic Faith. The lands of Asia, most notably the Philippines, also produced an extraordinary number of converts to the Faith. This unparalleled period of evangelization is highlighted by the apparition of Our Lady of Guadalupe, whose appearance served as a moving sign and offered hope to the New World, and the rest of the world, that her Son, in words of St. John Paul II, is the "Lord of history."

VOCABULARY

ACT OF SUPREMACY
Proclaimed King Henry VIII the supreme leader of the Church in England, which meant that the pope was no longer recognized as having any authority within the country, and all matters of faith, ecclesiastical appointment, and maintenance of ecclesiastical properties were in the hands of the king.

BONZES
Japanese Buddhist monks who saw St. Francis Xavier and his missionaries as a danger to their established influence; they worked to oust him from Japan.

CONSUBSTANTIATION
A term describing Christ's co-existence in the Eucharist. Luther taught that the Eucharist was not truly Christ, but that He was present in it as heat is in a hot iron. Accordingly, the substance of Christ's body co-exists with the substance of the bread and his blood with the wine.

DE PROPAGANDA FIDE
Congregation founded by Pope Gregory XV to promote and establish apostolic missions.

FIRST COVENANT
Document drawn up and signed by Scottish lords that adopted a Calvinist profession of faith and abolished the power of the pope, establishing Presbyterianism in Scotland.

INSTITUTES OF THE CHRISTIAN RELIGION
Written by John Calvin, it contained four books which codified Protestant theology. Among these beliefs were the ultimate authority of the word of God, the depravity of man, and his belief that the Bible is the only source of Revelation.

PILGRIMAGE OF GRACE
Catholic uprising in England in 1569 that tried to restore the Catholic religion, drive Protestant leadership from London, and acknowledge Mary Stuart as England's rightful heir.

PLURALISM
Within the Church, a bishop having control over more than one diocese.

POLITIQUES
French political faction with no strong religious ties that tried to manipulate political divisions in France for its own political gain.

PREDESTINATION
A doctrine of Calvin which taught that salvation depended solely on God's pre-determined decision. According to this principle, those who are saved (the elect) are chosen by God through no effort of their own. God also chooses others to be damned. This damnation is necessary to show God's great justice.

SCRUPULOSITY
The habit of imagining sin when none exists, or grave sin when the matter is not serious.

SOLA SCRIPTURA
"Scripture alone." It is the belief that all man needs for salvation is the Bible. This is a tenet for most Protestants.

SPANISH ARMADA
Attempting to remove Elizabeth from the throne of England, Philip II sent this "invincible" fleet of ships in 1588. The invasion was unsuccessful.

SPANISH FURY
During the occupation of the Low Countries by Philip II's forces, the Spanish army mutinied after not having received pay. During the subsequent rampage, these Spanish troops pillaged and murdered over six thousand people in Antwerp.

SPIRITUAL EXERCISES
During a year of intense prayer, St. Ignatius was inspired to write this guide for spiritual perfection, which is divided into reflections and meditations meant to help the believer emulate Christ.

VOCABULARY Continued

ST. THOMAS CHRISTIANS
Group of Christians in India who are descended from the original missionary activity of St. Thomas the Apostle.

STADTHOLDER
Local prince who led the provinces of the Low Countries during times of trouble. Otherwise business and politics in the region were carried out locally and independently.

THIRTY-NINE ARTICLES
Issued by Elizabeth I, these provided for the foundation of the Anglican Church, maintaining all the outward appearances of Catholicism, but implanting Protestant doctrine into the Church of England.

TILMA
Cloak worn by Indians in Mexico. It was on his tilma that Our Lady of Guadalupe left her image to St. Juan Diego.

TRANSUBSTANTIATION
The change of the substance of bread and wine into the Body and Blood of Christ with only the accidents (properties) of bread and wine remaining.

STUDY QUESTIONS

1. What abuses in the Church required reform?

2. What was the name of the document that Martin Luther nailed to the door of the Wittenberg cathedral? On what date did this happen?

3. What abuse initially captured Luther's attention and compelled him to write the document he nailed on the cathedral door?

4. What two sacraments did Luther retain?

5. What is consubstantiation?

6. Where and at what meeting did Luther answer charges before Emperor Charles V?

7. Where did Luther go to escape capture by the emperor?

8. What text did Luther translate from the original Greek into German while at Wartburg?

9. What was the key passage from St. Paul in Romans 1:17 that led Luther to the theological idea of "justification through faith alone"?

10. What book of the New Testament did Luther especially reject?

11. What relationship to secular authority did Luther and Lutheranism develop?

12. What was the Augsburg Confession (1530)?

13. Who developed the Reformed tradition in the Protestant Reformation?

14. What was the name of Calvin's most important work?

15. In what ways did Calvin go beyond Luther's theology?

16. What was Calvin's teaching regarding predestination?

17. In which city did Calvin establish a theocracy?

18. What work did Henry VIII of England write against Luther's ideas?

19. What was the state of the Catholic Church in England at the beginning of Henry VIII's reign?

20. What was the Act of Supremacy? When was it issued?

21. Who were two of the most important martyrs during Henry VIII's reign?

22. What happened to Church lands and religious houses in England?

23. How was the Church of England that Henry VIII started theologically different from the Catholic Church?

24. What book did Thomas Cranmer, Archbishop of Canterbury, publish under King Edward VI's reign?

25. Under whose reign did the Church of England truly accept the ideas of the Protestant reformation?

26. What are the Thirty-nine Articles?

27. What were some of the challenges posed by a Church council being called?

28. When did the Council of Trent occur?

29. What topics did the Council of Trent address?

30. At what important battle were the Turks defeated by European forces?

31. Who was the holy bishop of Milan who implemented the reforms of the Council of Trent?

32. Who helped reform the Carmelite order?

33. What important book did St. Ignatius of Loyola write that is still used for retreats today?

34. What kind of work did the Society of Jesus (Jesuits) do?

35. What was the name given to the Muslims who lived in Spain?

36. How did Philip II deal with these Muslim people in Spain?

37. What was the economic foundation of the Low Countries?

38. What did William of Orange and the Count of Egmont protest? Were they successful?

39. What actions taken by Calvinists in the Low Countries enraged Philip?

40. What was the "Spanish Fury"?

41. Whom did Philip send to replace the Duke of Alba? Was he more effective?

42. How were the Low Countries divided in 1578?

43. What cities were affected when the English aided the Netherlands?

44. What three factions battled over control of French politics after the death of Henry II?

45. Who was the most influential politique?

46. How did Catherine de Medici use marriage to further her political ends?

47. Why did Catherine de Medici instigate the St. Bartholomew's Day Massacre?

48. What famous statement did Henry of Navarre make shortly before being crowned King Henry IV of France?

49. How did the Edict of Nantes help Catholic-Protestant relations in France?

50. During the reign of Louis XIII, who really held power in France?

51. How did Cardinal Richelieu deal with the religious divisions in the country?

52. Who founded Presbyterianism in Scotland?

STUDY QUESTIONS Continued

53. What was the First Covenant?

54. How did Cardinal William Allen help the Catholic Church in England?

55. Why was Mary, Queen of Scots, a threat to Elizabeth I?

56. How did Francis Walsingham acquire evidence to convict Mary?

57. Who were the "Sea Dogs"?

58. How did Elizabeth I set about ridding Ireland of Catholicism?

59. What treaty ended the Thirty Years War?

60. How did the Church respond to new opportunities for conversion?

61. What were some obstacles faced by the missionaries?

62. Where did St. Francis Xavier carry on his missionary work?

63. Who carried on evangelization in India, and how did he do it?

64. Who evangelized in China, and what was his approach?

65. What hindered evangelization in Japan?

66. What delayed the spread of the Faith in Africa?

67. To whom and where did Our Lady of Guadalupe appear?

68. What was the direct result of Mary's appearance?

69. How many missions were established between 1610 and 1767 in Spanish lands?

70. Who founded the California missions, and how many did he found?

In 1590 King Henry IV of France held the south and west, and the Catholic League the north and east. The new king knew that he had to take Paris if he stood any chance of reuniting the kingdom. Paris was besieged, but the siege was lifted with Spanish support. Realizing that there was no prospect of a Protestant king succeeding in fanatically Catholic Paris, Henry with the famous phrase *"Paris vaut bien une messe"* (Paris is worth a mass) announced his conversion to the old faith and was crowned at Chartres in 1594.

PRACTICAL EXERCISES

1. Martin Luther developed four major theological principles: sola Scriptura, sola fide, sola gratia, and solo Christo (Scripture alone, faith alone, grace alone, and Christ alone). Each of Luther's four main theological principles was conceived in reaction to what he believed were false teachings of the Church. Using the Scholastic method, construct a Catholic rebuttal to Luther's ideas.

2. The lives of John Calvin and St. Thomas More reveal two distinct understandings of how Christ's life and teachings apply to living as a Christian. By comparing these two men, explain how their lives reflect their theological understanding of Christianity. (Use the teachings of the Council of Trent and Calvin's Institutes of the Christian Religion as a guide.)

3. What kind of Europe did Philip II inherit from his father Charles V? What were some of the divisions and problems he had to deal with? How did his faith help him? How did it hurt his ability to rule?

4. Cardinal Richelieu and Catherine de Medici had two different approaches to establishing order in France. How did they differ? How were they the same? Was the stability Richelieu established in France worth his use of negative methods?

5. England was particularly harsh in its treatments of Catholics. Why did Elizabeth I see Catholics as a severe threat? What countries today repress religious groups, including Catholics?

6. What were the major obstacles, physical and cultural, to Catholic missionary activity? How did the missionaries overcome these obstacles?

7. Choose a contemporary culture, either in the United States or elsewhere, and explain how a missionary could adapt his or her lifestyle in order to earn that culture's trust. Choose a Gospel story, and retell it in a way suited to that specific culture.

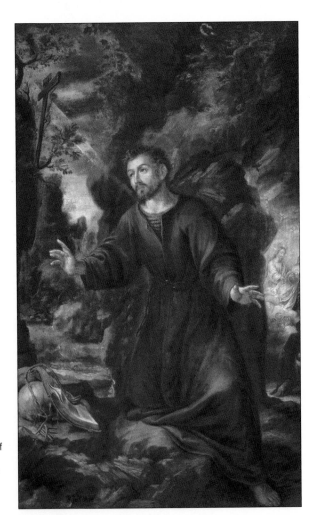

After St. Ignatius of Loyola made a general confession at the shrine of Our Lady of Montserrat, he laid his sword and dagger at the feet of Our Lady, and exchanged clothes with a poor beggar.

He then lived a year in the seclusion of a cave near the town of Catalunia, called Manresa. For an entire year, he knelt everyday for seven hours at a time, completely absorbed in prayer.

FROM THE CATECHISM

818 "However, one cannot charge with the sin of the separation those who at present are born into these communities [that resulted from such separation] and in them are brought up in the faith of Christ, and the Catholic Church accepts them with respect and affection as brothers.... All who have been justified by faith in Baptism are incorporated into Christ; they therefore have a right to be called Christians, and with good reason are accepted as brothers in the Lord by the children of the Catholic Church" (UR 3 § 1).

819 "Furthermore, many elements of sanctification and of truth" (LG 8 § 2) are found outside the visible confines of the Catholic Church: "the written Word of God; the life of grace; faith, hope, and charity, with the other interior gifts of the Holy Spirit, as well as visible elements" (UR 3 § 2; cf. LG 15). Christ's Spirit uses these Churches and ecclesial communities as means of salvation, whose power derives from the fullness of grace and truth that Christ has entrusted to the Catholic Church. All these blessings come from Christ and lead to him (cf. UR 3), and are in themselves calls to "Catholic unity" (cf. LG 8).

836 "All men are called to this catholic unity of the People of God.... And to it, in different ways, belong or are ordered: the Catholic faithful, others who believe in Christ, and finally all mankind, called by God's grace to salvation" (LG 13).

838 "The Church knows that she is joined in many ways to the baptized who are honored by the name of Christian, but do not profess the Catholic faith in its entirety or have not preserved unity or communion under the successor of Peter" (LG 15). Those "who believe in Christ and have been properly baptized are put in a certain, although imperfect, communion with the Catholic Church" (UR 3). With the Orthodox Churches, this communion is so profound "that it lacks little to attain the fullness that would permit a common celebration of the Lord's Eucharist" (Paul VI, Discourse, December 14, 1975; cf. UR 13-18).

849 The missionary mandate. "Having been divinely sent to the nations that she might be 'the universal sacrament of salvation,' the Church, in obedience to the command of her founder and because it is demanded by her own essential universality, strives to preach the Gospel to all men" (AG 1; cf. Mt 16:15): "Go therefore and make disciples of all nations, baptizing them in the name of the Father and of the Son and of the Holy Spirit, teaching them to observe all that I have commanded you; and Lo, I am with you always, until the close of the age" (Mt 28:19-20).

856 The missionary task implies a respectful dialogue with those who do not yet accept the Gospel (cf. RMiss 55). Believers can profit from this dialogue by learning to appreciate better "those elements of truth and grace which are found among peoples, and which are, as it were, a secret presence of God" (AG 9). They proclaim the Good News to those who do not know it, in order to consolidate, complete, and raise up the truth and the goodness that God has distributed among men and nations, and to purify them from error and evil "for the glory of God, the confusion of the demon, and the happiness of man" (AG 9).

905 Lay people also fulfill their prophetic mission by evangelization, "that is, the proclamation of Christ by word and the testimony of life." For lay people, "this evangelization... acquires a specific property and peculiar efficacy because it is accomplished in the ordinary circumstances of the world" (LG 35 § 1, § 2).

> This witness of life, however, is not the sole element in the apostolate; the true apostle is on the lookout for occasions of announcing Christ by word, either to unbelievers... or to the faithful. (AA 6 § 3; cf. AG 15)

FROM THE CATECHISM Continued

2104 "All men are bound to seek the truth, especially in what concerns God and his Church, and to embrace it and hold on to it as they come to know it" (DH 1 § 2). This duty derives from "the very dignity of the human person" (DH 2 § 1). It does not contradict a "sincere respect" for different religions which frequently "reflect a ray of that truth which enlightens all men" (NA 2 § 2) nor the requirement of charity, which urges Christians "to treat with love, prudence and patience those who are in error or ignorance with regard to the faith" (DH 14 § 4).

2105 The duty of offering God genuine worship concerns man both individually and socially. This is "the traditional Catholic teaching on the moral duty of individuals and societies toward the true religion and the one Church of Christ" (DH 1 § 3). By constantly evangelizing men, the Church works toward enabling them "to infuse the Christian spirit into the mentality and mores, laws and structures of the communities in which [they] live"

(AA 13 § 1). The social duty of Christians is to respect and awaken in each man the love of the true and the good. It requires them to make known the worship of the one true religion which subsists in the Catholic and apostolic Church (cf. DH 1). Christians are called to be the light of the world. Thus, the Church shows forth the kingship of Christ over all creation and in particular over human societies (cf. AA 13; Leo XIII, Immortale Dei 3, 17; Pius XI, Quas primas 8, 20).

2308 All citizens and all governments are obliged to work for the avoidance of war.

However, "as long as the danger of war persists and there is no international authority with the necessary competence and power, governments cannot be denied the right of lawful self-defense, once all peace efforts have failed" (GS 79 § 4).

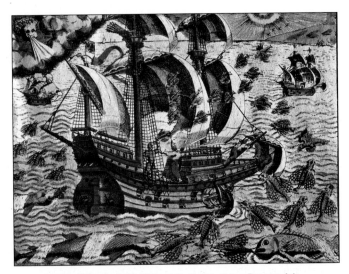

Ferdinand Magellan (1480-1521) was the first to sail from Europe to Asia, the first European to sail the Pacific Ocean, and the first to lead an expedition for the purpose of circumnavigating the globe. Though Magellan was killed in an attack by Philippine natives and never returned to Europe, eighteen members of his crew and one ship of the fleet returned to Spain in 1522, having circled the globe.

The Church And The Age Of Enlightenment

Out of the rubble of the religious wars rose strong monarchs who desired absolute control of their realms. Intellectuals focused on the individual and reason, challenging traditional philosophy and the Church.

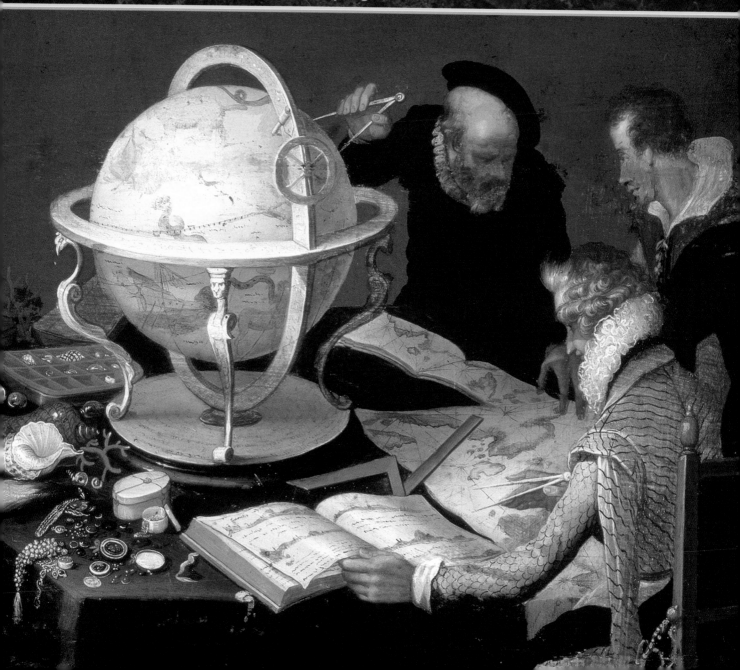

CHAPTER 7

The Church And The Age Of Enlightenment

The Reformation, and the wars that followed, brought to a close an era of a united Western Christendom. Out of the rubble of religious wars rose strong monarchs who looked to solidify control before their realms slipped back into internal turmoil. Typified by Louis XIV of France, monarchs began reorganizing their nations and assuming absolute power over their domains. Their efforts would unleash new tensions between kings and subjects, resulting in the emergence of constitutional monarchies together with various new political philosophies.

These new philosophies in significant part found their origins in the Renaissance and Reformation. They focused on the rights of the individual and the power of reason as a replacement for religious beliefs, which had caused so much tension in the past. Beginning with the scientific revolution in the seventeenth century, which significantly contributed to the eighteenth-century Age of Enlightenment, rulers, scientists, and philosophers throughout Europe challenged political authority, traditional philosophy, and the value of the Church. The proponents of the Enlightenment would conceive philosophies that would dismiss the guiding light of divine revelation and the Church's teaching authority. These new ideas, some of which were divorced from Christian principles, would give rise to revolutions that would do enormous harm to the Catholic Church.

The Church, in the aftermath of Trent, suffered over the wars of religion and the challenges of implementing the conciliar reforms. Throughout Europe, traditional beliefs and authority were being called constantly into question. The Church would have to contend with the increasing influence of civil rulers on Church matters and the influence of new ideas that eventually challenged the whole deposit of the Catholic Faith. Amid rising trends of atheism, agnosticism, and secularism, the Church would have to stand by her anchor, so well stated by St. John Paul II: "Jesus Christ alone is the adequate and final answer to the supreme question about the meaning of life and history!"

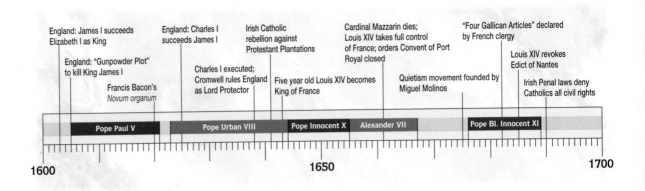

England: James I succeeds Elizabeth I as King

England: "Gunpowder Plot" to kill King James I

Francis Bacon's *Novum organum*

England: Charles I succeeds James I

Charles I executed; Cromwell rules England as Lord Protector

Irish Catholic rebellion against Protestant Plantations

Five year old Louis XIV becomes King of France

Cardinal Mazzarin dies; Louis XIV takes full control of France; orders Convent of Port Royal closed

Quietism movement founded by Miguel Molinos

"Four Gallican Articles" declared by French clergy

Louis XIV revokes Edict of Nantes

Irish Penal laws deny Catholics all civil rights

Pope Paul V | Pope Urban VIII | Pope Innocent X | Alexander VII | Pope Bl. Innocent XI

1600   1650   1700

PART I
King Louis's France

By the end of the Thirty Years War, France, too, was politically fragmented due to the recent religious conflicts and found herself composed of some three hundred feudal provinces. Against these obstacles, Richelieu worked to unify the country. He broadened the powers of the Bourbon kings and ended the toleration of Protestants. Henry IV's Edict of Nantes, he argued, created a state within a state, and for Richelieu, only strict loyalty to the King of France could provide effective cohesion in the realm. His policies cultivated a political environment ripe for a king to rule with absolute power over the entire country.

LOUIS XIV, THE SUN KING

Louis XIV ascended the throne in 1643 at the age of five. Too young to rule, power fell to another regent, Richelieu's successor, Cardinal Mazzarin. Mazzarin was so unpopular among the nobility that while Louis was still young, the nobility tried to rally against the king's rising power. The nobles came together to form an opposition group called the Fronde (French for "rebellion"). However, the Fronde was not a unified body, and Mazzarin was able to use the internal divisions between the nobles to suppress the rebellion. Rather than loosening the control of the king, the Fronde proved in

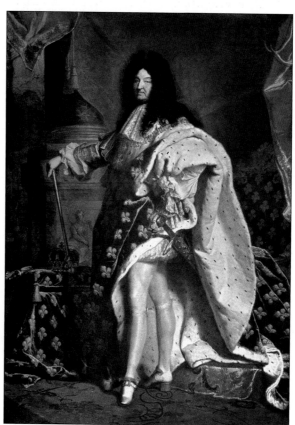

Louis XIV "The Sun King" (1638-1715) reigned as King of France and King of Navarre from May 14, 1643, until his death. As monarch, Louis saw himself as king and high priest, subject only to God. He felt a particular devotion to the Rosary and often made retreats in monasteries. On Holy Thursdays, Louis would kneel down, wash the feet of the poor in imitation of Christ, and serve them a meal. This famous portrait of Louis is by Hyacinthe Rigaud and records for us to see the extremes of power and vanity.

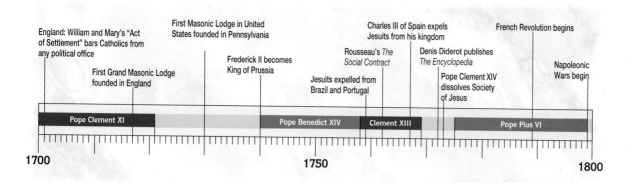

England: William and Mary's "Act of Settlement" bars Catholics from any political office

First Grand Masonic Lodge founded in England

First Masonic Lodge in United States founded in Pennsylvania

Frederick II becomes King of Prussia

Jesuits expelled from Brazil and Portugal

Rousseau's *The Social Contract*

Charles III of Spain expels Jesuits from his kingdom

Denis Diderot publishes *The Encyclopedia*

Pope Clement XIV dissolves Society of Jesus

French Revolution begins

Napoleonic Wars begin

Pope Clement XI | Pope Benedict XIV | Clement XIII | Pope Pius VI

1700   1750   1800

the mind of the young king the necessity to control powerful noble factions. When Mazzarin died in 1661, the twenty-three-year-old Louis took tight hold of the reins of power and for the next fifty-four years kept France firmly under his thumb.

To secure his power, Louis first dismissed all the great lords of France and anyone who could claim power through noble birth. The king freed these nobles from taxation in a shrewd move that in effect removed them from any interference in the affairs of his government. Instead, he turned the affairs of government over to persons belonging to minor families. Without any prior hope for such esteemed positions, these lower nobles felt eternally indebted to the king, assuring the king unfailing loyalty. He replaced the traditional feudal power structure with a central bureaucracy centered around himself.

GALLICANISM

Since the conflict between Pope Boniface VIII and King Philip IV in 1303, the relationship between the Church and the kings of France became strained. Throughout the Middle Ages, French kings attempted to control the affairs of the Church in France and appoint their own bishops. Philip IV asserted the independence of the French Church from Rome, and his successor Charles VII formally declared this independence with the Pragmatic Sanction of Bourges in 1438. Although in 1516 Pope Leo X persuaded Francis I to abolish the Pragmatic Sanction, the principles of an independent national or "Gallican" Church of France were deeply entrenched in the country. Louis XIV, who was strongly affected by the Gallican tradition, was a strong proponent of an independent Church in France.

Not surprisingly, as Louis XIV moved to control every aspect of French society, he especially tried to exert his influence over the Church in France. As monarch, Louis saw himself as king and high priest, subject only to God. This belief manifested itself in both his policies and his personal life. He was devoted to his faith and attended daily Mass. He felt a particular devotion to the Rosary and often made retreats in monasteries. On Holy Thursdays, Louis would kneel down, wash the feet of the poor in imitation of Christ, and serve them a meal. His actions were not a mere political show, but rather prompted by true religious sentiment. Louis exemplified an authentic spirituality that was rare for a king at the time.

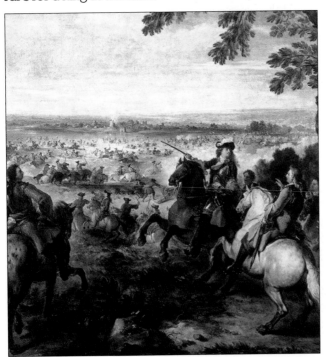

King Louis's difficulties with the Church arose over administration, not from matters of doctrine and spirituality. King Louis believed that everyone in France should be subject to his reign, both lay and clergy. He believed that his authority extended into matters of Church supervision and even doctrinal issues. In spite of his authoritarian disposition, Louis XIV tried to keep a delicate balance between his directives and those coming from the ecclesiastical authorities in Rome. Nevertheless, his relations with the Church often alternated between submission and schism.

The army of Louis XIV crosses the Rhine to attack the Netherlands in 1672. In a coalition with Charles II, France and England declared war on the Seven United Provinces (the Netherlands). Louis gained more territory in the Low Countries and regained the Franche-Comté (the former County of Burgundy) which France had lost to Spain in the 1668 Treaty of Aix-la-Chapelle.

It was not until 1693 that a compromise was reached. Louis XIV agreed to disavow the declarations of 1682 and end the mandatory teaching of the "Four Gallican Articles." In return, Bl. Innocent XI agreed to appoint all of the bishops Louis had nominated for the vacant sees in France. Despite this compromise, which respected the authority of Rome, the principles of Gallicanism continued to dominate the ecclesiastical community in France until the French Revolution in 1789, and would be resurrected again to a lesser degree within the Organic Articles of the 1801 Concordat.

JANSENISM

There were a number of heresies that were popular in France during the reign of Louis XIV, but none affected the nobility as profoundly as Jansenism. Jansenism is named after its founder

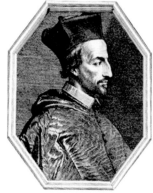

Cornelius Jansen (1585-1638), the Bishop of Ypres (Belgium). Early in his life, Jansen applied for entrance into the Jesuit order, but was rejected. A brilliant scholar, he nonetheless went on to become a priest and devoted himself to studying the works of St. Augustine of Hippo.

During his studies, Jansen became attracted to what he thought was a new way of understanding St. Augustine's understanding of grace. Believing he uncovered an overlooked truth of Catholicism, Jansen dedicated his life to formulating his own theory of grace and recording his ideas in his monumental work *Augustinus*.

The ideas of Jansen seemed to adapt a rigid Calvinist approach to Catholic teaching. According to the five principles of *Augustinus*, man was entirely free in the state of innocence and his will tended to do what was right. But original sin made man a slave to sin and all his actions

Cornelius Jansen

reflected a sin-ridden soul. His only hope was God's grace, which could save him. But Jansen taught that God only granted salvific grace to a small number of people. According to Jansen, Christ did not die for all men, since most people were predestined to damnation. The austere theology that grew out of these teachings eventually denied the validity of the Sacrament of Penance and taught that only the "just" or predestined should receive Holy Communion.

During his life, Jansen's ideas were unknown and the thinker himself never intended to contradict the Church's teachings. He shared his ideas with his close friend, Jean-Ambroise Duyegier, the Abbot of St. Cyran, and left his book to his friend for publication upon his death with the disclaimer to accept

whatever decision the Church made concerning his book. After Jansen died, Jean-Ambroise promoted his friend's work, and it soon became very popular throughout France and Belgium. Antoine Arnauld (1612-1694), a French philosopher who wrote his doctoral thesis on space, was closely associated with the famous convent which housed nuns of Jansenist persuasion, Port Royal, for three years. He effectively promoted the theology and thought of Cornelius Jansen. It is interesting to note that the celebrated French mathematician Blaise Pascal (1623-1662) wrote anonymously in defense of the spirit of Port Royal. In his writings he attacked the casuistry – at least according to his perception – of the Jesuits and advocated a more effective relationship with Christ.

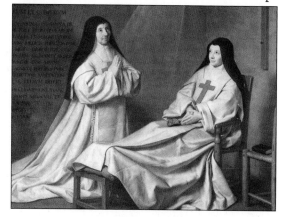

The Jansenist artist Philippe de Champaigne had two daughters educated at the Convent of Port Royal. One daughter, Catherine, remained there as a nun. This painting portrays the healing of his daughter's paralysis in 1661 by the prayers of the prioress, Mère Agnes Arnauld.

In 1653 Pope Innocent X condemned Jansenism and pointed to the teachings of the Council of Trent on God's grace to support his position. Innocent insisted that the Church teaches that God wills for everyone to be saved. God gives sufficient grace to each person for salvation, and everyone is given a free will which is designed to cooperate with God's grace. Trent taught that the Sacrament of Penance conferred sufficient grace to forgive all sins and that Holy Communion purifies the soul from venial sin and strengthens it against mortal sin.

Despite official condemnation, Jansenism continued to spread in France. After Pope Innocent X condemned Jansenism as heresy, Louis XIV saw the Jansenists as schismatic and threatening to his royal authority. He responded swiftly and strictly at the administrative and intellectual center of Jansenism, the Convent of Port Royal. As an extreme measure to erase the example of Port Royal and prevent the site from becoming a center of Jansenist pilgrimage, Louis ordered the entire convent razed in 1709 and had the bodies of the cemetery of the convent exhumed and placed in unmarked graves.

QUIETISM

Another heresy that developed during the reign of Louis XIV was Quietism. Founded around the year 1675 by a well-known confessor, Miguel Molinos, Quietism advocated absolute passivity during prayers and contemplation. The soul, according to Molinos, should be indifferent to everything, including temptation, and should simply rest perpetually in God. Unlike Jansenism, asceticism was not necessary, since it was sufficient for the soul to humble itself in order for God to accept someone with sins. Some Quietists even taught that God allowed demons to make persons perform sinful acts. One must make no effort to fight sin, they would say, but rather let the demon have his way. By stressing total abandonment in God, without the need for personal effort, the Quietist's spirituality leaned towards excessive comfort. Personal prayer and the Sacraments were unnecessary for the Quietist who believed merely in immersing oneself in God in order to find complete spiritual tranquility. Both King Louis XIV and Bl. Innocent XI condemned Quietism in 1687.

REVOCATION OF THE EDICT OF NANTES

In addition to suppressing the Jansenist and Quietist movements in France, King Louis XIV put a stop to the last vestiges of autonomy held by the Huguenots under the 1598 Edict of Nantes. Although Cardinal Richelieu had reduced the rights held by Protestants in France, Louis XIV demanded the abolition of all heretical movements. In 1681, Louis XIV granted special privileges to those who renounced Calvinism, and he deprived the Huguenots of many rights and privileges. Many insurrections broke out over Louis's actions, and although Bl. Innocent XI tried to encourage the king to be tolerant to Protestants living within France, Louis XIV saw the Huguenots as disloyal subjects and attempted to force conversion to the Catholic Faith. He revoked the Edict of Nantes in 1685 and prohibited the Huguenots from practicing their religion. Huguenot churches and schools were destroyed and congregations were banished from France. Many Huguenots fled to Prussia, England, and the Low Countries to escape Louis's persecution. Louis's actions resulted in retaliation against Catholics in countries like Ireland, England, and Holland, which were dominated by Protestant rulers.

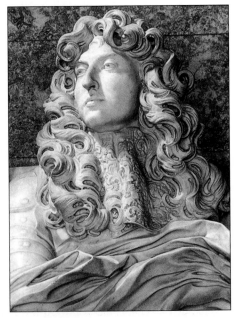

In October 1685, King Louis XIV issued the Edict of Fontainebleau, which revoked the 1598 Edict of Nantes.

PART II

The Stuart Kings of England

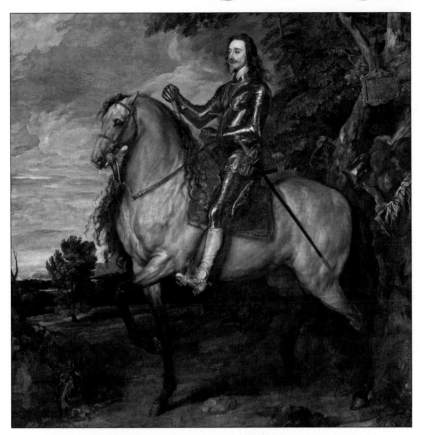

Charles I was king of England, Scotland and Ireland from March 27, 1625, until his execution on January 30, 1649. He engaged in a struggle for power with Parliament. He was an advocate of the divine right of kings. His struggles with ecclesiastical affairs–denying episcopal rights to the Scots and the victorious English parliamentarians–brought about his execution.

JAMES I AND CHARLES I

The death of Elizabeth I ended the Tudor line, and the son of Mary Queen of Scots, James I (a Stuart), succeeded Elizabeth to the throne in 1603. Despite his mother's fervent Catholic faith, James was raised a Protestant by Mary's half brother, and any question of James's affection for the Catholic Church was soon dispelled after the famed "Gunpowder Plot" of 1605. In the Gunpowder Plot, Guy Fawkes, a Catholic, plotted to blow up the king and Parliament. He failed, and in retribution, James renewed persecution of Catholics throughout England. Like Louis XIV, religion was very important to the English king as a means to solidify his authority. Under James I, Catholic education at home and abroad was totally prohibited. It was against the law to serve as a priest, and heavy fines were imposed on anyone who missed Anglican Sunday services.

Equally threatening to the king's power was the growing influence of Calvinism in England. James tolerated Puritan churches, but tithes had to be paid to the Anglican Church (to show loyalty to the English crown). Disgruntled by this taxation, a small band of Puritan separatists, called Pilgrims, left England during the reign of James I and set up a colony in the New World in September 1620.

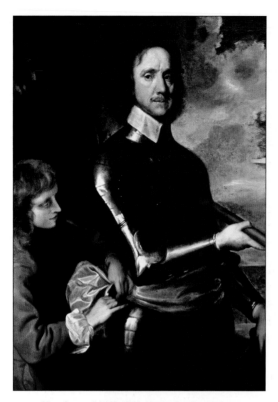

Oliver Cromwell (1599-1658). After leading the overthrow of the British monarchy and executing King Charles I, Cromwell ruled England, Scotland, and Ireland as Lord Protector until his death. During his ten year reign, a genocide was attempted against the Catholics of Ireland.

Catholics would also take advantage of the religious toleration that the New World offered, and in 1634 George Calvert received royal permission to create a colony in the New World as a refuge for Catholics. That colony, Maryland, was populated by more Catholics than any other English colony in the New World.

Charles I succeeded his father James in 1625. Unlike James, who was considered a foreigner from Scotland, Charles had been born in England, and he thought he could use the advantage of his English heredity to expand the limits of royal authority. Charles tried to increase royal revenues and centralize the English bureaucracy around the crown. However, without guarantees of religious toleration, the Calvinist-dominated Parliament refused to grant Charles enough money to carry out his policies. Charles responded by ruling on his own without Parliament for twelve years. When a war with Scotland broke out, Charles was forced to convene Parliament to help raise much-needed troops. The war did not go well for the king, and after attempting to force Anglican uniformity on his Scottish and Puritan subjects, the English Civil War of 1642-1649 broke out. Out of the war rose the Calvinist dictator Oliver Cromwell who seized power, established a harsh puritanical regime, and beheaded King Charles I.

Cromwell ruled England as "Lord Protector" from 1648 to 1658. His inability to come to terms with both the King and Parliament forced him to establish his own rule in the form of a military dictatorship based on Puritan principles. During his decade-long reign, Catholic faithful throughout the British Isles were persecuted with great vigor, and especially the people of Ireland suffered terribly.

PERSECUTION OF THE IRISH

Catholics in Ireland had suffered persecution ever since the time of Henry VIII. As English Protestant rulers worked to secure their power, they promoted successive policies designed to eradicate the Catholic population from the Emerald Isle. Irish bishops and priests were executed and exiled, access to even the most elementary of educations denied, lands seized, famine frequent, Masses and the sacraments illegal, and the Irish language (Gaelic) forbidden.

The situation in Ireland grew even worse under James I who established the first "Plantations" on the island. Plantations were large areas in the northeastern part of the island that were cleared of Catholics (without compensation for the lands) and resettled by Scottish Protestants. The idea was that the Protestants would eventually "breed-out" the Catholics. The effects of this policy are still felt today as both Catholic and Protestant Irish feel that they have a hereditary right to the land in Northern Ireland, thus making peace in the region terribly difficult. In 1641, rebellion broke throughout Ireland in retaliation to the Protestant "Planters," and about three thousand Protestants were killed.

After Oliver Cromwell defeated Charles I in 1648, he led a military campaign throughout Ireland. Cromwell entered Ireland with ten thousand troops, and at Drogheda and Wexford, his forces massacred every defender. Entire towns were destroyed, and properties were confiscated and given to the Protestants. Cromwell planned to create a huge plantation that covered most of Ireland. He sought to kill one-third of all Catholics in Ireland and enslave another third, forcibly raising their children Protestant. The remainder of Ireland, the most destitute portion, was to become a penal colony. Although Cromwell failed to destroy the Catholic Faith in Ireland, his invasion turned the country into a wasteland.

In 1691, the Irish Penal Laws attempted to destroy the Catholic Faith by enslaving the Irish population. Catholics were denied education, land ownership, and medical practice and treatment. Catholics were not allowed to enter the legal profession nor could they hold government offices. These harsh and oppressive regimes brought about a greater unity among the Irish and increased their loyalty to the Church of Rome. The Irish continued to suffer official persecution until the nineteenth century.

RISE OF PARLIAMENTARY DEMOCRACY IN ENGLAND

After the death of Oliver Cromwell in 1658, Parliament returned power to the sons of Charles I. Learning from his father's failed attempts to impose absolutist rule, Charles II ruled England with tact and care. He was sympathetic to Catholics because he spent most of his exile in France, under the protection of Louis XIV. As king he tolerated the Catholic religion, but kept his measures discreet so as not to agitate the still prevalent anti-Catholic sentiment. Charles II allowed Catholics to practice their Faith in the privacy of their own homes and let some prominent Catholics become his advisors.

In 1678, a group of Protestants led by Titus Oates accused the Catholic minority of plotting a French invasion of England and with it the massacre of all prominent Protestants. Although completely fabricated, the imagined "Popish Plot" brought pressure on Charles to renew persecution of Catholics in England, and a wave of anti-Catholic witch-hunts spread through England.

In 1685, Catholics became hopeful when Charles II died without an heir. His brother, James II, had converted to the Catholic Faith while in exile in France, and many Catholics hoped his rise to the throne might reestablish Catholicism in England. The Protestant-dominated Parliament was wary of Catholic succession, and they only allowed the elderly James to claim the crown because his daughter and successor, Mary, was Protestant.

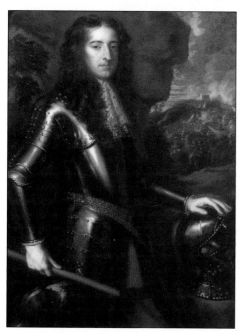

In 1688 James II's young, Catholic wife gave birth to a son who was baptized Catholic. This new successor, a threat to the Protestant claim to the crown, provoked Parliament to take direct measures to protect England against Catholic succession. They responded by claiming the "right to revolution" put forth in John Locke's Two Treatises on Government. According to this principle, Locke argued that whenever a monarch violated the social contract with his subjects, the people had the right to replace the ruler with someone of their own choosing. Claiming that James II had violated the social contract, the English launched the bloodless "Glorious Revolution" of 1688, in which James II was forced to abdicate

William III of England (1650-1702), also known as William III of Orange-Nassau, was a Dutch aristocrat and the Holy Roman Empire's Prince of Orange from birth. Born a member of the House of Orange-Nassau, William III won the English, Scottish and Irish Crowns following the Glorious Revolution, during which his uncle and father-in-law, James II, was deposed. He ruled jointly with his wife, Mary II, until her death in 1694. He is affectionately known as "King Billy" among Protestants in Scotland and Northern Ireland.

the throne and place power in the hands of William of Orange, his son-in-law, and Mary, his Protestant daughter. To help strengthen the new monarchy, the English Parliament allowed itself to be taxed and then used the funds to help centralize the government around the new rulers. In the English Bill of Rights of 1689, Parliament agreed to share power with the king, creating a governmental system called a "Constitutional Monarchy" that blended the monarchical and republican (parliamentary) systems.

William and Mary worked to ensure that the crown remained free from Catholic possession. In 1701, they passed the "Act of Settlement" which barred Catholics from politics and prohibited Catholics from sitting on the throne. Later "Test Acts" would add that no Catholic could practice a profession or even attend university within the British Isles. Over time, these laws would virtually remove any Catholic presence in England.

PART III

The Scientific Revolution and the Age of Enlightenment

The great scientific discoveries of the seventeenth century laid the foundation for what is known as the Age of Enlightenment. This intellectual movement sprang up from a wholehearted enthusiasm for, and faith in, scientific progress. As scientific discoveries began to prove the effectiveness of human reason and show that scientific knowledge could be useful in many areas of human life, many began to believe that the study of science and nature could help correct all the problems of society, including poverty, disease, and war.

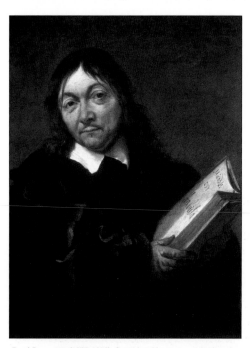

René Descartes (1596-1650). Considered by many as the founder of modern philosophy and the father of modern mathematics, he influenced generations of philosophers

But with this deep-rooted belief in the potential of scientific thought came a new skepticism. Soon, everything that did not fall under the umbrella of scientific explanation was dismissed or regarded with disdain. For the thinkers of the Enlightenment, what could not be proved could not be called true. Rationalism took precedence over faith, and reason became the guiding principle of this new philosophy.

DESCARTES AND BACON

The Frenchman René Descartes was a brilliant mathematician whose achievements include, among others, the invention of coordinate geometry (called "Cartesian geometry" in his honor). He had a superb mathematical mind, which ultimately led him to consider the universe in mechanistic terms. In his writings, Descartes would describe the world mathematically, hoping to attain for philosophy the same kind of absolute certainty provided by the clarity of mathematical demonstration. He proposed to sweep away traditional learning and replace it with a new system based on logical reasoning and certain proof.

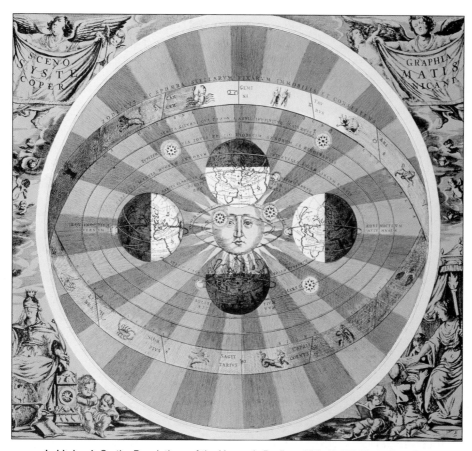

In his book *On the Revolutions of the Heavenly Bodies* published in 1543, Nicolas Copernicus postulated a heliocentric (sun-centered) system of the universe. His theory inaugurated the scientific revolution.

In 1637, Descartes published his celebrated treatise called Discourse on Method in which he advanced his principle of "systematic doubt." Given the subjective knowledge of every individual, Descartes questioned the possibility of achieving knowledge with absolute certainty. Human knowledge was flawed, Descartes argued, since it was never assured of clear certainty. Only the awareness of one's own existence was certain because even if one doubts his existence, he knows that he exists in order to be able to doubt. "Cogito ergo sum," he famously posited, "I think, therefore I am" (cf. Discourse on Method, chapter 4). By dismissing the validity of any understanding that was not based on empirical, provable data, Descartes unwittingly placed a huge wedge between Faith and reason.

Another thinker who contributed to the growth of scientific inquiry was the Englishman Sir Francis Bacon. Like Descartes, Bacon held that reason provided a true and reliable method of knowledge. Bacon advocated that this knowledge would help man control nature, and contribute to the wealth and comfort of civilization. Bacon described his new method of acquiring knowledge in his Novum organum, published in 1620. Moving away from the Aristotelian view of knowledge through logical deduction proceeding from general principles, Bacon posited that knowledge must originate from specific observations to a more general theory. This new "inductive" method involved the collection of vast quantities of empirical data from which general principles could be derived. Known as empiricism, this new philosophy gathered knowledge through observation and experience as a way of understanding how things worked. Bacon's methods showed how knowledge could produce many practical advancements to improve the quality of life.

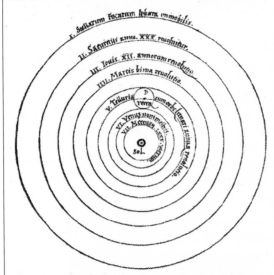

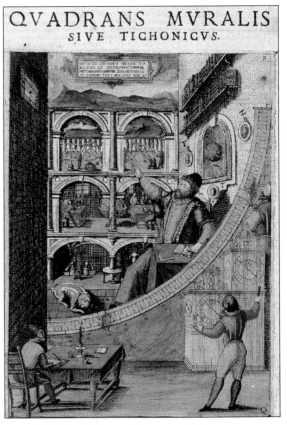

The diagram that shook the world, in chapter 10 of Book I of Copernicus's "On the Revolutions of the Heavenly Bodies" (*De revolutionibus orbium coelestium*). In the Copernican system the Earth is given three distinct motions: a daily axial rotation, an annual rotation about the Sun, and a third motion related to precession.

A tinted engraving from Tycho Brahe's 1598 publication *Astronomiae instaurata mechanica*. The illustration shows Tycho and his Great Quadrant at Uraniborg. The accuracy of this instrument, based on comparison with eight reference stars, has been estimated to 34.6 seconds of arc.

A NEW UNDERSTANDING OF THE UNIVERSE

All the way through the Medieval Era, people had been satisfied with the Greek Ptolemaic (earth-centered) view of the universe that believed that all the heavenly bodies revolved around the earth. This model of the universe, with the earth at its center, squares well with observations from earth and a Scriptural-Christian understanding of Heaven and earth. It also accurately explains the movement of the stars, sun, and planets of the cosmos. As thinkers challenged traditional explanations and based knowledge on observation, small errors began to be discovered which made the Ptolemaic model untenable. The Polish priest and astronomer Nicolas Copernicus suspected that the Ptolemaic model was erroneous after having made mathematical analyses and calculations of the rotation of the earth. In his book On the Revolutions of the Heavenly Bodies published in 1543, he postulated that the sun, rather than the earth, was the center of the universe. Although he believed the earth to be the actual, physical center of the universe, Copernicus argued that a sun-centered model made it much easier because it was easier to calculate planetary motions than in the Ptolemaic model. A seemingly small matter, the Copernican model would elicit a debate that would change the way man perceived the universe.

In the spirit of Bacon and Descartes (observation and mathematical demonstration), two scientists' work seemed to theoretically prove the Copernican model. From 1576 until his death in 1601, Danish astronomer Tycho Brahe devoted his life to plotting the movements of the stars, modifying the Ptolemaic (earth-centered) model along the way. Through his meticulous observations, Brahe discovered that the planets moved in elliptical, not circular, orbits. Following Brahe's death in 1601, his assistant, German astronomer and mathematician Johannes Kepler, devised a mathematical formula that described planetary motion, thereby verified the Copernican model. Kepler's theories translated the concrete world of matter into mathematical form; thus, Brahe's observations and Kepler's interpretations gave birth to modern scientific observation and experimentation (the "scientific method").

GALILEO GALILEI AND THE SCIENTIFIC METHOD

The future of scientific development was reinforced by the work of the Italian scientist Galileo Galilei. Prior to Galileo, theorists simply made observations to form general principles. Galileo, however, seeing science as a useful tool for solving practical matters, applied the principle of experimentation to reach verifiable conclusions. Through his experiments, Galileo began to offer hard evidence for the theories of other scientists. He combined observation, experimentation, and application into a new "scientific method" that standardized the study of the different areas of natural science.

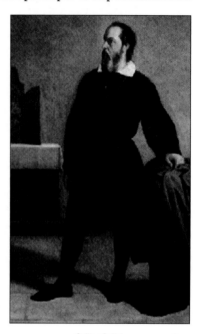

Galileo Galilei

Galileo's use of the scientific method allowed him to draw many verifiable conclusions about the workings of the natural world. Through his use of the telescope (developed by Dutch lens grinders in 1604), Galileo observed that the planets were constructed from the same material as earth. Galileo also proved the validity of the Copernican system that claims identical conclusions for both the earth and heavenly bodies. He was increasingly popular among the people since he could explain complex scientific breakthroughs in a simple manner. Galileo's new methodology and his findings would pave the way for Newton's laws of motion.

Unfortunately, Galileo's new discoveries came at a time when many churchmen were growing increasingly defensive and wary of science. During the Protestant Reformation, the Church had come under attack for advocating human reason and Scholastic education to the neglect of the study of Sacred Scripture. The great patron and supporter of education in all intellectual pursuits, the Church, was now trying to give greater emphasis to using Scripture to explain her origins. Balancing the pressure to remain faithful to the gospel with new and challenging scientific advancements would prove to be a difficult task, resulting in some unfortunate decisions by several churchmen.

Some of Galileo's observations contradicted prevalent interpretations of Scripture, and his theories brought him into conflict with ecclesiastical authority. Attempting to demonstrate faithful adherence to Sacred Scripture, ecclesiastical authorities condemned the theories of Galileo and required him to abandon his ideas. Galileo agreed to the condemnation under protest and continued to pursue his studies in astronomy. Despite the scientist's defiance, Pope Paul V and his successor Gregory X continued to support Galileo.

In 1632, Galileo presented his greatest work: Dialogue on the Two Chief Systems of the World. In it he defended the Copernican theory of the universe and ridiculed the geocentric (earth-centered) position. (Pope Urban VIII understood the geocentric fool "Simplicio" to be himself.) Ecclesiastical authorities again objected to Galileo's writings, and they asked that he present his findings as a hypothesis rather than a declaration. Galileo refused, and he was arrested and held in confinement at palaces in Siena and Florence. During this confinement, Galileo pursued his work and research.

PART IV

The Protagonists of the Enlightenment and its Effects

The Enlightenment would dominate the intellectual culture of Europe throughout the eighteenth century as thinkers and rulers alike would endeavor to implement ideas derived from the Enlightenment. The proponents of this new philosophy, called the philosophes, would become authorities on virtually all issues. Their work and influence would lay the foundation for the cultural, social, and political revolutions that would blossom in the late eighteenth and nineteenth centuries.

DEISM AND MASONRY

The greatest setback to the Church during the Enlightenment was the philosophes' rejection of Divine revelation and supernatural religion. The philosophes believed that all knowledge ought to be based on demonstration by the light of human reason. In keeping with the rationalistic position, the philosophes came up with a notion of God and his relationship to the world called Deism. Deism is a rationalist philosophy that accepted the principle of a first cause (similar to a creator) but denied divine intervention or providence in the world. These Deists saw God as a kind of great watchmaker who created the universe with laws and guiding principles that were "wound up," and then left to man's discovery and domination.

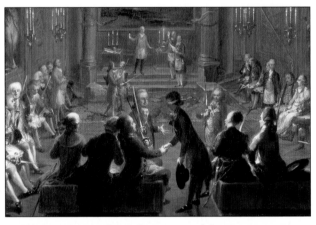

This painting depicts the initiation of Mozart into a lodge of the Freemasons. Mozart's last opera, *The Magic Flute,* includes Masonic themes and allegory. He was in the same Masonic Lodge as Joseph Haydn.

Deists believed that God did not demand faith, nor require prayers. God does not intervene in the world, and graces and blessings seen as expressions of God's loving providence should be considered absurd and impossible. Only reason – not divine assistance – is necessary to guide an individual through a life of decency, generosity, and honesty.

By 1717, many Deists had organized into a secret fraternal organization known as the Freemasons. Freemasonry quickly became an efficient vehicle for spreading rationalistic ideas, and many eighteenth-century leaders were members (including Americans George Washington and Benjamin Franklin, Britain's Edmund Burke, the Frenchman Voltaire, and Italian nationalists Giuseppe Mazzini and Giuseppe Garibaldi). Masonry is a Deistic sect that sees God as the grand architect of the universe and bases its practices, rules, and organization on Enlightenment philosophy and reason. More than simply dismissing Christian beliefs, Freemasons secretly have worked to destroy the Catholic Church and undermine her influence. Especially in the past, they have directly opposed the Church in many areas and are overtly antagonistic to organized religion. For example, Masons often cremated their dead as a way of flouting the Christian concept of the resurrection of the body, daring God to put back together what they had destroyed. Pope Clement XII in 1738 and Pope Benedict XIV in 1751 condemned Masonry, as well as has seven popes since; in 1884 Pope Leo XIII wrote the lengthy encyclical Humanum genus (The Race of Man) in condemnation of Freemasonry.

VOLTAIRE

France emerged as the intellectual center of the Enlightenment, and it produced the most influential thinkers of the time. Francois-Marie Arouet, better known as Voltaire, was one of the most renowned writers of the Encyclopedia, and became one of the period's most prominent thinkers associated with the Enlightenment.

Voltaire was Jesuit-educated, but as he grew older, his writing grew increasingly more anti-religious, and his hatred for Christianity became one of the main driving forces in his works. He habitually attacked Catholic dogma, the priesthood, Sacred Scripture, and even Christ himself. In his writings, Voltaire wrongly attributed to Christianity some of the greatest historical atrocities. Above all, his hatred of intolerance fueled Voltaire's attacks against the Church, and his fierce reaction to Catholicism was propelled by what he saw as the intolerance of the Church in France. He loved England, on the other hand, where he saw many different religions co-existing side by side.

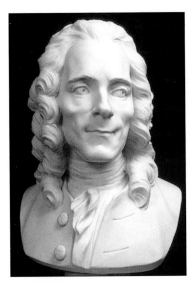

Francois-Marie Arouet (1694-1778), known by the pen name Voltaire, was an influential French Enlightenment writer, satirist, Deist and philosopher.

Voltaire thought that belief in God and the discernment between good and evil arose from reason alone, and he argued for natural religion and natural morality. For Voltaire, Christianity was a foolish and absurd religion that developed only to keep the masses quiet. He was the first to present a purely secular view of world history, presenting Christianity and other religions of the world as merely human invention and opinion.

As far as personal religious beliefs were concerned, Voltaire remained an enigmatic character throughout his life. He criticized Catholicism severely in his works, but built a Catholic chapel on his property, attended Mass, and had sermons read to him during solitary meals. Voltaire even belonged to a Catholic lay order and requested a Catholic burial after his death. Even though he could boast as one of Christianity's most bitter opponents, Voltaire allegedly repented at the end of his life. In spite of everything, his love for toleration did not exclude those good works and ideas of members of the Church, and he was partially won over by the intellectual and pious Pope Benedict XIV. Voltaire even dedicated one of his works to Benedict with the epitaph, "To the vicar of the God of Truth and meekness."

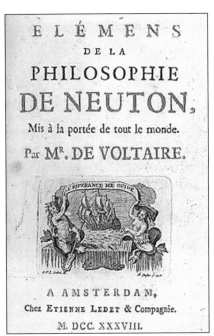

ELÉMENS
DE LA
PHILOSOPHIE
DE NEUTON,
Mis à la portée de tout le monde.
Par Mʳ. DE VOLTAIRE.

A AMSTERDAM,
Chez ETIENNE LEDET & Compagnie.
M. DCC. XXXVIII.

Voltaire's *Elements of the Philosophy of Newton* (1738) was the most important conduit for Newton's new system of natural philosophy in France. Voltaire's admiration for Newton is also evident in his letters on Newton in *Letters Concerning the English Nation.*

ROUSSEAU

Jean-Jacques Rousseau was born in 1712 to a lower-class Swiss family. Rousseau complained throughout his life that he was misunderstood and neglected as a child. As an adult, Rousseau was quite resigned to having no social status and no money. Instead of marrying, he had a mistress who bore him five children whom he deposited into an orphanage. By the age of forty, Rousseau

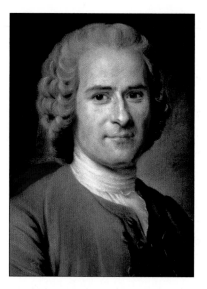

Jean-Jacques Rousseau

was still poor and unknown. Only after his work was discovered did he skyrocket into popular acclaim and thereby considered as one of the most profound writers of his age.

Rousseau drew much of his work from his own life experiences. He blamed society for all of man's difficulties. "Man was born free," said Rousseau, "but everywhere he is in chains" (cf. Social Contract, I.1). Rousseau believed society created rules to subjugate individual freedom. He saw man as naturally good, but society forced him to be a creature of violence and falsehood. If man were restored to his original liberty and equality, he believed, every human being would flourish. Rousseau imagined a primitive state of nature in which man was happy and innocent.

Rousseau's chief work, The Social Contract, espoused his principles of liberty and equality. He argued that individuals should not be subject to anyone, and any subjection to authority was contrary to man's nature. However, for the sake of protection, people agreed to form societies. Since the people allowed themselves to be governed, Rousseau reasoned that political authority came from the people, not from God. Free individuals living in a society created a "social contract" through which the people would choose an authority whose task was to rule and legislate.

FEBRONIANISM AND JOSEPHINISM

Protestantism offered European princes an ideological foundation for their expansive ambitions. Having neither legal nor religious ties to the Catholic Church, Protestant princes could now control and influence all aspects of society. It was much more difficult for Catholic leaders to have absolute domination within their territory since the ecclesiastical hierarchy wielded significant moral authority. To achieve greater independence from Rome, both secular and Church leaders embraced a Gallican view of the Church. Long condemned by the Church, these Gallican ideas spread throughout Catholic states in part because they seemed to offer a viable way for Catholic rulers to compete with their Protestant neighbors. Furthermore, in an age of burgeoning nationalism, Gallicanism offered the possibilities of greater independence on both the secular and ecclesiastical fronts.

Gallican influence entered Germany through the writings of Johann Nikolaus von Hontheim, the auxiliary bishop of Trier, who wrote under the pen name of Febronius. Febronius argued that the pope was merely an administrative head of the Church who did not have the power to legislate laws. He denied both the primacy of the pope over other bishops and his authority to speak definitively on matters of Faith and morals. Febronius rehashed arguments from conciliarism that stated that the ultimate authority of the Church rests on ecumenical councils and not the bishop of Rome. He urged the German bishops to assert their independence from Rome and called upon the secular authorities to abandon their allegiance to the pope and seize jurisdictional authority of their churches and ecclesiastical landholdings.

Pope Clement XIII was quick to condemn the writings of Febronius, and in 1764, he urged the German bishops to reject his teachings and suppress their diffusion. Febronius made a halfhearted retraction in 1778, but his writings continued to be quite influential, especially in inspiring German nationalism within the Church. A few of the German bishops employed arguments taken from Febronius's work to assert their independence from Rome, but their dissention did not take a strong hold among the majority of the German bishops. Eventually, all but one bishop pledged their fidelity and allegiance to Rome. Febronius reconciled himself with the Church before his death in 1790.

Joseph II's mother, Maria-Theresa, was responsible for many reforms in Austria. Maria-Theresa was a devout Catholic, and her court is widely viewed as the most moral in Europe. Just, efficient, and patient, she unified the loose-knit Austrian territories through a well-maintained bureaucracy that abolished internal tariffs and created the largest free trade zone in Europe. She improved the situation of the serfs in her country by passing laws to protect them against abuses of their rights and limited their service. Her good rule and sensible reforms helped maintain stability in Austria after a series of conflicts with neighboring German princes.

Joseph II of Austria regrettably espoused the ideas of Febronius, and the state of Austria would eventually suffer for it. Contrary to Maria-Theresa's prudence and good sense, her son, Joseph II, was impulsive and impatient and resented the slow pace of reform. He thought his mother was unnecessarily cautious and believed that he could change the Austrian state much more quickly. Much of Joseph's headstrong behavior was a result of an education imbued by principles of the Enlightenment. Seeing himself as a philosophe and encouraged by the success of Frederick the Great of Prussia, Joseph embraced the principles of Febronianism and set out to establish progressive policies in Austria.

Joseph II launched massive reforms to bring uniformity into the Austrian empire. He abolished local governments, removed privileges from nobles and free cities, and created one of the first secret police forces. Moreover, he mandated that the German language be spoken by all his subjects, a policy that alienated the Hungarians under his rule. Irritated with the slow progress of his mother's reforms, Joseph II attempted to free them with a single stroke of the pen. This quick remedy to the problem of serfdom in fact brought economic disaster to Austria. Although there was a certain wisdom in Joseph's reforms, the lack of prudence and sensitivity with which he instituted them alienated the nobility and angered his subjects.

Joseph's desire to exercise absolute, enlightened authority prompted him to dominate the Church in almost every area of its competence and jurisdiction. He insisted that all papal documents be approved by his office before publication and forbade the bishops of Austria to communicate directly with Rome, forcing them to take an oath of allegiance to the king. Joseph was especially influential in the seminary system of his

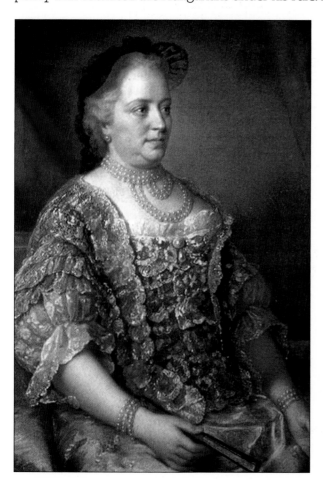

Maria Theresa (1717-1780), Holy Roman Empress.
A Habsburg by birth and one of the most powerful women of her time, she ruled over most of central Europe. Maria Theresa was married to Francis Stephen of Lorraine with whom she had sixteen children, six daughters (all named "Marie" including the future Queen of France, Marie Antoinette) and five sons surviving to adulthood (including the future emperors Joseph II and Leopold II). She recognized Joseph II, her eldest son, as co-regent and emperor, but allowed him only limited power because she felt he was rash and arrogant.

country. He required all prospective priests to study in Austrian seminaries under his control. The seminarians were required to use a watered-down catechism that Joseph authorized, and the seminary professors were restricted to preaching on moral subjects and barred from teaching Catholic doctrine. Monasteries that Joseph thought served no practical purpose were suppressed, and religious communities were cut off from their superiors in Rome. Joseph micro-managed the Austrian Church to the extreme extent of determining the number of candles used for Mass.

Unfortunately for Joseph II and Austria, the emperor's reforms began to unravel before his death. The emperor recognized his mistakes and tried to rectify the situation, but in many cases it was too late. In one instance, much to his embarrassment, when the Austrian Netherlands rose in rebellion, Joseph II was forced to turn to the pope in the hopes that he could persuade the Belgians to return to their original allegiance with Joseph. Despite Joseph's promises to withdraw his restrictions on the Church, it was too late to save Austrian control of the Netherlands. Joseph II recognized his incompetent leadership, and tragically wrote his own epitaph: "Here lies a prince whose intentions were pure, but who had the misfortune to see all his projects fail" (quoted in Harney, The Catholic Church through the Ages, 1974, p. 452). He died alone, after a ten-year reign, in 1790, the same year as Febronius.

SUPPRESSION OF THE JESUITS

As secular rulers rose to power, they sought to suppress all opposition that could seriously hinder the exercise of their authority. Any groups associated with the old order of European rule were seen as a danger to progress and prosperity. The Jesuit order had long been influential in Europe. They served as advisors to all the Catholic rulers and noble houses throughout Europe and held

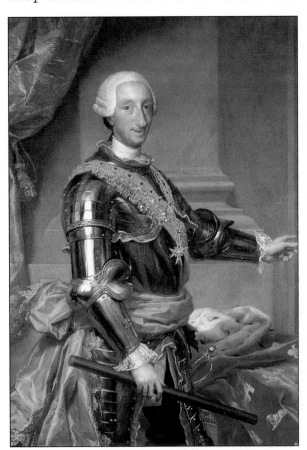

a large number of key positions at the major universities. Founded to help counteract the Protestant Reformation, the Jesuits were well educated, well connected, and well established. The order was dedicated to the service of the pope, and their missionary success brought millions to the Church of Rome. In short, there was no other Catholic order or group that could seriously counteract the rationalist ideology Enlightenment as the Jesuits. As the philosophes grew increasingly dominant, the Jesuits became more and more the object of severe hatred for their intellectual prowess and loyalty to the pope.

Typically, the Jesuits were accused of all types of criminal intrigue. All of the major ministers of Europe at the time were disciples of the Enlightenment and had at their disposal the military and police power of the state. They controlled the press and helped shape public opinion against the Church and the Jesuit Order. By 1767, through the actions of these powerful secular authorities, the Jesuit Order

Charles III (1716-1788), King of Spain, was an "enlightened despot." He expelled the Jesuits from Spain and South America in 1767.

was banished from Portugal, France, Spain, and the Kingdom of Naples. French and Italian princes threatened Pope Clement XIII, but he did not support them in their general antagonism against the Jesuits, remaining firm in his support of the order until his death.

Prime Minister Pombal of Portugal was the first to attack and banish the Society of Jesus. Educated in London and trained in the philosophy of the Enlightenment, Pombal was avidly anti-Christian and believed the Church was a threat and hinderance to his secular leadership in Portugal. He was not entirely misled. The Jesuits had strongly opposed Pombal's foreign policy and for a long time attacked Portugal's leading role in the slave trade. However, the lucrative reward of suppressing the order was far more enticing than the moral counsel the Jesuits offered. Portugal had gained territory from Spain in 1754 near the Jesuit missions in Paraguay and Brazil, and the Portuguese now desired to extend their territory and wealth by annexing lands protected by the Jesuit missionaries. When the Guarani tribes of Paraguay launched fierce resistance against the Portuguese, burning their lands rather than turning them over, Pombal blamed the Jesuits for inciting the Guarani rebellion. This was only one of the many national tragedies that were pawned off on the Jesuits. After an attempted assassination of the King of Portugal, Pombal accused prominent Jesuits of plotting the assassination. Without trial, many Jesuits were condemned to life imprisonment, many dying of illness and neglect. Although the pope protested, Pombal banished the papal nuncio and had an eighty-year-old Jesuit who protested that action strangled and then burned alive.

France and Spain were quick to follow the lead of Portugal. By 1754, Gallicans, Jansenists, self-proclaimed philosophes, and even the mistress of Louis XV worked to suppress the Jesuits in France. In 1767, D'Aranda, the president of the council of Castile and a close friend of Voltaire, convinced King Charles III of Spain that the Jesuits were inciting riots and were spreading rumors of the King's illegitimacy. Using evidence planted by agents of D'Aranda, Charles III condemned and banished all the Jesuits from his kingdom. He confiscated all Jesuit properties throughout Spain and South America, leaving more than five hundred thousand faithful in the missions without priests. Nearly six thousand Jesuits were forced to leave Spain.

After the suppression of the Jesuits in Spain, a campaign spread against the entire order. In 1768, French troops took over Avignon, and Neapolitan troops took over papal duchies in central Italy. With mounting military and political pressure at his doorstep, the pope was being threatened with deposition if he did not take actions against the Jesuits. Clement XIII refused to give in to the Bourbon demands, but the resistant pontiff died in February 1769. The new pope, Clement XIV, was faced with new ultimatums from Spain to destroy all religious orders throughout its realm and cut off the Church in Spain entirely from the Holy See. The pope delayed action for two years, hoping that he could restore peace and security within the Church. Finally, in 1773, under heavy pressure, Clement XIV issued his brief Dominus ac Redemptor that dissolved the Society of Jesus. The pope, and others in the Church, saw the action as merely an administrative measure meant to restore peace and tranquility to the Church. No blame was placed on the Jesuits and it did not impugn the orthodoxy of their doctrines. Jesuit priests simply became part of the diocesan clergy and were allowed in some places to continue as professors of universities. However, the execution of the dissolution was left to the local bishops, resulting in widely varied treatment of the Jesuits (Livingstone, The Oxford Dictionary of the Christian Church, 1997, p. 498).

Unfortunately for Clement, the suppression of the Society of Jesus did not restore tranquility to the Church. Confident of their success against the Jesuits, secular rulers continued to make demands upon the papacy. Although Clement's successor, Pius VI, tried to restore order, the ensuing revolution in France made that impossible. During the French Revolution, forty-four Jesuits were martyred, and of those, twenty-three are now beatified. Former Jesuit priests continued their work despite the suppression, and in 1814, forty years after their suppression, Pope Pius VII solemnly restored the Society of Jesus throughout the world.

PART V

From Revolution to Republic

THE OLD RÉGIME: THREE ESTATES

Before the revolution, French society was legally divided into three "estates" or classes. These three main social divisions included the clergy, nobility, and the commoners (everybody else). Clearly, these class distinctions were a remnant of the Medieval age and were no longer compatible with the political and economic changes of the time.

By 1789, there were about 100,000 clerics in France out of a total population of 24,000,000. Nonetheless, the Church played a significant role as both guardian and guide for society. For instance, the Catholic Church was connected to virtually every charitable institution, from orphanages and hospitals to schools and universities. The Church also took responsibility for unemployment compensation and distribution of food to the destitute. All these services were a costly endeavor, and understandably required tithes from the people. In addition to the tithe, landholdings provided a vast source of wealth for the ecclesiastical hierarchy charged with Church administration. By 1789, the Church of France was the largest landholder in the kingdom, owning approximately one-fifth of the total lands available.

In addition to serving the many who were in need, some of the clergy served as regents to the kings and advisors to the nobility, making themselves available for spiritual guidance and political advice. Although the special services given to the king and the aristocracy gave those particular clerics special honor and prestige, it tended to shift their loyalties more to the state than to the Church.

This **First Estate**, comprised of clergy, was itself divided between wealthy and influential clerics and the great majority of poor parish priests. Most of the priests lived simple and impoverished lives no different from the people to whom they ministered. This great disparity within the Church in France showed the urgent need for reform. Unfortunately, the excessive resistance of kings, nobles, and wealthy clerics to the mandates of the papacy severely compromised the implementation of the Tridentine Reforms.

The **Second Estate** consisted of about 400,000 nobles. Since the death of Louis XIV, these noble aristocrats enjoyed a resurgence of power, and again they began to exercise some of their traditional feudal privileges. They exempted themselves from taxation and blocked every attempt at modernizing France's economic structure. Because of those self-serving exemptions, France's tax coffers remained empty, despite being the wealthiest country of eighteenth-century Europe.

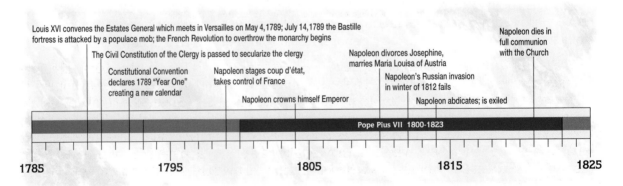

Louis XVI convenes the Estates General which meets in Versailles on May 4, 1789; July 14, 1789 the Bastille fortress is attacked by a populace mob; the French Revolution to overthrow the monarchy begins

Napoleon dies in full communion with the Church

The Civil Constitution of the Clergy is passed to secularize the clergy

Napoleon divorces Josephine, marries Maria Louisa of Austria

Constitutional Convention declares 1789 "Year One" creating a new calendar

Napoleon stages coup d'état, takes control of France

Napoleon's Russian invasion in winter of 1812 fails

Napoleon crowns himself Emperor

Napoleon abdicates; is exiled

Pope Pius VII 1800-1823

1785   1795   1805   1815   1825

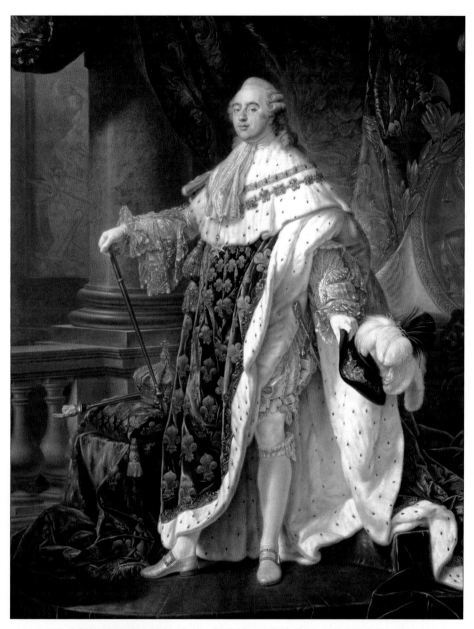

Louis XVI (1754-1793) was King of France until his arrest and execution during the French Revolution.
King Louis XVI was guillotined in front of a cheering crowd on January 21, 1793. His wife, Marie Antoinette,
followed him to the guillotine on October 16, 1793. Beloved by the people at first, Louis's indecisiveness and
conservatism led the people to reject and hate him and associate him with the tyranny of former kings of France.
Today, some historians see him as an honest man with good intentions but who was unfit for the huge task of
reforming the monarchy. He was tragically used as a scapegoat by the Revolutionaries.

The **Third Estate** (the remaining ninety-seven percent of the population) consisted of an absurdly disparate portion of society. Wealthy bankers, lawyers, merchants, and other elite members of society who could not claim nobility from birth composed the bourgeoisie. The bourgeoisie held great political and economic power and were constantly in conflict with the nobility. They resented the nobility's parasitic drain on the society's economy and their unwarranted legal privileges. At the same time, the bourgeoisie, who could have easily paid taxes, exempted themselves as well. It logically followed that the poor masses were left to shoulder the burden of the taxes, fueling a dark future for France.

THE FINANCIAL CRISIS

France's financial crisis, which led to the political turmoil of 1789, was the result of nearly a century of economic mismanagement and abuse typified by Louis XIV's lavish lifestyle and careless wars. Obviously, irresponsible expenditures had produced a severe strain on the economy. In 1739, France spent thirty-six percent of her annual income on paying off the debt incurred by Louis XIV's wars. In addition, the cost of Versailles and the monarchy's lifestyle cost ten percent of the entire national budget. Compared to the eight percent delegated to social programs and pensions, it was clear that economic priority was inordinately given to the kings' whims and caprices. By 1763, the debt reached sixty-two percent of the annual income, and after France supported the American Revolution, debt consumed one hundred percent of the entire national income.

Surprisingly, France's monumental debt was not much larger than most European countries in the late eighteenth century. What made France's situation worse were the severe inequities heaped on the meager financial resources of the poor. The nobility and bourgeoisie did not pay taxes; therefore, the entire sum fell on the lowest classes of society. These poor farmers and city workers simply had nothing with which to pay the debt.

Both Louis XV and Louis XVI realized that their country was in a dire economic situation and tried to reform the system of taxation. Unfortunately, the nobility opposed whatever reforms the kings tried to pass. The nobility's motives were twofold: they wanted to remain free from taxation, but more importantly, they hoped economic constraints on the kings would insure their own political power. They pressured Louis XVI to call the Estates General in order to fix the debt problem. The nobles hoped to use that legislative body to force concessions from the king on their behalf and establish for themselves long-term influence in the affairs of France. Backed into a corner, Louis XVI agreed, and convened the Estates General in 1788.

THE ESTATES GENERAL

The Estates General had not been convened since 1614, and reconvening it was not a simple task. Each Estate hoped that through the Estates General they could further their own cause and influence. The nobility hoped the body would organize as it was in 1614 with each of the three Estates having one vote and sitting in separate chambers. However, both the First and Third Estate rejected this organization, claiming that it was out of date and inadequately represented the French people. Clearly, the nobility had worn out its welcome, and the French people were quite eager for a dramatic change.

In response to the convocation of the Estates General, the clergyman Abbé Sieyès wrote a pamphlet called "What is the Third Estate?" In it the clergyman argued that the Third Estate by itself represented the people of France. Sieyès believed that since the Third Estate best represented the majority of France, its interests were in fact the interests of France. He saw no need to include any other minorities in the future government of the country. Sieyès's pamphlet became immensely popular and roused the general population to support the aboli-

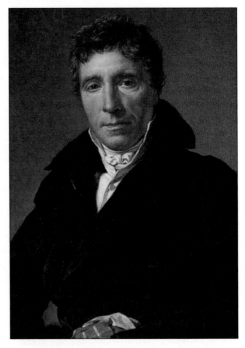

Emmanuel Joseph Sieyès (1748-1836) was a French abbé (abbot) and one of the chief theorists of the revolutionary era. He renounced his faith during the Cult of Reason, voted for the death of King Louis XVI, and defended his conduct with the ironical words "I lived."

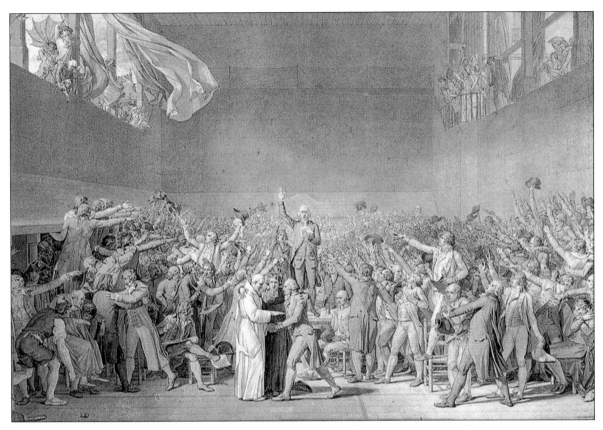

The Tennis Court Oath (*serment du jeu de paume*) was a pledge signed by 577 members of France's Third Estate on June 20, 1789.
King Louis XVI had locked the deputies of the Third Estate out of their meeting hall so they met instead in a nearby tennis court.
The Tennis Court Oath is often considered the moment of the birth of the French Revolution.

tion of the First and Second Estates. Amid growing public pressure, the king responded by allowing the Third Estate to bring twice as many representatives to the Estates General. This enraged the nobility, but delighted the French public who found new hope. When the Estates General finally met on May 4, 1789 at Versailles, popular unrest and social tensions were high.

In Versailles, the Third Estate immediately tried to exert its popular demand. They requested that the three-chamber distinction between the Estates be abolished and that the legislature meet as a single body. A number of clerics and bishops from the First Estate who sympathized with the plight of the poor masses supported this motion and joined the Third Estate in their chamber. The Third Estate understood itself as the only true representative body in France, and so on June 17, the Third Estate proclaimed itself the "National Assembly," assuming sovereign power and free jurisdiction over France.

Predictably, the nobility rejected the National Assembly and pressured the king to suppress the new legislature. On June 20, King Louis XVI acceded to the nobility's wishes and had the National Assembly locked out of the meeting hall. Rather than discouraging the new legislature from further action, the Assembly simply moved to a nearby tennis court where they promised to stay in session until a new constitution was drafted.

The king was fearful of the popular power held by the National Assembly. He tried to reach a compromise and agreed to limit his authority if the three Estates continued to sit separately in the Estates General. However, his provisions came too late. The National Assembly rejected his proposal and continued to meet. With the situation out of his hands and revolution immanent, the king ordered 20,000 troops to Versailles and Paris.

THE BASTILLE

On July 12, riots broke out in Paris over the food shortages. Mobs of poor, hungry commoners took to the streets demanding food, and French troops, wary of firing on their fellow countrymen and starting a full-scale revolt in Paris, withdrew to the outskirts of the city. Mobs began looting stores and warehouses. They burned tariff houses and sacked the convent of Saint-Lazare in hopes of finding food.

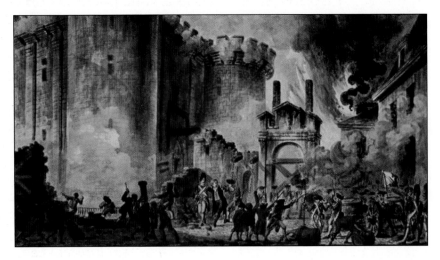

On July 14, 1789, a mob attacked the Bastille, a Medieval fortress used as an arsenal and a prison, and seized 40,000 muskets and a dozen pieces of artillery. A skirmish ensued between the mob and the Bastille guards that left a hundred rioters and a half-dozen soldiers dead. Violence spilled into other parts of Paris, and the governor and a number of officials were killed or maimed. Still unsure about marching against their fellow countrymen, the troops on the outskirts of Paris did not intervene.

This day, July 14, 1789, is remembered as Bastille Day, the beginning of the French Revolution, because it marks the beginning of the common people's role in the overthrow of the French monarchy. The attack tipped the balance of power and frightened both the king and the nobility into making concessions to the people. The king recognized a citizens' committee that had been formed in Paris as the new municipal government. He disbanded the armies at Paris and urged the First and Second Estates to join the National Assembly. To restore order in Paris and other cities, the bourgeoisie in the National Assembly set up a force called the "National Guard." The tri-color flag that these forces adopted would become the symbol of the revolution.

THE DECLARATION OF THE RIGHTS OF MAN AND CITIZEN

The proliferation of farmers' revolts throughout France complicated the political situation in Versailles. The National Assembly, which was largely made up of bourgeois leaders, was forced to deal with these riots and promote peace by meeting the demands of the peasants. In order to respond quickly, the Assembly convened a meeting with a small group of liberal nobles

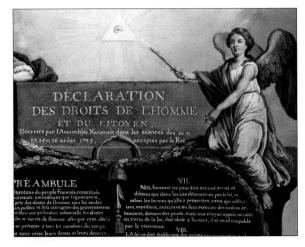

during the night of August 4, 1789, hoping the odd hour would discourage high attendance and consequently simplify the passage of legislation. Their plan worked, and the Assembly was able to pass radical legislation that ended the feudal obligations of peasant serfs and eliminated most of the special rights and privileges of the nobility. The Assembly issued a decree that summarized the resolutions of the "night of August 4" that read simply: "feudalism is abolished" (quoted in Palmer, et al., History of the Modern World, 2002, p. 371).

With these far-reaching provisions in place, the National Assembly set out to construct a new order in France. On August 26, 1789, the Assembly issued The Declaration of the Rights of Man and Citizen, declaring the following principles of the revolution: all men were born equal and held rights to liberty, property, security, and resistance. Influenced by Rousseau's "social contract."

The Declaration was particularly vague on matters of religion. The only article relating to religion alluded to religious tolerance as long as religious beliefs did not "disturb the public order established by law" (translated by Robinson, Declaration, art. 10). Although this clause seemed to secure toleration for all religions, it would soon serve as a pretext to squelch the Church's freedom. Since the Catholic Church was associated with the Old Régime that robbed the people of their rights and welfare, the article opened the road to persecution of the Church.

On October 6, the mob stormed the palace grounds, captured the king, and forced him and his queen, Marie Antoinette, to accompany them back to Paris. After that episode, the National Assembly established a single chamber for the governing body called the Legislative Assembly that met in Paris together with the king.

Assault on Versailles, October 6, 1789

THE CIVIL CONSTITUTION OF THE CLERGY

With the king in Paris, the Legislative Assembly set about reorganizing the country's governing body as it tried to solve the ever-growing problems of debt, poverty, and widespread famine. Seen as a relic of the Old Régime, the Church was the first to fall victim to these new measures of financial reform. The Assembly hoped to balance the budget by seizing the Church's wealth and landholdings. They passed laws to confiscate all Church lands, disband monasteries and convents, and redistribute the land among the French people. The Church was the largest landowner in France, and within ten years, nearly ten percent of all the lands and buildings in France were passed to the French citizens in the form of paper bonds called Assignats. These paper bonds became so numerous that in some circles they circulated like paper currency. Unfortunately, rather than resolving the debt crises, this largest transfer of property in European history largely benefited the upper middle class bourgeoisie who dominated the Legislative Assembly. In addition, the massive confiscation of the Church's possessions put the incipient revolution in opposition to the very Church that was working to improve the situation of the country.

Underlying the motives of this grand-scale seizure of Church lands was the Legislative Assembly's desire to bring the Church in line with the principles of the revolution and establish a Gallican

THE FRENCH UNDERGROUND:
BL. WILLIAM JOSEPH CHAMINADE

Many priests refused to take the oath of The Civil Constitution of the Clergy, and as a result, were forced to take their priestly ministry underground. One of these priests was Bl. William Joseph Chaminade, a native of Périgueux, France who was ordained a priest in 1785. Just fours years after his ordination, the French Revolution broke out, and Chaminade moved to Bordeaux, where he would spend most of his life. In 1791, Chaminade refused to take the oath of The Civil Constitution of the Clergy, instead practicing his priestly ministry in secret, putting his life in constant danger.

Many recognized Chaminade's extraordinary Faith during this time of persecution in France, and in 1795, he was given the task of receiving back into the diocese those priests who had taken the oath. During this time he reconciled some fifty priests with the Church. Two years later, in 1797, The Directory came to power. A price was put on his head, and Chaminade was forced to flee France to Saragossa, Spain, where he lived for three years. While in Spain, Chaminade was inspired to found a family of religious and laity: the Society of Mary. He wished to return to France and begin to re-evangelize the country that had suffered so much under the tyrannies of the revolution.

After returning to Bordeaux in 1800, Chaminade asked for and received the title of "Missionary Apostolic" from Rome. He was going to be a new kind of missionary, one that reconverted those who had fallen away from the Church. On December 8, 1800, the Feast of the Immaculate Conception, Chaminade gathered twelve young Catholics to form the Marian Sodality, which would become the basis of his new evangelization. "You are all missionaries" he told them, called to "multiply Christians."

Chaminade strove to provide a solid religious formation to the members of his Sodality, hoping to make these groups the basis of the re-Christianization of France. Soon the Sodality of Bordeaux spread to other cities. Chaminade encouraged groups of young men and women who, desiring greater dedication, made private vows and dedicated themselves to the apostolate of the Sodality without leaving their secular work. His followers, called Marianists, dedicated themselves to teaching and opened primary and secondary schools throughout France. They also established a network of teachers' schools for Christian education. Continuous revolution, however, made long-term growth difficult. In the mid-nineteenth century the Marianists spread to Switzerland and the United States where they continued to establish schools and educate young people in the Faith.

The last years of Chaminade's life were difficult. Health problems, financial difficulties, the departure of some of his disciples, misunderstandings and distrust, and obstacles to the exercise of his mission as founder all tested Chaminade's Faith. Nonetheless, he faced these difficulties with great confidence in Mary, faithful to his conscience and to the Church, filled with faith and charity. He died peacefully in Bordeaux on January 22, 1850, and he was beatified by St. John Paul II on September 3, 2000.

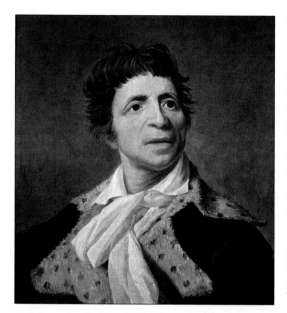

The infamous Jean-Paul Marat (1743-1793), was a member of the radical Jacobin faction during the Revolution. He helped launch the Reign of Terror. Marat composed the death lists from which the innocent and the guilty alike were executed. He was assassinated by Charlotte Corday, an aristocrat who supported the Girondists. She was sent to the guillotine four days later. Marat became a martyr for the Revolution, and busts of Marat replaced religious statues in the French churches.

Church that would merely serve as a social arm of the secular government. In July 1790, the Legislative Assembly passed The Civil Constitution of the Clergy, a piece of legislation designed to secularize the clergy, govern the Church in France, and separate all its administrative decisions from the papacy. Divided into four parts, The Civil Constitution dealt with everything from the number of bishops to the length of travel allowed to priests. In an effort to "democratize" the Church, priests would be chosen by local assemblies, and all citizens, including non-Catholics, would choose the hierarchy of the Church. The Assembly also reorganized the clergy's salary structure, reducing their status to state officials and their authority to that of simple civil servants. In order to separate the French Church from Rome, The Civil Constitution of the Clergy prohibited clergy from leaving their parishes for more than two weeks and outlawed the publication of any papal documents. This legislation placed the Catholic Church in France under the jurisdiction of the civil authorities. Diplomatic ties with the Holy See were severed in 1791.

THE FRENCH REPUBLIC

The Constitutional Convention met in September 1792. These popular, working class revolutionaries threw out the constitution drafted by the National Assembly and completely reorganized France's political structure. They created a strictly republican model of government, abolished the monarchy, and emphasized the jurisdiction of neighborhood clubs and assemblies in order to open the democratic process up to the ordinary citizen. Believing they had finally established a government with real equality with the lower classes, the Convention declared 1789 "Year One" of the new political age. The founding of the republic became known as the "second" French Revolution.

In that same month, French armies won their first victory over Prussian forces. The new government harnessed popular jubilation and called upon the people of France to join the army and help establish the new republic. The French army quickly swelled from 180,000 to 650,000 troops, and the massive army seemed unstoppable. French troops entered Belgium, the German Rhineland, and northern Italy. Established by the Constitutional Convention, the National Convention would serve as the main legislative body for the next three years.

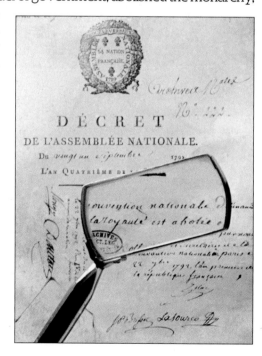

The National Assembly Decree abolishing the monarchy, September 22, 1789

PART VI

The Death of Louis XVI and the Age of the Revolutionary Republic

The new French Republic never achieved a stable government. Rather, as power shifted between various political factions and committees, France remained in a perpetual state of unrest and fear. Along with the establishment of the National Convention, came the power shift from the bourgeois party, called the Girondins, to the poor urban "sans-culottes," named after their working class pants. These "sans-culottes" represented the commoners of the cities and drew strength from both radical and popular elements. They worked to institute republican reforms and continued the policies of revolutionary expansion. These popularists never balked at using violence and brutality to better enforce and promote the principles of the revolution.

In December 1792, the National Convention, under the heavy influence of the san-culottes, put King Louis XVI on trial for treason. The king was condemned to death by a slim majority (361-360) and was guillotined on January 16, 1793. The execution of the king marked a new era of prolonged violence in France. Old problems, such as civil disorder, food shortages, and rising prices, continued to frustrate the lower classes. The poor began to doubt the principles of the revolution, which seemed only to bring about anarchy. Wishing to protect the revolution, the sans-culottes pressured the Convention to take more radical measures against dissent. They declared France to be in a state of emergency and formed the Committee of Public Safety to suppress all "counterrevolutionary" factions. This Committee began instituting a systematic policy of curbing violence through more frequent and persistent accusations and mass executions. Their rule during this period became known as "The Reign of Terror."

THE REIGN OF TERROR AND THE "DE-CHRISTIANIZATION" OF FRANCE

The Reign of Terror promoted by The Committee of Public Safety was meant to suppress counterrevolutionary tendencies and utilize all of France's resources to support the wars abroad. Control of the Committee was dominated by Maximilian Robespierre, a firm believer in the principles of the revolution. Out of a desire to promote civic virtue and create a society of good and honest citizens, Robespierre did not hesitate to use brutal and unjust means to achieve his ends.

As the Reign of Terror spread throughout the country, mob violence soon followed. Gangs of marauders, who believed they were acting in the best interest of the Committee, destroyed farms, houses, and churches. Mutinies broke out in the army and navy, and many nobles and political monarchists were forced into exile. During the Reign of Terror, no suspect was left unharmed, and many innocent were punished unjustly.

The Church in France was hit particularly hard by the Reign of Terror. Considering any religion counterrevolutionary, the Committee launched a program of "de-Christianization" in November 1793. "Missionary Representatives" were sent out into the countryside to close down churches, hunt down priests, and punish anyone accused of harboring clergy. The Cathedral of Notre-Dame de Paris was dedicated as a temple to the Goddess of Reason.

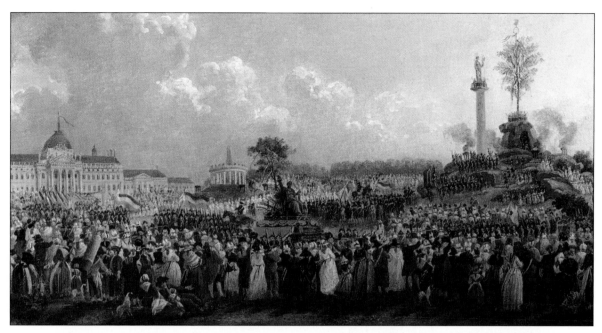

Robespierre and his colleagues decided to replace both Catholicism and the rival, atheistic Cult of Reason (promoted by the Hébertists) with the Cult of the Supreme Being. On May 7, 1794 he secured a decree from the Convention recognizing the existence of the Supreme Being. This worship of the Supreme Being or Godhead (a kind of Deistic God, rejecting a personal God) was based upon the ideas of Rousseau in *The Social Contract*. On June 8, 1794, the then still powerful Robespierre personally led a vast procession through Paris to the Tuileries garden in a ceremony to inaugurate the new religion. It was not a popular concept. Robespierre was guillotined with Saint-Just and other supporters on July 28, 1794.

Church buildings were vandalized; Gospel books and crucifixes burned; statues and relics of the Saints destroyed; and church bells and sacred vessels melted down for artillery pieces. Citizens were offered bounties for turning over priests who refused to take an oath of loyalty to the revolution. Furthermore, any priest found resisting the policies of the National Convention was ordered to be executed within twenty-four hours. Under the pretext of enforcing the Committee's policies, Catholics were killed publicly in cruel and gruesome ways. Mobs massacred entire monastic communities and Christian women and children were murdered in an effort to stop the spread of Christianity to future generations.

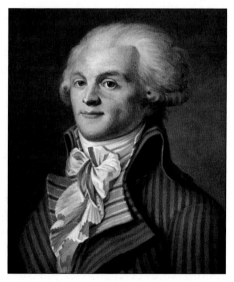

Maximilien Robespierre, (1758-1794) was a fanatical disciple of Rousseau and architect of the Cult of the Supreme Being.

In place of Christianity, the Committee of Public Safety set up a state-sponsored Deistic religion. The Mass was replaced with a civil ceremony celebrating the Goddess of Reason, and Paris's Notre Dame Cathedral was renamed the "Temple of Reason and Liberty." In the cathedral, wives and daughters of the revolutionaries took turns acting out the part of the Goddess of Reason on the altar. In addition to establishing new pagan cults, the Committee completely changed the calendar in an effort to suppress Christian worship. They eliminated the Lord's Day by instituting a ten-day week and exchanged saint and feast days for yearly celebrations of reason, liberty, and the republic. During the Reign of Terror all talk, practice, and promotion of religion was strictly and brutally repressed. The tomb of Genevieve, patroness of Paris, was replaced with a pantheon of France's great revolutionary men.

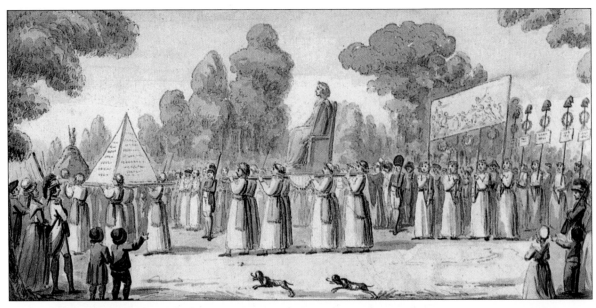

The Goddess of Reason procession. The Cult of Reason was a religion based on Deism devised by Jacques Hébert and Pierre Gaspard Chaumette in opposition to Robespierre's Cult of the Supreme Being. They considered Robespierre's cult a return to theism and in response advocated worship of Reason, personified as a goddess. Statues of the goddess were placed in the Cathedral of Notre Dame after the destruction of all Christian statues. She is considered by some to be the forerunner of "Marianne," the national emblem of France, personifying the triumph of Liberty and Reason. Her profile is on the official seal of the country, engraved on French Euro coins, and appears on French postage stamps.

THE DIRECTORY

In many ways, The Directory was a weak party formed in reaction to the extremists who had dominated the previous government. The Directory primarily consisted of bourgeoisie who had not only retained their influence during the volatile instability and anarchy of the revolution, but in fact profited from the chaos. Among the French people, loyalties were still scattered. Some hoped for the return of the monarchy with certain reforms of the old system. Others longed for the return to the revolutionary activism of Robespierre. Still others thought that Robespierre had been too moderate and formed a radical group known as the "Conspiracy of Equals." Although The Directory was active in suppressing all these factions, while in power, it did little to solve the ongoing, pervasive problems of hunger and inflation.

The Directory's policies were particularly hard on the Church. Although it claimed to promote republican liberalism, freedom, and toleration, oppressive laws were restored regarding priests who refused to take the Oath of the Republic. Hunting parties were organized throughout France to arrest recalcitrant priests. Consequently, thousands of priests were killed or deported to the penal colony in Guiana (northeast South America). Hoping that the Church might simply die out due to a lack of leadership, The Directory also refused to fill vacancies in dioceses where bishops died. Throughout the years of revolution, the Church was considered an obstacle to the revolution, and therefore outlawed aggressively.

THE ELECTION OF PIUS VII

Despite the sack of Rome and the eagerness of many French leaders to proclaim the Church extinct after the death of Pius VI, the cardinals assembled to elect a new pope. Before he died, Pius VI gave orders to elect the new pope in the city with the most cardinals. On November 30, 1799, the cardinals met in Venice, which enjoyed complete independence from French influence.

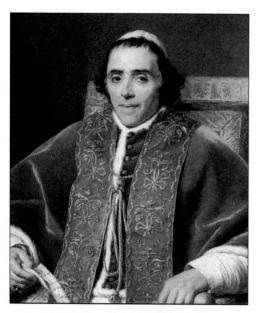

Pope Pius VII was born Giorgio Barnaba Luigi Chiaramonti on August 14, 1740. He was Pope from March 14, 1800, until August 20, 1823.

The conclave at Venice was divided. Some cardinals supported the wishes of the late Pius VI to elect a successor who would espouse moderate political views. Others, influenced by the Austrian monarchy, hoped for a pope who would favor the monarchical rule of the past. The debate continued for three months, and in the end, the supporters of Pius VI helped lead the College of Cardinals to a unanimous decision. They elected Barnaba Chiaramonti who took the name Pius VII.

Cardinal Chiaramonti, who had a strong personality, wanted to see the life of the Church restored in France as well as the rest of Europe. He understood how deeply the Faith was still rooted in the French people and for this reason believed in the possibility of a Christian revival. However, far from siding with old monarchical regimes, Chiaramonti was a progressive thinker who sympathized with the plights of the masses in France and their desire to establish liberty and equality in their country. He never condemned the principles of democracy outright, but rather the unjust means through which some of the revolutionaries sought them. Throughout the revolution, Chiaramonti had insisted that God preferred no particular form of government and that Democracy was not contrary to the Gospel. Nevertheless, he distinguished himself from the revolutionaries in France by arguing that liberty and equality were ideals that could only be achieved in Christ. Therefore, a Democracy required people of virtue and upright character that could only be made possible with the help of divine grace. Pope Pius VII clearly showed that the Church was open to a changing political climate but would always resist ideas or laws that would compromise her mission and violate her freedom. On July 3, 1800, Pius VII arrived in Rome with courage and faith to push Christ's kingdom forward amid cheering crowds.

PART VII

Napoleon Bonaparte

Napoleon Bonaparte was born in Corsica in 1769 to a family of minor nobility. During the days of the monarchy, he attended French military schools and proved to be an outstanding student. Despite his extraordinary gifts, there would have been little hope for advancement up the military chain of command during the Old Régime; the revolution changed that. Napoleon was already an officer before the revolution, but after 1789 he quickly rose through the ranks of the army. He was made a brigadier general during the Reign of Terror and, in 1796, received command of an army in which he proved his superior military skill. Crossing the Alps, Napoleon drove the Austrians from Northern Italy and began governing the region on his own. Like many of the French generals of the time, Napoleon acted independently of the government in Paris.

The civilian government on their own never had firm enough control to implement both their domestic and foreign policies, and therefore became increasingly more reliant on their generals to enforce their policies. Napoleon set up a republic in northern Italy and counseled the government in Paris. When the 1797 election ushered in a more conservative government, the weak, expansionist

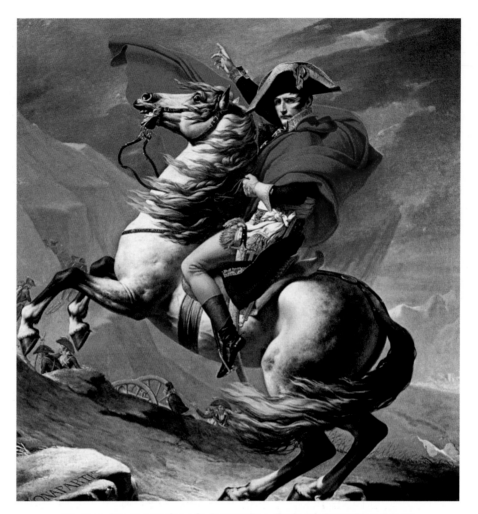

Napoleon Crossing the Great St. Bernard Pass. The Great St. Bernard Pass is the most ancient pass through the Western Alps, bordering Switzerland and Italy. Travel through the pass dates back to the Bronze Age. Hannibal crossed with elephants in 217 BC; Julius Caesar crossed in 57 BC; Emperor Augustus built a road across the pass and built a temple to Jupiter at the top; Charlemagne crossed in AD 800 following his coronation in Milan. In May 1800, Napoleon led 40,000 troops over the pass into Italy.

In 1049, St. Bernard of Menthon founded a hospice on the pass for weary and harassed travelers. The hospice, which still functions today, became famous for its St. Bernard dogs. The rescue dogs were bred by the monks to be large enough to handle the deep snow and to scent out lost persons.

government in Paris gladly accommodated the wishes of the French victor. Given his proven abilities as a leader, Napoleon was chosen to serve as the First Consul (1799) in the new government. Napoleon's ascent to power managed to stabilize the country, thereby ending the revolution in France. Out of the chaos of the preceding years, Napoleon would set up a new French Empire that blended the revolutionary idealism of 1789 with the power and control of an absolute monarch.

THE CONSULATE AND THE CONCORDAT OF 1801

As Napoleon began his term as First Consul (a term that was supposed to last for ten years), he set about reorganizing the French Republic and began to restore peace and order. A vital part of stabilizing France after ten years of near anarchy was to restore religious freedom to the French people and rebuild a severely persecuted Church. Napoleon understood how deeply rooted the Catholic Faith was in the hearts of most French people and also realized that the revolution's violent

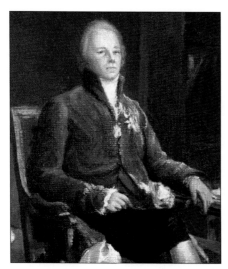

The French diplomat Charles Maurice de Talleyrand (1754-1838) is regarded by many historians as one of the most versatile and influential diplomats in European history.

suppression of religion was a key factor in fostering strong desires for a return to the Old Régime. Part of restoring the Catholic Church would involve re-establishing favorable relations with the pope.

Napoleon began normalizing relations between the government and the Church by securing a commitment of fidelity to the laws of France among priests who had refused to take the Oath to the French Republic. Once the priests assured patriotic loyalties to France, they were again able to carry out their priestly ministry publicly. He reopened the churches in France and released any imprisoned priests. Napoleon discarded the ten-day week and reestablished a nationwide day of rest. His policies immediately won the confidence of the French people, and most especially, the trust of French Catholics.

Napoleon sent his secretary of state, the famous revolutionary and former bishop Charles Maurice de Talleyrand, to meet with the illustrious Vatican diplomat, Cardinal Ercole Conslavi. In 1801, the two worked on drawing up a concordat that would create a new legal framework between the Church in France and the papacy. This concordat occasioned a repeal of revolutionary laws that were harmful to the Church. After a series of rejected proposals that attempted to create a Gallican national French church under the authority of Napoleon, Pius VII agreed to a final version of the Concordat on August 15, 1801.

Outlining the new policies in seventeen articles, the Concordat guaranteed the free and public practice of Catholicism in France. Civil authorities could only intervene in Church matters in instances of "public safety." In return, the Church agreed to the realignment of the French dioceses according to the new geographical breakdown of the country. This territorial reconfiguration occasioned a reduction in the number of French bishops from one hundred thirty six to sixty. The Pope also agreed to ask bishops who had lost their sees because of this realignment to resign from their offices. As for the appointment of new bishops, the pope agreed to allow Napoleon to nominate candidates, but it was ultimately up to the pope to give his final word. The Concordat rejuvenated Christian life throughout France. All the cathedrals and churches were reopened, and the government of France agreed to compensate for the loss of Church property by providing suitable salaries to the clergy. The dark days of religious suppression seemed to be over.

THE ORGANIC ARTICLES

The renewal of relations between France and the pope in Rome brought about great rejoicing for Catholics in France and around the world. But the joy did not last long. Soon after the signing of the Concordat, the French government passed a series of legislative restrictions limiting the Church's independence. Appealing to the provision in the Concordat regarding intervention in the Church's affairs in the interest of "public safety," the legislature passed the Organic Articles. These articles are best summed up as a combination of the Gallicanism prevalent during the reign of Louis XIV and the restrictions of The Civil Constitution of the Clergy. The worst of both worlds, the Organic Articles forbade the publication of all papal documents, decrees of the councils, or the convocation of any synod without the consent of the government. The new French government introduced a Gallican Catechism to be taught in all French seminaries, limited the administrative powers of the bishops in France; promoted civil marriages; and suppressed religious orders.

The Articles nullified whatever apparent liberty was granted to the Church by the Concordat of 1801, and they re-asserted the authority of Napoleon over the Church of France. It was clear that there was still strong animosity toward the Church, and these articles sought to appease the anti-Catholic forces by imposing damaging restrictions on the Catholic Church.

THE CORONATION OF NAPOLEON I

By 1802, thanks to the successful establishment of the Consulate, the Revolution was over. The French political scene had been finally pacified with the emergence of the strong Consulate, and Napoleon's power over Europe continued to grow. As First Consul, Napoleon soon made peace with the pope, Britain, and all the continental powers. This period of peace, which lasted from 1802 until 1803, was called the "Peace of Amiens" (Amiens being the city in which the treaty was signed), and it made Napoleon very popular. During the peace, Napoleon quietly advanced his interests, reorganized France's possessions, and annexed a number of small German principalities. In August 1802, Napoleon's popularity was so great that he named himself consul for life. Two years later in 1804, Napoleon had himself named emperor.

As soon as Napoleon was named emperor, despite his revolutionary pretenses, he surrounded himself with a lavish court and took on all the pomp of nobility. He desired to have himself crowned in a dazzling ceremony and exquisite pageantry. In keeping with the long tradition of the French monarchy dating back to Charlemagne, Napoleon wanted the pope to crown him. Napoleon sent word to the pope, requesting that Pius VII crown him in the cathedral at Notre Dame in Paris on December 2, 1804.

The pope was cautioned that a rejection of Napoleon's request might prove detrimental to the recent friendly relations between Rome and France since the Concordat of 1801. Since those relations, although much improved, were far from ideal, Pius VII still hoped to convince the emperor to revoke some of the provisions of the Organic Articles. The pope therefore felt that his involvement in the coronation of Napoleon might work to further the freedom of the Church in France. Pope Pius VII graciously assented to the invitation. However, before leaving for Paris, he signed a conditional act of abdication that provided for the election of a new pope in the event that Napoleon prevented his return to Rome.

In Paris, the pope tried to use his visit to influence Napoleon's policies and retain some authority over the French church that now was controlled by the new emperor. Pope Pius VII established a moral advantage over Napoleon by objecting to the emperor's marriage to Josephine, which was not celebrated according to the Church's specifications. The pope refused to attend the coronation until the marriage was preformed validly. Napoleon reluctantly conceded and was married in private on December 1, the night before the coronation.

The next day Napoleon would be crowned emperor. However, before the pope could crown Napoleon, he snatched the crown from the pope's hands and placed it on his own head. Napoleon wanted to acknowledge publicly that his authority did not come from the pope, but rather from himself. After crowning himself emperor, Napoleon crowned his wife empress.

Pius VII was never able to secure from Napoleon needed concessions for the Catholic Church in France. Napoleon ignored most of the pope's requests, in part to show that his authority would not be influenced by the Roman pontiff. To prevent relations from completely souring, Napoleon did agree to replace the calendar of the revolution (with 1789 recognized as year one) with the traditional, Gregorian calendar. With only this small concession in place, Pius VII left Paris very displeased with the emperor.

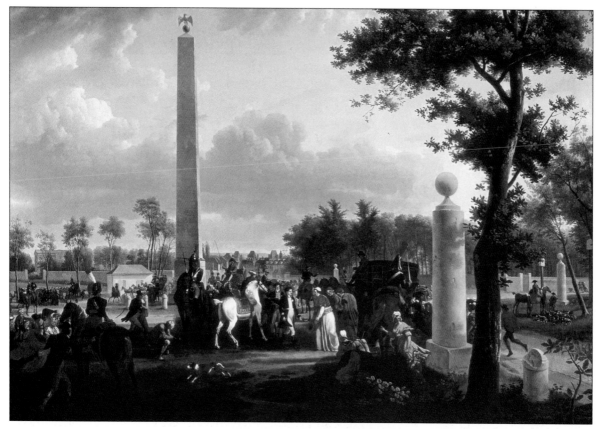

Napoleon Meets With Pope Pius VII.
Napoleon seized huge portions of the Papal States and assumed jurisdiction over the power of the pope. After Pius VII excommunicated Napoleon, Napoleon had the pope arrested on July 5, 1805 and taken to Savona, in France, where he was imprisoned for six years.

EMPEROR NAPOLEON AGAINST PIUS VII

In the years that followed his coronation, Napoleon extended his interests throughout Europe. Through an unprecedented series of military victories, the French empire expanded across the continent. With each new area he conquered, Napoleon enforced his legal code, called the "Napoleonic Code," which introduced the emperor's typical mix of revolutionary and traditional ideas. The Code provided for equality among religious denominations and freedom of religious practice, but it also introduced civil marriage and divorce and placed heavy restrictions on the Church. In the region of Italy under his control, Napoleon and the pope came into conflict once again, this time over the marriage of Napoleon's brother Jerome.

In 1805, Napoleon asked Pius VII to annul his brother's marriage. The emperor wished his brother to remarry for political reasons, and the pope refused to grant the dispensation. Pius VII also refused to go along with Napoleon in joining the Continental System. Angered by the pope's rejection, Napoleon threatened to abolish priestly celibacy throughout Europe, suppress more religious orders, and establish a French patriarch to oppose the pope's authority over the Church in France. Pius VII still refused to compromise the position of the Church on marriage. Frustrated with the pope's resistance, Napoleon ordered his troops to march on Rome.

As emperor, Napoleon claimed succession from Charlemagne, and with that, he claimed the right to revoke the "donation of Pepin," which established the Papal States in 756. Napoleon then seized huge portions of the Papal States in 1808 and assumed jurisdiction over the pope. These moves involved a rejection of the pope's temporal authority and transferal of the Papal States to French rule. Rome was made the second city of the Empire, and the pope was issued a salary. The pope's authority was restricted to the supervision of the papal palaces. Although not totally clear, it is generally agreed that Pius VII responded by excommunicating the responsible parties with the bull Quum memoranda and possibly Napoleon himself. Napoleon in turn had the pope arrested on July 5 and taken to Savona (France) where he was imprisoned for six years.

In 1809 Napoleon divorced his wife Josephine, hoping to build an alliance with Austria and secure an heir by marrying Maria Louisa, the daughter of the Hapsburg emperor. Although Napoleon had his marriage to Josephine dissolved by the French Senate, the Austrian court would not accept the senate's authority over such matters. They insisted that the emperor have his marriage annulled by the Church. Knowing that Pius VII would refuse to annul the marriage, Napoleon turned to the Gallican Church Court of Paris which gladly granted a dispensation. Despite vehement protests of Pius VII from his prison, Napoleon married Maria Louisa on April 1, 1810.

Many rejected the authority of the Gallican Church Court and its decision to annul Napoleon's marriage. In protest, thirteen cardinals refused to attend the wedding ceremony. Napoleon reacted by having these cardinals arrested and their properties confiscated. They were forbidden to wear their red cardinalatial robes, and forced to wear the plain garb of ordinary clerics. These dissenting cardinals, as a result, became known as the "black" cardinals.

THE FRENCH COUNCIL OF 1811
AND THE CONCORDAT OF FONTAINEBLEAU

Despite his imprisonment, the pope continued to issue Papal Bulls that rejected many of Napoleon's policies. The emperor wanted a remedy to the situation, and in 1811 called for a national council of French bishops in an effort to gain authority over all ecclesiastical affairs.

Despite Napoleon's intentions, the council remained loyal to the pope and refused to grant Napoleon's requests. Rather than grant authority to the emperor to make ecclesiastical appointments in the pope's absence, at the advice of Pius VII, the council agreed to allow the archbishop of a province to appoint new bishops in the event of a papal absence lasting more than six months. As an assertion and endorsement of the pope's authority, the installation was to be performed in the name of the absent pope. Napoleon was outraged at the decision of the council. He closed the council and arrested three bishops involved with the decisions. Failing to gain the support of "his council," as he called it, Napoleon tried to pressure the pope into submission.

Before leaving for his Russian military campaign in 1812, Napoleon moved Pius VII from Savona to the palace of Fontainebleau. Cut off from the contact of his supporters, sick and alone, the pope was pressured to comply with the emperor's wishes. After Napoleon's return from Russia and under tremendous pressure, Pius VII agreed to preliminary discussions over the issue of Napoleon's authority in making ecclesiastical appointments. Before the pope gave any formal agreement to the measures under study, Napoleon had these discussions published. This forced "agreement" in 1813 was called the Concordat of Fontainebleau, and if it had been allowed to stand, it would have placed all French and Italian bishops under the control of the Emperor.

One benefit of the Concordat of Fontainebleau was that it allowed the "black" cardinals to visit with the pope. As soon as these loyal servants met with Pius VII, the "black" cardinals suggested that the pope publish his rejection of the Concordat of Fontainebleau. Pius formally rejected the Concordat of Fontainebleau two months after its publication and sent letters disavowing the signature he had given and voiding all of the recent episcopal appointments. Although Napoleon ordered this letter kept secret, news of the pope's retraction spread throughout Europe.

THE FALL OF NAPOLEON

Napoleon's empire began to collapse with the loss of his army in his failed invasion of Russia in the winter of 1812. Encouraged by Napoleon's defeat, a renewed coalition between Austria, Prussia, Russia, and England marched towards Paris and forced the emperor's abdication. With Napoleon's defeat in 1814, Pius VII was free to return to Rome. The people cheered as Napoleon's great adversary returned to the Eternal City.

Despite the difficulties between Napoleon and the Church, after his downfall, Pope Pius VII took measures to protect the former emperor's family from any harsh retribution. Pius also interceded on Napoleon's behalf when he learned that the former emperor sought the services of a Catholic priest while in captivity on the Island of St. Helena. Pius VII continued to show charity to Napoleon and his family, and he did not abandon the former emperor during his captivity. During the end of his life, Napoleon spoke of Pius VII as "an old man full of tolerance and light". "Fatal circumstances," he added, "embroiled our cabinets. I regret it exceedingly" (quoted in Goyau, "Napoleon I [Bonaparte]," The Catholic Encyclopedia, vol. X, 1911). Napoleon was eventually restored to full communion with the Church before he died in his confinement on May 5, 1821.

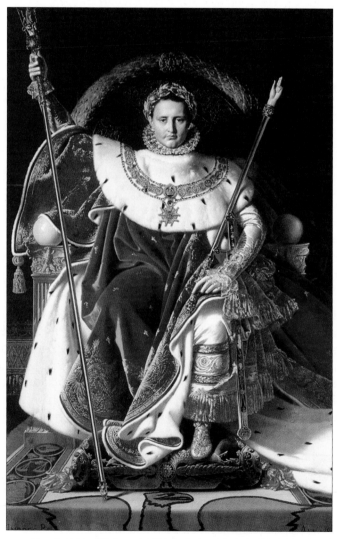

Napoleon I on His Imperial Throne by Jean Auguste Dominique Ingres

CONCLUSION

Although his rise to power ended the revolution, Napoleon's death marked the close of the revolutionary era. The storm of revolutionism, the ideas of secularism, and the passions that fueled the upheaval of the old European regimes had crisscrossed the continent for over thirty years. Nations had fallen and new ideologies had taken root in the popular imagination of almost every nation. Although the nations that toppled Napoleon would attempt to restore the old order, the principles of revolution had already begun to erode the old political order.

In 1814, members of all the European nations met in Vienna to determine the aftermath of the Napoleonic era. Napoleon's France had restructured most of Europe, and representatives at the Congress of Vienna, as the meeting was called, sought to reorganize the continent. There was an immense amount of reconstruction to be done, especially for the Church. All over Europe dioceses had been redrawn and Church properties redistributed. Religious orders had been decimated, seminaries were closed, and communication with Rome was, in many regions, destroyed. The Church would dedicate much of its work throughout the nineteenth century to recovering the losses from the period of Napoleonic conquest. The example of Pius VII had impressed many nations and would help the Church as it negotiated with European powers. Nonetheless, in the face of new ideologies and emerging nationalism and industrialization, the road ahead for the Church would not prove easier than the road it left behind.

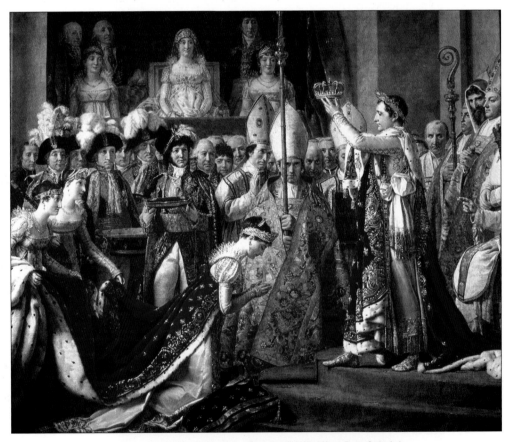

Napoleon crowned himself Emperor on December 2, 1804 at Notre-Dame Cathedral.
Napoleon then crowned his wife Joséphine as Empress. On May 26, 1805,
in Milan's Cathedral, Napoleon was crowned King of Italy, with the Iron Crown of Lombardy.

VOCABULARY

AGE OF ENLIGHTENMENT

Intellectual movement which sprang up from a whole-hearted enthusiasm for, and faith in, man's use of reason and scientific progress. Enlightened man believed that the study of science and nature could help correct all the problems of society, including poverty, disease, and war.

ASSIGNATS

Paper bonds. After the Legislative Assembly passed laws to confiscate all church property, the lands were redistributed to the people in the form of Assignats.

BLACK CARDINALS

Cardinals who were forced to wear the same black vestments as priests instead of their usual red as a punishment by Napoleon for refusing to recognize his marriage to Maria Louisa.

BOURGEOISIE

French upper middle class composed of mostly wealthy bankers, merchants, and lawyers.

CONSTITUTIONAL MONARCHY

System of government established in England in 1689 which blended the monarchical and parliamentary systems.

DEISM

Rationalist philosophy which accepted the principle of a first cause, but denied Divine intervention or Providence in the world. Deism understood God as a great watchmaker who created the universe with laws and guiding principles, but then left the world to man's discovery and domination.

ESTATES GENERAL

Legislative body of the Old Régime in France. Although it had not been called since 1614 and was widely held as misrepresentative, Louis XIV convened it in 1788 to respond to the growing financial crisis in France.

FEBRONIANISM

"Gallican" movement that influenced the Church in Germany. It argued that the pope was merely an administrative head of the Church who did not have the power to legislate. According to this, ultimate authority of the Church is found in the national leader. It further denied the primacy of the pope over bishops and the pope's authority to speak definitively on matters of Faith and morals.

FREEMASONRY

A major vehicle in the spreading of rationalist ideas, this secret, fraternal organization bases all its practices, rules, and organization on Enlightenment philosophy and reason. Many eighteenth-century European and American leaders were members of this organization that sought (and still seeks) to destroy the influence of the Church.

GLORIOUS REVOLUTION

Bloodless revolution in England in which James II was forced to abdicate the throne and power was placed in the hands of his children, William and Mary.

JANSENISM

Developed by Cornelius Jansen, erroneous belief that man was entirely free in the state of innocence and his will tended to do what was right. According to him, original sin made man a slave to sin and all his actions corrupted him. His only hope was God's grace, which could save him. Jansen taught that God only granted salvific grace to a small number of "predestined" people.

NAPOLEONIC CODE

Napoleon's code of law which blended revolutionary and traditional ideas. It provided for equality and freedom of religion, but it also introduced civil marriage and divorce and placed heavy restrictions on the Church.

VOCABULARY Continued

PHILOSOPHES

French word describing the proponents of Enlightenment philosophy who arose as the new authorities on virtually all matters. They rejected divine revelation and supernatural religion, rather than believing that all knowledge ought to be based on demonstration through human reason.

PLANTATIONS

Large areas in the northeast of Ireland that were cleared of Catholics by James I and resettled by Scottish Protestants in an effort to "breed out" the Catholics.

QUIETISM

Movement founded by Miguel Molinos which advocated absolute passivity during prayers and contemplation. The soul, according to Molinos, should be indifferent to everything, including temptation, and should simply rest perpetually in God. Asceticism was not necessary, since it was sufficient for the soul to humble itself in order for God to accept someone with sins. Quietists taught people to make no effort to avoid sin nor cooperate with God's grace for his salvation.

REIGN OF TERROR

Describes rule under the Committee of Public Safety in which the committee instituted a systematic policy of curbing violence through frequent and persistent accusations and mass execution in the interest of suppressing counterrevolutionary tendencies.

STUDY QUESTIONS

1. What belief of Jansenism made it heretical?

2. Why did the Church condemn Quietism?

3. Who was Guy Fawkes?

4. Who was the "Lord Protector"?

5. Who founded the colony of Maryland and why?

6. How does a decree of James I still affect Ireland today?

7. William and Mary passed which laws against Catholics?

8. What movement in the seventeenth century helped lead to the Age of Enlightenment?

9. How did Enlightenment philosophy affect the religious convictions of Europeans?

10. What supposition did René Descartes and Sir Francis Bacon make regarding human reason?

11. Why did Galileo Galilei find himself in conflict with the Church?

12. How did the Enlightenment threaten the Church?

STUDY QUESTIONS Continued

13. What is Deism?

14. Who were/are the Freemasons?

15. Who was Voltaire? What did he think about the Catholic Church?

16. How did Jean-Jacques Rousseau differ from other Enlightenment thinkers?

17. Who was Febronius? On what matters did he disagree with the Church?

18. What were some differences between Maria-Theresa and her son Joseph II?

19. How were the classes structured within the "Old Régime"?

20. Why was the Estates General reconvened?

21. What is the significance of the Bastille?

22. What were the major principles held by The Declaration of the Rights of Man and Citizen?

23. What was The Civil Constitution of the Clergy, and why was it passed?

24. What is the "second" French Revolution?

25. Who were the "sans-culottes"?

26. What was the Reign of Terror? Who were its main supporters?

27. Who was Robespierre?

28. What happened to the Church during the Reign of Terror?

29. Who belonged to The Directory, and who was its most famous leader?

30. What was Pope Pius VII's attitude towards democracy?

31. What were the Organic Articles?

32. Who crowned Napoleon emperor?

33. Who were the black cardinals?

34. Which event led to the collapse of Napoleon's empire?

35. How did Napoleon's reign affect the rest of Europe?

36. How did Napoleon's reign affect the power of the Church?

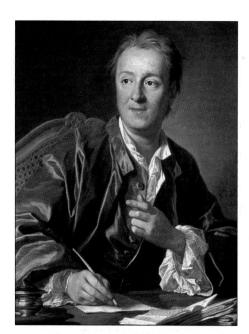

Denis Diderot (1713-1784) was the Editor-in-Chief of the influential Encyclopedia.

PRACTICAL EXERCISES

1. Jansenism and Quietism are two heresies with almost opposite understandings of piety and faith. They offered opposing exaggerations of aspects of Christianity. Why did these heresies appear at around the same time? What was appealing to believers about each of these heresies?

2. The First Amendment to the United States Constitution (1789) states in part: "Congress shall make no law respecting an establishment of religion." In light of the political developments in France and England during the seventeenth and eighteenth centuries, why were the founders concerned with drafting this position?

3. How did scientific rationalism employed in the work of thinkers like Descartes, Bacon, and Galileo differ from St. Thomas Aquinas and other Scholastics? How were they similar? Why should Christians be wary of the claim that human reason can provide absolute certainty?

4. The Enlightenment was a philosophical reaction to the Reformation and the Wars of Religion of the preceding centuries. In what way is this statement true? In what way is it false? Why did Enlightenment thinkers voice so much opposition to religion?

5. From a Christian perspective, was the French Revolution justified? (Consider the situation of each social class before, during, and after the revolution.)

6. Why did the revolution work to "de-Christianize" France? What were the political motives? What were the ideological motives?

7. How was Napoleon Bonaparte like a monarch? How was he a proponent of the revolution? How did the way Napoleon combine these two roles make recovering from Napoleonic rule so difficult?

FROM THE CATECHISM

50   By the natural reason man can know God with certainty, on the basis of his works. But there is another order of knowledge, which man cannot possibly arrive at by his own powers: the order of divine Revelation (cf. Dei Filius: DS 3015). Through an utterly free decision, God has revealed himself and given himself to man. This he does by revealing the mystery, his plan of loving goodness, formed from all eternity in Christ, for the benefit of all men. God has fully revealed this plan by sending us his beloved Son, our Lord Jesus Christ, and the Holy Spirit.

1952   There are different expressions of the moral law, all of them interrelated: eternal law–the source, in God, of all law; natural law; revealed law, comprising the Old Law and the New Law, or Law of the Gospel; finally, civil and ecclesiastical laws.

1953   The moral law finds its fullness and its unity in Christ. Jesus Christ is in person the way of perfection. He is the end of the law, for only he teaches and bestows justice of God: "For Christ is the end of the law, that every one who has faith may be justified" (Rom 10: 4).

The Church Gives Witness In Wars And Revolutions

During this century of rapid political and cultural change, the Church began to speak on behalf of the working class and would be strengthened by the leadership of two celebrated popes.

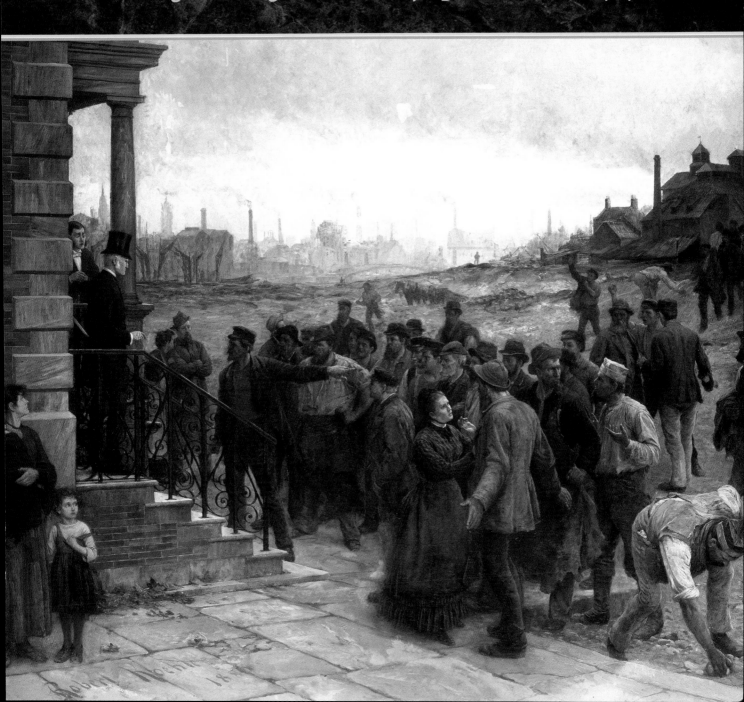

CHAPTER 8

The Church Gives Witness In Wars And Revolutions

After the fall of Napoleon, the victorious nations met in Vienna to restore the balance of power in Europe. European leaders hoped to restore peace by reestablishing the monarchy in France and conservative governments throughout Europe. However, the events of the previous decades proved irreversible. Although the diplomats who gathered in Vienna drew new political boundaries and supported traditional regimes, the inertia of radical social and economic developments already left a permanent mark on the cultural landscape of Europe.

Despite the Congress of Vienna's efforts to reinstate the regimes of the past, widespread Liberalism would effectively counteract any endeavor to turn back the political clock. Widely embraced by the professional and business class who had risen to prominence during the age of the revolution, Liberalism was a political philosophy that strove to create an enlightened society marked by freedom and equality. As these self-made men tried to improve the organization of society and its relationship to its governing body, economic and technological innovations would powerfully weigh in as a new social order was formed. Liberalization of government, accompanied by the emergence of industrialization, in significant part defined the nineteenth century.

During nineteenth century, the economies of Europe and the United States rapidly moved from agricultural commerce towards mechanized manufacturing and industry. This rapid industrialization had tremendous social and economic effects on the world, transforming centuries-old ways nations operated and people lived within the course of a few years. The economic changes caused by industrialization occasioned the birth of a number of new ideologies and philosophies. Economic ideologies such as capitalism and Marxism, and political orientations such as nationalism, and imperialism all enjoyed a strong connection with the Industrial Revolution. These monumental changes prompted the Church to expand her doctrinal base and develop her social teachings. Popes responded to the different philosophies spawned by both the Enlightenment and Industrialization. The Church worked to assist those who were victims of the rapid social changes brought about by the Industrial Revolution. The popes spoke of the dangers of a materialistic view of work and the human person.

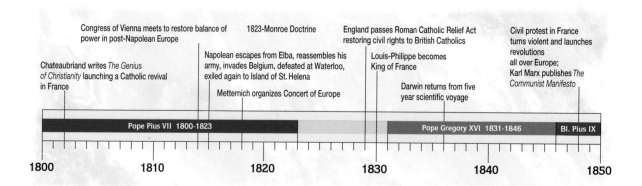

As the industrialization of society gave rise to abuses of human rights, the Church began to speak on behalf of the working class. During this century of political, economic, and cultural change, the Church became vulnerable to virulent attacks and persecutions, which would violate her own rights of free expression. Lastly, the nineteenth century would see the long pontificates of two celebrated popes, Bl. Pius IX and Leo XIII, whose leadership and authority would make the Church stronger through the First Vatican Council and well-crafted social doctrine at the service of human rights.

PART I
The Post-Napoleonic Era

The Congress of Vienna met in 1814 to restore the balance of power in Europe offset by fifteen years of Napoleonic domination. Representatives of the four nations that made up the victorious alliance–Britain, Prussia, Austria, and Russia–wanted to make sure that their countries remained strong and prepared to defend themselves against any future aggression.

The mastermind of the Congress was the Austrian diplomat, Clement von Metternich. Metternich began directing Austria's foreign affairs in 1809 (at the height of Napoleon's power) and would retain control for nearly forty years. In Vienna, he worked to extend Austria's domains into northern Italy and block Prussia and Russia from gaining too much power during the new division of Europe. With Napoleon defeated, Russia's increasing military strength under Czar Alexander I posed a new threat. After months of debate, new boundaries were drawn, and the three major European powers, Austria, Prussia, and Russia, all came out strong.

METTERNICH'S EUROPE: 1815-1830

The arrangements made at the Congress of Vienna beginning in 1814 were briefly interrupted by Emperor Napoleon I's remarkable escape from the island of Elba in March 1815. Returning to France and retaking power, the emperor made one last attempt to restore his rule. Napoleon invaded Belgium and was met there by the British commander, the Duke of Wellington, who soundly defeated the emperor at Waterloo aided by the arrival of 30,000 Russian troops. This second threat thwarted, the nations of Europe reconvened to make certain that peace would not again be disturbed.

Late in 1815, Russian Czar Alexander I proposed the creation of a "Holy Alliance" which promised to uphold Christian principles of charity and peace. Russia, Prussia, and Austria joined the Holy

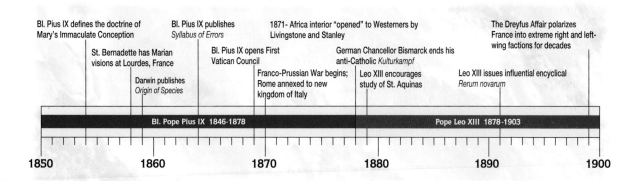

Bl. Pius IX defines the doctrine of Mary's Immaculate Conception

St. Bernadette has Marian visions at Lourdes, France

Darwin publishes *Origin of Species*

Bl. Pius IX publishes *Syllabus of Errors*

Bl. Pius IX opens First Vatican Council

Franco-Prussian War begins; Rome annexed to new kingdom of Italy

1871- Africa interior "opened" to Westerners by Livingstone and Stanley

German Chancellor Bismarck ends his anti-Catholic *Kulturkampf*

Leo XIII encourages study of St. Aquinas

The Dreyfus Affair polarizes France into extreme right and left-wing factions for decades

Leo XIII issues influential encyclical *Rerum novarum*

Bl. Pope Pius IX 1846-1878   Pope Leo XIII 1878-1903

1850   1860   1870   1880   1890   1900

Alliance, but Pope Pius VII and Great Britain refused to join. Despite Alexander's pious intentions, the Holy Alliance did not outline an effective program to ensure peace and was thus not taken seriously by its members.

Metternich, who remained suspect of Alexander's intentions, sought to balance Russian power by warming Austria's relations with the other European powers. Disregarding the Holy Alliance as a reliable treaty or a binding coalition, Metternich tried to forge a more stable alliance. He helped restore the Bourbon family to the throne of France and included them in a conservative coalition of European powers that included France. Through a series of Congresses at Aix-la-Chapelle in 1818, Troppau in 1820, and Verona in 1822, Metternich established the "Concert of Europe" which aimed at dismantling the reforms institutionalized by Napoleon and crush any liberal revolution. The arrangement left Austria–and Metternich–as the main arbiter of European affairs.

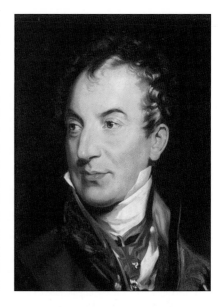

Clement von Metternich (1773-1858) was an Austrian statesman and perhaps the most influential diplomat of his era. He was the mastermind at the Congress of Vienna and established the anti-liberal, anti-revolution "Concert of Europe."

Metternich's conservative Concert soon provoked sharp reaction. Secret societies were founded in Spain, Italy, and Germany to overturn the monarchies. In Greece and Poland, patriots fought to restore their independence. During the time of the French Revolution, Latin American states had won their independence from Spain, and they now wanted to keep that independence. Metternich, fearing any successful defiance, worked with his conservative coalition to put down all threats.

In 1820, members of the Italian secret political society, the Carbonari (charcoal burners) led a successful revolution against the King of Naples, the Bourbon monarch Ferdinand I. During that same year, the Spanish government also fell to revolutionaries who forced King Ferdinand VII to adopt a liberal constitution. Metternich considered these revolutions the beginnings of a larger movement, and at Troppau, Austria, on December 8, 1820, he convinced the Concert to take strong and immediate action against the revolutionaries. An army entered Naples and suppressed the

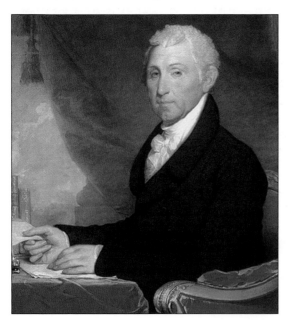

Italian revolutionaries, restoring Ferdinand I to the throne. In 1822, Metternich convinced the Concert of Europe to intervene in Spain and restore the government of Ferdinand VII.

The next step for the Concert was to stop the revolutions in Latin America. Before that happened, United States president James Monroe interceded by issuing the Monroe Doctrine in 1823. The Monroe Doctrine announced that the Western Hemisphere was closed to further European colonization and that any attempt by

James Monroe (1758-1831) was the fifth President of the United States (1817-1825). Monroe is best known for the Monroe Doctrine devised by his Secretary of State, John Quincy Adams. Monroe delivered the Doctrine in a message to Congress on December 2, 1823. Not only must Latin America be left alone, he warned, but also Russia must not encroach southward on the Pacific coast. "…the American continents, by the free and independent condition which they have assumed and maintain, are henceforth not to be considered as subjects for future colonization by any European Power."

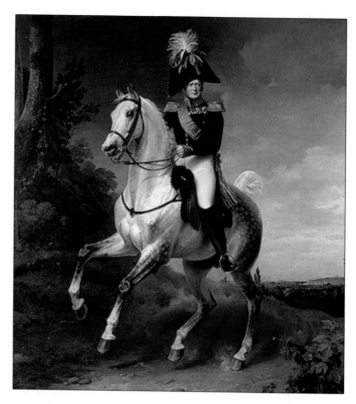

Czar Alexander I of Russia (1777-1825), Emperor of Russia (1801-1825), King of Poland (1815-1825). Alexander was one of the most important figures in the 19th century. His relationships with European rulers fluctuated back and forth between cooperation and hostility. His complex nature was a result of his early environment and education. Raised in the free-thinking atmosphere of the court of Catherine the Great, he was immersed in the principles of Rousseau by his Swiss tutor. From his military training, he acquired the traditions of Russian autocracy. His father, Emperor Paul I, taught him to combine a theoretical love of mankind with a practical contempt and distrust of men.

European states to intervene in the affairs of Latin America would be considered an act of war against the United States. Britain had already established economic interests in the Western Hemisphere during Napoleon's reign and to maintain them supported the United States' isolationist policy. As a result, the Americas would remain independent of European political developments during the nineteenth century.

THE BREAKDOWN OF THE CONCERT OF EUROPE: 1830-1848

Metternich's coalition began to break down after the death of Czar Alexander I in 1825. Alexander was succeeded by Nicholas I who, while maintaining his predecessor's desire to expand Russian influence, did not share Alexander's policy of unanimously supporting traditional regimes. In 1821, Alexander I had refused to support the Greek revolution against the Ottoman Empire. However in 1830, Nicholas I assisted the Greeks to victory, thus extending Russia's influence further west. The Greek revolution marked a turning point for the Concert of Europe.

The fatal blow to the Concert came from France after the Bourbon king, Louis XVIII, died in 1824. Louis's successor, Charles X, introduced a number of counterrevolutionary policies, including an indemnity to be paid to those who lost their land during the revolution and the death penalty for those who committed sacrilege in church buildings. Opposition against the king immediately broke out and newspapers and political leaders criticized his actions. Finally, in July 1830, revolution broke out. Charles X fled to England, and the revolutionaries set up a constitutional monarchy, choosing Louis-Philippe of Orléans as their new king. He would rule France for the next eighteen years.

The successful revolution in France encouraged similar uprisings in Poland and Belgium. Poland had been restored by the Congress of Vienna in 1814 but was under the direct rule of the Russian Czar. In 1830 Polish nationals rebelled, but Russia moved in and crushed the resistance. At the Congress of Vienna, Belgium was united with Holland, and now Belgian nationals hoped to win independence. Thanks to the support of Louis-Philippe and the new regime in France, the Belgian revolution was successful. After Greece and Belgium won independence, the counterrevolution launched by Metternich and the Concert of Europe seemed destined to fail.

PART II
The Church in the Post-Napoleonic Era

GERMANY AND FRANCE

After 1815, Germany was dominated by the northern, predominately Protestant state of Prussia. Seeking to impose rigid unity over the other German states, Prussia began to introduce policies designed to undermine Catholic influence in Germany. In 1825, Prussia passed a law requiring children to be raised in the father's religion. Prussian executives were then sent into Catholic German states with the purpose of marrying young Catholic girls. They hoped to establish a Protestant leadership in these Catholic states through effective breeding.

In response to the Prussian law, Pius VIII required that all Catholics who married outside of the Faith instruct their children in the Catholic Faith, thus directly opposing the Prussian law. Catholics throughout Germany responded to the pope's request by condemning the Prussian law and refusing to follow the anti-Catholic guidelines. In 1837, the Archbishop of Cologne, Clement Droste von Vischering, was arrested by Prussian authorities for supporting the Papal directive. As persecution continued, Catholics in Germany began to unify behind the pope.

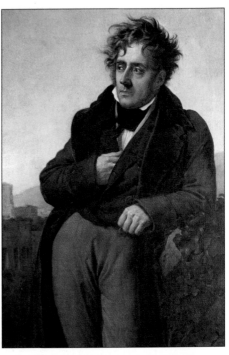

François-René de Chateaubriand (1768-1848), a French writer and diplomat, is considered the father of Romanticism in French literature. He began a post-revolution Catholic revival in France with *The Genius of Christianity*, written in 1802. His refusal in 1830 to swear allegiance to King Louis-Philippe put an end to his political career.

In the years following Napoleon's defeat, a Catholic intellectual revival took place in France, which generated enthusiasm toward their Catholic identity. In part, this renewal was prompted by the French writer François-René de Chateaubriand whose The Genius of Christianity, written in 1802, defended Catholic dogma against liberal and atheistic attacks. After that publication, a number of Catholic French intellectuals worked to counteract anti-Catholic sentiment arising from both liberal and conservative sectors of society.

THE UNITED STATES

Shortly after the independence of the United States was recognized in the Treaty of Paris (1783), Baltimore became the first diocese within the thirteen original states in 1789. Immigrants began to flock to the United States, and this immigration created the need for a well-structured Church in America. In 1808, Pope Pius VII erected the Dioceses of Boston, New York, Philadelphia, and Bardstown (which eventually moved to Louisville), and named Baltimore a metropolitan see. In 1820 the Dioceses of Charleston and Richmond were added, and in 1821, the Diocese of Cincinnati.

The first immigrants from Ireland and Germany began to flood into the United States in 1820, and immigration continued throughout the century. By 1850 immigrants from Germany, Italy and Eastern Europe made Catholicism one of the largest Christian denominations in the country. This massive influx of Catholic immigrants frightened the Protestant-American public and led to a fierce anti-Catholic backlash. Books and pamphlets were distributed that attacked the morals and uprightness of priests and nuns; Churches were burned down; and some Catholics were lynched. Political cartoons depicted the Irish as monkeys or wild-eyed terrorists, and the Catholic Church was accused of sending papal spies to America. Political parties, such as the infamous Know-Nothing Party, became popular on nativist, anti-Catholic, and anti-immigrant platforms.

To protect each other, Catholics developed support networks that centered on parish life and parochial schools. Immigrants also built Catholic orphanages, hospitals, and nursing homes as a way of living out their Christian vocation and preservering their Catholic Faith.

THE BRITISH ISLES

Catholic persecution persisted in Britain since the time of the Reformation. Catholics could not vote, sit in Parliament, nor hold civil offices. In 1778 and 1791, the British passed reform bills that helped bring about the revocation of many anti-Catholic laws in Great Britain and Ireland. In 1801, British parliament was considering freedom of Catholic worship in Ireland but unfortunately dropped the idea. Moreover, the British government dissolved the Dublin parliament and declared Anglicanism as the official religion of Ireland. Consequently, Irish Catholics were forbidden to hold public office and denied a right to vote. Nonetheless, the support of England by Pope Pius VII during the Napoleonic wars helped ease ill feelings towards Catholics in Britain, and to avert an Irish uprising, Parliament passed the Catholic Relief Act in 1829, thereby granting emancipation to Catholics. Lastly, the life of the Church in the British Isles would be largely affected by industrialization, since many of the laborers employed in many of the new factories would be Catholic.

PART III

The Industrial Revolution

As political revolution was changing the ruling structures of continental Europe, at the same time an economic revolution was occurring all over Europe, but especially in Great Britain, whose effects would be felt throughout the world. Toward the end of the eighteenth century, some key social changes and technological innovations would turn Britain to change rapidly from an agricultural to an industrial economy. This change – traditionally called the Industrial Revolution – would dramatically affect the culture and life style of British society.

The Industrial Revolution in Great Britain was closely linked to its agricultural developments. During the late seventeenth and eighteenth centuries, farmers and landowners in Britain began experimenting with various technological and scientific improvements in farming, including new breeding techniques and methods of cultivation. In order to implement these new agricultural improvements, the landowners began to accumulate farming plantations by buying up many small farms. Unlike other parts of Europe, which were still ruled by powerful monarchs, these wealthy British landowners were extremely influential in the English Parliament and used this influence to obtain a number of land reforms. Landowners acquired new farmlands formally held in common by towns or villages and worked to bring all of the farming in England under private ownership. As a result, peasant farmers who used to work on common lands or small farms were now displaced from their lands and needed to look for other ways to make a living. These farmers were hired by the wealthy landowners for a daily wage. This created a large, mobile workforce that was dependent on wages.

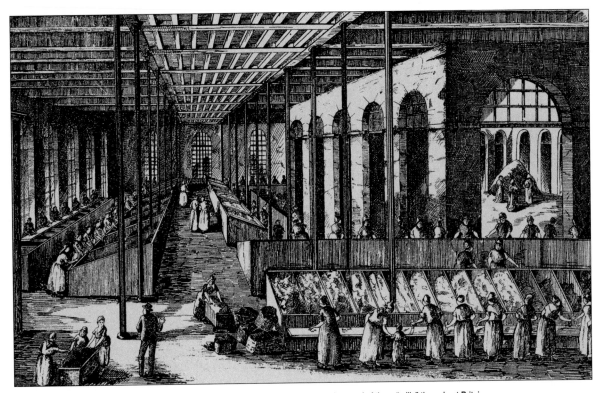

A nineteenth century textile factory. By 1823, there were ten thousand of these "mills" throughout Britain.

As these agricultural changes were occurring, those involved with Britain's already prosperous textile trade were also looking for new ways to increase their profits. New technologies, such as the fly shuttle, spinning jenny, and water frame, led to the development of a power loom, which could produce more cloth and material than ever before. Other explorations into ways of powering these new machines produced the steam engine, and with it, a greater reliance on burning coal for energy. Factories, or "mills," were built in towns and cities to house the new machines and the volume of production immediately grew. The first steam loom factory opened in Manchester in 1806, and by 1823 there were more than 10,000 throughout Britain. As jobs proliferated in the factories, many farm workers headed to cities to find work in the mills.

SOCIAL CONSEQUENCES OF INDUSTRIALIZATION

As cities grew, so did the population. Between 1750 and 1850, the population of England tripled to over thirty million. Nonetheless, the population explosion in no way signified a rising standard of living among the masses. Life for the common worker became increasingly difficult.

During industrialization, cities became densely packed and overcrowded industrial centers where poor workers earned very meager wages in the factories. Skilled workers lost their jobs to new, more efficient technologies. Out of desperation to support themselves and their families, people were forced to work in factories or mines under dangerous conditions, sometimes for fourteen or more hours a day. Women and children, sometimes better suited for jobs because of size or familiarity with looms, worked similar hours for even lesser wages.

City life also changed familial relationships. On the farm, family members worked and lived together, complementing each other's roles and skills. But in urban centers, families were apart for long hours, and employment was often necessary for every member of the family. Large families became beneficial to bring home extra wages as children as young as six worked along side grown men, enduring

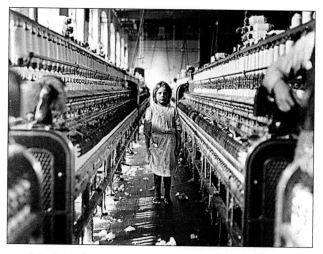

In the mid-nineteenth century, more than twenty percent of all employees in textile mills and coal mines were under the age of ten years old.

the same conditions and long hours. Mine owners employed children to pull coal carts in the small recesses of the mineshaft, and mill owners used children to crawl into tight spaces. Child wages were the lowest and loss of life was frequent. In the mid-nineteenth century, more than twenty percent of all employees in textile mills and coal mines were under the age of ten years old.

Urban life was typically squalid and destitute. For a great number of people in most cities, services were poor due to a lack of city planning. Families crammed together in poorly-built tenement houses, sometimes sharing just a single room. Sanitary conditions were awful, and fresh water was rare. At the time, most buildings and factories burned coal for heat and fuel, producing black soot that clouded the air and stained buildings. Diseases such as tuberculosis, cholera, and dysentery were rampant in working-class districts. Life expectancy was low among the working class. A study conducted by the British Parliament in 1842 found that in Manchester the average age of death was thirty-eight for professional classes, twenty for shopkeepers, and seventeen for the working class.

FROM ECONOMIC TO POLITICAL REVOLUTION

At the end of the eighteenth century, political power in Britain rested in the hands of about five hundred wealthy landed gentry. This gentry class pushed for many of the land reforms that helped bring about the Industrial Revolution. However, rapid economic and social developments quickly caused the country's political organization to become obsolete. As cities grew, new industrial leaders gained wealth and influence, and they pressed for political reform.

Representation in British Parliament had not been altered since 1688. At that time, large cities like Manchester and Birmingham did not exist, and so despite their growth, they lacked real political representation. Adding to the discontent of the powerful, city-based industrialists, the landed gentry continued to pass laws that taxed imports, thus restricting free economic exchange. These laws, known as the Corn Laws, angered industrialists who sought to minimize their expenses and maximize their profits by following laissez-faire economic principles. Political unrest began to build, and fearing similar civil disorder that plagued continental Europe, Parliament passed the Great Reform Bill of 1832. This re-apportioned representation in England and brought about a shift in power that would eventually help "free-trade" legislation pass through Parliament. The Corn Laws would be overturned in the 1840s.

These new reforms also helped end centuries of government- sanctioned Catholic oppression. In 1829, thanks to the support of the British Home Secretary Robert Peel, the Roman Catholic Relief Act was passed which granted Catholic emancipation and enabled Catholics to hold Parliamentary seats. The Irish activist Daniel O'Connell became the first Irishman to represent his people in London. Daniel O'Connell had worked to organize Irish Catholics for political representation since 1800. He had instituted "Catholic Rent," gathering as little as a penny a month from poor Irish Catholic families to help finance his political organization and unite Catholics behind a common cause. O'Connell went on to become a major figure in the House of Commons, prominent in the struggles for prison and law reform, free trade, the abolition of slavery, and universal suffrage.

PART IV

Bl. *Pio Nono* and the Rise of Nationalism

In June 1846, a conclave met to choose Gregory XVI's successor. The cardinals picked the fifty-five-year-old Cardinal Giovanni Maria Mastai-Ferretti, who took the name Pius IX, or Pio Nono as he would be affectionately called throughout the world. Bl. Pio Nono was young, popular among Italians, poor (he borrowed money to afford the trip to the conclave), and sympathetic to the liberal cause. His election gave new hope to revolutionaries throughout Europe, especially in Italy, while worrying Metternich and other conservatives who feared a liberal pope could tip the balance of the continent towards revolution.

Metternich was right to worry. One of the earliest acts by the new pope was to threaten the Austrian leader with excommunication unless Austrian troops withdrew from Ferrara in northern Italy. Metternich complied, and this tough diplomacy made Bl. Pio Nono immensely popular in Italy. Some even hoped the pope might become president of a new Italian republic.

In Rome, the new pope took his pastoral mission very seriously. He visited hospitals and schools, made improvements to the city, and allowed for greater toleration of Roman Jews. As ruler of the Papal States, he created an assembly with lay representatives to help govern, granted amnesty to revolutionaries in the Papal States, helped to introduce tax reform, and established an agricultural institute to provide advice and assistance to farmers. Bl. Pio Nono's generous reforms won support from Catholics, Protestants, and secular liberals alike. Nevertheless, in 1848, Bl. Pio Nono's popularity dwindled. Revolution once again erupted all over Europe, and Bl. Pio Nono found himself pulled from every side to join in the violence.

THE REVOLUTIONS OF 1848

By 1848, Metternich's Europe – the tight conservative grip that kept unhappy peasants and unruly revolutionaries at bay – was slowly weakening. After thirty years of mounting unrest, revolution erupted throughout the continent. Once again, revolution started in France. In February 1848, an accidental shot fired into a protesting mob sparked violence and turned the protest into a full-scale insurrection. Barricades were set up in the streets and King Louis-Philippe, fearing for his life, fled to Great Britain.

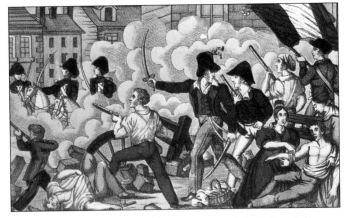

In Paris, France, February 1848, a shot fired into a mob of protestors set off a year of anti-conservative revolutions across Europe.

In France a group of bourgeois liberals set up a provisional government. The new government harnessed the support of poor urban workers by employing them in communal workgroups. But the Parisian bourgeoisie underestimated the rural French who used the elections held in April of that year to swing support behind candidates who would establish a conservative republic. The newly elected government dissolved the workgroups, and the urban workers once again took to the streets in protest. During the month of June 1848, hundreds of people were killed and hundreds more sent overseas to French colonial prisons. Civil unrest continued throughout the year, and in December, elections were held again. This time Louis-Napoleon Bonaparte, the nephew of Napoleon, won an overwhelming majority. It would take this new Bonaparte only three years to seize total control of France in a coup d'état and proclaim himself Napoleon III. Tragically, the 1848 revolution only helped widen an ever-growing cultural divide between rural and urban French.

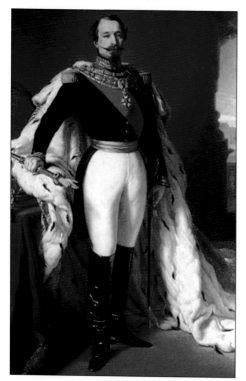

Napoleon III, (1808-1873), Emperor of France, sent French troops to drive out Italian revolutionaries and restored control of the Holy City and the Papal States to Bl. Pope Pius IX.

News of the Parisian insurrections reached the German-speaking world in early March 1848. Liberal students immediately took to the streets, demanding an end of Metternich's undemocratic system. The uprising gained momentum, and Metternich was forced to flee for his life.

Unlike France, the spirit of revolution in central Europe was linked to a latent desire for national unity. Protests quickly spread to the capitals of Hungary and Bohemia where nationalists met to discuss the establishment of new, independent states. In May, over eight hundred delegates from all over the Germanophone world met in Frankfurt in order to draft a constitution that could consolidate the Hapsburg and Prussian empires into a new German state. Debates between Protestant Prussia and the Catholic South prolonged the meeting for eleven months. During a delay in the congress, the reigning Austrian government managed to suppress the rebellion in Vienna and regain an authoritative hold on the country. After Czar Nicholas I mobilized his army to win Hungary back for the Austrians, Prussia also backed out of the convention in Frankfurt. The liberals' effort to unify Germany had failed.

In Italy, Bl. Pius IX faced growing pressure to declare war on Austria on behalf of Italy. Italians wanted to win back the regions of Lombardy and Venice that Austria seized during the Congress of Vienna. Because of the pope's popular liberal policies, many had hoped that the pope would actually lead in the initiative to fight Austria. Not surprisingly, the pope refused to involve the papacy in a war against another Catholic nation. He condemned the idea of a federal Italy led by the pope and urged the Italian people to stay faithful to their respective princes.

In the eyes of the people, Bl. Pio Nono's opposition to the revolution made him an enemy. On November 15, 1848, Bl. Pius IX's prime minister was murdered as he attempted to open the Parliament, and mobs over-ran the assembly. The endangered pope was forced to flee the city. Insurrections sprang up throughout the peninsula as the nationalist movements led by Giuseppe Manzzini (a Freemason) and his "Young Italians" and the liberal Freemason and revolutionary Giuseppe Garibaldi gained momentum.

With the pope out of Rome, Manzzini and Garibaldi proclaimed a new Roman Republic, and for nearly a year, revolutionaries had control over the Holy City. Finally, Bl. Pius IX called on the Catholic powers of Europe to restore his temporal rule over the papal states. French troops sent by the new Emperor Napoleon III retook the city and the Papal States, and on April 12, 1850, Bl. Pius IX returned to Rome. He was no longer the beloved pope of the people, and having protested the excesses of the revolution in Italy, Bl. Pius IX was no longer seen as a friend to the liberal cause.

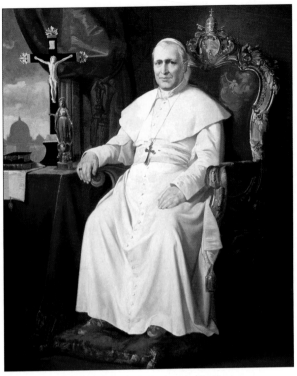

Pope Blessed Pius IX or affectionately, *Pio Nono,* born Giovanni Maria Mastai-Ferretti (1792-1878), was pope for a record pontificate of over 31 years, from June 16, 1846 until his death. Pope Pius IX was the last pope to hold temporal powers.

The revolutions of 1848 and his exile from Rome not only changed Bl. Pius IX's political position, but also the focus of his papacy. As liberalism was spreading throughout Europe, Italian unification, which was spreading across most of the peninsula, now threatened the independence of the Papal States. If those lands were lost, the pope thought, so would be the freedom of the Church. To defend his sovereign territory, Bl. Pius IX raised an international army of volunteers.

Leadership of the newly unified Italy now passed to the Piedmont king Vittorio Emmanuelle and his Freemason premier Count Camillo Cavour. Bl. Pius IX privately admired Emmanuelle as a champion of Italy, but was very apprehensive over Cavour's revolutionary tendencies and his policies. In 1854, Cavour had all the monasteries and convents in Piedmont closed, a move that made Bl. Pius IX increasingly suspicious and fearful of the unification movement's effect on the life of the Church.

ULTRAMONTANISM

The ongoing liberal revolutions of the nineteenth century divided Catholics. Some believed that anti-clericalism was implicit in Liberalism and that revolutions would threaten to unleash a new period of prolonged religious persecution. Others hoped that Catholicism and Liberalism could find common ground. After the exile of Bl. Pius IX, Catholics were uneasy and divided as to what should be the Church's next step.

During the nineteenth century, two schools of Catholic thought developed over the idea of Liberalism, and two German universities became the centers of these ideological discussions and deliberations. In Mainz, thinkers believed that liberal ideas were too secular, rational, and anti-clerical. They began to look to the pope as the last defender of the Catholic cause, the final bulwark against a liberal world. These Catholics became known as the ultramontanists (over the mountains) because as they looked to the pope for support and leadership, emphasizing his centrality and authority more than ever before.

In Munich, another Catholic school recognized an inevitable trend of European governments towards liberal democracy and sought to build bridges of mutual understanding between the Church and democratic regimes. These thinkers were optimistic about modern culture and believed that Church leaders could co-exist with liberal ideas and that dialogue with the modern world was beneficial for the future of the Church. The German theologian Johann Mohler proposed a number of reforms, like the use of the vernacular in the liturgy, some of which would eventually be adopted following the Second Vatican Council.

In response to the ultramontanists, the famous Anglican convert John Henry Cardinal Newman worried that by bypassing the diocesan ordinaries, the ultramontanists were creating a "Church within a Church" subservient exclusively to Rome. He criticized their immoderate dismissal of

BL. JOHN HENRY CARDINAL NEWMAN

Catholics in England had been disliked and persecuted ever since the Reformation, and were considered second-class citizens within English society. The Penal Laws that tried to wipe out Catholicism in England were quite successful. While the nineteenth century also saw the development of rights for Catholics in England, society at large was still suspect of all so-called "papists." After such a long period of oppression, by this century the Catholic minority in England was scorned and hated by the Protestant majority.

It was under these conditions that the unthinkable happened. The Reverend John Henry Newman, the most famous and influential Anglican preacher in all of England, a writer of incomparable ability, converted to Catholicism. His life was then dedicated to leading thousands of other English Protestants down the same path, and to this day, his writings still bring many back into the Church.

Born in 1801 to Anglican parents, Bl. John Henry Newman grew up holding the traditional English ideas towards Roman Catholicism—that the Catholic Church taught superstitious doctrine contrary to the gospels. From an early age he exhibited great potential. A highly gifted student, at the age of fifteen he went to Oxford University, and was later ordained in the Anglican Church, establishing himself as a great preacher. He began to study the teachings of the Church Fathers, and to his surprise discovered that many doctrines taught in the early Church—apostolic succession and the Sacraments, for example—were still found in the Catholic Church but had been long abandoned by his own Anglican Church. He soon joined the "Oxford Movement," a group of Anglicans who attempted to reestablish these lost doctrines back into the Anglican Church.

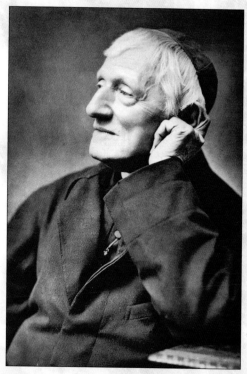

Bl. John Henry Newman, the leader of the Oxford Movement in the Church of England, was received into the Catholic Church in 1845. He is considered a sensitive Christian thinker, and his influence brought many converts to the Church in England. He was named a cardinal in 1879 and beatified in 2010.

While Bl. John Henry Newman's extraordinary gifts established him as the leading spokesman for this cause, he eventually came to the realization that what he was defending could be found in its entirety in the Catholic Church. This realization led to his conversion to Catholicism, after which he was ordained a priest, later in life being named a cardinal by Pope Leo XIII. Bl. John Henry Newman died on August 11, 1890. Some of his greatest works published during his Catholic years include *The Idea of University* (1852), *An Essay in Aid of a Grammar of Assent* (1870), and *Apologia pro Vita Sua* (1864).

liberal ideas, saying, "we are shrinking into ourselves, narrowing the lines of communication, trembling at freedom of thought, and using the language of dismay and despair at the prospect before us" (quoted in Gilly, *Newman and His Age*, 1990, p. 344). As the gap between these two Catholic opinions widened, some Catholics seemed to have experienced a growing identity crisis.

THE IMMACULATE CONCEPTION

Ironically, it was a religious proclamation, not a political one, that would bring the questions of Liberalism and papal authority to the forefront of debate within the Church. In 1854, four years after his return to Rome, Bl. Pius IX solemnly defined the doctrine of Mary's Immaculate Conception.

Throughout the history of the Church, Mary had been venerated as the Immaculate Conception, and the theological foundations of this title go back to the early centuries. Many of the Church Fathers referred to Mary as the "new Eve" (Eve was also created without original sin), and St. John of Damascus argued that the sinlessness of Mary was implicit in her title "*Theotokos*" (literally, "bearer of God"). Although the feast of her Immaculate Conception had been celebrated since the seventh century, debate over the issue continued during the twelfth century. St. Bernard of Clairvaux and St. Thomas Aquinas were not sure concerning the doctrine of the Immaculate Conception, but Bl. John Duns Scotus defended it. In 1439, the Council of Basel ruled that the Immaculate Conception was a pious opinion in accordance with Faith, reason, and Scripture. Over one hundred years later, the Council of Trent specifically excluded Mary from its decree that all have inherited the stain of original sin. After these conciliar decisions, the issue was generally defended, but the exact nature of the Immaculate Conception was never officially defined as a dogmatic statement of the Church.

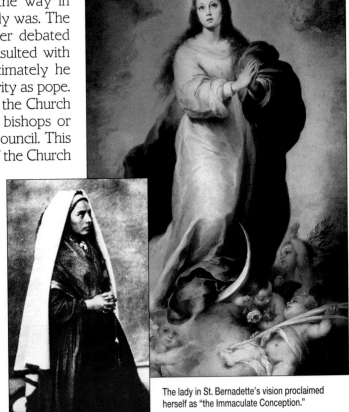

Although the dogma of the Immaculate Conception was not a surprising proclamation, the way in which Bl. Pius IX proclaimed it certainly was. The Immaculate Conception was no longer debated theologically, and Bl. Pius IX had consulted with bishops before his definition, but ultimately he defined this tenet of Faith on his authority as pope. Furthermore, he spoke as the voice of the Church and certainly not as the first among bishops or within the context of an ecumenical council. This bold move implied that the authority of the Church on doctrinal and moral matters lay within the competence of the papal office. Ultramontanists rejoiced at this victory for papal centrality, but others feared the implications of Bl. Pius's pronouncement.

Four years later, in 1858, at the grotto of Massabielle, in Lourdes, France, a young girl named Bernadette Soubirous had a vision. Mary appeared to the girl, proclaiming in the ninth vision, "I am the Immaculate Conception." It seems that she was pleased with Bl. Pius's solemn declaration.

The lady in St. Bernadette's vision proclaimed herself as "the Immaculate Conception."

OUR LADY OF LOURDES

The appearance of Our Lady of Lourdes to St. Bernadette is one of the most famous of all Marian apparitions. The story began on Thursday, February 11, 1858, when Bernadette, 14, a poor, uneducated peasant girl in Southern France, went to a nearby river with her sister Marie and a friend to gather firewood. After these two crossed the river, leaving St. Bernadette alone, she heard what sounded like a storm coming from a nearby grotto called Massabielle. Looking inside the grotto she saw a golden cloud, and shortly thereafter a beautiful lady with a rosary draped over her right arm. St. Bernadette fell to her knees and began to pray the rosary with the lady (although the lady only recited the Our Father and the Gloria). After completing the rosary, the lady disappeared into the grotto without telling St. Bernadette who she was.

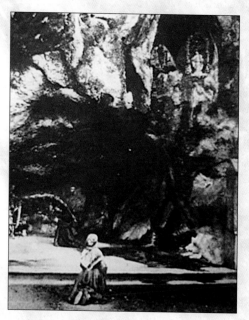

St. Bernadette kneeling at the grotto in Lourdes taken in 1862, three years after the Marian apparitions.

St. Bernadette herself later wrote of this first apparition:

> While I was saying the Rosary, I was watching as hard as I could. She was wearing a white dress reaching down to her feet, of which only the toes appeared. The dress was gathered very high at the neck by a hem from which hung a white cord. A white veil covered her head and came down over her shoulders and arms almost to the bottom of her dress. On each foot I saw a yellow rose. The sash of the dress was blue, and hung down below her knees. The chain of the rosary was yellow; the beads white, big and widely spaced.

This was the first of many apparitions. As word spread, many people would accompany St. Bernadette to the grotto, but only St. Bernadette was able to see the lady. During these apparitions the lady would tell St. Bernadette to pray for sinners and on one occasion asked her to dig and scratch the ground and drink from the spring that flowed forth. This spring was later discovered to contain miraculous healing powers. At the request of the village Curé, St. Bernadette asked the lady who she was. On the Feast of the Annunciation, March 25, the lady told St. Bernadette, "I am the Immaculate Conception." St. Bernadette repeated these words, which she probably did not even understand, to the astounded Curé. (The dogma of the Immaculate Conception had been solemnly defined only four years prior to this apparition.)

In all, St. Bernadette received eighteen visitations from Mary over a six month period. The Church declared the apparitions authentic in 1862, and today Lourdes is one of the world's most popular pilgrimage sites. The miraculous spring has healed thousands of people from all over the world.

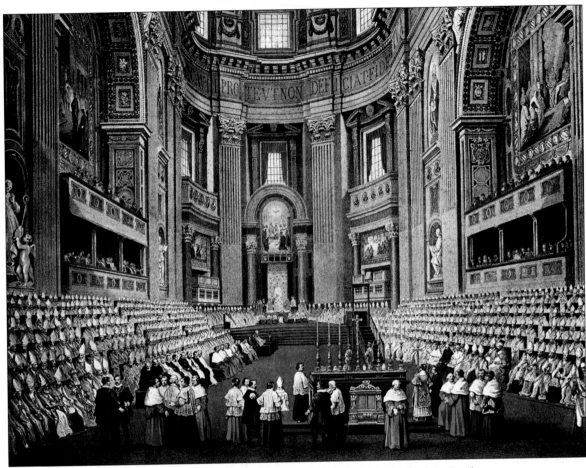

On December 8, 1869, the Feast of the Immaculate Conception, Pope Pius IX opened the first Vatican Council.
The decrees issued from the council condemned modern-day materialism, atheism, and declared papal infallibility.

THE FIRST VATICAN COUNCIL

Bl. Pius IX continued to assert his opposition to the liberal world. In 1864, Bl. Pius IX issued the encyclical *Quanta Cura* with its Syllabus of Errors. In this encyclical, the Pope attacked many ideologies and opinions that challenged Church authority, which included socialism, Gallicanism, rationalism, and the separation of Church and state. Many ultramontanists were calling for an all out denouncement of liberal thought, and they urged the Pope to reprimand those Catholics sympathetic to liberal democracy. This desire was fulfilled by the publication of *Quanta Cura*, which would widen the rift between the liberals and ultramontanists.

The Syllabus condemned many errors prevalent in nineteenth-century Europe, including pantheism; naturalism; rationalism, whether absolute or moderate; false tolerance in religious matters; socialism; communism; secret societies; errors regarding the Church and her rights, especially in relation to the state; and errors regarding Christian Matrimony. Many of the faithful received the Syllabus well. It was essentially a compilation of errors which Bl. Pius IX had been addressing for almost two decades. The enemies of the Church nevertheless received it as an affront to the modern state and a rejection of modern culture.

For centuries Popes had written encyclicals for the express purpose of counseling and instructing members of the Church on certain aspects of her teaching. However, in the wake of the declaration of the Immaculate Conception, many ultramontanists erroneously believed that every papal pronouncement stood as official Church doctrine. Specifically, they declared that all the contents of Bl. Pius's Syllabus must be followed unquestioningly since "all papal declarations were infallible."

At the time, all Catholics generally agreed that the pope taught infallibly. Like the Immaculate Conception, this belief had never been solemnly defined, and as a result, Catholics held diverse opinions on the subject. Some argued that the pope spoke as the first among all bishops and that his role as leader did not mean that Church authority lay exclusively in the pope himself. Others argued that as the Vicar of Christ, the pope himself was infallible and that all his letters, encyclicals, and teachings stood as official Church doctrine.

On December 8, 1869, the Feast of the Immaculate Conception, Bl. Pius IX opened the First Vatican Council to help reconcile these growing divisions between members of the Church. The council met over eleven months in three sessions approving just two constitutions: the "Dogmatic Constitution on the Catholic Faith" and the "First Dogmatic Constitution on the Church of Christ." The "Faith" constitution spoke about proof for the existence of God, revelation, Faith, and the role of Faith and reason while at the same time condemning contemporary errors on those topics. The second constitution dealt with the main issue of the council: papal infallibility.

The chief arguments against papal infallibility – as specific and distinct from the Church's infallibility – involve instances wherein popes stand accused of teaching heresy. The most common among these arguments pertains to Popes Liberius, Honorius, and Vigilius in the early centuries of the Church and the Galileo affair in the seventeenth century. Pope Liberius, however, whether an Arian or semi-Arian as critics claim, at worst acted under duress and coercion. This lack of freedom certainly does not allow a pope to teach ex cathedra (from the chair [of St. Peter]). Pope Honorius is accused of both teaching the Monothelite heresy and being condemned by the Third Ecumenical Council of Constantinople. Based on his letters to the heretic Sergius, he was most likely imprecise in his theological terminology about the question as to whether Christ had two wills or one. As for the condemnation of the Third Council of Constantinople, St. Leo II, who ratified the decrees, noted that Honorius was condemned for his lack of papal zeal in combating heresy, not for teaching heresy himself. Pope Vigilius simply wavered in the face of a controversy about whether to condemn three contentious letters as containing heresy. As for the Galileo affair, the Holy Office – the Roman congregation that advises the pope on doctrinal questions – handled the inquiry and meted out the punishment. Although, from a modern perspective, this matter should have been handled better, the silencing of Galileo was a disciplinary measure and not a doctrinal one. It bears repeating: disciplinary actions do not fall within the context of infallibility.

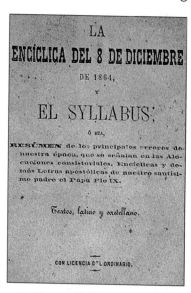

The title page of Bl. Pius IX's *El Syllabus*, December 1864

Proof in favor of papal infallibility can be found in both Scripture and Tradition. Sacred Scripture includes three specific proofs. Matthew 16:18 records Christ's words to St. Peter: "You are Peter, and on this rock I will build my church, and the powers of death shall not prevail against it." This text contains the promise that St. Peter was to be the rock-foundation of the Church, and it follows that his successors are heirs to this promise. Luke 22:31-32 records Christ saying to St. Peter: "Simon, Simon, behold, Satan demanded to have you, that he might sift you like wheat, but I have prayed for you, that your faith may not fail; and when you have turned again, strengthen your brethren." This prayer of Christ was specifically for St. Peter as head of the Church. John 21:15-17 recounts the post-Resurrection triple command of Christ to St. Peter, culminating with: "'Simon,

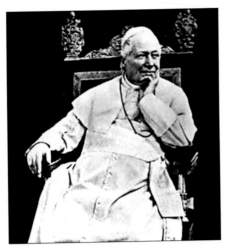

Bl. Pius IX never accepted the "Law of Guarantees" declaring himself a "prisoner of the Vatican."

son of John, do you love me?'…And he said to him, 'Lord, you know everything; you know that I love you.' Jesus said to him, 'Feed my sheep.'" The whole of Christ's flock is thus entrusted to St. Peter and his successors.

Sacred Tradition offers several proofs. The letter of St. Clement I in the first century–even while St. John, one of the Twelve, was still alive–was written to correct the Corinthians' behavior. St. Irenaeus claimed that conformity with the Roman bishop was proof of Apostolicity of doctrine (cf. Adv. hær., III, iii). History has recorded many statements in almost every century to the effect of "Peter has spoken through ___" (whoever was the reigning pope at the time). St. Augustine famously denounced the Pelagian heresy in a sermon after the receipt of St. Innocent I's letter: "Rome's reply has come: the case is closed" (Serm. 131, c. x). Specific or indirect reference to papal infallibility is even found in many councils before Vatican I, including the Councils of Ephesus (431), Chalcedon (451), Constantinople III (680-681), Constantinople IV (869-870), and Florence (1438-1445).

The bishops debated the issue intensely, and in June 1870, a draft entitled "On the Infallibility of the Roman Pontiff" was presented to the bishops for discussion. In a particularly dramatic moment, the Dominican theologian Cardinal Guidi, Archbishop of Bologna, criticized the title of the draft, insisting that the pope was not infallible, but rather the pope's teaching was. He warned against the dangers of rashly proclaiming infallibility because although his solemn teachings are considered true, the person of the pope is certainly not impeccable. The ultramontanists protested Guidi's argument, and even Bl. Pius IX admonished the cardinal for his comments. In the end, Guidi's understanding proved to be in line with Catholic teaching, and the final draft of the definition of papal infallibility made the distinction between infallible teaching and the assurance of moral integrity of the pope. It read, under the title "On the Infallible Teaching Authority of the Roman Pontiff":

> We teach and define as a divinely revealed dogma that when the Roman Pontiff speaks ex cathedra, that is, when, in the exercise of his office as shepherd and teacher of all Christians, in virtue of his supreme apostolic authority, he defines a doctrine concerning faith and morals to be held by the whole Church, he possesses, by the divine assistance promised to him in blessed Peter, that infallibility which the divine Redeemer willed his Church to enjoy in defining doctrine concerning faith or morals. Therefore, such definitions of the Roman Pontiff are of themselves, and not by the consent of the Church, irreformable (Constitutio prima de Ecclesia [First Dogmatic Constitution on the Church of Christ], 1870, 4.9).

This definition, approved by Bl. Pius IX, set specific parameters for infallible papal teachings. Therefore, without the necessary conditions for infallibility, encyclicals, letters, and homilies are simply ranked as ordinary teachings of the pope. Although these papal writings still enjoy very high authority of opinion, they are not to be considered infallible teachings of the Catholic Church on their own authority.

THE ROMAN QUESTION

During the Franco-Prussian War, Germany sought to dominate northern Europe. Italian revolutionaries took advantage of France's wartime weakness, and King Vittorio Emmanuelle resumed the Italian political revolution and modernization called the Risorgimento. On September 19, 1870, he took Rome, and Bl. Pius IX, driven from his palace in the Quirinale, took refuge in the Vatican.

In November 1870, Italy passed the "Law of Guarantees" to regulate the new relations between Church and state. (A similar offer had been rejected by Bl. Pius IX before the conquest of Rome.) The law provided that the pope would retain all of the honors and immunities of a sovereign. It gave the pontiff use of the Vatican, the Lateran, and Castel Gandolfo, the papal residence in the hills southwest of Rome, and allotted him three and a half million lire each year as compensation for his territorial losses. Significantly, the law also stated that the pope would appoint all the Italian bishops (the highest concentration of bishops in the world). Before this time, papal appointment of bishops was not an assumed or guaranteed privilege. Paradoxically, by losing control of the Papal States, the pope gained greater moral authority in administering the Church as a whole.

Bl. Pius IX refused to accept the "Law of Guarantees." Instead, he locked himself inside the Vatican palace, declaring himself a "prisoner of the Vatican." The Popes' official status would remain that of a prisoner until 1929, when Italy, under Mussolini, agreed to an independent Vatican city-state and granted the pope possession of his palaces (not just "use" as the "Law of Guarantees" had stated), resolving this "Roman Question," as it came to be called.

In the meantime, the pope was at the mercy of the Italian state, and consequently, Church and state were at odds. The Italian government seized Church properties, and took responsibility for education away from religious orders. Monasteries were suppressed and religious orders abolished. Those who protested these measures were either thrown in prison or exiled from the country.

In 1868, Bl. Pius IX had issued the decree *Non expedit* which forbade Catholics from participating in the Italian political process, either by voting or running for office. Catholics, who comprised the vast majority of the Italian population, became second-class citizens in their own country. Somehow the Italians, who were used to living under foreign rule, learned to discretely keep a foot in both worlds, Church and state, without allowing the two to mix.

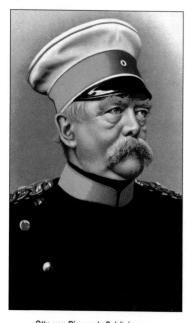

Otto von Bismarck-Schönhausen, (1815-1898). As Prime Minister of Prussia from 1862 to 1890, he engineered the unification of the numerous states of Germany. He then served as the first Chancellor of the German Empire from 1871 to 1890. Following unification, Germany became one of the most powerful nations in Europe.

GERMAN UNIFICATION AND THE *KULTURKAMPF*

The Franco-Prussian War, which allowed Italy the opportunity to seize the Papal States, was the culmination of a long process of German unification under the leadership of the master Prussian diplomat Otto von Bismarck.

Bismarck became chancellor to the Hohenzollern king, Wilhelm I, in 1873. Wilhelm I assumed leadership in 1861 after his older brother Frederick Wilhelm IV stepped down due to failing mental stability. Unlike his romantic and idealistic brother, Wilhelm I was determined to strengthen the Prussian military and expand the country's influence throughout the continent. However, he lacked the necessary political skills, and so he turned to his chancellor to lead the country. Bismarck, nicknamed the "Iron Chancellor," began an extended program of militarization and diplomatic manipulation through which he created a unified German Empire.

Bismarck's plan for German unification was supported by the general and awakened sentiment of German nationalism. The chancellor believed that the sense of nationalism was strong enough in Germany to overcome the traditional North-South, Protestant-Catholic divisions, which had previously prevented the formation of a unified Germany. With this in mind, Bismarck drew

Prussia into war with the surrounding countries in order to inspire the other German states to fight along side their fellow Prussian Germans. Bismarck went to war with Denmark in 1864, Austria in 1866, and finally France in 1870. With each conflict, more German states joined Prussia. Finally, on January 18, 1871, after the conclusion of the Franco-Prussian War, Bismarck met with the heads of twenty-five German states at Versailles where Wilhelm I was proclaimed emperor of a new, unified German Empire. Having defeated both Austria and France, the new German Empire now the dominant force on the continent.

Despite success in unifying Germany, Bismarck and Protestant Prussia still saw the Catholic Church as an obstacle to the advancement of the new Empire. German Catholics opposed Bismarck's militaristic and nationalistic regime, forming the Center Party in 1870, which allied itself with liberal critics of Bismarck. In 1872, Germany passed the "Falk Laws" (alternately known as the "May Laws" as they were passed in May 1873) in an effort to dismantle Catholic unity within Germany. These laws, named after the "minister of cults," Dr. Falk, subjected Catholic schools and seminaries to state control, prohibited religious orders from teaching, and expelled the Jesuit order from Germany. (Eventually every religious order would be expelled from Germany.) Furthermore, any priest or bishop who did not acknowledge state supremacy over the Church in Germany would be fined or imprisoned. These laws ushered in Bismarck's new internal policy, the Kulturkampf (culture struggle), whose aim was to rid Germany of Catholicism.

By 1876, there were no longer any bishops in Prussia, and more than a thousand priests were either exiled or imprisoned, leaving Catholics without access to the Sacraments. Bismarck even tried to create divisions between Catholics themselves, offering exemptions to those who cooperated with the newly established laws and by supporting those Catholics who rejected the decrees of the recent Vatican Council. Nonetheless, German Catholics would not comply with the Chancellor's policies. They published Catholic journals and joined the Center Party, which grew in strength in opposition to Bismarck. German bishops who had been driven from the country continued to serve their dioceses while in exile. Bl. Pius IX voiced opposition to Bismarck's policies, stating that no Catholic in Germany was obliged to obey any of the Falk Laws.

Bismarck eventually realized that his anti-Catholic program was not working, and, as the new Socialist Party gained strength in Germany, he knew he would need Catholic support to preserve the empire. The death of Bl. Pius IX in 1878 provided Bismarck with an opportunity to abandon his Kulturkampf without the humiliation of giving in to papal pressure. On the day of Pope Leo XIII's election, Bismarck wrote the new pope a letter of apology. Bismarck ended his anti-Catholic policies, and shifted his support to the Catholic Center Party, which opposed the rising tide of socialism in Germany.

PART V

Imperialism

THE OPENING OF AFRICA

Although the coast of Africa had been part of the European trade network since the fifteenth century, prior to 1845, virtually all the expeditions into the African interior resulted in failure due to the outbreaks of malaria, yellow fever, typhus, and dysentery. Disease seemed to protect the African interior with an impenetrable barrier. However, the introduction of Quinine (a drug made from bark used to treat malaria) and the discovery of the causes of yellow fever eventually protected Europeans as they traveled deeper into the African interior.

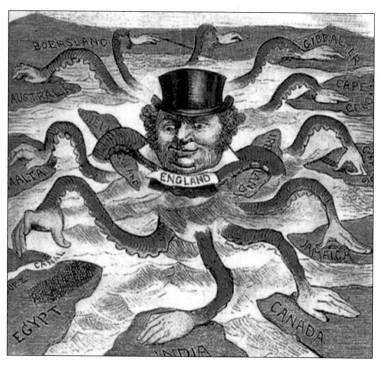

A political cartoon illustrates the extent of British expansion in the nineteenth century.

As had been the case with the explorations of the sixteenth century, Imperial expansion into Africa also brought about a great missionary revival. This time, both Catholics and Protestants flooded the newly-opened African interior. Protestant missionaries traveled with European traders and often had native tribes learn western cultural habits. On the other hand, Catholic missionaries in Africa continued to learn local languages and assimilate African ways of life and so better adapt the Faith to cultural subtleties. Unfortunately, because of this assimilation, many European nations saw the Catholic presence in Africa as a threat to colonization. Although Britain was generally tolerant of both Catholic and Protestant missionaries, King Leopold of Belgium forbade Catholic missionaries from entering the Congo, and the Portuguese colonies of Angola and Mozambique had relatively little Christian presence. At first, France welcomed Catholic missionaries and worked with them in the administration of their colonial possessions. However, after the establishment of the Third Republic in 1871, the French government's support for the Catholic missions dwindled.

As they had done in the past, Catholic missionaries worked at putting into place self-sufficient Catholic communities in Africa with native clergy and an African ecclesiastical hierarchy. The acquisition of native clergy would occur slowly at first, and large numbers of priests would not be ordained until well into the twentieth century. The first native African bishop since the Muslim expansion into North Africa was Laurean Cardinal Rugambwa, who was appointed in 1953. The African clergy founded schools to help maintain and develop the Church in Africa. As a result, most African Catholics

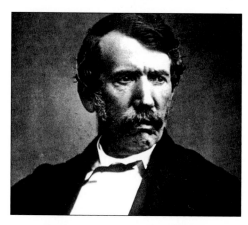

David Livingstone (1813-1873) was a Scottish missionary and explorer of the Victorian era. In 1852-56, he explored the African interior, discovering Victoria Falls (which he named after his monarch, Queen Victoria). Livingstone was one of the first Westerners to cross the African continent.

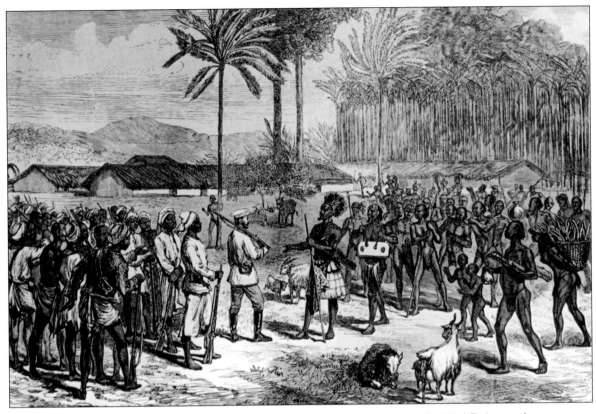

A sketch by Henry Morton Stanley (1841-1904) depicts his arrival to the village of Manyema (Kenya, East Africa). The journeys of Livingstone and Stanley opened Africa to Christian missions. Stanley was instructed in 1869 by the owner of his newspaper to "Find Livingstone!" Stanley traveled to Zanzibar and outfitted an expedition with the best equipment and 2,000 porters. He located Livingstone on November 10, 1871 near Lake Tanganyika (present-day Tanzania), and greeted him by saying "Dr. Livingstone, I presume?"

owed their conversions to black catechists who had been trained to preach the gospel, and this effort produced a huge increase of African Catholics. In southern Nigeria, for example, the Catholic community grew from five thousand in 1900 to seventy-four thousand by 1912. The success of these early missionary efforts is reflected today in the strong and vigorous Catholic communities that are still thriving and growing in Africa.

MISSIONARY APOSTOLATE IN THE FAR EAST

Missionary efforts in the Far East would prove more difficult than in Africa. In China, apart from admitting a small number of Christian missionaries and European traders in the sixteenth century, for three thousand years the country remained isolated from the rest of the world. During the early part of the nineteenth century, China seemed interested in preserving this isolation, but Great Britain, determined to tap into the huge Chinese market, found ways to introduce the highly addictive drug opium into the country. The Chinese attempted to block the importation of opium, and between 1839 and 1841, China fought two wars with Britain over the sale of the drug. Britain won the Opium Wars, and in the Treaty of Nanking (1842), Britain obtained long-term access to the port city of Hong Kong – the first step towards open trade throughout all of the coastal Chinese ports. Soon, every European nation established "Spheres of Influence" in that country, i.e., regions in which the colonizers traded freely and administered under their own laws.

Before the opening of China, missionaries were subject to severe persecutions, and many were exiled and even killed. After the European nations established their Spheres of Influence, the Chinese government restored properties seized from Christians and protected churches from violence. Nevertheless, missionaries were still seen as representative of Western expansion, and popular violence against them continued. Two examples of these violent persecutions took place in 1866 when two bishops and seven priests were decapitated, and in 1870, when twenty-two Christians were executed, including the French consul, the chancellor, an interpreter, his wife, and ten sisters of St. Vincent de Paul. Persecution and general rejection of the Western missionaries never ceased, nor did the overall precarious situation of the Church in China improve in the twentieth century.

In Japan, since 1640, after the Tokugawa Shogunate drove the last Europeans from the Japanese mainland, Japan had been closed to foreigners. In 1853 an American warship, commanded by Commodore Matthew Perry, forced a trade agreement with the Tokugawa leadership that reopened Japan to the West. In 1868 the Tokugawa were overthrown, and the new imperial house of Meiji took power. The new emperor began a rapid and remarkable policy of modernization in an effort to compete with Western powers and prevent future Western domination of their country. In just thirty years, Japan underwent an incredible period of change during which it adapted aspects of its business, legal system, and military to that of the United States, France, and Great Britain. Japan's extraordinary modernization was evident by 1901 when it defeated Russia in the Russo-Japanese War.

Japanese missionary activity resumed with the new access into Japan after 1853. At first, French missionaries, arriving in 1859, resided in open ports for the service of foreigners. In March 1865, in Nagasaki, fifteen Japanese Christians discreetly approached the French missionaries. They were careful not to disclose their full identity until they questioned the missionaries about three unique aspects of Catholicism. Some of the Japanese who were converted by the original Jesuit missionaries in the seventeenth century, had passed the Faith down from generation to generation, and looked to see if the new missionaries believed in loyalty to the authority of the Roman pontiff, the veneration of the Blessed Virgin, and celibacy of the clergy. When the fifteen were convinced that the French missionaries shared their same beliefs, over fifty thousand Japanese Christians came forth to support the missionaries. Unfortunately, the sudden appearance of the Japanese Christians drew the attention of the authorities, and persecution resumed. In July 1867, 40,000 faithful were exiled to various provinces. However, the restoration of the emperor in 1868 established a policy of toleration for Christians, and in 1873, persecution ceased and the exiles were allowed to return to their homes.

PART VI

Leo XIII (1878-1903): The Church Confronts a Changing World

Bl. Pius IX died on February 7, 1878, after thirty-two years as pope, the second-longest reign ever. (St. Peter, the first pope, reigned for about thirty-five years.) During his pontificate, the world and the Church's situation had changed dramatically. The new pope would not inherit the Papal States, and he would have to minister to a Church suffering persecution and marginalization in many European countries. At the same time, thanks to the First Vatican Council and changes in Italy, the pope would enjoy a position of greater moral authority, universally recognized as the focal

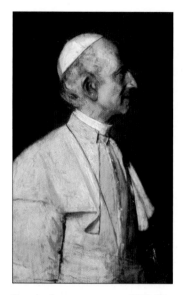

point of unity in the Catholic world and the one responsible for the appointment of bishops throughout the world.

At the conclave, the cardinals chose the relatively unknown Bishop of Perugia, Gioacchino Pecci, who took the name Leo XIII. The choice of Leo XIII was surprising not only because he came from the small and obscure see of Perugia, but also because Gioacchino Pecci had been somewhat unsuccessful in his career in the papal service (he was removed as nuncio from Belgium after mishandling a delicate political situation). In addition, Pecci was made Camerlengo (the person who oversees economic affairs and the convocation of the conclave for the papal election) just a few months before Bl. Pius's death. Usually due to age, the Camerlengo is not elected pope, and this appointment by the ailing pontiff may have signified Bl. Pius's desire to prevent Pecci from becoming pope.

There were a number of reasons why Pecci was elected. He had the reputation of being more traditional, and his opinions had helped form the content of Bl. Pius IX's Syllabus of Errors. Yet Pecci was also a successful and popular diocesan bishop who had published a series of pastoral letters that spoke positively about the possibilities of a modern society and the advances of science. Indeed, the successor of Bl. Pius IX would have the task of addressing a changing and hostile Europe, tackling the many new schools of thought that were shaping the future of the Western world. The election of Leo XIII placed a strong pastoral leader in the chair of St. Peter, a firm defender of the Faith who could mend rifts and speak positively about the contemporary world. During his twenty-five year pontificate, Leo XIII served as a teacher, issuing eighty-seven encyclicals, addressing almost every major issue of the day.

THE BIRTH OF SECULAR HUMANISM

The nineteenth century saw the beginning of a new humanistic and philosophical mind-set devoid of any spiritual or religious component. This new humanism, called Secular Humanism, became perhaps the most comprehensive and influential general ideology since the Enlightenment. Growing nationalism, blind faith in the "progress" of civilization, and exaltation of man as a replacement for God, all gave rise to notions of the human person divested of any relationship with the Divine. Secular humanism better describes a general sentiment and spirit of thought more than a unified school. What binds these thinkers is their increasingly materialistic understanding of the human person. As philosophy drifted even further from notions of God and religion, many began to argue that the world does not reflect the eternal wisdom and law of God and, therefore, standards for governing what is right and wrong do not apply, or, at best, they are relative. Instead of God, man became the subject of study, and his motives and desires were believed to be quantifiable and calculable. This premise, which influenced nearly every discipline from science to politics, posed major challenges to the Church. The encyclicals of Leo XIII responded to these erroneous ideas with explanations that presented the human person, society, and politics from a Christian perspective.

CHARLES DARWIN AND THE SURVIVAL OF THE FITTEST

From 1831 to 1836, the British naturalist Charles Darwin sailed around the world, studying the wide variety of species of plants and animals found in the many corners of the globe. Besides surveying species in South America, Australia, and Asia, Darwin recorded observations about the abundant rare species found on the Galapagos Islands in the Pacific Ocean. As Darwin compared the many species, he believed he found similarities that led him to startling conclusions.

Darwin observed how some species, such as those living on the Galapagos Islands, seem to resemble species in other lands in every way except for a few peculiar characteristics – such as a lizard that swims or a bird which cannot fly. Darwin concluded that this was the result of the species' gradual adaptation to their specific environment. Over time, he argued, two animals living in two different places would develop into two entirely different species by way of accidental mutations, which better equip each organism to survive in its specific environs. Darwin called this process "natural selection" since nature seemed to determine which members of a species were better equipped for survival. Darwin theorized that, over the course of thousands – if not millions – of years, the process of natural selection causes various species to "evolve" from a single species. This theory of evolution proposed that every living thing originated from a distant source: man from apes, birds from dinosaurs, frogs from fish, and the like.

Besides creating an entirely new field of scientific research, Darwin's theories greatly influenced nineteenth and twentieth century social thought. Although Darwin was never concerned with the social and religious implications of his theories, others took his theories and applied them to many other branches of thought such as anthropology, philosophy, and economics.

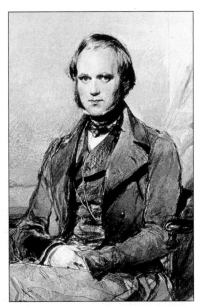

Charles Robert Darwin (1809-1882) was a British naturalist who achieved lasting fame as originator of the theory of evolution through natural selection. He wrote his theories after a five year voyage on the ship H.M.S. Beagle.

Natural selection, for instance, weeded out the weak, the poor, and the lower classes who were not strong enough to survive in harsh social environments. Wealthy industrialists believed their success reflected their "natural selection" in the continuation of the human species. (The full title of Darwin's best-known work is On the Origin of Species by Means of Natural Selection, or the Preservation of Favoured Races in the Struggle for Life.) No matter how unjust society became, they claimed that the future of humanity is determined by the "survival of the fittest," and economic or racial superiority leads to the advance and perfection of the human species.

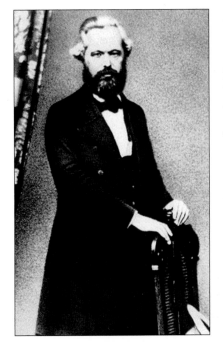

KARL MARX AND THE POLITICS OF ATHEISM

Karl Marx (1818-1883) was born in Alsace (on the border between France and Germany) into a particularly violent and volatile world. He spent much of his life working as a writer and journalist in Germany and France where he witnessed firsthand both political and economic revolution. He saw the massive social problems brought about by industrialization, including the emergence of a large urban working class, the widening gap between the wealthy and the poor, and the miserable situations experienced by workers marginalized by laissez-faire economics. In response to these, Marx wrote articles that criticized capitalism, liberal democracy, and religious beliefs and practices referred to as the "the opiate of the masses." Instead of these systems, he proposed a social-political structure called communism, which, he argued, would inevitably emerge as the dominant force in the world.

More than a political system, communism was envisioned by Marx as a necessary historical development, the culmination of human history. Marx posited that throughout history the majority of people have suffered in society due to wealth and property being controlled by a few ruling elite. But history also shows, he said, that these elite have been continuously overthrown through violent rebellion and replaced by those citizens lower down the social ladder. He said the French Revolution, which succeeded feudal power with rule by the bourgeoisie, perfectly illustrated this historical process.

For Marx, history was approaching a new era because the working class (proletariat), who represented the lowest and most numerous members of society, were the next social class poised for rebellion. Instead of simply seizing control of wealth and property and taking the place of the ruling elite, Marx argued that this exploited class would establish, through revolution, a new socio-economic system in which social classes no longer existed. In theory, this system (called communism) offered a Utopian vision: the proletariat held all wealth and property in common, creating a society based on absolute equality in which the government provided everyone with whatever they needed.

Marx believed history and society were based primarily on material motives and not on transcendental forces. (He called religion "the opiate of the masses" since it made the lower classes content with their rotten state.) Based on his scientific examination of the laws of economics, Marx argued that the proletariat would rise up in a last, bloody, worldwide revolution, finally overthrowing the owners of capital and destroying the principle of private property. Although Marx's theories found fertile ground among those members of society who had been hurt and left behind by the proponents of laissez-faire economics, the communist regimes in reality have violated human dignity more than any other political system and has utterly failed in its attempt of promoting the rights and welfare of the workers and common people. Most communist countries began to take on more mercantilist or capitalist systems by the end of the twentieth century. By the dawn of the third millennium, only five countries could be described as communist, including the largest in population: China.

The Encyclicals of Leo XIII

Leo XIII was the first pope in over a millennium and a half not to exercise temporal power. Being divested of temporal authority gave this new pope the capacity to focus on the pastoral needs of the Church and formulate Catholic teaching applicable to the needs of the times. He put out a staggering eighty-seven papal encyclicals, which reflected a papacy free of the distractions of temporal rule and focused on the moral leadership of the Church..

Leo XIII's encyclicals touched on the many burning issues affecting society as well as the spiritual welfare of the person. His writings include various and sundry themes such as doctrinal formation, freedom, scripture, and the Rosary.

Inscrutabili Dei (April 21, 1878)

Leo XIII issued his first encyclical just two months after becoming pope, and it set the tone for his later teachings. Inscrutabili Dei (On the Evils of Society) stated briefly all the accumulated problems affecting contemporary society. Evils have oppressed the human race "on every side," he argues

Inscrutabili Dei summarizes over a hundred years of offences perpetrated by the revolutionary regimes whose excesses had plunged society into its present sorry state. The pope contends that these evils are a result of the setting aside of "the holy and venerable authority of the Church" (Inscrutabili Dei, no. 3). To support his argument, Pope Leo XIII quotes St. Paul who warned in

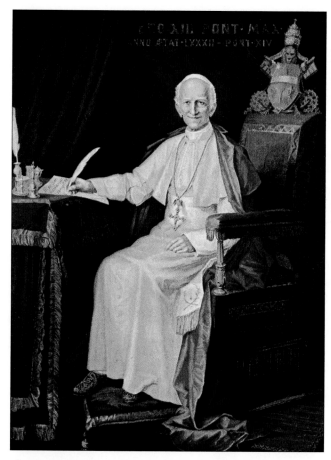

Pope Leo XIII, born Vincenzo Gioacchino Raffaele Luigi Pecci (1810-1903), succeeded Blessed Pius IX on February 20, 1878 and reigned until his death. Leo XIII worked to encourage understanding between the Church and the modern world. He firmly re-asserted the study of Scholastic philosophy, especially St. Thomas Aquinas, in his encyclical *Æterni Patris* (1880).

his letter to the Colossians: "Beware lest any man cheat you by philosophy or vain deceit, according to the tradition of men, according to the elements of the world and not according to Christ (Col 2:8)" (Inscrutabili Dei, no. 13).

Inscrutabili Dei is an effective introduction to both Leo XIII's papacy and his extensive teachings. As if drawing a line in the sand, Leo identifies the problems of the age, illustrates their opposition to the Church, and argues that fidelity to the Christian message expressed through the Catholic Church is the only hope for restoring and curing society.

Picking up where Bl. Pius IX left off, Leo XIII strongly emphasized the important role of papal authority in preserving the future of the Church. The encyclical also shows that Leo XIII understood papal teaching as a central aspect of the church's mission. He illustrated in later encyclicals that the church guidance and mission will never be compromised by any kind of political regime governing a nation.

In the closing paragraphs of Inscrutabili Dei, the pope offers a hopeful solution to overcoming contemporary difficulties, stating that a healthy society is possible as long as "each member will gradually grow accustomed to the love of religion and piety, to the abhorrence of false and harmful teaching, to the pursuit of virtue, to obedience to elders, and to the restraint of the insatiable seeking after self-interest alone, which so spoils and weakens the character of men" (Inscrutabili Dei, no. 15).

Immortale Dei (November 1, 1885)

Leo XIII's encyclical Immortale Dei (On the Christian Constitution of States) exemplifies the pope's careful efforts to show understanding for liberal political movements while clearly transmitting the Church's doctrine on the dynamics and role of civil society. Leo XIII begins the encyclical by restating the Church's belief that God is the root and source of all political authority and that both civil and divine authority have a duty and responsibility to God. "For, men living together in society," he argues, "are under the power of God no less than individuals are, and society, no less than individuals, owes gratitude to God who gave it being and maintains it and whose ever bounteous goodness enriches it with countless blessings" (Immortale Dei, no. 6). Because civil authority is ultimately an expression of God's plan, Pope Leo warns against those who may incite revolution against civil government.

Nonetheless, Leo XIII did not seek to separate the Church from legitimate political change and modernization. He devotes the closing section of his encyclical to insisting that the Church "most gladly welcomes whatever improvements the age brings forth" (Immortale Dei, no. 23). Neither does he endorse any specific form of government, such as a monarchy with the union of throne and altar. These were welcoming words to political progressives and provided some resolution to the ideological struggle between the Church and the modern world. Finally, the pope closes with an invitation to Catholics to participate in the new democratic societies that recently emerged.

Rerum Novarum (May 15, 1891)

Among the eighty-seven encyclicals written by Leo XIII, none was so widely received, praised, and influential as Rerum novarum (On Capital and Labor), his encyclical on social justice. This encyclical is perhaps Leo XIII's most unique work since it outlines for the first time the principles of Catholic Social Teaching that would remain in force throughout the late nineteenth and twentieth centuries.

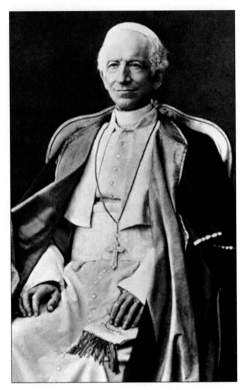

A large part of this encyclical is dedicated to a refutation of the principles of socialism which proposes a society that holds all property in common to be administered by the state. Leo XIII condemned socialism as an attack on human freedom and dignity, arguing that the worker would be the first to suffer from such a regime. "Remunerative labor," the pope says, is "the impelling reason and motive of . . . work [to obtain property]" (Rerum novarum, 5). Acquisition of private property is an intrinsic right of every human being who is called by God to use the material resources for his own benefit and welfare. The worker gains private property as the fruit of his labor "Man not only should possess the fruits of the earth," the pope writes, "but also the very soil, inasmuch as from the produce of the earth he has to lay by provision for the future" (Rerum novarum, 7).

Leo XIII also argues that the loss of private ownership would cause harm to the human family. "That right to property," he says, "must in like wise belong to a man in his capacity of head of a family . . . The contention, then, that the civil government should at its opinion intrude into and exercise intimate control over the family and the household is a great and pernicious error" (Rerum novarum, 13-14).

"And if human society is to be healed now, in no other way can it be healed save by a return to Christian life and Christian institutions."

— Pope Leo XIII, *Rerum novarum*, 27

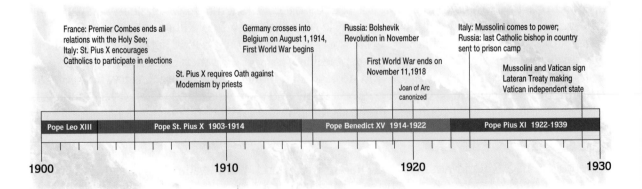

France: Premier Combes ends all relations with the Holy See; Italy: St. Pius X encourages Catholics to participate in elections

St. Pius X requires Oath against Modernism by priests

Germany crosses into Belgium on August 1, 1914, First World War begins

Russia: Bolshevik Revolution in November

First World War ends on November 11, 1918

Joan of Arc canonized

Italy: Mussolini comes to power; Russia: last Catholic bishop in country sent to prison camp

Mussolini and Vatican sign Lateran Treaty making Vatican independent state

Pope Leo XIII   Pope St. Pius X 1903-1914   Pope Benedict XV 1914-1922   Pope Pius XI 1922-1939

1900   1910   1920   1930

Although he clarifies the evils of socialism, Pope Leo did not praise the capitalist economy of the Industrial Age, which he said had laid upon the poor "a yoke little better than that of slavery" (Rerum novarum, 3). Pope Leo referred instead to the Gospel. "If Christian precepts prevail," he argues, "the respective classes will not only be untied in the bonds of friendship, but also in those of brotherly love" (Rerum novarum, 25). Pope Leo saw Christianity, with its foundation in fraternal love, as the only solution to the problems of modern society. Only when there is recognition of our common Father, who is God, can a just society be formed, since justice is perfected by charity. The pope went on to rebuke the wealthy who by their unjust and uncharitable exploitation of the working classes ignore the words of Christ: "'It is more blessed to give than to receive' (Acts 20:35)" (Rerum novarum, 22).

Leo XIII also addressed the erroneous belief that the wealthy and working classes were intended by nature to live in mutual conflict. The pope maintained that this view was directly contrary to the truth, and that it was "ordained by nature that these two classes should dwell in harmony and agreement, so as to maintain the balance of the body politic" (Rerum novarum, 19). The employer provides the capital required for producing the goods and services and the employee provides the labor to turn the capital into the goods and services. One cannot exist without the other.

Both classes, however, have duties to the other that must be followed. The worker, for example, must fully and faithfully "perform the work which has been freely and equitably agreed upon" and "never to resort to violence in defending their own cause, nor to engage in riot or disorder" (Rerum novarum, 20). On the other hand, the employer is bound "not to look upon their work people as their bondsmen" and "never to tax his work people beyond their strength, or employ them in work unsuited to their sex and age" (Rerum novarum, 20). Additionally, although the employer and employee are free to bargain as to wages, the employer always has a duty to pay his workers a just wage sufficient "to support a frugal and well behaved wage-earner" (Rerum novarum, 45).

PART VII

St. Pius X (1903-1914)

The first pope elected in the twentieth century was St. Pius X. St. Pius X was born Giuseppe Sarto at Riese, Upper Venice, on June 2, 1835. His father was a postman, and his mother a seamstress. A man of simple origins, after discovering his vocation, Giuseppe Sarto wished only for a simple life of servitude as a country priest. After studying at the seminary in Padua, he was ordained on September 18, 1858, and for the next nine years served as a rural parish priest. Sarto's intellectual

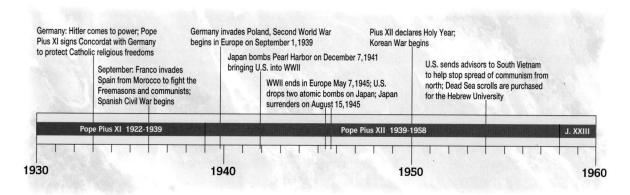

Germany: Hitler comes to power; Pope Pius XI signs Concordat with Germany to protect Catholic religious freedoms

September: Franco invades Spain from Morocco to fight the Freemasons and communists; Spanish Civil War begins

Germany invades Poland, Second World War begins in Europe on September 1, 1939

Japan bombs Pearl Harbor on December 7, 1941 bringing U.S. into WWII

WWII ends in Europe May 7, 1945; U.S. drops two atomic bombs on Japan; Japan surrenders on August 15, 1945

Pius XII declares Holy Year; Korean War begins

U.S. sends advisors to South Vietnam to help stop spread of communism from north; Dead Sea scrolls are purchased for the Hebrew University

Pope Pius XI 1922-1939   Pope Pius XII 1939-1958   J. XXIII

1930   1940   1950   1960

gifts and exceptional spiritual depth were recognized by his superiors, and in 1875 he was asked to be chancellor of the Diocese of Treviso and spiritual director of its seminary.

In Treviso, Sarto worked tirelessly, taking on more jobs than was required of the priest. He restored the church, provided for the enlargement and maintenance of the hospital by his own means, and devoted himself to ministering to the poor and those who were suffering from cholera, which was especially widespread at the time. As rector of the seminary, Sarto was dedicated to teaching the Faith. He became well known as an excellent instructor of adults and worked to make it possible for students in public schools to receive religious instruction.

In 1884, Pope Leo XIII appointed him Bishop of Mantua, and nine years later Pope Leo named him Patriarch of Venice and a cardinal. In both places, he showed himself to be a hard-working, pastoral bishop devoted to his priests and people.

THE PONTIFICATE OF ST. PIUS X

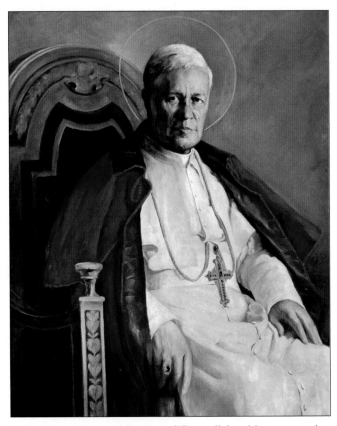

At the conclave after Pope Leo's death, because the Austrian Emperor Franz Joseph intervened to veto the selection of another candidate, the cardinals chose Cardinal Sarto as the next pope on August 4, 1903. Taking the name Pius X, the new pope adopted the motto "To Restore All Things in Christ" (Eph 1:10), and his pontificate was indeed dedicated to a renewal of the Church in the ways of Christ. St. Pius X set the tone of his pontificate by formally ending the custom by which the Holy Roman Emperor could intervene in papal elections. It was but the first step the new pope took to further the independence of the Church from civil intervention.

St. Pius X also did much to strengthen Catholic life and religious practice. One of his earliest official acts was to launch the updating and systematic compilation of the law of the Church. The result – the Code of Canon Law of 1917 – was published after his death, but most of the work was done in his pontificate. He reorganized the Roman Curia and, in encyclicals in 1905 and 1906, encouraged Catholic Action, an organization that was to become a key instrument of lay apostolate.

St. Pius X also took important steps in the area of liturgy and worship. New norms were published for liturgical music centering on encouragement of Gregorian

St. Pius X is considered one of the greatest of all popes. He issued decrees encouraging frequent, even daily, reception of communion by the laity. He relaxed the rules for reception of communion by the sick, and allowed children to receive First Holy Communion at an earlier age, arguing that the Body and Blood of Christ should be available to children at the earliest age of reason. He made known his hope that the Catholic laity would form action groups and play a greater role in the apostolic life of the Church. His encyclicals condemning Modernism and promoting the teaching of Christian doctrine are noteworthy. In 1917 a new compilation of the Code of Canon Law was completed as well. He encouraged the Confraternity of Christian Doctrine (CCD) in every parish worldwide to educate everyone in the Faith.

Chant. The revision of the Divine Office was begun. He fostered religious education, and in a 1905 encyclical, strongly encouraged the program of the Confraternity of Christian Doctrine in every parish to help with the education of the young in the Faith.

St. Pius X is probably best known, however, as the "Pope of the Eucharist." He issued decrees encouraging frequent, even daily, reception of communion. The pope said that in receiving the Eucharist, "union with Christ is strengthened, the spiritual life more abundantly sustained, the soul more richly endowed with virtues, and the pledge of everlasting happiness more securely bestowed." (Sacra Tridentina [On Frequent and Daily Reception of Holy Communion], 1905, no. 6). St. Pius X relaxed the rules for reception of communion by the sick, and allowed children to receive First Holy Communion at an earlier age, arguing that the Body and Blood of Christ should be available to children at the earliest age of reason (about 7 years old).

CHRISTIAN MODERNISTS

The movement known as Modernism originated in the late nineteenth century. Some Catholic intellectuals, out of a desire to address contemporary currents of thought, embraced trends in psychology, science, and philosophy and tried to adapt Christian thought to them.

Never very numerous, the Modernists were found in only a few countries, principally France. Lack of any clear organization makes it hard to describe the movement precisely, but certain characteristics stand out. Considering religion to be a matter of psychological experience rather than objective truth, Modernism was fundamentally relativistic. Taking its lead from popular ideas about biological evolution, it regarded all Church doctrines and structures as always subject to change. It rejected the thought of St. Thomas Aquinas and Scholastic philosophy at the very time the Church was promoting a revival of Thomism. It viewed the Bible, including the New Testament, as a record of its human authors' religious experience rather than a divinely inspired source of truth. All traditional truths were questioned.

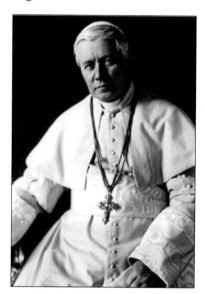

When World War I broke out, St. Pius X was devastated and died only days after the hostilities had begun.

St. Pius X called Modernism a "compendium of all heresies" and addressed the problem early in his pontificate. On July 3, 1907, the Vatican's doctrinal agency, the Holy Office, issued a decree called Lamentabili summing up the errors of Modernists in sixty-five propositions. The decree condemned modernist ideas such as revelation was "nothing other than the consciousness acquired by man of his relation to God" and Christ did not claim to be the messiah, found a Church, nor teach "a defined body of doctrine applicable to all times and all men." The sixty-fifth condemned proposition was the capstone of the rest: "Present day Catholicism cannot be reconciled with true science, unless it be transformed into a kind of nondogmatic Christianity, that is, into a broad and liberal Protestantism."

Modernism was, and is, a genuine and serious problem, and St. Pius X succeeded in eradicating outright declarations of its teachings. On September 1, 1910, St. Pius X issued a mandate requiring all priests to take a new Oath against Modernism. The Oath worked, but only to some extent; Modernist thinking went underground. Modernism was to resurface around the time of the Second Vatican Council when many of its proponents tried to reintroduce its relativistic principles. This would only produce confusion and dissent, but in the end it was the Holy Spirit guiding the Church through the decrees of Vatican II.

St. Pius X worked to keep the European powers from engaging in war until his death on August 20, 1914, just as World War I was getting underway. It is said he died of a broken heart because of this war. A man of great personal holiness, he was beatified by Pope Pius XII on June 3, 1951, and canonized by the same pope on May 29, 1954.

PART VIII

War, Revolution, and Persecution

POPE BENEDICT XV (1914-1922)

Born into an old family in Genoa on November 21, 1854, Giacomo della Chiesa received a doctorate in civil law at the University of Genoa in 1875, studied in Rome, and was ordained a priest in December 1878. He continued his studies at the Vatican's training academy for the papal diplomatic corps. From 1883 to 1887 he was an assistant to the Holy See's nuncio to Spain, Archbishop Mariano Rampolla, and when Leo XIII named Rampolla Secretary of State, della Chiesa returned to Rome to serve as his secretary. Della Chiesa was named Undersecretary of State in 1901, and he continued in that position under St. Pius X. The Pope appointed him Archbishop of Bologna in 1907 and named him a cardinal in May 1914, just a few months before the conclave. Three months later, when the cardinals gathered to elect a successor to St. Pius X, the ominous international scene caused them to turn to an experienced diplomat, Cardinal della Chiesa.

Although some expected the war to be a short affair, World War I dragged on four long years. "A disaster has visited the world," wrote Cardinal Desire Mercier of invaded, occupied Belgium on Christmas 1914. No one understood that better than Benedict XV.

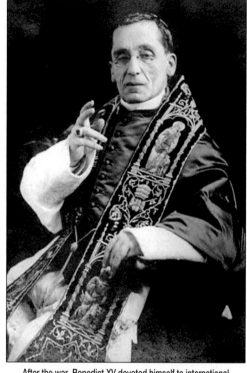

After the war, Benedict XV devoted himself to international reconciliation. France resumed diplomatic relations with the Holy See, warmed by the pope's canonization of Joan of Arc in 1920. Even Britain sent a chargé d'affaires to the Vatican in 1915, the first in 300 years.

As pope, Benedict XV, a compassionate and sensitive priest, protested the barbarity of the war, but took great care to maintain strict impartiality, a policy that brought criticism from both sides. Benedict hoped that by remaining impartial, the Vatican could better serve the peace process.

He outlined a seven-point peace program that he sent to the warring nations in August of 1917, but despite its basis for a just and stable settlement, the peace plan was ignored. Meanwhile, the pope acted vigorously to assist war victims. He sought humane treatment for the wounded and prisoners-of-war and carried on a large-scale charitable program without regard for nationality or religion.

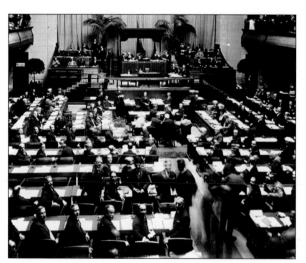

The first meeting of the League of Nations Assembly in Geneva, Switzerland in 1920. The League of Nations was an international organization founded after the First World War at the Paris Peace Conference in 1919. The League's goals included disarmament; preventing war through collective security; settling disputes between countries through negotiation and diplomacy; and improving global welfare. Because it had no real enforcement powers it failed to prevent a second World War. The United Nations replaced it after World War II and inherited a number of agencies and organizations founded by the League.

After the war, Pope Benedict hoped to be a party to the peace talks in Versailles, but the Italian government vetoed the idea. The pope's exclusion from the peace process marked an important transition in the role of the pope in the modern world. For over a century, the papacy had retreated from direct involvement in the political scene, and was now forbidden any official political capacity. The pope began to serve a new purpose in the world, issuing many encyclicals that addressed specific moral and ethical problems, and offered the Church's wisdom and understanding to the world. In this capacity, the popes of the twentieth century began to act as the world's moral conscience, witnessing history and guiding it through their words and actions. The unfortunate reality was, however, that political leaders rarely took the words of the pope very seriously.

THE RISE OF SOVIET COMMUNISM

Soviet-style Communism had its roots in the theories of Karl Marx (1818-1883), who in 1848 with Friedrich Engels (1820-1895), set out their key ideas in the Communist Manifesto. During World War I, popular unrest and mutinies in the Russian military forced Czar Nicholas II to abdicate in March 1917. A brief period of rule by a liberal government was followed by the Bolshevik Revolution of November 1917, which brought Communists to power under the leadership of Vladimir Lenin (1870-1924). Upon seizing power, the country's new masters set about cruelly suppressing political opposition and managed to establish tight socialist control over the country, including the brutal execution of the czar and his family. Out of this bloodshed and violence, the Soviet Union emerged. Around the same time, (October 1917) the Blessed Virgin Mary appeared to three peasant children at Fatima, Portugal. Offering a message of hope in the face of this political calamity in the East, Mary spoke of these events and urged prayer for the conversion of Russia, which she promised would eventually occur.

Skilled in propaganda, the Communists in the 1920s and 1930s convinced many Western intellectuals that the Soviet Union was a workers' paradise and a model for the world. However, the harsh reality of life in the Soviet Union was vastly different from the propagandists' idealized picture, and under Lenin's successor, Joseph Stalin (1879-1953), brutality and totalitarian oppression only grew worse. During Stalin's dictatorship, nearly fifty million supposed opponents of the regime were either executed or sent to the vast system of Siberian prison camps and penal colonies called the gulag.

Religious persecution was a major element of the Communist program. Both Catholic and Orthodox churches were destroyed or desecrated and put to other uses including dance halls, stables, museums of atheism, chicken coops, and public baths. The Russian Orthodox Church was seen as nationalistic as well as religious and was therefore allowed to exist; however, its priests and bishops made many compromises with the communist regime. Soviet authorities set out to eradicate the Catholic Church in Russia. Before 1917 there were 54,000 churches in Russia, 300 of which were Catholic; by 1939, there were fewer than 100 churches, only two of which were Catholic. In 1923 the last Catholic bishop in Russia, John Cieplak, was sentenced to ten years in a prison camp. Eventually, only one Catholic priest was permitted to minister in the country, and he was stationed at the French embassy in Moscow and restricted to serving the diplomatic community. By 1959, according to a study by the U.S. House of Representatives' Judiciary Committee, some two and a half million Catholics in the Soviet Union had lost their lives, and millions more had been imprisoned or deported.

The Church opposed Communism from the start. In 1891, Pope Leo XIII wrote his landmark encyclical Rerum novarum, which presented a Christian alternative to socialist and Marxist theories of economic and social life. Rerum novarum prophetically warned against socialism, arguing that despite its apparent protection of the poor man, "the working man himself would be among the first to suffer" from a socialist regime. Instead, Leo XIII urged the protection of individual dignity and emphasized mutual responsibility between workers and employers.

OUR LADY OF FATIMA

After making failed pleas for peace to the warring nations, Pope Benedict XV appealed directly to Mary. On May 5, 1917, he wrote a pastoral letter urging all Christians to ask Mary to bring peace to the world.

> To Mary, then, who is the Mother of Mercy and omnipotent by grace, let loving and devout appeal go up from every corner of the earth-from noble temples and tiniest chapels, from royal palaces and mansions of the rich as from the poorest hut-from blood-drenched plains and seas. Let it bear to Her the anguished cry of mothers and wives, the wailing of innocent ones, the sighs of every generous heart: that Her most tender and benign solicitude may be moved and the peace we ask for be obtained for our agitated world.

Mary's response came only one week later. On May 13, she appeared to three children in the small village of Fatima, Portugal. The three children, St. Jacinta, St. Francisco, and Lucia (ages 7, 9, and 10, respectively) had been visited by an angel the previous year in preparation for Mary's visit. In Lucia's own words, they saw "a lady, clothed in white, brighter than the sun, radiating a light more clear and intense than a crystal cup filled with sparkling water, lit by burning sunlight." The lady told them she had come from heaven and that she would appear to them in the same place on the 13th of every month for the next 6 months. She asked them to say the rosary, offer themselves to God, and bear suffering as an act of reparation for the conversion of sinners.

Over the next few months, the children received a visit from the Blessed Virgin on the 13th of every month. During the July visit, she promised that in October she would tell them who she was and perform a miracle for all to see and believe. The children were also shown a vision of hell, and were told how God wished to save souls from eternal damnation through devotion to her Immaculate Heart. She also warned of another great war, the persecutions of the Church and the Holy Father, and asked for prayers for the conversion of Russia.

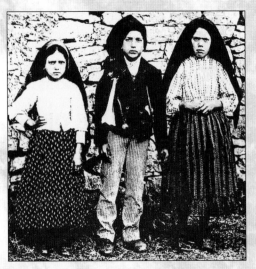

On October 13, 1917, despite a terrible storm, speculation of a public miracle attracted tens of thousands of pilgrims to Fatima. With many onlookers present, Mary again appeared to the children, finally telling them who she was: "the Lady of the Rosary." Then, more than 70,000 people witnessed a true miracle. The grey clouds suddenly parted, and, according to a journalist from an atheist newspaper who was there:

> One could see the immense multitude turn towards the sun, which appeared free from clouds and at its zenith. It looked like a plaque of dull silver and it was possible to look at it without the least discomfort. It might have been an eclipse which was taking place. But at that moment a great shout went up and one could hear the spectators nearest at hand shouting: "A miracle! A miracle!" Before the astonished eyes of the crowd, whose aspect was Biblical as they stood bareheaded, eagerly searching the sky, the sun trembled, made sudden incredible movements outside all cosmic laws—the sun "danced" according to the typical expression of the people.

Sts. Jacinta and Francisco were canonized by Pope Francis on February 13, 2017. Lucia passed away in 2005 at the age of 97; in 2017 she was given the title Servant of God, the first major step toward her canonization.

Pope Pius XI's encyclical Divini Redemptoris, published in 1937, was a powerful critique of Communism. Soviet Communism, the pope warned, "aims at upsetting the social order and at undermining the very foundations of Christian civilization." Pius XI's assessment would become more and more haunting as the abuses of the Soviet regime were fully discovered and documented. Unfortunately, it would take fifty more years for the Soviet Union to crumble and for Communism to fall in Eastern Europe.

POPE PIUS XI (1922-1939)

The end of the First World War, "the war to end all wars," in no way brought an end to violence and difficulty. Benedict XV lived to see the rise of Communism in Russia. After the pope's death, the Church would suffer further persecution, not only in Russia, but in Mexico and Spain as well. Indeed, when Pius XI, a strong-minded and determined pope, was elected to the head of the Church, he did not foresee the end of war. He would reign during an era of crisis marked by global economic collapse, the spread of totalitarianism, and increasing international conflict. Nazism, an ideology and a political movement fundamentally opposed to Christianity, came to power in Germany and threatened the peace of Europe and the world.

The future Pope Pius XI, Achille Ratti, was born May 31, 1857, near Milan. His father was a factory manager. Following ordination in 1879, Ratti pursued graduate studies in Rome and taught at the seminary in Padua. An excellent scholar, he worked from 1888 to 1911 at the Ambrosian Library in Milan. In 1911 he joined the staff of the Vatican Library as pro-prefect, and in 1914 became its prefect (director). In 1918, Pope Benedict XV sent Ratti to Poland on a diplomatic mission and later appointed him Nuncio to that country. While stationed in Warsaw, Ratti showed exemplary courage and dedication to his ministry when he refused to leave the city in the face of a threatened Bolshevik attack in August 1920. The following year, Pope Benedict named him Archbishop of Milan and a cardinal. Following Benedict's death, Ratti was elected pope on February 6, 1922, and he took the name Pius XI.

One of the first problems to confront Pius XI was the "Roman Question," that is, the difficulties that continued to arise over the relationship between the Vatican and the Italian government. Since the seizure of the Papal States in the nineteenth century, the popes declared themselves "prisoners of the Vatican," protesting their loss of the traditional lands ruled by the pope. In 1922, a Fascist government came to power under Benito Mussolini, and for the sake of national unity, Mussolini sought to improve relations with the pope. In 1929, they signed the Lateran Treaty, which recognized Vatican City as an independent state and reimbursed the Vatican for the loss of territory. Mussolini accepted Roman Catholicism as the established church of Italy and allowed religious instruction in the schools. In return, the Holy See recognized Italy's sovereignty with Rome as its capital. Despite the Lateran Treaty, the papacy and the Church were in growing conflict with the Fascists. In 1931, Pope Pius XI would vigorously protest their attacks in the encyclical Non Abbiamo Bisogno (On Catholic Action in Italy).

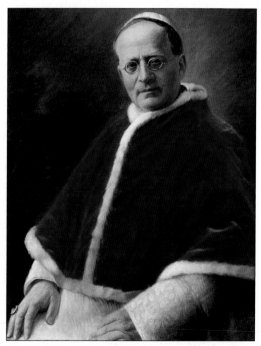

As soon as he became pope, Pius XI worked to resolve the relationship between the Vatican and the Kingdom of Italy. The Lateran Treaty with Mussolini was signed on February 11, 1929.

THE ENCYCLICALS OF PIUS XI

Pius XI published many notable encyclicals on various topics. Divini illius magistri (On the Christian Education of Youth), written in 1929, spelled out the rights and duties of parents, the state, and the Church in education. The right of parents to guide their children's education, Pope Pius said, "has precedence over any right of civil society and of the state, and for this reason, no power on earth may infringe upon it."

In 1931, Pius's encyclical Quadragesimo anno (The Fortieth Year: i.e., since the publication of Leo XIII's Rerum novarum) further expanded the Church's social teaching. This encyclical appeared at the height of the Great Depression, a global economic crisis that produced widespread unemployment and heightened social tensions in many countries, and presented a comprehensive vision of the economic structuring of a just society. Pius XI made a powerful case against totalitarianism, and particularly noteworthy was the statement of the principle of subsidiarity:

> A community of a higher order should not interfere in the internal life of a community of a lower order, depriving the latter of its functions, but rather should support it in case of need and help to coordinate its activity with the activities of the rest of society, always with a view of the common good.

Subsidiarity proved to be a valuable principle in an era of totalitarian governments and over-centralized state authority.

Pope Pius's encyclical on Christian Matrimony, Casti connubii (1930), reaffirmed Christian teaching on Matrimony and family life and restated the Church's condemnation of contraception. Declaring that some, "openly departing from the uninterrupted Christian tradition…recently have judged it possible solemnly to declare another doctrine regarding this question," Pope Pius said:

> [A]ny use whatsoever of matrimony exercised in such a way that the act is deliberately frustrated in its natural power to generate life is an offence against the law of God and of nature, and those who indulge in such are branded with the guilt of a grave sin.

Pope Pius also championed Catholic Action, making it the subject of his first encyclical, Ubi arcano Dei consilio, in 1922. Catholic Action was for many years the Church's principal form of organized lay apostolate. The idea that lay people should play an active role in the mission of the Church is present also in documents of Pope Leo XIII and St. Pius X, but Pius XI took up the cause vigorously and became known as "the Pope of Catholic Action."

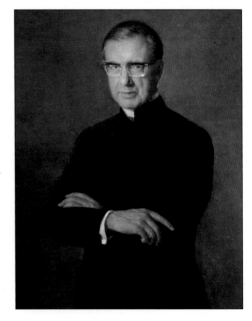

With encouragement from popes and bishops, the Catholic Action movement spread rapidly in Europe, the United States, and other places. Canon (later Cardinal) Joseph Cardijn of Belgium (1882-1967), founder of the Young Christian Workers and other groups for the formation of the laity, helped tremendously with the growth of Catholic Action. On October 2, 1928, St. Josemaría Escrivá was inspired by a charism that would give lay people a greater awareness of their call to holiness and evangelization in the midst of the

St. Josemaría Escrivá (1902-1975) was a Spanish Catholic priest and founder of the Prelature of the Holy Cross and Opus Dei. St. John Paul II's decree *Christifideles Omnes* on Escrivá's virtues said that "by inviting Christians to be united to God through their daily work, which is something men will have to do and find their dignity in as long as the world lasts, the timeliness of this message is destined to endure as an inexhaustible source of spiritual light, regardless of changing epochs and situations."

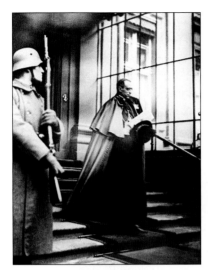

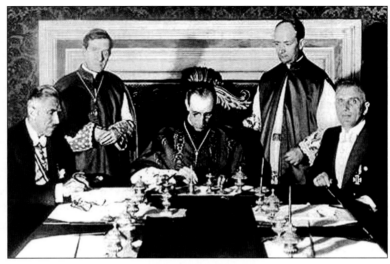

Left: Eugenio Pacelli, Apostolic Nuncio to the German Weimar Republic, in 1929 leaving the Presidential Palace in Berlin.
Right: The signing of the Concordat with Germany (The *Reichskonkordat*) on July 20, 1933. Left to right: German Vice-Chancellor Franz von Papen, representing Germany, Giuseppe Pizzardo, Cardinal Pacelli, Alfredo Cardinal Ottaviani, German ambassador Rudolf Buttmann. Today, the Concordat is still valid in Germany. Article 1 of the Concordat protects the right to freedom of religion. Article 31 protects Catholic organizations and religious practice. Article 21 allows for the Catholic religion to be taught in schools.

world. With this special grace, he formed Opus Dei, whose members would model themselves after the very first Christians. These new developments in the understanding of the lay vocation and the laity's role in the world would form part of the Church's teaching at the Second Vatican Council (1962-1965).

THE CHURCH AND THE RISE OF NAZISM

One of the most critical challenges facing Pope Pius XI was the rise of Adolf Hitler (1889-1945) to power and the National Socialist (Nazi) party in Germany.

Deeply resenting the terms of the peace settlement after World War I, Germany was in political and economic turmoil when Hitler came to power in 1933. Working to consolidate power at home and win influence and favor abroad, one of the dictator's first acts was to seek a new concordat with the Church. On July 20, 1933, Germany and the Vatican signed an agreement.

The principal negotiator of the Concordat with Germany was Pius XI's Secretary of State, Cardinal Eugenio Pacelli, the future Pope Ven. Pius XII. Pacelli was especially concerned with the independence of the Church in Germany, and recognizing the potential radicalism of Hitler's regime, he wished to preserve religious freedom for German Catholics. The Concordat provided that the German clergy be subject to canon law and gained special privileges for Catholic schools and organizations. In exchange, the Vatican agreed to encourage the German clergy to temper their political resistance to Hitler. Although the Concordat did allow the Church to stay independent in Hitler's Germany, and therefore conduct many efforts to save those persecuted by the Nazi regime, the Concordat led to the self-disbanding of the once powerful Catholic Center Party, which may have helped with early resistance against the Nazi dictator. The members were urged to join the Nazi party.

Pius XI had no illusions about the intentions of the Nazi leader, but hoped, he said, to "safeguard the freedom of the Church" in Hitler's Germany. Despite the agreement, Hitler and the Nazis violated the concordat from the start. As systematic oppression began, the Pope sent thirty-four separate notes of protest to the German government between 1933 and 1936. Hitler did not heed his policies.

On March 14, 1937, Pope Pius XI published the encyclical *Mit Brennender Sorge* (With Burning Worry), a powerful indictment of Nazism and the Nazi regime. At his direction, the encyclical was read from the pulpit of every Catholic Church in Germany. Charging the regime with repeated violations of the concordat and an open attack on the Church, the pope said:

> None but superficial minds could stumble into concepts of a national God, of a national religion; or attempt to lock within the frontiers of a single people, within the narrow limits of a single race, God, the Creator of the universe, King and Legislator of all nations before whose immensity they are "as a drop of a bucket" (Isaiah xl, 15). (no. 11)

Infuriated by the pope's criticism, the Nazis launched a campaign of propaganda against the Church. The Concordat could no longer hide the animosity between Nazis and Catholics. The conflict was now in the open, and there would be no turning back.

PERSECUTION IN MEXICO AND SPAIN

During the pontificate of Pius XI, persecution of Catholics was not limited to the Soviet Union and Germany. Traditionally Catholic Mexico and Spain had broken into civil war, and Pius XI was forced to confront, as he described in his 1937 encyclical on Communism, Divini Redemptoris, the "indiscriminate slaughter" of bishops, priests, and men and women religious, as well as thousands of lay people.

The situation in Spain had been deteriorating for years, as forces of the "left" and the "right" competed for power. After King Alfonso XIII was forced to leave the country, a republic was proclaimed in 1931. The government disestablished the Church, secularized education, and sanctioned the burning of churches. In 1936, a leftist government of Socialists, Anarchists, and Communists called the Popular Front came to power in an election. Many feared that a revolution by the radical left was now imminent.

In July that year, Spanish army units in Morocco rebelled, and soon Spain was engulfed in a civil war. As Spain divided, European powers backed each side, mimicking the alliances they would soon build during World War II. The Nationalist forces, led by General Francisco Franco, had military support from Italy and Germany, while the Republicans were aided by the Soviet Union and leftist "international brigades."

For years before the civil war, leftists and Freemasons had waged attacks on the Church. Churches were sometimes sacked and burned, and clerics were assassinated. The civil war brought a reign of terror on a much larger scale. Between July 18 and July 31, 1936, fifty priests were killed in Madrid and a third of the city's one hundred fifty churches were sacked or burned. In August, more than two thousand priests and religious were killed in the Republican zone of the country.

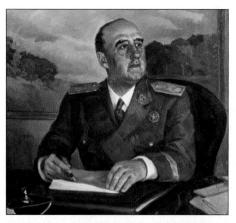
Francisco Franco (1892-1975) was ruler of Spain from 1939 until his death in 1975.

The killings declined as Franco's government gained greater control of the country, but they continued sporadically until the war's end. In all, 6,832 priests and religious and thirteen bishops were martyred from 1936 to 1939. One out of seven Spanish diocesan priests and one out of five male members of religious orders were killed. There is no telling how many lay people lost their lives because of their Catholic Faith. Some executions occurred after hasty trials by "people's courts"; other victims were simply lynched. Pope Pius XI called this bloodbath "the natural fruit of a system which lacks all inner restraint."

One million people died in the brutal struggle from which the Nationalists emerged victorious in 1939. Franco's authoritarian regime suppressed opposition and executed opponents, but it maintained stability, ended much of the violence against the Catholic Church, and kept Spain out of World War II.

Events in Mexico followed a similar pattern. Mexico had been a Catholic country since colonial times, but revolutionaries, Freemasons, and various political "reformers" frequently turned on the Church after the coming of independence in the nineteenth century. A revolution in 1917 made Mexico the world's first officially socialist, anti-religious, constitutional revolutionary republic. The Church could not own property, and any privileges it previously held were removed. Anti-Christian sentiments were so high that the governor of the Tabasco province, a particularly brutal persecutor of religion, named his children Lenin, Lucifer, and Satan.

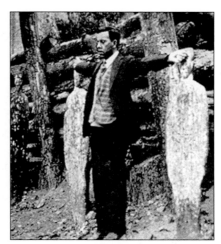

Bl. Miguel Pro held his arms out
in the sign of the cross
just before the shots were fired at his execution.

Violence was common in Mexico, particularly under the regime of Plutarco Calles (1924-1928), and persecution eventually led to an armed rebellion by Catholics called Cristeros. The rebellion was quickly put down, and a well-known martyr of the rebellion, Bl. Miguel Pro, S.J., was executed by a firing squad on November 23, 1927. Just before his death, he cried out "Viva Cristo Rey!"–Long Live Christ the King. Bl. Miguel Pro was beatified by St. John Paul II in 1988, and in 2000 the same Pope declared several of the Cristeros saints. His feast day is celebrated on November 23.

During the years after the rebellion, the government killed 250,000-300,000 people, most of them Catholics. Between late 1931 and early 1936, 480 churches, schools, orphanages, and hospitals were closed or used for other functions such as movie theaters, garages, and shops.

Beginning around 1940, there was a gradual easing of persecution in Mexico as authorities relaxed their enforcement of anticlerical laws. However, more than half a century still had to pass before the religious rights of the Church and the Mexican people were restored.

PART IX

The Pontificate of Ven. Pius XII
(1939-1958)

THE POPE AND THE WORLD CRISIS

Eugenio Pacelli, a lawyer's son, was born in Rome on March 2, 1876. He studied for the priesthood in Rome and was ordained in April 1899. Two years later he entered the service of the Holy See and from 1904 to 1916 worked on the project that resulted in the 1917 Code of Canon Law. He also taught international law at the training academy for Vatican diplomats.

In April 1917, Pope Benedict XV named Pacelli an archbishop and appointed him Nuncio to Bavaria. Two years later he was named Nuncio to the new German republic, remaining in that post until 1929. When he returned to Rome, Pacelli was named a cardinal and became Secretary of State under Pope Pius XI. In the 1930s he traveled to a number of countries, and in 1936 visited the United States and conferred with President Franklin D. Roosevelt. Many saw Pacelli as an obvious

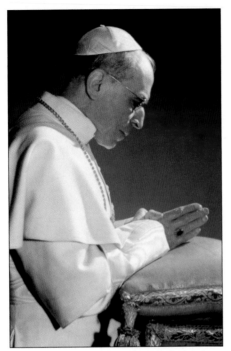

choice for the next pope. Even Pius XI said that the reason he sent Pacelli all over the world was "so that he may get to know the world and the world may get to know him" (quoted in Duffy, Saints and Sinners: A History of the Popes, 2002, p. 346). Pacelli was elected on March 2, 1939, and took the name Pius XII.

When Pius XII was elected pope, all-out war in Europe was already thought inevitable. Nonetheless, Pope Pius XII worked strenuously to promote peace and try to prevent World War II. Once war broke out, he continued to appeal for peace. Unlike Benedict XV's untiring efforts to promote peace during World War I, Pius XII knew that World War II was a different kind of war and that the Vatican could not be satisfied with simply acting as a voice of peace. The Holy See remained officially neutral, but the pope privately offered to serve as a channel for communication between anti-Hitler elements in Germany and the Allies. Through his diplomacy, he won for the city of Rome status as an "open city," exempt from military attacks. Repeatedly he appealed for peace, especially in a series of Christmas radio addresses from 1939 to 1942. Pius XII laid out a five-point peace plan of his own, and through the Pontifical Aid Commission, he directed a large-scale program of assistance to war victims and prisoners-of-war.

In 1943, after the fall of Mussolini's government and the occupation of Rome by German troops, church institutions throughout the city, acting at the pope's direction, sheltered thousands of Jewish and non-Jewish refugees. Many also took refuge at the papal summer residence at Castel Gandolfo, and others were sheltered in Vatican "safe houses" throughout the city of Rome. Hundreds of thousands of Jews' lives were saved through the efforts of Pope Pius and other Vatican officials working under the shelter of neutrality. After the war, Pope Pius XII won the praise of many prominent Jews and Jewish groups for his assistance during Nazi occupation. Remarkably, the Chief Rabbi of Rome, Israel Zolli, largely through the example of selfless risk and extraordinary charity exhibited by Vatican agents during the war, became a Catholic, taking as his baptismal name Eugene out of gratitude to Pius XII (Eugenio Pacelli).

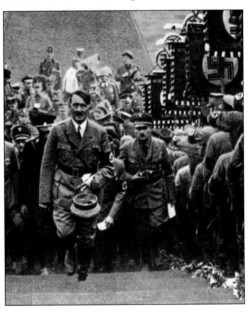

TWO SAINTS OF THE NAZI PERSECUTION

Although the policy of Jewish genocide by the Nazis was a devastation, Jews were not the only people who suffered. Gypsies also were targets of genocide, and historian Franciszek Piper estimates that the Nazis killed as many as 1.9 million non-Jewish Poles, a majority of those at the Auschwitz prison camp. Throughout these persecutions, many Catholics sacrificed themselves for their Faith and fellow man, and many were martyred. Among these, two figures typify the carnage and the heroism of this era: St. Maximilian Kolbe and St. Teresa Benedicta of the Cross, whose name by birth was Edith Stein.

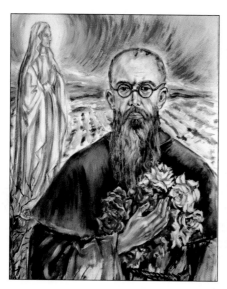
St. Maximilian Kolbe

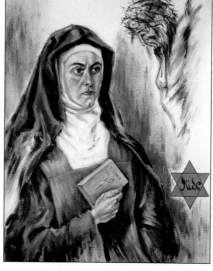
St. Teresa Benedicta of the Cross

Maximilian Kolbe (1894-1941), priest and martyr, was a Polish Conventual Franciscan. Devoted to the Blessed Virgin, he founded a group called the *Militia of Mary Immaculate*, edited its magazine, and established an international center of Marian devotion. After the fall of Poland, he was arrested by the Nazis, released, and then re-arrested in 1941 for assisting Jews and members of the Polish underground. Sent to Auschwitz, he was treated brutally because he was a priest. When ten of his fellow prisoners were marked out for execution in reprisal for a prison escape, Father Kolbe voluntarily took the place of one of them, who was a married man. He died on August 14, 1941, and St. John Paul II canonized him in 1982. His feast day is celebrated on August 14.

Edith Stein (1891-1942) was born into a Jewish family and at an early age declared herself an atheist. A brilliant student, she studied philosophy under the renowned philosopher Edmund Husserl and became identified with the philosophical school called phenomenology. During her studies, and after beginning her career as a teacher and writer, she was led towards the Catholic Faith. After reading the autobiography of Saint Teresa of Avila, she was moved to convert, and was baptized on January 1, 1922. In 1934 she joined the Carmelites in Cologne, taking the religious name Teresa Benedicta of the Cross. As the Nazi campaign against Jews intensified, she was smuggled to the Netherlands in 1938. In 1942 she was arrested as part of the Nazi reaction to the Dutch bishops' condemnation of Nazism and sent to Auschwitz, where she was killed in the gas chamber on August 9, 1942. St. John Paul canonized her in 1998. Her feast day is celebrated on August 9.

THE TEACHING OF PIUS XII

Along with being active in world affairs, Pope Pius XII produced a significant body of teaching, much of it is contained in a series of important encyclicals that helped set the stage for the Second Vatican Council.

Mystici corporis Christi (The Mystical Body of Christ) in 1943 draws on the teaching of St. Paul to present the Church as a communion whose members play complementary roles in continuing the mission of Christ. This encyclical makes clear both the Church's hierarchical structure, involving specific offices and authority, and her "charismatic" dimension whereby God gives individuals gifts to be used in the service of all. All the members of the Church are united to Christ, the head of the Church, in a relationship analogous to the connection of the organs of a physical body to the head.

Divino afflante Spiritu (Inspired by the Holy Spirit) in 1943 gave encouragement to Biblical studies. Scholars were told to respect the literal sense of Scripture while making use of historical-critical methods in order to understand the literary forms used by the inspired human authors and the historical circumstances in which they wrote.

Mediator Dei (Mediator of God) in 1947 endorsed the movement for liturgical renewal. Liturgical changes approved during the pontificate of Pius XII included the revision of the Holy Week rites, the reduction of the Eucharistic fast, and permission for afternoon and evening Masses.

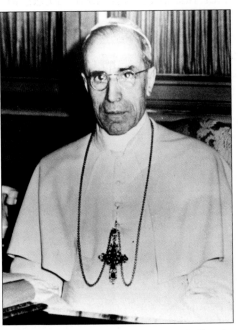

Humani generis (The Human Race) in 1950 warned against emerging theological errors of the day contrary to the Christian tradition. In the various positions condemned by Pope Pius XII one can see a resurgence of Modernist thinking condemned four decades earlier by St. Pius X.

Pope Pius declared 1950 a Holy Year and capped the observance by infallibly declaring the Assumption of Mary to be a dogma of Faith. The apostolic constitution Munificentissimus Deus (The Most Bountiful God) of Pope Pius XII (November 1, 1950) declared:

> …we pronounce, declare, and define it to be a divinely revealed dogma: that the Immaculate Mother of God, the ever Virgin Mary, having completed the course of her earthly life, was assumed body and soul into heavenly glory.

Like Pius IX and Leo XIII, Pius XII was devoted to the Blessed Virgin Mary. In 1950, he declared a Holy Year, bringing millions of pilgrims to Rome. He closed the Holy Year in Fatima, Portugal, one of the great Marian shrines of the Catholic world.

The definition of the Assumption is important not only as a contribution to teaching about the Blessed Virgin but for rejecting the idea of body-soul dualism.

THE CHURCH AND THE COMMUNIST EMPIRE

Military victory in World War II and the postwar settlement among the allies left the Soviet Union the master of Eastern Europe. The Soviets supported Communist puppet governments and stationed troops throughout the region. An Iron Curtain, as British Prime Minister Winston Churchill called it, descended across Europe, dividing the democratic West from the Communist East.

Pope Pius XII worked to rally Catholics against the threat of Communist takeover in the West. Looking to crucial elections in Italy, the Vatican's Holy Office in 1949 warned that Catholics who joined or supported Communist parties would be excommunicated.

"Communism is materialistic and anti-Christian," it said, and Communist leaders are "enemies of God, of the true religion, and of the Church of Christ." Although Communism would not spread to any other European countries, the Iron Curtain divided Europe for another 40 years.

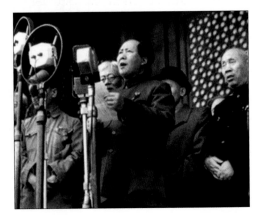

Mao Tse-Tung (1893-1976) declared the formation of the People's Republic of China at Tiananmen Square on October 1, 1949. Mao developed his own version of communism based on the theories of Hegel and Marx. The ideology of Maoism has influenced many communists around the world, including third world revolutionary movements such as Cambodia's Khmer Rouge, Peru's Shining Path, the revolutionary movement in Nepal, and the Revolutionary Communist Party in the United States.

International Communism was on the march outside Europe. The number of Catholics and other Christians in China was comparatively small, but the Church there had been making progress for several decades. That changed dramatically when the Communists under Mao Tse-tung took over mainland China in 1949. Foreign missionaries were expelled; many priests, religious, and lay people were imprisoned and forced to do slave labor; religious schools and institutions were closed; and Catholic movements were banned for alleged "counterrevolutionary activities."

The Communists concentrated on separating Chinese Catholics from the Holy See and creating a state-controlled national church. For this purpose, a Chinese Catholic Patriotic Association was established, and the government began choosing puppet bishops. Despite this state-sponsored nationalistic church, loyal bishops, priests, religious, and laity maintained an underground Church in communion with Rome. In response to the Chinese puppet church, Pope Pius XII underlined the universal nature of the Catholic Church and rejected the idea of national churches in his 1954 encyclical *Ad Sinarum gentem* (To the Chinese People).

CONCLUSION

In every period of history, the Church works to transmit the wealth of her wisdom. During this age of political, economic, and social change, together with persecution and suppression, the Church emerged once again as a strong moral force. It can be argued that the papacy, especially

in the person of Leo XIII, not only plays the role of promoting unity in the Catholic Church, but also more and more becomes a champion of human rights and a defender of human dignity. As of the end of the nineteenth century, the pope not only serves as Holy Father for the Church, but as a common father for all humanity.

Pius XII died on October 9, 1958. By that point in the twentieth century, the Catholic Church had weathered two world wars, numerous revolutions, and social turmoil, and had emerged as a strong, united community of Faith. However, it had serious external enemies. Secular humanism of two kinds posed a powerful threat to all religion – Marxist humanism, which dominated the Soviet Union, Eastern Europe, and China, and the materialistic, hedonistic secular humanism of the consumer societies of the West. Responding to these challenges would occupy the Church in the decades ahead.

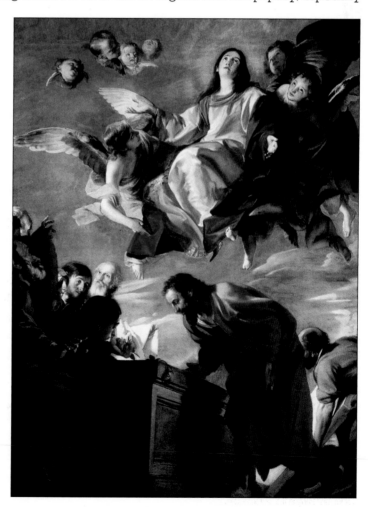

Assumption of the Virgin by Juan Martin Cabezalero

VOCABULARY

CATHOLIC ACTION
An organization encouraged by Popes St. Pius X and Pius XI that was to become a key instrument of the lay apostolate.

CHRISTIAN MODERNISM
Originated in the late nineteenth century, some Catholic intellectuals, out of a desire to address contemporary currents of thought, embraced trends in psychology, science, and philosophy and tried to adapt Christian thought to them.

COMMUNISM
As envisioned by Karl Marx, more than a political system, this was a necessary historical development, the culmination of human history. The exploited proletariat would establish, through revolution, a new social-economic system in which social classes no longer existed. In theory, this system offered a Utopian vision: the proletariat held all wealth and property in common, securing a society based on absolute equality in which the government provided everything that everyone needed.

CONCERT OF EUROPE
Alliance established by Metternich which sought to dismantle the reforms brought about by Napoleon and crush any liberal revolution. This arrangement left Austria, and Metternich, as the main arbiter of European affairs beginning in 1815.

CRISTEROS
This Catholic group led an armed rebellion under the regime of Plutarco Calles in Mexico. They sought to resist anti-Catholic persecution but were quickly put down. Several of the fighters are martyrs and saints.

GULAG
A vast system of Siberian prison camps and penal colonies set up during Stalin's dictatorship in which many thousands of opponents of the regime served long sentences or were executed.

HOLY ALLIANCE
In 1815, Czar Alexander I of Russia proposed the creation of this alliance (including Russia, Prussia, and Austria) which promised to uphold Christian principles of charity and peace. Despite Alexander's pious intentions, the Holy Alliance did not outline a program effective enough to ensure peace and was not taken seriously by its members.

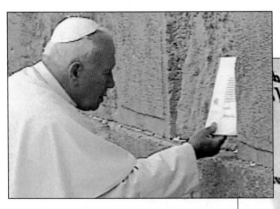

St. John Paul II places a prayer for the people of the Covenant in the Wailing Wall of the Temple in Jerusalem during his pilgrimage there in 2000.

God of our fathers,
...ose Abraham and his descendants
... bring your Name to the Nations:
we are deeply saddened
by the behaviour of those
who in the course of history
...ve caused these children of yours to suffer,
and asking your forgiveness
we wish to commit ourselves
to genuine brotherhood
with the people of the Covenant.

VOCABULARY Continued

INDUSTRIALIZATION

The rapid transformation from an agricultural to an industrial economy which altered the way people lived and dramatically changed how countries did business toward production of goods through mechanization.

KULTURKAMPF

Bismarck's policy of ridding Germany of Catholicism. It subjected Catholic schools and seminaries to state control, forbade religious orders to teach, and banned every religious order in Germany. Furthermore, any priest or bishop who did not acknowledge state supremacy over the Church in Germany was fined or imprisoned.

LIBERALISM

Put generally, this ideology approved of everything that was modern, enlightened, efficient, and reasonable. Based on the principles of natural law, liberals saw monarchies as unjust, out-of-date, and not properly representative of the people.

MONROE DOCTRINE

American President James Monroe's isolationist announcement in 1823 that the Western Hemisphere was closed to further European colonization and that any attempt by European states to intervene in the affairs of Latin America would be considered an act of war against the United States.

NAZISM

A blend of nationalist totalitarianism, racism aimed especially at Jews, neo-paganism, and the moral nihilism of the nineteenth century German philosopher Friedrich Nietzsche, this political party, headed by Adolf Hitler, seized power in 1933 and initiated policies that sought to strengthen and unify Germany in order to bring about an expansive New World Order based on Nazi ideals.

OATH AGAINST MODERNISM

In an encyclical issued on September 1, 1910, St. Pius X required all Catholic priests to uphold Catholic teaching against modern heresies. Because of the Oath, much Modernist thinking in the Church went underground.

PAPAL INFALLIBILITY

The dogma that the pope cannot make an error, when speaking ex cathedra (when in the exercise of his office as shepherd and teacher of all Catholics) and defining a doctrine concerning Faith and morals to be held by the whole Church.

SECULAR HUMANISM

Nineteenth-century intellectual movement in which thinkers described an increasingly mechanical understanding of the human person. As philosophy drifted even further from notions of God and religion, many began to argue that the world is essentially amoral and that the guidelines for governing what is right and wrong no longer apply.

ULTRAMONTANISM

Literally "over the mountains." Catholics who looked to the pope for support and leadership, emphasizing his centrality and authority more than ever before.

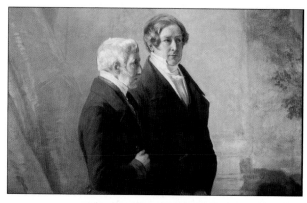

The Duke of Wellington with Sir Robert Peel.
As British statesmen they both supported reforms to end oppression.

STUDY QUESTIONS

1. What alliance established by Metternich dominated the European political sphere for fifteen years?

2. Why was the Monroe Doctrine respected by the European powers?

3. How did the Prussians seek to eliminate Catholic influence in the southern German States? How did Pope Pius VIII respond to this policy?

4. What positions helped the nativist Know-Nothing Party gain popularity?

5. What economic developments preceded the Industrial Revolution?

6. What changes did industrialization bring to family life?

7. What event caused Bl. Pio Nono to grow suspicious of liberal reform?

8. What two Marian titles best express the Church Fathers' belief that Mary was immaculately conceived?

9. What miraculous event reinforced Bl. Pius IX's proclamation of the Immaculate Conception?

10. What did Quanta cura and the Syllabus of Errors address?

11. What event forced the disbanding of the First Vatican Council?

12. What was the Roman Question?

13. How did Bismarck successfully unite the German States?

14. What three teachings did Japanese Christians use to verify the orthodoxy of French missionaries?

15. Karl Marx believed that history and society was primarily driven by what?

16. Leo XIII was the first pope in over a millennium and a half to lack what papal power upon his election?

17. According to Leo XIII's encyclical Inscrutabili Dei, what will help a healthy society emerge?

18. According to Leo XIII's encyclical Immortale Dei, who is the root and source of all political authority?

19. Leo XIII's Rerum novarum particularly condemns what nineteenth century political system and ideology?

20. Who was the first pope elected in the twentieth century?

21. What was the motto of St. Pius X?

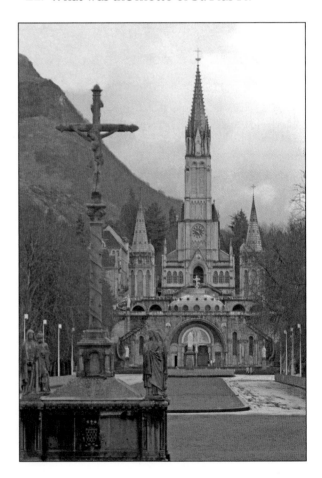

The Basilica at Lourdes, France. This immense concrete church was built above the grotto in 1958 to accommodate the ever increasing number of pilgrims. It replaced the original basilica built in 1876. The basilica seats 20,000. The pilgrimage season lasts from April through October, with the main pilgrimage day being August 15, the Marian Feast of the Assumption. Four to six million pilgrims visit the shrine each year. It is estimated that more than 200 million pilgrims have come to Lourdes since 1860.

STUDY QUESTIONS Continued

22. At the beginning of his pontificate, St. Pius X launched the updating and systematic compilation of what Church document?

23. Why is St. Pius X known as the "Pope of the Eucharist"?

24. How did Modernists view religion?

25. Why did St. Pius X refer to Modernism as a "compendium of all heresies"?

26. What did the election of Giacomo della Chiesa as Pope Benedict XV imply?

27. What dominating political regime rose to power after World War I?

28. What happened in Fatima?

29. Why did Russia need so many prayers?

30. Who founded Opus Dei?

31. What was decided by the 1933 Concordat between Germany and the Vatican?

32. How did civil war in Spain affect Spanish Catholics?

33. Who were the Cristeros of Mexico?

34. Whose name did the chief rabbi of Rome take when he was baptized a Catholic after World War II?

35. How many Catholics died in Auschwitz?

36. Who was St. Maximilian Kolbe?

37. Who was Edith Stein?

38. Which were Pius XII's major encyclical works?

39. In what year did Pius XII define the Assumption of Mary a matter of dogma?

40. What was the Chinese Catholic Patriotic Association?

PRACTICAL EXERCISES

1. Through a comparison of Pius VII and Leo XIII, explain how the events of the nineteenth century changed the role of the pope both in the world and in the Church. What specific events led to the shift?

2. What effects did industrialization and imperialism have on European and non-European countries?

3. What problems did the three exemplary secular humanist thinkers pose to the Church? How have their ideas affected today's society?

4. The two major ideologies of the twentieth century, Communism and Fascism, represent two opposite ends of the political spectrum, and yet, their attitudes towards religion and the Church are comparable. Based on what you have read in previous chapters about the birth of these ideologies and the Enlightenment principles which underlie their ideas, explain why both have such a negative understanding of the role of God and religion in the world.

5. Pius XII is often accused of being "silent" in the face of the Nazi atrocities during World War II. How did the silence of the Vatican enable the Church to aid those suffering under the Nazi regime?

FROM THE CATECHISM

852 Missionary paths. The Holy Spirit is the protagonist, "the principal agent of the whole of the Church's mission" (John Paul II, RMiss 21). It is he who leads the Church on her missionary paths. "This mission continues and, in the course of history, unfolds the mission of Christ, who was sent to evangelize the poor; so the Church, urged on by the Spirit of Christ, must walk the road Christ himself walked, a way of poverty and obedience, of service and self-sacrifice even to death, a death from which he emerged victorious by his resurrection" (AG 5). So it is that "the blood of martyrs is the seed of Christians" (Tertullian, Apol. 50, 13: PL 1, 603).

1882 Certain societies, such as the family and the state, correspond more directly to the nature of man; they are necessary to him. To promote the participation of the greatest number in the life of a society, the creation of voluntary associations and institutions must be encouraged "on both national and international levels, which relate to economic and social goals, to cultural and recreational activities, to sport, to various professions, and to political affairs" (John XXIII, MM 60). This "socialization" also expresses the natural tendency for human beings to associate with one another for the sake of attaining objectives that exceed individual capacities. It develops the qualities of the person, especially the sense of initiative and responsibility, and helps guarantee his rights (cf. GS 25 § 2; CA 12).

1883 Socialization also presents dangers. Excessive intervention by the state can threaten personal freedom and initiative. The teaching of the Church has elaborated the principle of subsidiarity, according to which "a community of a higher order should not interfere in the internal life of a community of a lower order, depriving the latter of its functions, but rather should support it in case of need and help to coordinate its activity with the activities of the rest of society, always with a view to the common good" (CA 48 § 4; cf. Pius XI, Quadragesimo anno I, 184-186).

2107 "If because of the circumstances of a particular people special civil recognition is given to one religious community in the constitutional organization of a state, the right of all citizens and religious communities to religious freedom must be recognized and respected as well" (DH 6 § 3).

2314 "Every act of war directed to the indiscriminate destruction of whole cities or vast areas with their inhabitants is a crime against God and man, which merits firm and unequivocal condemnation" (GS 80 § 3). A danger of modern warfare is that it provides the opportunity to those who possess modern scientific weapons – especially atomic, biological, or chemical weapons – to commit such crimes.

2425 The Church has rejected the totalitarian and atheistic ideologies associated in modern times with "communism" or "socialism." She has likewise refused to accept, in the practice of "capitalism," individualism and the absolute primacy of the law of the marketplace over human labor (cf. CA 10; 13; 44). Regulating the economy solely by centralized planning perverts the basis of social bonds; regulating it solely by the law of the marketplace fails social justice, for "there are many human needs which cannot be satisfied by the market" (CA 34). Reasonable regulation of the marketplace and economic initiatives, in keeping with a just hierarchy of values and a view to the common good, is to be commended.

2437 On the international level, inequality of resources and economic capability is such that it creates a real "gap" between nations (cf. SRS 14). On the one side there are those nations possessing and developing the means of growth and, on the other, those accumulating debts.

CHAPTER 9

Vatican II And The Church In The Modern World

An anti-authoritarian spirit of rebellion revolutionized and secularized society. The Church faced controversies over the interpretation of the Second Vatican Council.

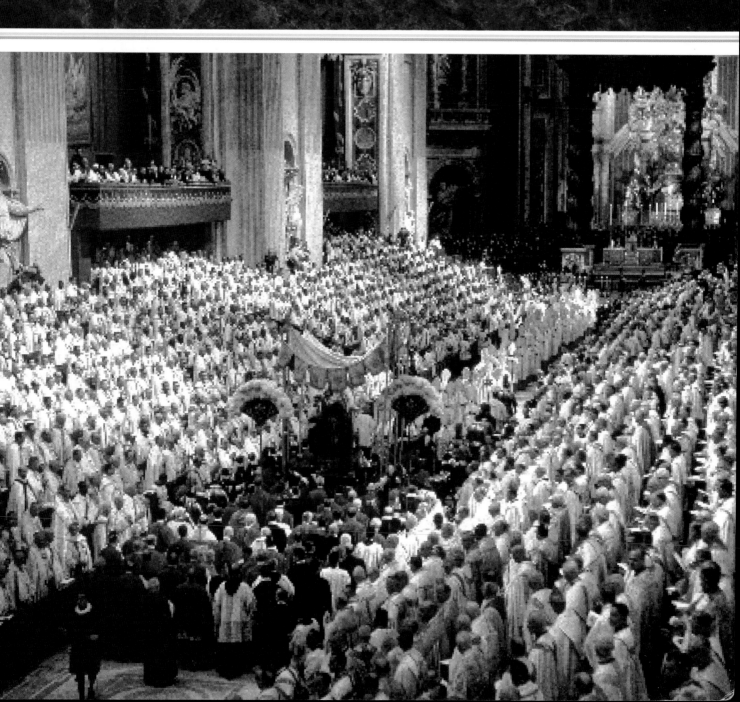

CHAPTER 9

Vatican II And The Church In The Modern World

Midpoint in the twentieth century, the Catholic Church was united in doctrine, worship, and loyalty to the Pope and bishops. The Catholic population was growing rapidly in many places, especially the Third World. Priestly and religious vocations flourished, and lay movements were strong and enthusiastic. Overall, the Church seemed strong despite frequently confused and troubled times the world had been experiencing.

At the same time, the Church faced different challenges. Living under the threat of nuclear extinction in the Cold War, Catholics along with everyone else wrestled with the moral dilemmas of nuclear deterrence and modern warfare. Totalitarian regimes in the Soviet Union, Eastern Europe, and China persecuted religion, and the "Church of Silence," as the Church in China became known, produced many martyrs. The gap between rich and poor nations broadened, and demands for recognition of human rights, especially within the women's and civil rights movements, placed new pressures on old patterns of behavior both within and without the Church.

In the twentieth century, increasingly secular attitudes towards Matrimony and sexuality changed the way the family and society understood itself. The practice of birth control by means of contraception was spreading, spurred by new oral contraceptives and the sexual permissiveness they encouraged, and by propaganda about a largely fictitious "population explosion." Abortion already was legal in some places, and efforts were underway to bring about its legalization elsewhere. Marriage also came under assault from the growing acceptance of divorce.

Few people at mid-century anticipated how great an upheaval in ideas, values, and behavior lay ahead. In wider society, the sixties brought an anti-authoritarian spirit of rebellion, especially among the youth, and social movements would revolutionize the way life was lived in contemporary society. For the Church, much of the upheaval is associated with the Second Vatican Council, with controversy over how the Council's decisions should be interpreted and carried out, and with the dissent and defections from the clergy and religious life during and after the council. Vatican II itself did not encourage or cause these things, but the winds of change it occasioned contributed to bringing them about.

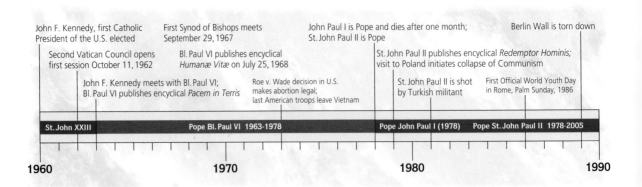

John F. Kennedy, first Catholic President of the U.S. elected

First Synod of Bishops meets September 29, 1967

John Paul I is Pope and dies after one month; St. John Paul II is Pope

Berlin Wall is torn down

Second Vatican Council opens first session October 11, 1962

Bl. Paul VI publishes encyclical *Humanæ Vitæ* on July 25, 1968

St. John Paul II publishes encyclical *Redemptor Hominis*; visit to Poland initiates collapse of Communism

John F. Kennedy meets with Bl. Paul VI; Bl. Paul VI publishes encyclical *Pacem in Terris*

Roe v. Wade decision in U.S. makes abortion legal; last American troops leave Vietnam

St. John Paul II is shot by Turkish militant

First Official World Youth Day in Rome, Palm Sunday, 1986

St. John XXIII   Pope Bl. Paul VI 1963-1978   Pope John Paul I (1978)   Pope St. John Paul II 1978-2005

1960   1970   1980   1990

PART I

St. John XXIII and the Council

THE CARETAKER POPE

Angelo Giuseppe Roncalli was born on November 25, 1881, into a family of peasant farmers in Sotto il Monte, an Italian village near the town of Bergamo. He studied for the priesthood at the Bergamo diocesan seminaries and the St. Apollinare Institute in Rome and was ordained in 1904. From 1904 to 1914 he was secretary to the Bishop of Bergamo and taught Church history at one of the local seminaries. In World War I, Father Roncalli was drafted into the Italian army and served as a hospital orderly and chaplain.

After the war, Pope Benedict XV named Roncalli Italian president of the Society for the Propagation of the Faith, an organization that supported missionary work. He wrote studies on the history of the Bergamo diocese and on St. Charles Borromeo (1538-1584), the Archbishop of Milan who was a leader of the Catholic Counter-Reformation. While researching at the Ambrosian Library in Milan, he met Achille Ratti, and after Ratti was elected Pope Pius XI, he named Roncalli an archbishop and appointed him apostolic visitor to Bulgaria and, in 1934, apostolic delegate to Turkey and Greece. Much of Roncalli's experience as an archbishop would highlight his ecumenical understanding of the universal Church and his strong background in Church history, especially of the Counter-Reformation period.

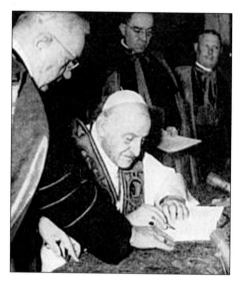

During his time as a delegate in the East, Archbishop Roncalli developed good relations with the Orthodox Church, and during World War II, he worked to assist Jews and other refugees. In December 1944, Pius XII named him apostolic nuncio to France where Roncalli had to deal with

St. John XXIII signing his encyclical *Pacem in Terris* (Peace on Earth) that captured the world's attention during a time of extremely dangerous tensions between the world's two superpowers.

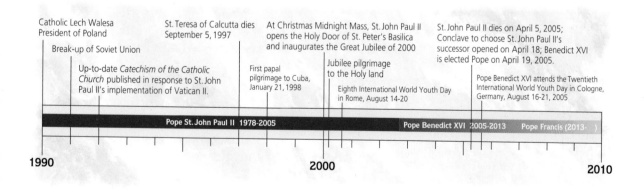

Catholic Lech Walesa President of Poland

Break-up of Soviet Union

Up-to-date *Catechism of the Catholic Church* published in response to St. John Paul II's implementation of Vatican II.

St. Teresa of Calcutta dies September 5, 1997

First papal pilgrimage to Cuba, January 21, 1998

At Christmas Midnight Mass, St. John Paul II opens the Holy Door of St. Peter's Basilica and inaugurates the Great Jubilee of 2000

Jubilee pilgrimage to the Holy land

Eighth International World Youth Day in Rome, August 14-20

St. John Paul II dies on April 5, 2005; Conclave to choose St. John Paul II's successor opened on April 18; Benedict XVI is elected Pope on April 19, 2005.

Pope Benedict XVI attends the Twentieth International World Youth Day in Cologne, Germany, August 16-21, 2005

Pope St. John Paul II 1978-2005

Pope Benedict XVI 2005-2013

Pope Francis (2013-   )

1990

2000

2010

a number of difficult problems. He negotiated with the new government over the appointment of bishops and aid to church-sponsored schools; he worked out arrangements for seminarians who had served in the German army and were now prisoners of war to continue their theological studies; he dealt with the problem of bishops who had collaborated with the unpopular French Vichy government during the German occupation. In 1952, he was appointed the Holy See's representative at the United Nations Educational, Scientific, and Cultural Organization.

In June 1953, Pope Pius XII named Roncalli a cardinal and Patriarch of Venice, just as St. Pius X had been five decades earlier. In Venice, he became a popular figure known for pastoral zeal and an informal style. At seventy-six, Roncalli was seen as a popular choice for Pope, a well-loved man of the people who could offer a smooth transition between Pius XII and Roncalli's own successor.

Following his election as Pope, one of St. John XXIII's first acts was to abolish the rule dating back to the sixteenth century which set the number of cardinals at seventy. Thereafter he took steps to increase the size of the College of Cardinals and make it a more international body. It was a bold and progressive move, but it was only the start for the seventy-six-year-old historian Pope.

On January 25, 1959, St. John XXIII announced to the world three projects for his pontificate: a diocesan synod for Rome, the drafting of a new Code of Canon Law, and an ecumenical council – the first such gathering of the world's bishops since Vatican Council I (1869-1870) and only the twenty-first ecumenical council in the Church's history. Preparatory commissions and secretariats for the council were established in June 1960, and a commission responsible for revising the Code of Canon Law was appointed in March 1962.

St. John XXIII was a man of faith and piety whose friendly manner won him fame as "Good Pope John." He cracked jokes and visited prisoners and hospital patients. He took ground breaking ecumenical steps, including establishing a Vatican office for Christian unity.

St. John XXIII published several notable encyclicals. *Ad Petri Cathedram* ("To the Chair of Peter"), written in 1959, discussed the unity of the Church. *Mater et Magistra* ("Mother and Teacher"), 1961, developed Catholic social teaching and stressed the duty of developed nations to provide assistance to underdeveloped ones.

This champion of peace died of stomach cancer on June 3, 1963, after the first session of his most lasting legacy, the Second Vatican Council. St. John Paul II beatified him in 2000, and Pope Francis canonized him in 2014.

St. John XXIII, "Good Pope John." born Angelo Giuseppe Roncalli (1881-1963), reigned as Pope from October 28, 1958, until his death in 1963. St. John XXIII was a man of traditional faith and piety whose friendly manner won him fame as "Good Pope John."

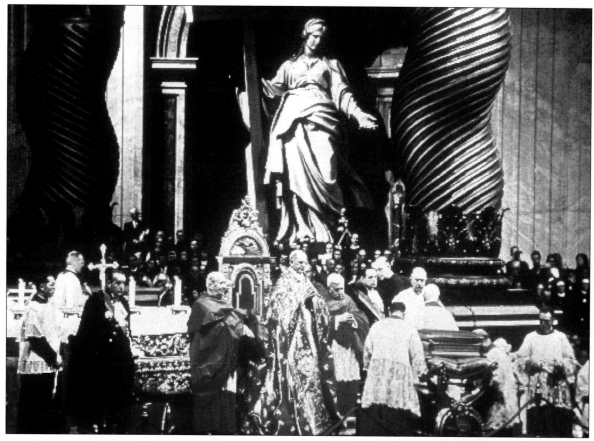

Pope Paul VI opened the second session of the Second Vatican Council on September 29, 1963. Pope Paul's opening address stressed the pastoral nature of the Council, and set out four purposes: to more fully define the nature of the Church and the role of the bishops; to renew the Church; to restore unity among all Christians; and to start a dialog with the contemporary world.

THE SECOND VATICAN COUNCIL

Why did St. John XXIII convene the Second Ecumenical Council of the Vatican? Although he certainly had a number of purposes in mind, one stood out especially.

In the apostolic constitution *Humanæ Salutis* ("For the Salvation of Men") of December 25, 1961, formally convoking the Second Vatican Council, he spoke of a "twofold spectacle"–the secular world in "a grave state of spiritual poverty" and the Church, "so vibrant with vitality." The Church, he noted, was strong in faith and enjoyed an "awe-inspiring unity." Through an Ecumenical Council, she hoped to update herself in order to meet the urgent spiritual needs of the world.

The Second Vatican Council took place in four sessions: October 11–December 8, 1962; September 29–December 4, 1963; September 14–November 21, 1964; and September 14–December 8, 1965. General congregations were held in St. Peter's Basilica. About 2860 of the world's bishops attended some or all of the Council; 274 bishops did not attend because of age, health, or some other reason (including the refusal of Communist governments in some places to permit them to go). Representatives of other Christian churches and religious bodies also attended, along with selected priests, deacons, religious, and lay people.

Extensively covered by secular and religious media, the Second Vatican Council was one of the major media events of the 1960s. It became the focus of an enormous amount of speculation, hope, anxiety, pressure, and debate. Vatican II is widely considered to have been the most important event in the Church's life in the twentieth century.

In a hope-filled speech at the opening session, St. John denounced "prophets of gloom who are always forecasting disaster, as though the end of the world were at hand." He insisted a "new order of human relations" was emerging, which would allow the Church to make her contribution.

Less than eight months later he died. On June 21, 1963, the cardinals elected Cardinal Montini of Milan, who took the name Paul VI and immediately announced that the council would continue. (Recall an Ecumenical Council must be presided over by the Pope or his legate, so if Paul VI had not continued it, the council would have disbanded or continued as a local (i.e., not Ecumenical) council.

The substantive work of the Second Vatican Council is embodied in sixteen documents. There are four "constitutions" (on the Church, on Divine Revelation, on Liturgy, and on the Church in the Modern World), nine "decrees" (on the pastoral office of bishops, on missionary activity, on ecumenism, on the Eastern Catholic Churches, on the ministry and life of priests, on priestly formation, on the appropriate renewal of religious life, on the apostolate of the laity, and on the instruments of social communication or media), and three "declarations" (on religious freedom, on the Church and non-Christian religions, and on Christian education).

The four constitutions are the central documents of Vatican II and provide the theological basis and vision for the rest.

THE DOGMATIC CONSTITUTION ON THE CHURCH

Lumen Gentium ("Light of Nations") uses scriptural images like the Body of Christ and People of God to present the Church as *communio*. The Church is a hierarchically structured community of faith whose members possess a fundamental equality in dignity and rights while having different but complementary roles in her mission. The constitution describes collegiality, according to which the bishops, in union with and under the Pope, share in teaching and governing the Church. Chapter V, "The Call to Holiness," teaches that all members of the Church, including lay people, are called to be saints. Chapter VIII, "Our Lady," contains the Council's principal treatment of the Blessed Virgin Mary.

THE DOGMATIC CONSTITUTION ON DIVINE REVELATION

Dei Verbum ("The Word of God") treats Sacred Scripture and Sacred Tradition as God's divinely inspired Word with approval of the responsible use of contemporary scholarly methods for understanding its historical context and literary forms. Scripture and Tradition are not two independent sources of Revelation but are intimately and inextricably linked: "Sacred Tradition and Sacred Scripture make up a single sacred deposit of the Word of God, which is entrusted to the Church." It also stresses that the "authentic interpretation" of God's Word "has been entrusted to the living teaching office [Magisterium] of the Church alone."

THE CONSTITUTION ON THE SACRED LITURGY

Sacrosanctum Concilium ("The Sacred Council") recognized the liturgy as "the summit toward which the activity of the Church is directed, at the same time it is the font from which all her power flows." In a key passage, it called for "full, conscious, and active participation" by all members of the Church, especially in the Eucharistic liturgy, or Mass. It opened the door to expanded use of vernacular languages and to liturgical adaptations suited to the needs of particular groups, provided these had the approval of Church authority, and called for other steps to foster "active participation."

THE PASTORAL CONSTITUTION ON THE CHURCH IN THE MODERN WORLD

Gaudium et Spes ("Joy and Hope") was the Council's most direct response to St. John 's desire that the Church be more directly at the service of the world. Its famous opening words declare: "The joy and the hope, the griefs and the anxieties of the men of this age, especially those who are poor or in any way afflicted, these are the joys and hopes, the griefs and anxieties of the followers of Christ." Topics include the dignity of the human person in light of Christ, the causes of atheism, the nature of the common good, social justice and economic life, marriage and the family, the evangelization of culture, work, private property, politics, war and peace, and the sanctity of human life.

The official document declaring the completion of the Second Vatican Council was read at the closing ceremonies in 1965. Pope Paul VI summed up the Council thusly:

> It was the largest in the number of Fathers who came to the seat of Peter from every part of the world....It was the richest because of the questions which for four sessions have been discussed carefully and profoundly. And finally it was the most opportune, because above all it sought to meet pastoral needs, bearing in mind the needs of the present day, and...has made a great effort to reach not only Christians still separated from the Holy See but also the whole human family.

PART II

Pope Paul VI and the Postconciliar Years

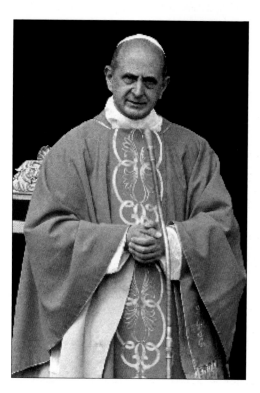

The Pope who saw Vatican II to its successful conclusion, Paul VI, also conscientiously directed its implementation. Despite his best efforts, however – and to his increasing sorrow – the optimism of the Council years was soon replaced by some confusion, misinterpretations, and dissent.

He was born Giovanni Battista Montini on September 26, 1897, near the city of Brescia. His father was a lawyer, editor, and member of parliament. The studious young man prepared for the priesthood at the diocesan seminary, was ordained in 1920, and pursued graduate work in Rome. In 1922 he joined the Vatican Secretariat of State where, except for serving briefly in Warsaw in 1923, he was to remain for the next thirty-two years. He was active as a chaplain to Catholic students and taught at the training academy for Vatican diplomats.

Pope Paul VI became the first Pope to visit all five* continents, earning him the nickname "the Pilgrim Pope." He was also the last Pope to be crowned. Paul VI donated his Papal Tiara to the Basilica of the National Shrine of the Immaculate Conception in Washington, D.C.

* The Vatican considers North and South America as one continent.

Monsignor Montini held key posts in these years. In 1937 he became assistant to Cardinal Eugenio Pacelli, the Secretary of State, whose close collaborator he remained after Cardinal Pacelli was elected Pope Pius XII in 1939. In 1944, he was named head of the section of the Secretariat of State responsible for internal Church affairs, and in 1952 he became Pro-Secretary of State, or the second in charge of the department.

Pope Pius XII appointed Montini to be Archbishop of the huge Archdiocese of Milan in 1954. There he worked to resolve social tensions and win over industrial workers alienated from the Church; he also took a number of ecumenical initiatives. St. John XXIII named him a cardinal in 1958, and he had an active role in preparations for the ecumenical council.

Paul VI was strongly committed to Christian unity and pursued this cause through meetings with the leaders of other churches and religious bodies. During his trip to Jerusalem in January 1964, he met with the Ecumenical Patriarch Athenagoras I, and on

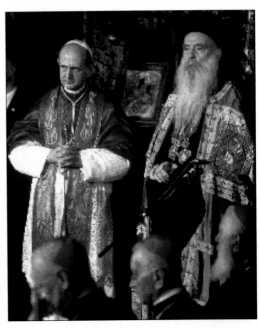

During his trip to Jerusalem in January 1964, Paul VI met with the Patriarch of Constantinople, Athenagoras I.

December 7, 1965, the Pope and the patriarch issued a joint statement withdrawing the mutual excommunications that had formalized the Catholic-Orthodox split in the year 1054. He met with two Archbishops of Canterbury (Ramsey in 1966, Coggan in 1977) and again with Patriarch Athenagoras in Constantinople (1967). International bilateral commissions were established for Catholic dialogue with Anglicans, Lutherans, and others.

Pope Paul VI moved vigorously to carry out the decisions of Vatican Council II. New commissions and other structures were established and detailed documents were issued spelling out steps to take in the reform of the liturgy, the restoration of the permanent diaconate, and other areas. He approved the New Order of the Mass (that is, the new rite of the Eucharistic liturgy in the Western Church) and published a reformed liturgical calendar.

HUMANÆ VITÆ

The document of Pope Paul VI that had the greatest impact was his encyclical *Humanæ Vitæ* (On Human Life), published July 25, 1968, in which he reaffirmed that the use of artificial contraception is intrinsically wrong. In *Humanæ Vitæ*, the Pope wrote that "the Church, nevertheless, in urging men to the observance of the precepts of the natural law, which it interprets by its constant doctrine, teaches that each and every marital act must of necessity retain its intrinsic relationship to the procreation of human life" (no. 11).

It had been long expected that the Pope would speak out definitively on this subject. In 1964 he had announced that St. John XXIII several years earlier set up the Papal Commission for the Study of Problems of the Family, Population, and Birth Rate with bishops, theologians, and specialists in several fields as members. Paul VI continued and expanded this body, which came to be popularly called the "Birth Control Commission."

Pressure for approval of artificial contraception came from revisionist theories of some moral theologians, anxiety about the supposed "population explosion," the growing use of oral contraceptives, and the fever for change then existing among a good number of Catholics. Already the sexual revolution of the 1960s had tried to reject the traditional morality in favor of permissiveness:

why not the Catholic Church? Thus, the stage was set for Paul VI's encyclical declaring that there could and would be no change in Catholic doctrine on this matter. He taught:

> This particular doctrine, often expounded by the magisterium of the Church, is based on the inseparable connection, established by God, which man on his own initiative may not break, between the unitive significance and the procreative significance which are both inherent to the marriage act. (HV 12)

Prophetically, the Pope warned of an even broader breakdown of morality if this teaching were rejected.

A CULTURE OF DISSENT AND DEFECTION

Along with dissent from *Humanæ Vitæ*, other factors made for troubled conditions in the Church beginning in the late 1960s. While some dissent and defections from the priesthood and religious life were increasing, and controversies over the interpretation of Vatican II were now becoming increasingly common.

Joseph Cardinal Ratzinger – the future Pope Benedict XVI – said, "dissension…seems to have passed over from self-criticism to self-destruction." Especially destructive, he added, was the tendency to turn away from what the council actually taught, in favor of a so-called spirit of Vatican II – in reality, a "pernicious anti-spirit." ("How many old heresies have surfaced again in recent years that have been presented as something new!" he exclaimed.)

Reflecting on the turmoil of these years, Pope Paul VI said in a homily on June 29, 1972, that "the smoke of Satan" seemed to have entered the Church (Homily, June 29, 1972). Worn out by the long struggle to establish order and defend orthodoxy, he died on the Feast of the Transfiguration, August 6, 1978.

PART III

The Restoration of Confidence and Hope

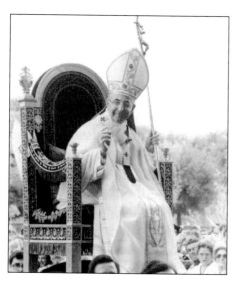

Pope John Paul I is seated on the *sedia gestatoria,* the portable papal throne which was carried on the shoulders of twelve footmen. This allowed the Pope to be seen above the heads of the crowd. The *sedia* has since been replaced by the white "Pope-mobile."

In the conclave that followed the death of Pope Paul VI, the cardinals chose the Patriarch of Venice, Cardinal Albino Luciani, as Pope on August 26, 1978. He took two names – John Paul – to signify continuity with his immediate predecessors.

Born October 17, 1912, John Paul I had been a bishop since 1958 and had been Patriarch of Venice since 1969. His friendly manner won him the nickname "the smiling Pope." Barely a month after his election, on September 28, 1978 the world was shocked to learn that he had died of a heart attack.

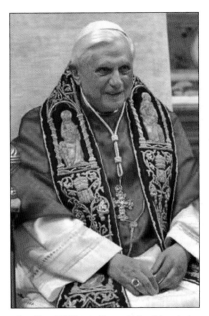

Pope Benedict XVI, one of the most influential academic theologians of the late twentieth century, had served as Archbishop of Munich, Prefect of the Congregation for the Doctrine of the Faith, and Dean of the College of Cardinals. He was a trusted friend and ally to St. John Paul II.

Beginning in 1981, St. John Paul II's principal collaborator in dealing with issues of faith and dissent was Joseph Cardinal Ratzinger – the future Pope Benedict XVI. Under his direction the Congregation for the Doctrine of the Faith issued important statements on liberation theology, the ordination of women, homosexual unions, the duties of Catholic politicians and citizens, and the role of Christ in salvation and the Catholic Church.

St. John Paul II brought to completion and in 1983 published the new *Code of Canon Law* for the Western Church, a project begun by St. John XXIII. The new compilation of Church law had been thoroughly revised in light of the Second Vatican Council. Its innovations included giving far more attention than ever before to the duties and rights of lay people, with a whole section devoted to the members of the Church in general and the laity in particular. A first-ever *Oriental Code of Canon Law* for the Eastern Rites of the Catholic Church was published in 1990.

Responding to a suggestion at the 1985 Synod of Bishops, St. John Paul II commissioned the first new, universal catechism of Catholic doctrine since the sixteenth century. The *Catechism of the Catholic Church*, an up-to-date statement of Faith incorporating clarifications and teachings since the Ecumenical Council of Trent, was published in 1992. Since then it has had a central role in efforts to establish uniform, solid, and reliable content for Catholic religious education.

St. John Paul II traveled frequently. His pastoral visits were more than occasions for outdoor Masses and colorful ceremonies that drew huge crowds; they were key tools by which he exercised his authority as the Bishop of Rome, acting as universal pastor of the Church, in order to foster unity and bolster every Catholic's faith. Along with a willingness to innovate, St. John Paul II had strong traditional devotions, especially to the Blessed Virgin Mary. In October 2002 he surprised many by adding the five Luminous mysteries to the Rosary, which are based on Christ's public life.

Despite his age and declining health, as the new millennium got underway, St. John Paul II continued to travel and to launch initiatives. Among the latter was the proclaiming of a 2004–2005 Year of the Eucharist for the entire Church. The public witness of his perseverance in the face of personal suffering was an inspiration to countless people. Finally, on April 2, 2005, worn out by the debilitating effects of Parkinson's disease, he died in his apartment in the Apostolic Palace. He was 84.

A remarkable worldwide outpouring of grief and expressions of admiration greeted the news of death of a man universally recognized as one of the towering figures of modern times. American president George W. Bush called him "one of history's great moral leaders and a hero for the ages." Hundreds of world leaders – heads of state from Afghanistan to Zimbabwe – attended St. John Paul II's funeral, as did religious leaders such as the Orthodox Patriarch Bartholomew I of Constantinople; Anglican Archbishop Rowan Williams of Canterbury; heads of numerous Protestant bodies; and many representatives of Jewish, Muslim, Buddhist, Sikh, and Hindu groups.

POPE BENEDICT XVI AS UNIVERSAL PASTOR

A few days after presiding at the funeral of St. John Paul II, Joseph Cardinal Ratzinger was elected Pope, taking the name Benedict XVI. He visited many countries around the world in his role as Chief Shepherd of the Catholic Church. Much of the focus of his pontificate was on evangelization and ecumenism.

T. JOHN PAUL II AND HIS ASSASSIN

On the afternoon of May 13, 1981, John Paul II was struck by three bullets while being driven in a slow-moving convertible through St. Peter's Square, where 20,000 people had gathered to see the pontiff. The Pope later recalled that, immediately after his assassination attempt, he had a "strange feeling of confidence" that he would live. Some see his survival as a miraculous event. His would-be assassin, an international terrorist wanted for murder in his native Turkey, was no amateur, and he had fired from point-blank range. The bullet that entered the Pope missed his main abdominal artery by a mere fraction of an inch. According to the Pope himself, "one hand fired, and another [the Blessed Virgin Mary's] guided the bullet." The Pope later publicly forgave his would-be assassin for his actions soon after the event.

Almost as remarkable was the meeting on December 27, 1983, between the Pope and his would-be assassin, Mehmet Ali Agca. Photographs of this meeting show the two seated in the corner of Agca's cell. During this encounter, Agca explained to the Pope his fears that Our Lady of Fatima was going to have her revenge on him for his assassination attempt. (The Pope was shot on May 13, the anniversary of the apparition of Our Lady of Fatima, and Mary is venerated by many Muslims.) Agca believed that "the Goddess of Fatima" saved the Pope and was now going to kill him. St. John Paul patiently listened to Agca's concerns and finally explained to him that the Blessed Virgin Mary is the Mother of God and loves all people, and he should not be afraid.

Fifteen years after the shooting, St. John Paul II met with the mother of Mehmet Ali Agca. Aided by the personal intervention of the Pope, Agca was eventually pardoned for his crime and, in 2000, was extradited to Turkey, where he remains imprisoned for other crimes.

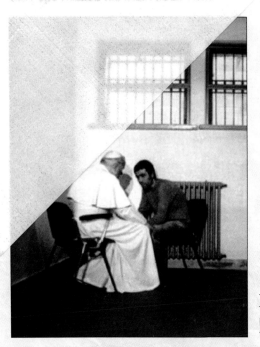

The remarkable meeting of St. John Paul II and Mehmet Ali Agca in 1983. They spoke quietly in Italian for twenty minutes.
In 2005 Mehmet Ali Agca asked Turkish authorities permission to attend the funeral of St. John Paul II. The request was denied.

In 2010 Pope Benedict XVI inaugurated the Pontifical Council for Promoting the New Evangelization, which coordinates efforts for renewing the Faith in regions that have been increasingly secularized. This council continues the call of St. John Paul II for a new evangelization of what was once called Christendom, where, according to Pope Benedict, the Faith "still shows signs of possessing vitality and profound roots among entire peoples."

Pope Benedict XVI also reached out to Eastern Orthodox and Protestant Christians, especially to the leaders of the Greek and Russian Orthodox Churches. In 2006 Archbishop Christodoulos of Athens made the first official visit to the Vatican by a Greek Orthodox bishop since the Great

Schism of the eleventh century. In 2008 Pope Benedict met with Patriarch Bartholomew of Constantinople. Together they celebrated Vespers of the Feast of St. Andrew the Apostle who, according to tradition, founded the local church in Constantinople. The next morning Pope Benedict attended the Divine Liturgy celebrated by Patriarch Bartholomew.

Pope Benedict XVI, who grew up in Germany, expressed a special affinity for the Lutheran tradition and desired a reunion of all separated Christians. In 2009 he established a Personal Ordinariate for Anglicans who wish come into full communion with the Catholic Church, and in 2010 he beatified Bl. John Henry Newman, a convert who led many from Anglicanism to Catholicism (see page 363).

Like his predecessors, Pope Benedict XVI traveled to every continent and was greeted by large crowds. During his travels he met with representatives of local churches, movements to renew the Faith, international organizations, nations, and universities. He continued St. John Paul II's initiative to meet with young people at World Youth Day, where Catholics and young people of other faith traditions meet in a different city around the world every two to three years.

Shortly after his election Pope Benedict paved the way for the canonization of his predecessor. This was announced on May 13, 2005, the Feast of Our Lady of Fatima – twenty-four years since the 1981 attempt on his life (see page 411), who credited Our Lady of Fatima for saving him from the bullet.

The Church's canonization process requires that two miracles be attributed to the intercession of the person whose cause is being promoted. After confirmation of the first such miracle, the individual can be beatified, after which he or she is called "Blessed"; after confirmation of the second miracle, the individual can be canonized, meaning he or she is affirmed to be in Heaven and is called "Saint." In order to be confirmed, an alleged miracle must be thoroughly and carefully documented and examined by a panel of theologians and other experts – including medical doctors, in the case of a miraculous healing – in order to rule out any natural causes or medical explanations. The findings must then confirmed by the Congregation for the Causes of Saints.

St. John Paul II was declared "Venerable" in 2009; this designation affirms that an individual lived a life of heroic virtue and is worthy of further consideration for sainthood. In 2011 the congregation confirmed the miraculous healing of a French nun suffering from Parkinson's disease attributed to the intercession of John Paul II, and he was beatified later that year. Two years later a miraculous healing of a Costa Rican woman was approved, clearing the path for his canonization.

On Divine Mercy Sunday, April 27, 2014, Pope Francis – Pope Benedict XVI's successor – canonized Popes John Paul II and John XXIII in a joint ceremony. It is estimated that half a million people attended the canonizations in St. Peter's Square.

Several other causes for sainthood involving holy men and women with ties to the Church in the United States were advanced during the reign of Pope Benedict XVI. These include the following:

Mother Marianne Cope (1838–1918), who worked with St. Damien of Moloka'i in Hawaii to care for people suffering from leprosy, was canonized in 2012.

Mother Theodore Guerin (1798–1856), who founded the Sisters of Providence of Saint Mary-of-the-Woods in Indiana, was canonized in 2006.

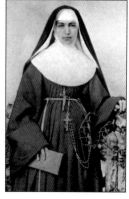

Brother Andre Bessette (1845–1937), a lay brother from the Congregation of the Holy Cross who spread devotion to St. Joseph and was the inspiration for St. Joseph's Oratory in Montreal, was canonized in 2010.

Kateri Tekakwitha (1656–1680), the first Native American saint from the United States, was canonized in 2012 (see page 413).

"I am hungry for the work and I wish with all my heart to be one of the chosen Ones, whose privilege it will be, to sacrifice themselves for the salvation of the souls of the poor Islanders.... I am not afraid of any disease, hence it would be my greatest delight even to minister to the abandoned 'lepers.'" (St. Marianne Cope, responding to a request to work with leprosy patients.)

POPE BENEDICT'S ABDICATION

Pope Benedict XVI surprised the world in February 2013 when he announced that he would resign from the papacy later that month. "I have come to the certainty that my strengths, due to an advanced age, are no longer suited to an adequate exercise of the Petrine ministry," he said in explaining his decision. The news was unexpected because Popes traditionally serve until death and no pope had resigned the office in nearly 600 years. As a cardinal and head of the Vatican's doctrinal congregation, Pope Benedict had been a close friend and advisor to St. John Paul II and had been at his side during the final years of his pontificate. Just as St. John Paul II shepherded the Church humbly and courageously during his declining years and offered a profound witness to the redemptive power of suffering, so, too, did Pope Benedict act with humble courage in resigning the office with the knowledge that the Church needed a strong and vibrant Pope to guide the faithful through the challenges of the modern era.

After his resignation Pope Benedict led a relatively secluded life and made few public appearances so as to not interfere with the papal responsibilities of his successor.

THE ELECTION OF POPE FRANCIS

Two weeks after Pope Benedict's resignation, the cardinal-electors met in conclave and elected a new Pope: Jorge Cardinal Bergoglio, Archbishop of Buenos Aires. His election was a "first" in several ways: He is the first pontiff to take the name Francis, which he did in honor of St. Francis of Assisi; he is the first Jesuit to assume the papacy; and, as a native of Argentina, he is the first Pope to come from the Americas.

From the first moments of his papacy, Pope Francis set a tone of simplicity, humility, and poverty. Stepping out onto the balcony of St. Peter's Basilica to meet the gathered crowd, he wore a simple white cassock rather than the full, traditional papal garments. He prayed with the crowd below and then asked for their blessing: "Before the bishop blesses his people, he asks that you pray to the Lord to bless me, the prayer of the people for the blessing of their bishop," he said as he bowed his head and clasped his hands for a period of silent prayer.

In Argentina Cardinal Bergolio had lived in a simple apartment rather than the official archbishop's residence; as Pope Francis he chose to reside in the Vatican guesthouse rather than take up residence in the papal apartments, expressing his desire not to be isolated from others. Just as he used to mingle and minister among the poor in the worst slums of Argentina, his humility is expressed also in his common touch with the people he meets on the streets of Rome and in the cities he visits around the world. As Pope he has continued his usual practice as archbishop of Buenos Aires in celebrating the Holy Thursday Mass of the Lord's Supper in chapels where he ministers to the marginalized such as imprisoned youth. "I want a poor Church, and for the poor," Pope Francis has said in what could be called a byword for his papacy.

Before the papal conclave the cardinals had expressed a desire for the next Pope to reform the Vatican Curia, which is a sort of administrative branch for the Holy See. Following these wishes, Pope Francis formed a group of eight cardinals from throughout the world to advise him on how to go about such a reform of the various Vatican offices; among these advisers was Sean Cardinal O'Malley, Archbishop of Boston. One of the first concerns of these reforms was the financial transparency and revision of the Vatican Bank.

Just a few months after his election, Pope Francis published his first encyclical, *Lumen Fidei* ("The Light of Faith"), in June 2013. The encyclical had been begun by Pope Benedict XVI, and its collaborative nature was acknowledged by Pope Francis in the opening paragraphs: He expressed his gratitude to Pope Benedict for an almost completed draft. The encyclical discusses salvation history from the Old Testament through the New Testament and presents faith as the light for both every human person and for all human society.

Pope Francis published an apostolic exhortation, *Evangelii Gaudium* ("The Joy of the Gospel"), in November 2013, focusing on the Church's mission of evangelization. Among its various themes, he wrote about the obligation of all Christians to serve the poor and marginalized and to work for economic and political systems that support justice, uphold human dignity, and promote the common good.

In addition to emphasizing evangelization and the needs of the poor, Pope Francis spoke numerous times on abortion and the right to life, stewardship of the environment, the great evil of sexual abuse and human trafficking, the important role of women in the Church, and the need for mercy and forgiveness. He stressed the immense graces available to Catholics in the Sacrament of Penance and Reconciliation. His simplicity and personal style has won Pope Francis much admiration both within and outside the Catholic Church, opening new opportunities by which he can lead the faithful in teaching the truths of our Faith in the midst of a world in desperate need of the Good News of salvation.

PART IV

The Church in the United States: The Colonial Era

Before the founding of the United States of America, "Catholic identity" was not an issue. The Spanish and French explorers, conquerors, and colonizers who came to the New World were Catholics. Accompanying them were priests – Jesuits, Dominicans, Franciscans – who provided them with pastoral care and worked to convert the native peoples to Christianity.

These missionaries preached the gospel with great courage and dedication. Outstanding figures included the Franciscan Juan Padilla, Servant of God, martyred by Indians in Kansas around 1540, and six French Jesuit priests and two lay assistants, known as the North American Martyrs, who were killed by the Iroquois between 1642 and 1649 in parts of present-day northern New York and Ontario. These latter were canonized by Pope Pius XI in 1930.

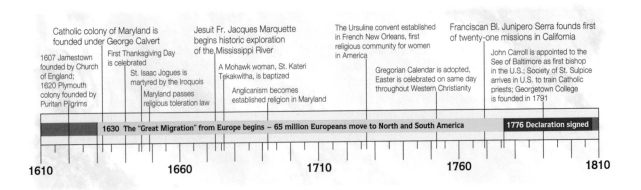

Catholic colony of Maryland is founded under George Calvert

Jesuit Fr. Jacques Marquette begins historic exploration of the Mississippi River

The Ursuline convent established in French New Orleans, first religious community for women in America

Franciscan Bl. Junipero Serra founds first of twenty-one missions in California

1607 Jamestown founded by Church of England; 1620 Plymouth colony founded by Puritan Pilgrims

First Thanksgiving Day is celebrated

St. Isaac Jogues is martyred by the Iroquois

Maryland passes religious toleration law

A Mohawk woman, St. Kateri Tekakwitha, is baptized

Anglicanism becomes established religion in Maryland

Gregorian Calendar is adopted, Easter is celebrated on same day throughout Western Christianity

John Carroll is appointed to the See of Baltimore as first bishop in the U.S.; Society of St. Sulpice arrives in U.S. to train Catholic priests; Georgetown College is founded in 1791

1630 The "Great Migration" from Europe begins – 65 million Europeans move to North and South America

1776 Declaration signed

1610   1660   1710   1760   1810

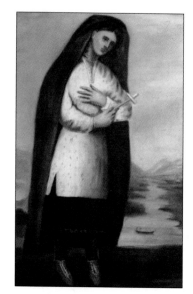

Called "The Lily of the Mohawks." St. Kateri Tekakwitha (1656-1680) was the daughter of a Mohawk warrior and a Christian Algonquin woman. St. Kateri was converted in 1676 and received instruction from Fr. Jacques de Lamberville, a Jesuit. At her baptism, she took the name "Kateri," a Mohawk pronunciation of "Catherine." This image of St. Kateri was painted after her death by Fr. Claude Chauchetiere, a missionary priest at Sault Saint-Louis where she spent her final years. He was inspired to paint the portrait after having a radiant vision of St. Kateri. It hangs at the Saint Francis Xavier Mission at Kahnawake, Quebec.

Probably the best known of these heroic martyrs was the Jesuit priest St. Isaac Jogues, who died in 1646. In an account of his final days, he calls the opportunity to convert the Iroquois "the bond of his captivity." The narrator explained: "He would have escaped a hundred times if providence had not checked him, by offering him… the means of opening the gates of paradise to some poor soul" (quoted in "The Jesuit Relations: The Sufferings and Martyrdom of Isaac Jogues, S.J." *Readings in Church History*, ed. Barry, 1985, pp. 812-813). Others like the Spanish Franciscan priest Bl. Junipero Serra devoted their lives to the spiritual and temporal advancement of the native peoples. Bl. Junipero Serra founded nine of the twenty-one Franciscan missions in present-day California and was president of the missions until his death in 1784. He was beatified by St. John Paul II in 1988; his feast day is celebrated on July 1.

Thanks to the zeal of such missionaries, many of the native peoples did become Christians. St. Kateri Tekakwitha, a young Mohawk woman, was baptized in 1676 and died four years later at the age of twenty-four; she was canonized by Pope Benedict XVI in 2012; her feast day is celebrated on July 14.

The early presence of Catholics in parts of the present-day United States of America has left a distinctive mark on many parts of the country. Founded by the Spanish in 1565, the city of St. Augustine in Florida was the first permanent settlement in the United States of America and the site of the first parish, established the same year. The French Jesuit Jacques Marquette accompanied Louis Joliet on a historic exploratory voyage of the Mississippi River in 1673. Other missionaries also played important roles to open up and develop the Southeast and Southwest.

By contrast, in the English colonies on the Eastern seaboard, Catholics were generally excluded by penal law. The exceptions to this exclusion were Quaker Pennsylvania and, especially, Maryland, which was granted to George Calvert (Lord Baltimore) in 1632 and settled by Catholics and Protestants beginning in 1634. Two Jesuits, Andrew White and John Altham, accompanied the first settlers and, besides serving the settlers' spiritual needs, began to evangelize the native peoples.

In 1649 Maryland's General Assembly adopted an unprecedented act of religious toleration providing that, for the sake of "quiet and peaceable government" and "mutual love and unity among the inhabitants," no Christian in Maryland was to be "troubled, molested, or discountenanced" for

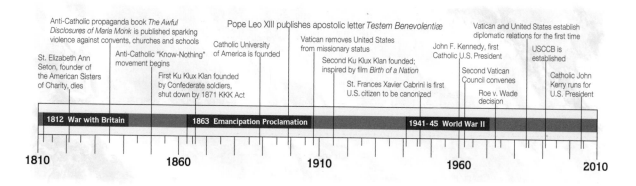

Anti-Catholic propaganda book *The Awful Disclosures of Maria Monk* is published sparking violence against convents, churches and schools

Pope Leo XIII publishes apostolic letter *Testem Benevolentiæ*

Vatican and United States establish diplomatic relations for the first time

St. Elizabeth Ann Seton, founder of the American Sisters of Charity, dies

Anti-Catholic "Know-Nothing" movement begins

Catholic University of America is founded

Vatican removes United States from missionary status

John F. Kennedy, first Catholic U.S. President

USCCB is established

First Ku Klux Klan founded by Confederate soldiers, shut down by 1871 KKK Act

Second Ku Klux Klan founded; inspired by film *Birth of a Nation*

Second Vatican Council convenes

Catholic John Kerry runs for U.S. President

St. Frances Xavier Cabrini is first U.S. citizen to be canonized

Roe v. Wade decision

1812 War with Britain | 1863 Emancipation Proclamation | 1941-45 World War II

1810 | 1860 | 1910 | 1960 | 2010

his or her faith or forced to practice another religion. Except for a four-year interval of Puritan control, religious toleration remained the rule until 1688, when Maryland was made a crown colony. In 1692 Anglicanism became the established religion in that English colony.

PART V

Catholicism and the Birth of a Nation

THE REVOLUTIONARY YEARS (1775-1783)

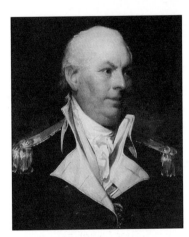

Commodore John Barry, USN, (1745-1803), an Irish Catholic, was commander of the first ship commissioned by Congress after the Revolutionary War, the frigate *United States*. The U.S. Navy has named four destroyers in honor of him. He is the "Father of the American Navy."

Catholics, though few, played a considerable role in the emergence of the United States of America. Charles Carroll of Maryland was among the signers of the Declaration of Independence, and he and his cousin, Fr. John Carroll, accompanied an official delegation sent to Canada by the Continental Congress to secure Canadian neutrality in the Revolutionary War. As many as fifty percent of George Washington's troops had Irish surnames, although certainly some percentage of these were not Catholics. Catholic officers from abroad, including the French Lafayette and the Polish Pulaski and Kosciusko, served with Washington. John Barry, an Irish Catholic and commander of the first ship commissioned by Congress, is considered the Father of the American Navy. Catholic France provided crucial military and naval support, and Catholic Spain helped with money and by remaining neutral. Two Catholics–Daniel Carroll of Maryland and Thomas FitzSimmons of Philadelphia–signed the U.S. Constitution.

In a letter to Catholics, Washington spoke of the "patriotic part" they had played in the Revolutionary War and of the "important assistance" received from a nation–France–"in which the Roman Catholic faith is professed." The First Amendment to the U.S. Constitution rejected the idea of an established national church and guaranteed the free exercise of religion.

THE POST-REVOLUTIONARY PERIOD

At the close of the Revolutionary War there were about 25,000 Catholics, mostly in Maryland and Pennsylvania, out of a total population of four million. They were served by twenty-four priests. Father Carroll was named "Superior of the Mission in the Thirteen United States" on June 9, 1784. In 1789 Baltimore was designated the first diocese of the new country, and Fr. Carroll was elected its bishop after a vote by the priests. (This was the first and only time in the New World a bishop was appointed by vote.) At its founding the Diocese of Baltimore covered all thirteen states.

Soon a number of Catholic institutions were founded in the United States. Georgetown University, the oldest Catholic institution of higher learning in the United States, was established in 1789. The first seminary, St. Mary's in Baltimore, was established in 1791. The first Catholic women's school was founded by Visitation nuns in Washington, D.C., in 1799. In 1808 the Diocese of Baltimore

THE CARROLL FAMILY AND THE FOUNDING OF THE UNITED STATES

John Carroll was probably the most influential Catholic figure in the establishment of the Church in America. Appointed the first bishop in this country, he faced the difficult task of finding a place for the Faith in a new political order, a task most agree he handled with great skill. In addition to his own contributions during the American Revolution, other members of the Carroll family played prominent roles: his brother Daniel was one of two Catholic signers of the 1787 Constitution, and his cousin Charles Carroll, a signer of the Declaration of Independence.

Born in 1735, John received his education from the Jesuits at Bohemia Manor in Maryland. Because there were no schools for the training of seminarians in the colonies during this time, he went to St. Omer's College in French Flanders to continue his education. He entered the Society of Jesus in 1753, and after studying in Liege was ordained in 1769. After the suppression of the Jesuit order in Europe, he returned to America in 1774, only one year before the onset of the Revolutionary War.

In 1776 a committee composed of Benjamin Franklin, Samuel Chase, and Charles Carroll of Carrollton was elected by the Continental Congress to be sent to Canada to ask for their neutrality during the war. By a special resolution, John Carroll was asked to accompany this committee to "assist them in such matters as they shall think useful." He accepted this task, and spent the winter in Canada. While there he developed a close friendship with Benjamin Franklin, earning his admiration and respect.

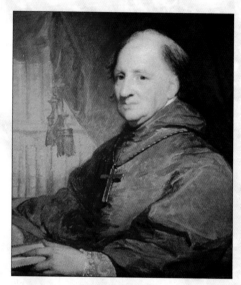

Archbishop John Carroll painted by the most famous portrait artist of the American Revolution period, Gilbert Stuart.

Partly due to the recommendation of Benjamin Franklin, on June 9, 1784 the papal nuncio established Father Carroll as the Superior of the Mission in the Thirteen United States. He became the first bishop of Baltimore in 1790, his diocese covering the whole of the United States. As bishop he dealt with all the major issues of his time, including the controversy over lay trustees. Under his watch the U.S. Catholic population grew from 25,000 to 200,000. The influence of John Carroll over his fellow Americans cannot be overstated. For example, the four states that adopted constitutions allowing Catholics complete equality with other citizens (Pennsylvania, Delaware, Virginia, and Maryland) were all located nearest to Father (later Archbishop) John Carroll's area of ministry.

became an archdiocese with Bishop Carroll as its archbishop, and four new dioceses were created: Boston; New York; Philadelphia; and Bardstown, Kentucky (the present-day Archdiocese of Louisville). During the following century, the United States was considered a missionary territory, and the Church was supervised by the Holy See.

The first half of the nineteenth century saw a number of outstanding Catholic figures. St. Elizabeth Ann Seton (1774-1821), a convert from Episcopalianism and widowed mother of five, began the Sisters of Charity in the United States and was canonized in 1975. Her feast day is celebrated on January 4.

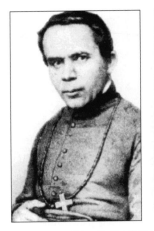 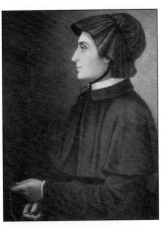

Bishop St. John Neumann and St. Elizabeth Ann Seton were pioneers in the parochial school movement.

The French-born St. Rose Philippine Duchesne (1769-1852) established the first U.S. convent of the Religious of the Sacred Heart in Missouri in 1818 and was canonized in 1988. Her feast day is celebrated on November 18. Bishop St. John Neumann (1811-1860), a native of Bohemia, was the fourth Bishop of Philadelphia and was canonized in 1977. His feast day is celebrated on January 5. Sts. Elizabeth Ann Seton and John Neumann were pioneers in the parochial school movement, which is still to this day one of the outstanding features of the Church in the United States. Fr. Michael J. McGivney founded the Knights of Columbus in 1882. The Knights are Catholic men who work to make their communities better places while enhancing their faith.

PART VI

A Church of Immigrants

Massive Catholic immigration from Europe to the United States began early in the nineteenth century and continued well into the twentieth century. The newcomers were attracted by the promise of work, land, and religious and political freedom. Of the nearly three million Catholic migrants who came between 1830 and 1870, most came from Ireland, Germany, and France. The 1880s saw more than one million additional Catholic immigrants, with Catholics from Eastern

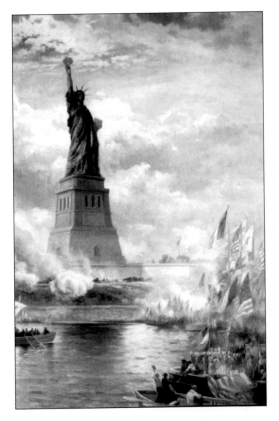

President Grover Cleveland joined the celebration dedicating the Statue of Liberty in New York Harbor on October 28, 1886. Built on a colossal scale, the statue has become one of the most potent symbols of human freedom and is an icon to immigrants coming to America. "Liberty Enlightening the World," was a gift from the people of France to the people of the United States. Conceived by the French sculptor Frédéric de Bartholdi, it celebrated a century of friendship between the two Republics.

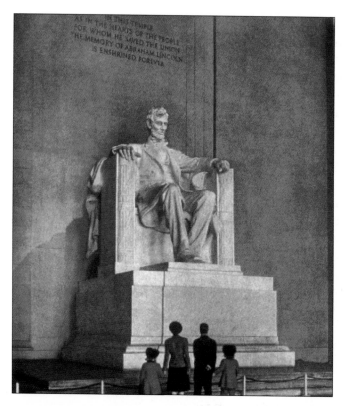

The Lincoln Memorial in Washington D.C.–By 1860, there were 4.5 million slaves in the United States. Two major milestones marked slavery's final abolition during the war years: the Emancipation Proclamation and the Thirteenth Amendment to the Constitution. President Abraham Lincoln issued the Emancipation Proclamation on January 1, 1863, declaring that "all persons held as slaves . . . are and henceforward shall be free." Of the over four million slaves emancipated in 1863, an estimated one hundred thousand were Catholics.

and Southern Europe–Poles, Slovaks, Ukrainians, Italians, and others–joining the influx. These immigrants quickly fanned out from the East to many other parts of the expanding nation, so much so that new cities like Chicago, Milwaukee, and St. Louis became important Catholic population centers.

Due to immigration and higher birth rates, the growth of American Catholicism was remarkably rapid. Church leaders made heroic efforts to provide personnel and parishes, schools, monasteries, and other institutions to keep up with the expansion. By 1840, there were fifteen dioceses in the country and 663,000 American Catholics served by 500 priests, many of them foreign-born. The Catholic Church was the largest religious body in the country by about the 1860s.

THE RISE OF ANTI-CATHOLICISM

Although the United States government is committed by its Constitution to religious toleration, starting in the 1830s Catholic immigration and rapid Catholic population growth were greeted by the rise of anti-Catholic Nativism.

Aiding the popularity of anti-Catholic sentiment, *The Awful Disclosures of Maria Monk*, a book full of lurid tales of convent life, was published in 1835, and it became a best-seller second only to the Bible in American religious publishing history. Purporting to be the work of an ex-nun, it was written by Protestant ministers. The book helped fuel anti-Catholic violence throughout the United States. The year before it was published, an Ursuline convent in Charlestown, Massachusetts, was attacked and burned by a mob. In 1844, thirteen people were killed, and two churches and a school were burned in Nativist riots in Philadelphia. The 1850s brought the Know-Nothing movement (so named because members were instructed to say they knew nothing about its activities), which sought to exclude foreigners and Catholics from public office. Abraham Lincoln once remarked to a friend that if the Know-Nothings got power, the Declaration of Independence would have to be rewritten to read, "All men are created equal except negroes, foreigners, and Catholics."

The Know-Nothings were a significant political force until about 1860. Catholic political strength also grew during these years, especially in urban areas of the East and Midwest where the Irish proved skillful at political organization. However, anti-Catholicism remained a factor in American life throughout the rest of the century and much of the century that followed. Other noteworthy anti-Catholic groups included the virulently hostile American Protective Association, founded in 1887, and the Ku Klux Klan, which was also anti-black and anti-Jewish. In a famous incident in 1884, a

Republican campaign speaker's attack on the Democrats as the party of "Rum, Romanism, and Rebellion" (in other words, anti-prohibition, anti-Catholic, and pro-Confederacy) tipped the election in favor of the Democratic presidential candidate, Grover Cleveland.

PART VII

Growth and Conflict

American Catholicism continued its remarkable expansion after the Civil War, with dioceses, parishes, educational institutions at all levels, hospitals, and other organizations and programs multiplying rapidly.

From 1829 to 1849, the bishops had addressed the needs of the growing Catholic community in a series of decision-making assemblies called provincial councils. (At the time, the country had only one ecclesiastical "province"–the Archdiocese of Baltimore–to oversee the other dioceses).

The provincial councils were followed in 1852, 1866, and 1884 by plenary councils, also held in Baltimore, which legislated for the needs of the expanding Church. The Third Plenary Council, the best known of these gatherings, took steps that led to the writing of the famous Baltimore Catechism, the normative text for Catholic religious education in the United States for some seventy-five years, and the founding of the Catholic University of America in Washington, D.C.

Chief Catholic figures during these decades included two who came to represent the opposing sides of a debate then taking shape over Catholic cultural assimilation: Isaac Hecker and Orestes Brownson.

Isaac T. Hecker (1819-1888) was a convert to Catholicism who first became a Redemptorist priest, then founded a new religious community, the Missionary Priests of St. Paul the Apostle (Paulists), committed to the conversion of Protestant America. In order to evangelize effectively, Hecker argued, the Church in the United States had to be fully and unreservedly American. Speaking to the bishops at the plenary council of 1866, he said:

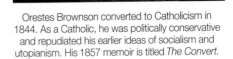

Orestes Brownson converted to Catholicism in 1844. As a Catholic, he was politically conservative and repudiated his earlier ideas of socialism and utopianism. His 1857 memoir is titled *The Convert*.

> Here, thanks to the American Constitution, the Church is free to do her divine work. Here, she finds a civilization in harmony with her divine teachings. Here, Christianity is promised a reception from an intelligent and free people, that will give forth a development of unprecedented glory.

Apparently it was the French edition of a biography of Father Hecker by one of his Paulist disciples, and especially its introduction by a French priest, that prompted Pope Leo XIII to condemn "Americanism" in his apostolic letter *Testem Benevolentiæ*.

Orestes Brownson (1803-1876), the leading Catholic intellectual of his day, had been part of the New England philosophical and religious movement called Transcendentalism before becoming a Catholic in 1844, the same year as his friend Hecker. A writer and social critic, he was editor of a periodical called *Brownson's Quarterly Review*.

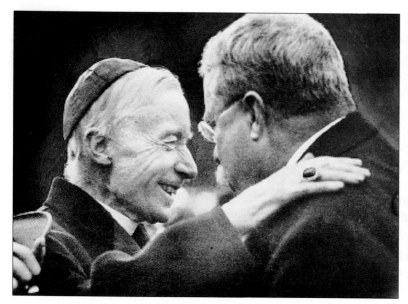
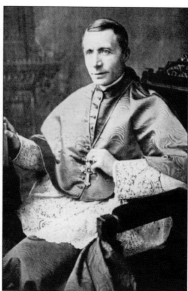

President Theodore Roosevelt said to James Cardinal Gibbons, "Taking your life as a whole I think you now occupy the position of being the most respected and venerated and useful citizen of our country." In 1869, then Bishop Gibbons went to Rome as the youngest prelate at the First Vatican Council. As Archbishop he succeeded to the see of Baltimore in 1877, and was made a Cardinal in 1886. In his long episcopacy, he played an important role in improving Church-State relations, integrated great waves of immigrants into American society, defended the poor, preached morality, coped with the turbulence of World War I, and championed the rights of labor.

Brownson at first shared Hecker's views about the need to "Americanize" Catholicism, but the Civil War shook his faith in American democracy, and as he grew older, he became increasingly skeptical that the secular culture of the United States could provide a congenial environment for the Church. Brownson, one historian remarked, "wanted to be fully Catholic, and he wanted to remain fully American, and it was becoming more and more difficult to be both" (quoted in O'Brien, *Public Catholicism*, 1989, p. 60).

The two leading figures in the hierarchy in this era – Cardinal Gibbons of Baltimore (1834-1921) and Archbishop Ireland of St. Paul (1838-1918) – were "Americanizers" who favored the full and rapid integration of Catholicism and Catholics into the surrounding culture. Speaking in France in 1892, Ireland declared his ardent patriotism as a Catholic American:

> By word and act we prove that we are patriots of patriots. Our hearts always beat with love for the republic. Our tongues are always eloquent in celebrating her praises. Our hands are always uplifted to bless her banners and her soldiers.

Others were not so sure rapid Americanization was a good idea. German Catholics in particular favored a slower approach that would allow immigrants to retain their own language and their German Catholic culture; they sought the appointment of German bishops in proportion to the number of Germans in the Catholic population and backed the establishment of German parishes. The argument came to a head over "Cahenslyism." This was a movement taking its name from Peter Paul Cahensly, a German layman who became alarmed about the spiritual state of the immigrants and petitioned Pope Leo XIII on their behalf.

Although it was often said that Pope Leo's *Testem Benevolentiæ* spoke of problems that were non-existent in American Catholicism, conflicts and controversies like these undoubtedly provided at least part of the background for the Pope's rejection of Americanism. Among the central tenets of this error, he said, was this:

> In order to more easily attract those who differ from her, the Church should shape her teachings more in accord with the spirit of the age and relax some of her ancient severity

and make some concessions to new opinions. Many think that these concessions should be made…in regard to doctrines which belong to the deposit of the faith.

The Pope, of course, thought this would not be a good idea. The Americanizers also insisted they wanted nothing of the sort.

PART VIII

The Twentieth Century

By the year 1900, Catholics in the United States numbered 12,000,000 out of a total population of 76,000,000. They lived in eighty-two dioceses and were served by 12,000 priests and many thousands of religious men and women who staffed a large and growing network of Catholic schools and other institutions. Catholic immigration remained high. One notable figure of this era was the Italian-born St Frances Xavier Cabrini (1850-1917). Mother Cabrini founded the Missionary Sisters of the Sacred Heart, who worked among Italian immigrants in Chicago and other cities. She became an American citizen in 1909 and, in 1946, became the first U.S. citizen to be canonized. Her feast day is celebrated on November 13.

THE GREAT WAR AND YEARS OF DEPRESSION

During World War I, American Catholics in large numbers once again fought for their country. During the war, the bishops took the important step of establishing a new organization – the National Catholic War Council – to coordinate programs for military personnel. After the war, despite opposition from bishops concerned about possible interference in diocesan affairs and initial reservations on the Vatican's part, the hierarchy continued the organization, now renamed the National Catholic Welfare Conference. The NCWC was the bishops' vehicle for cooperative national-level action in social action, education and youth work, communications, and other fields.

In 1919 the bishops published their famous Program of Social Reconstruction, a postwar plan for the nation that advocated economic and social measures well ahead of their time. The document was largely the work of Msgr. John A. Ryan (1869-1945), a priest who served for years on the NCWC staff; he came to be known as "Monsignor New Dealer" for his support of President Franklin D. Roosevelt's Depression-era policies.

During the 1920s and 1930s, many Catholic organizations and movements were established to reflect the Catholic Action movement championed by Pope Pius XI to encourage lay involvement in social and political activity. The Liturgical Movement for renewal of the liturgy also became an important presence among American Catholics during these years.

In 1928 the Democratic Party nominated former New York governor Al Smith as its candidate for president. It was the first time a Catholic had run for the nation's highest office. There was little chance of any Democrat being elected president that year, but Smith's candidacy occasioned a resurgence of anti-Catholicism, and he lost badly.

With the Great Depression and the New Deal in the 1930s, Catholics swung more strongly than ever behind the Democrats. There also was another Catholic response to the economic and social crisis – the Catholic Worker movement, founded by Dorothy Day and Peter Maurin. The Catholic Worker movement was a sometimes controversial group committed to a radical brand of Catholicism that

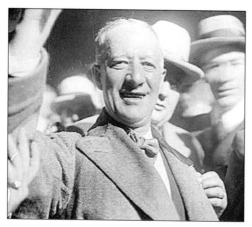

Irish Catholic Al Smith (1873-1944) was Governor of New York and a U.S. presidential candidate in 1928.

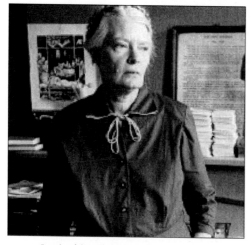

Founder of the Catholic Worker Movement in 1933, Dorothy Day (1897-1980) was a social activist for the homeless and impoverished.

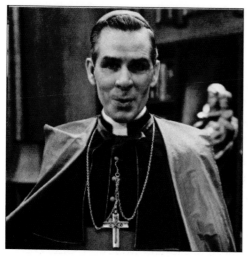

In the early 1950s, Bishop Ven. Fulton Sheen (1895-1979) became the first significant television preacher. Sheen's program *Life Is Worth Living* was highly regarded and received an Emmy award. Sheen remained on television until 1968.

advocated social justice, aid to the poor, and pacifism. Although never large in numbers, the Catholic Worker movement helped shape the attitudes of many Catholic intellectuals and activists.

WORLD WAR II AND AFTER

When the United States entered World War II in 1941, many American Catholics again responded with patriotic fervor, though some Italians and Germans refused to fight their old-countrymen. With the return of peace, fervent anti-Communism, intensified by the Soviet-backed Communist takeover in Eastern Europe and the persecution of the Catholic Church there, soon put Catholics at the forefront of the national mobilization during the Cold War. Catholics also served in large numbers in the Korean War (1950-1953), fought by the U.S. and its allies under United Nations auspices to repel Communist aggression from Communist Red China and North Korea.

Meanwhile the Church in the United States was experiencing profound changes because of postwar socio-economic developments. Catholics flocked to college with the assistance of the GI Bill, a government program that paid military veterans' education costs. More education and increased prosperity fostered Catholics' upward mobility and accelerated their entry into the social mainstream. A vast movement of population – out of old inner-city ethnic neighborhoods, often focused on parish churches, into booming new suburbs – led Catholics to mix and mingle more freely than ever before with people of diverse religious and ethnic backgrounds.

In these years, too, churchmen like Francis Cardinal Spellman, the powerful Archbishop of New York; the convert and author turned Trappist monk, Thomas Merton; television preacher Bishop Ven. Fulton Sheen; and Church-state theologian John Courtney Murray, S.J., became national figures. Catholic personalities and Catholic themes were featured in popular films and other media. Catholic numbers continued to grow rapidly, and Catholic schools at all levels expanded dramatically. Catholicism was on its way to becoming a dominant force in shaping American culture. A rise in anti-Catholicism was one predictable result, reflected in the book American Freedom and Catholic Power (1949) by writer Paul Blanshard.

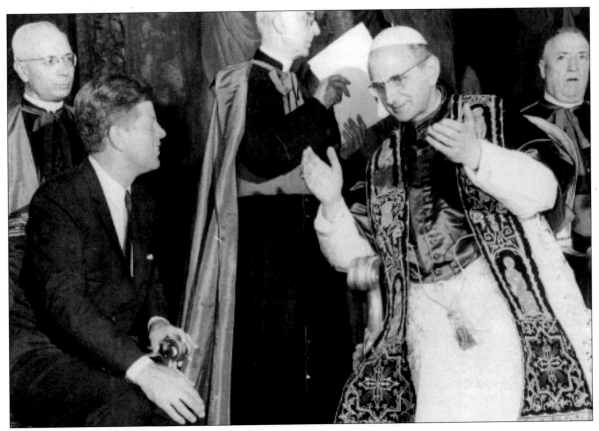

In July 1963, Pope Paul VI met with President John F. Kennedy, the first Catholic president of the United States. The audience was originally to have been with St. John XXIII, but he died before the meeting. Kennedy would be assassinated only months later on November 22. This photo captures what could have been: "the most powerful man in the world" and "the parish priest of the world" working together.

Against this background, the election in 1960 of Massachusetts Senator John F. Kennedy as the first Catholic President of the United States was a watershed event–a definitive defeat for anti-Catholicism. On the other hand, it came at a price. During the campaign, Kennedy gave a famous speech to Protestant ministers in Houston, Texas, assuring them that, if elected, he would not let his religion influence his performance in office. In doing so, he established a pattern–certainly not an integrated, Catholic approach–that many Catholic politicians would adopt in the decades that followed.

VATICAN II AND THE AMERICAN CHURCH

American Catholics were generally enthusiastic about the Second Vatican Council (1962-1965), and implementation of its decisions seemed to go well at first. Responding to a Vatican II mandate, the bishops organized themselves as an episcopal conference–the National Conference of Catholic Bishops–replacing the old, more loosely structured NCWC. They also created a sister organization, the United States Catholic Conference, to collaborate with priests, religious, and laity in number of fields. (The NCCB and USCC were combined in 1991 into a single structure, the United States Conference of Catholic Bishops.)

Problems soon arose. New candidates for the priesthood and religious life began to drop sharply, and there was a continuing stream of defections. Enrollment in Catholic elementary and secondary schools plummeted. Though some remained staunchly faithful, many Catholic colleges and universities distanced themselves from the Church. Pope Paul VI's 1968 encyclical *Humanæ Vitæ*, reaffirming the Church's condemnation of artificial birth control, met with organized dissent. Unauthorized liturgical experiments became commonplace. Mirroring the anti-authoritarian mood of the 1960s and growing opposition to the Vietnam War, authority in the Church came under attack. According to opinion polls, many Catholics rejected the doctrinal and moral teaching of the Church on numerous issues.

Perhaps the most damaging and disheartening development in the American Catholic Church was the disclosure of rampant sexual abuse of minors among some American clergy. During the early years of the twenty-first century, it was discovered that some priests had been sexually abusing minors, most cases going as far back as the 1960s and 1970s; many churchmen had hushed the abuse to avoid scandal. Decades of suppression of these clerical sins only contributed to the humiliation when these incidents were revealed in the media. Because of abuse, American dioceses paid settlements totaling hundreds of millions of dollars, even to the point of bankruptcy. Still, these financial penalties were insignificant compared to the Church's overall loss of moral credibility and public esteem in the United States.

CONCLUSION: PRESENT AND FUTURE

St. John Paul II called often for a "new evangelization" in formerly Christian regions–notably Western Europe–where faith and religious practice have declined in the face of affluence, pleasure-seeking, and the secularist mentality arising from the rationalism of eighteenth-century Enlightenment philosophy and the scientism of the nineteenth century. Only Christianity, he noted, has convincing, satisfying answers to perennial questions about life's meaning–"Who am I? Where have I come from and where am I going? Why is there evil? What is there after this life?" This human need for meaning provides the starting-point for renewal of faith.

Although conditions in the Church stabilized and improved under St. John Paul II, the crisis of dissent that began in the 1960s persisted, especially in Western Europe and North America. Neo-Modernism made deep inroads. The result in a number of countries was a catechetical collapse leading to ignorance of the Catholic tradition among many Catholics. Programs for implementing the Catechism of the Catholic Church have begun to address these problems within the context of the New Evangelization.

A deeply disturbing aspect of secularism in the twentieth century was the rise of the culture of death–a worldview and value system expressed in things like contraception, population control, and abortion. Moreover, other forces of evil were presented as progress: euthanasia, the acceptance of homosexual acts, human cloning, the destruction of nascent human life for the sake of scientific experimentation, embryonic stem-cell research, and the threat of large-scale warfare by nuclear, chemical, or other means. The Church supports genuine human rights and the progress of scientific knowledge at the service of human needs. However, it is necessary to distinguish true rights and legitimate advances from policies and practices based on utilitarian "ends-justify-the-means" reasoning.

In the face of these and other challenges now present or yet to come, however, the Church continues her pilgrimage through history with serenity and hope. In his apostolic letter Novo millennio ineunte (At the Beginning of the New Millennium), published January 6, 2001, as a kind of inaugural greeting to a new era, St. John Paul II said the essence of faith is not "a magic formula" but a Person–Jesus Christ. "It is not therefore a matter of inventing a new 'program,'" added this highly innovative Pope.

> The program already exists: it is the plan found in the Gospel and in the living Tradition, it is the same as ever. Ultimately, it has its center in Christ himself...

Recent events have reopened the debate about whether American culture at its roots is or is not compatible with Catholic beliefs and values. Some hold that founding documents like the Declaration of Independence and the Constitution are grounded in the natural law tradition largely shaped by Catholic thinkers such as St. Thomas Aquinas; as a result, they say, American values offer a congenial setting for Catholicism. Others maintain that the founding documents are grounded in the rationalism of the eighteenth century Enlightenment: moral relativism, religious indifferentism, individualism, and the ethic of "choice" visible in today's American culture.

Whichever may be the case, the religious and secularist worldviews have both been part of the American experience from the time of the nation's founding. In recent decades the conflict between religion and secularism has become an ongoing "culture war"–a struggle over values and beliefs that shape American institutions and policies.

As the twenty-first century began, the Catholic Church in the United States faced a host of challenges bearing in one way or another upon the question of Catholic identity: What does it mean to be an American Catholic? Catholics not only are part of America's culture war but also engaged in their own intramural, ideological struggles over the future of the Church. Moreover, although American Catholics are more numerous today than ever, only about one out of three regularly attends Sunday Mass, and many reject Church teachings on important matters of belief and practice. Although the number of priests and religious has fallen in the past forty years, new vocations to the priesthood and religious life are showing much promise that is expressed in serious spirituality and vibrant pastoral zeal. A number of dioceses and religious orders throughout the United States are showing hope in the form of a small resurgence of priestly vocations.

The United States is the scene of a profound conflict between Americans who support religiously based values and secularized Americans who advocate a relativistic morality of individual "choice." Catholics can be found on both sides of this divide. In these new, and in some ways more difficult, circumstances, many American Catholics still face the old need to decide what it means to be both Catholic and American.

Throughout the pontificate of Benedict XVI, the joyful optimism of his predecessor, St. John Paul II, has been very much alive and well. Although the tensions between advocates of natural law, Judeo-Christian-based morality, and proponents of moral relativism strongly persist, Pope Benedict's teaching about the power of holiness and the charity of Christ will be the ultimate solution to these tensions. In a spirit of hope, at World Youth Day in Cologne during the summer of 2005, the Holy Father alluded to a spiritual "nuclear fission" that will extend Christ's kingdom of love, peace, truth, and justice as long as there are individuals who, like the early Christians, aspire to be great saints and evangelizers in their workplaces and in their families.

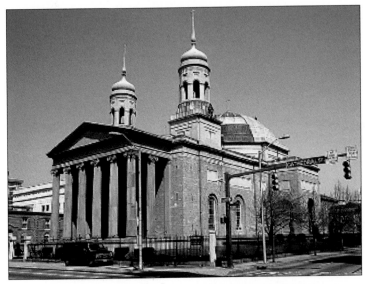

The Basilica of the National Shrine of the Assumption of the Blessed Virgin Mary in Baltimore, Maryland is considered the motherchurch of the United States.

The history of the Church has demonstrated throughout the centuries that the witness of holiness will push the Kingdom of God forward in the United States. Modern-day saints living and working for Christ in the world will show what it means to be a Catholic and an American.

VOCABULARY

AMERICANISM
Condemned by Pope Leo XIII, this movement sought a way to adapt the Catholic Faith within American principles and modern ideas. It questioned themes like passive and active virtues, the best form of religious life, and the correct approach to evangelization.

CARETAKER POPE
Refers to an aged Pope whom the College of Cardinals elects to serve as a pastoral figure who would make few changes. John XXIII was elected as a caretaker Pope but proved to be anything but.

DOCTRINE OF COLLEGIALITY
Set out by the Dogmatic Constitution of the Church published by the Second Vatican Council, this states that bishops, in union with and under the Pope, share in teaching and governing the Church.

LAY TRUSTEEISM
Partly to conform to American civil law, partly out of enthusiasm for democracy, and partly in imitation of the congregational system in American Protestantism, laymen became the owners of parish property, administered parish affairs, and in some places began hiring their own pastors in defiance of the bishop.

NATIONAL CATHOLIC WELFARE CONFERENCE
The NCWC was the bishops' vehicle in the early- and mid-twentieth century for cooperative national-level action in social action, education and youth work, communications, and other fields.

NATIONAL CONFERENCE OF CATHOLIC BISHOPS
(NCCB) Responding to a Vatican II mandate, the bishops organized themselves as an episcopal conference replacing the old, more loosely structured NCWC.

NEW EVANGELIZATION
Called by St. John Paul II, he hoped to reintroduce the Faith into formerly Christian regions – notably Western Europe – where religious practice had declined in the face of affluence, pleasure-seeking, and the secularistic mentality arising from the rationalism of eighteenth-century Enlightenment philosophy and the scientism of the nineteenth century.

QUEBEC ACT
Passed in 1774 by the British Parliament, it extended political and legal concessions to the inhabitants of Quebec and granted them religious freedom.

UNITED STATES CATHOLIC CONFERENCE
(USCC) A sister organization to the NCCB created to collaborate with priests, religious, and laity in a number of fields.

UNITED STATES CONFERENCE OF CATHOLIC BISHOPS
(USCCB) Single structure that replaced the NCCB and USCC in 1991.

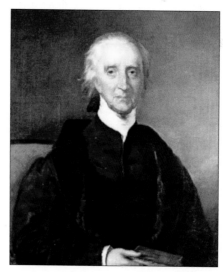

Charles Carroll (1737-1832), a lawyer from Maryland, was a delegate to the Continental Congress and later a United States senator. He was the only Catholic signer of the *Declaration of Independence*. Charles Carroll was a cousin of Archbishop John Carroll and Daniel Carroll.

STUDY QUESTIONS

1. What are St. John XXIII's nicknames? Why does each apply?

2. What were the three most progressive and long-lasting changes made by St. John XXIII?

3. What reasons did St. John XXIII give for calling the Second Vatican Council?

4. How long did Vatican II last? Where was it held?

5. What is Lumen gentium? Why was it significant?

6. What is Dei verbum? What Catholic teaching did it emphasize?

7. What does the document Sacrosanctum concilium discuss?

8. To what was the document Gaudium et spes written in response?

9. What Pope was elected during Vatican II and saw it through to the end?

10. How did Paul VI help improve relations with the Eastern Orthodox Church?

11. What steps did Paul VI take to implement the teachings of Vatican II?

12. What was so significant about Humanæ Vitæ?

13. Who was "the smiling Pope"?

14. At the time of St. John Paul II's election, how long had it been since a non-Italian was Pope?

15. With what powerful words did John Paul II open his pontificate?

16. What did St. John Paul II's first encyclical, Redemptor Hominis, emphasize as being the plan for his pontificate?

17. What two forms of secular humanism did St. John Paul II see as the biggest threat to Christianity in the modern world?

18. Who was St. John Paul II's "right-hand man" combatting matters of faith and dissent?

19. Who was St. Isaac Jogues?

20. What was the first Catholic parish in the New World?

21. What was the Quebec Act of 1774?

22. Name two Catholics who signed the Constitution.

23. What city was the seat of the first diocese in the United States?

24. What university is the oldest Catholic institution of higher learning in the United States?

25. Who is considered the founder of the American Navy?

26. How did lay trusteeism become a problem in America?

27. What book was written by some Protestant ministers to defame the Church?

28. Who were the Know-Nothings?

29. Why was the Democratic Party of the 1880s called the party of "Rum, Romanism and Rebellion"?

30. Who founded the Paulists?

31. Orestes Brownson edited what periodical?

32. What was particular about the German Catholics' experience in nineteenth-century America?

33. What Catholic leader worked to preserve good relations between the Church and labor unions?

STUDY QUESTIONS Continued

34. Who founded the Missionary Sisters of the Sacred Heart?

35. Why was the NCWC organized?

36. What organization did the NCWC eventually become?

37. Who was the first major party Catholic to run for President of the U. S.?

38. Who founded the Catholic Worker Movement?

39. Who was the first Catholic President?

40. What papal encyclical was widely ignored by American Catholics?

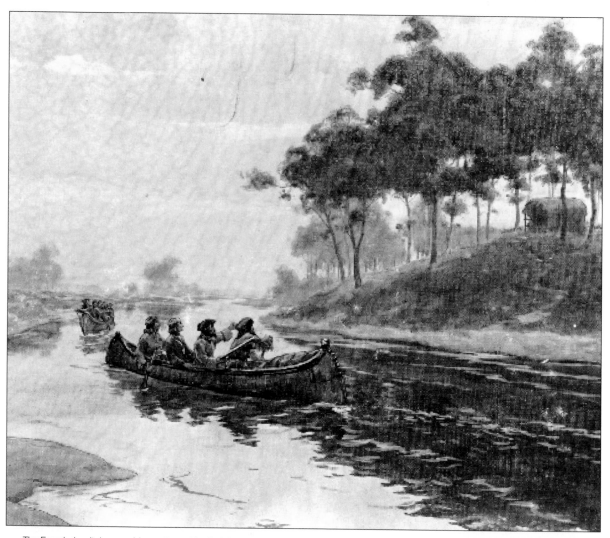

The French Jesuit Jacques Marquette and Louis Joliet on their historic exploratory voyage down the Mississippi River in 1673. Father Jacques Marquette, S.J. (1637-1675) and Louis Joliet, a French Canadian explorer, were the first Europeans to see and map the Mississippi River. They departed from Mackinac, Michigan with two canoes and five other explorers of French-Indian ancestry. They followed Lake Michigan to the Bay of Green Bay and up the Fox River. From there, they portaged to the Wisconsin River entering the Mississippi River near Prairie du Chien, Wisconsin. The Joliet-Marquette expedition traveled to within 435 miles of the Gulf of Mexico, but turned back at the mouth of the Arkansas River fearing contact with the Spanish. They returned to Lake Michigan by way of the Illinois River. After a visit to the mission of St. Francis Xavier in Green Bay, Fr. Marquette returned to the Illinois River in 1674 to found a mission on the shore of Lake Michigan. The mission would later grow into the city of Chicago.

PRACTICAL EXERCISES

1. Why did St. John XXIII call the Second Vatican Council? How did this council differ from others in the Church's history?

2. The 1960s and 1970s were a time of worldwide social change. Drawing from your knowledge of Church history, describe how those changes may have affected the Church had the Second Vatican Council not occurred.

3. How did St. John Paul II change the way the world saw the papacy? Choose a Pope from the Church's history that you believe was similar to St. John Paul II. In what ways were their papacies similar? How did they differ in their understanding of the papacy? What do their similarities and differences say about the role of the Church in the world?

4. At the founding of the United States of America, the drafters of the Constitution secured toleration for all religions in the United States. In Europe, on the other hand, the revolutions of the eighteenth and nineteenth centuries brought about fierce anti-Catholic persecution. What factors in Europe made the same toleration difficult to attain? What was different about the situation in America that allowed for Catholic toleration?

5. Throughout the history of the Church, from Constantine and Charlemagne to Louis XIV and Vittorio Emmanuelle, various nations have tried to assert their own national identities onto the Church in their countries. Using the history of the Church in the United States as a reference, explain why "Gallicanism" has been so prevalent in the Church throughout the ages.

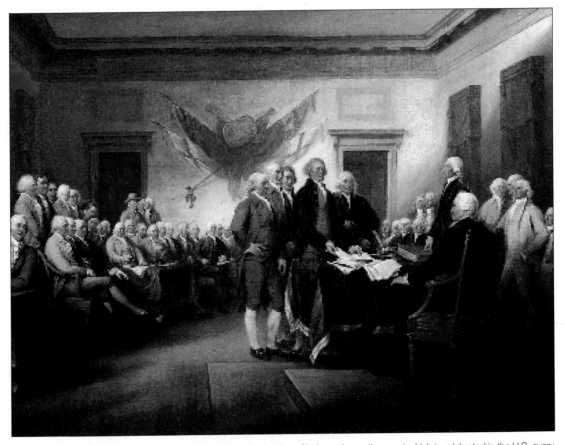

John Trumbull's famous painting depicts the signing of the *Declaration of Independence,* the event which is celebrated in the U.S. every July 4th. The independence of the American colonies was recognized by Great Britain on September 3, 1783, by the Treaty of Paris.

FROM THE CATECHISM

834 Particular Churches are fully catholic through their communion with one of them, the Church of Rome "which presides in charity" (St. Ignatius of Antioch, Ad Rom. 1, 1: Apostolic Fathers, II/2, 192; cf. LG 13). "For with this church, by reason of its pre-eminence, the whole Church, that is the faithful everywhere, must necessarily be in accord" (St. Irenaeus, Adv. haeres. 3, 3, 2: PG 7/1, 849; cf. Vatican Council I: DS 3057). Indeed, "from the incarnate Word's descent to us, all Christian churches everywhere have held and hold the great Church that is here [at Rome] to be their only basis and foundation since, according to the Savior's promise, the gates of hell have never prevailed against her" (St. Maximus the Confessor, Opuscula theo.: PG 91: 137-140).

882 The Pope, Bishop of Rome and Peter's successor, "is the perpetual and visible source and foundation of the unity both of the bishops and of the whole company of the faithful" (LG 23). "For the Roman Pontiff, by reason of his office as Vicar of Christ, and as pastor of the entire Church has full, supreme, and universal power over the whole Church, a power which he can always exercise unhindered" (LG 22; cf. CD 2, 9).

1905 In keeping with the social nature of man, the good of each individual is necessarily related to the common good, which in turn can be defined only in reference to the human person:

> Do not live entirely isolated, having retreated into yourselves, as if you were already justified, but gather instead to seek the common good together (Ep. Barnabae, 4, 10: PG 2, 734).

1913 "Participation" is the voluntary and generous engagement of a person in social interchange. It is necessary that all participate, each according to his position and role, in promoting the common good. This obligation is inherent in the dignity of the human person.

2104 "All men are bound to seek the truth, especially in what concerns God and his Church, and to embrace it and hold on to it as they come to know it" (DH 1 § 2). This duty derives from "the very dignity of the human person" (DH 2 § 1). It does not contradict a "sincere respect" for different religions which frequently "reflect a ray of that truth which enlightens all men," (NA 2 § 2) nor the requirement of charity, which urges Christians "to treat with love, prudence and patience those who are in error or ignorance with regard to the faith" (DH 14 § 4).

2127 Agnosticism assumes a number of forms. In certain cases the agnostic refrains from denying God; instead he postulates the existence of a transcendent being which is incapable of revealing itself, and about which nothing can be said. In other cases, the agnostic makes no judgment about God's existence, declaring it impossible to prove, or even to affirm or deny.

2128 Agnosticism can sometimes include a certain search for God, but it can equally express indifferentism, a flight from the ultimate question of existence, and a sluggish moral conscience. Agnosticism is all too often equivalent to practical atheism.

2188 In respecting religious liberty and the common good of all, Christians should seek recognition of Sundays and the Church's holy days as legal holidays. They have to give everyone a public example of prayer, respect, and joy and defend their traditions as a precious contribution to the spiritual life of society. If a country's legislation or other reasons require work on Sunday, the day should nevertheless be lived as the day of our deliverance which lets us share in this "festal gathering," this "assembly of the firstborn who are enrolled in heaven" (Heb 12: 22-23).

FROM THE CATECHISM Continued

2241 The more prosperous nations are obliged, to the extent they are able, to welcome the foreigner in search of the security and the means of livelihood which he cannot find in his country of origin. Public authorities should see to it that the natural right is respected that places a guest under the protection of those who receive him.

Political authorities, for the sake of the common good for which they are responsible, may make the exercise of the right to immigrate subject to various juridical conditions, especially with regard to the immigrants' duties toward their country of adoption. Immigrants are obliged to respect with gratitude the material and spiritual heritage of the country that receives them, to obey its laws, and to assist in carrying civic burdens.

2244 Every institution is inspired, at least implicitly, by a vision of man and his destiny, from which it derives the point of reference for its judgment, its hierarchy of values, its line of conduct. Most societies have formed their institutions in the recognition of a certain preeminence of man over things. Only the divinely revealed religion has clearly recognized man's origin and destiny in God, the Creator and Redeemer. The Church invites political authorities to measure their judgments and decisions against this inspired truth about God and man:

> Societies not recognizing this vision or rejecting it in the name of their independence from God are brought to seek their criteria and goal in themselves or to borrow them from some ideology. Since they do not admit that one can defend an objective criterion of good and evil, they arrogate to themselves an explicit or implicit totalitarian power over man and his destiny, as history shows (cf. CA 45; 46).

2246 It is a part of the Church's mission "to pass moral judgments even in matters related to politics, whenever the fundamental rights of man or the salvation of souls requires it. The means, the only means, she may use are those which are in accord with the Gospel and the welfare of all men according to the diversity of times and circumstances" (GS 76 § 5).

2304 Respect for and development of human life require peace. Peace is not merely the absence of war, and it is not limited to maintaining a balance of powers between adversaries. Peace cannot be attained on earth without safeguarding the goods of persons, free communication among men, respect for the dignity of persons and peoples, and the assiduous practice of fraternity. Peace is "the tranquillity of order" (St. Augustine, De civ. Dei, 19, 13, 1: PL 41, 640). Peace is the work of justice and the effect of charity (cf. Is 32:17; cf. GS 78 §§ 1-2).

2364 The married couple forms "the intimate partnership of life and love established by the Creator and governed by his laws; it is rooted in the conjugal covenant, that is, in their irrevocable personal consent" (GS 48 § 1). Both give themselves definitively and totally to one another. They are no longer two; from now on they form one flesh. The covenant they freely contracted imposes on the spouses the obligation to preserve it as unique and indissoluble (cf. CIC, can. 1056). "What therefore God has joined together, let not man put asunder" (Mk 10: 9; cf. Mt 19: 1-12; 1 Cor 7: 10-11).

2373 Sacred Scripture and the Church's traditional practice see in large families a sign of God's blessing and the parents' generosity (cf. GS 50 § 2).

2378 A child is not something owed to one, but is a gift. The "supreme gift of marriage" is a human person. A child may not be considered a piece of property, an idea to which an alleged "right to a child" would lead. In this area, only the child possesses genuine rights: the right "to be the fruit of the specific act of the conjugal love of his parents," and "the right to be respected as a person from the moment of his conception" (CDF, Donum vitæ II, 8).

DOCTORS OF THE CHURCH

Proclaimed by Pope Boniface VIII, September 20, 1295
1. St. Ambrose
2. St. Jerome
3. St. Augustine of Hippo
4. St. Gregory the Great

Proclaimed by St. Pius V, April 11, 1567
5. St. Thomas Aquinas

Proclaimed by St. Pius V, 1568
6. St. Athanasius
7. St. Basil the Great
8. St. Gregory of Nazianzus
9. St. John Chrysostom

Proclaimed by Pope Sixtus V, March 14, 1588
10. St. Bonaventure

Proclaimed by Pope Clement XI, February 3, 1720
11. St. Anselm of Canterbury

Proclaimed by Pope Innocent XIII, April 25, 1722
12. St. Isidore of Seville

Proclaimed by Pope Benedict XIII, February 10, 1729
13. St. Peter Chrysologus

Proclaimed by Pope Benedict XIV, October 15, 1754
14. St. Leo the Great

Proclaimed by Pope Leo XII, September 27, 1828
15. St. Peter Damian

Proclaimed by Bl. Pius VIII, August 20, 1830
16. St. Bernard of Clairvaux

Proclaimed by Bl. Pius IX, May 13, 1851
17. St. Hilary of Poitiers

Proclaimed by Bl. Pius IX, July 7, 1871
18. St. Alphonsus Liguori

Proclaimed by Bl. Pius IX, November 16, 1871
19. St. Francis de Sales

Proclaimed by Pope Leo XIII, July 28, 1882
20. St. Cyril of Alexandria
21. St. Cyril of Jerusalem

Proclaimed by Pope Leo XIII, August 19, 1890
22. St. John of Damascus

Proclaimed by Pope Leo XIII, November 13, 1899
23. St. Bede the Venerable

Proclaimed by Pope Benedict XV, October 5, 1920
24. St. Ephraem of Syria

Proclaimed by Pope Pius XI, May 21, 1925
25. St. Peter Canisius

Proclaimed by Pope Pius XI, August 24, 1926
26. St. John of the Cross

Proclaimed by Pope Pius XI, September 17, 1931
27. St. Robert Bellarmine

Proclaimed by Pope Pius XI, December 16, 1931
28. St. Albert the Great

Proclaimed by Pope Pius XII, January 16, 1946
29. St. Anthony of Padua

Proclaimed by St. John XXIII, March 19, 1959
30. St. Lawrence of Brindisi

Proclaimed by Pope Paul VI, September 27, 1970
31. St. Teresa of Avila

Proclaimed by Pope Paul VI, October 4, 1970
32. St. Catherine of Siena

Proclaimed by St. John Paul II, October 19, 1997
33. St. Therese of Lisieux

Proclaimed by Pope Benedict XVI, October 7 2012
34. St. John of Avila
35. St. Hildegard of Bingen

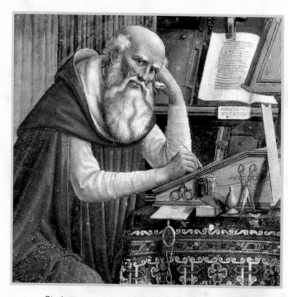

St. Jerome was proclaimed a Doctor of the Church
by Pope Boniface VIII on September 20, 1295.

THE POPES

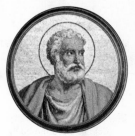

1. St. Peter

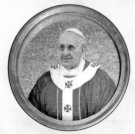

266. Francis

FIRST CENTURY
St. Peter (AD 33-67)
St. Linus (67-76)
St. Anacletus (76-88)
St. Clement I (88-97)
St. Evaristus (97-105)

SECOND CENTURY
St. Alexander I (105-115)
St. Sixtus I (115-125)
St. Telesphorus (125-136)
St. Hyginus (136-140)
St. Pius I (140-155)
St. Anicetus (155-166)
St. Soter (166-175)
St. Eleutherius (175-189)
St. Victor I (189-199)
St. Zephyrinus (199-217)

THIRD CENTURY
St. Callistus I (217-222)
St. Hippolytus (217-235)
St. Urban I (222-230)
St. Pontian (230-235)
St. Anterus (235-236)
St. Fabian (236-250)
St. Cornelius (251-253)
Novatianus (251)
St. Lucius I (253-254)
St. Stephen I (254-257)
St. Sixtus II (257-258)
St. Dionysius (259-268)
St. Felix I (269-274)
St. Eutychian (275-283)
St. Caius (283-296)
St. Marcellinus (296-304)

FOURTH CENTURY
St. Marcellus I (308-309)
St. Eusebius (309-310)
St. Miltiades (311-314)
St. Sylvester I (314-335)
St. Marcus (336)
St. Julius I (337-352)
Liberius (352-366)
Felix II (353-365)
St. Damasus I (366-384)
Ursinus (366-367)
St. Siricius (384-399)
St. Anastasius I (399-401)

FIFTH CENTURY
St. Innocent I (401-417)
St. Zozimus (417-418)
St. Boniface I (418-422)
Eulalius (418-419)

St. Celestine I (422-432)
St. Sixtus III (432-440)
St. Leo I (440-461)
St. Hilary (461-468)
St. Simplicius (468-483)
St. Felix III (II) (483-492)
St. Gelasius I (492-496)
Anastasius II (496-498)
St. Symmachus (498-514)
Laurentius (498-505)

SIXTH CENTURY
St. Hormisdas (514-523)
St. John I (523-526)
St. Felix IV (III) (526-530)
Boniface II (530-532)
Dioscurus (530)
John II (533-535)
St. Agapitus I (535-536)
St. Silverius (536-537)
Vigilius (537-555)
Pelagius I (556-561)
John III (561-574)
Benedict I (575-579)
Pelagius II (579-590)
St. Gregory I (590-604)

SEVENTH CENTURY
Sabinian (604-606)
Boniface III (607)
St. Boniface IV (608-615)
St. Deusdedit (615-618)
  or Adoedatus I
Boniface V (619-625)
Honorius I (625-638)
Severinus (640)
John IV (640-642)
Theodore I (642-649)
St. Martin I (649-655)
St. Eugene I (654-657)
St. Vitalian (657-672)
Adeodatus II (672-676)
Donus (676-678)
St. Agatho (678-681)
St. Leo II (682-683)
St. Benedict II (684-685)
John V (685-686)
Conon (686-687)
Theodore II (687)
Paschal I (687-692)
St. Sergius I (687-701)

EIGHTH CENTURY
John VI (701-705)
John VII (705-707)

Sisinnius (708)
Constantine (708-715)
St. Gregory II (715-731)
St. Gregory III (731-471)
St. Zachary (741-752)
Stephen II (752)
St. Paul I (757-767)
Constantine (767)
Philip (767)
Stephen III (768-772)
Adrian I (772-795)
St. Leo III (795-816)

NINTH CENTURY
Stephen IV (816-817)
St. Paschal I (817-824)
Eugene II (824-827)
Valentine (827)
Gregory IV (827-844)
John VIII (844)
Sergius II (844-847)
St. Leo IV (847-855)
Benedict III (855-858)
Anastasius III (855)
St. Nicholas I (858-867)
Adrian II (867-872)
John VIII (872-882)
Marinus I (882-884)
St. Adrian III (884-885)
Stephen V (VI) (885-891)
Formosus (891-896)
Boniface VI (896)
Stephen VI (VII) (896-897)
Romanus (897)
Theodore II (897)
John IX (898-900)

TENTH CENTURY
Benedict IV (900-903)
Leo V (903)
Christopher (903-904)
Sergius III (904-911)
Anastasius III (911-913)
Landus (913-914)
John X (914-928)
Leo VI (928)
Stephen VII (928-931)
John XI (931-935)
Leo VII (936-939)
Stephen VIII (IX) (939-942)
Marinus II (942-946)
Agapetus II (946-955)
John XII (955-964)
Leo VIII (963-965)

Benedict V (964-966)
John XIII (965-972)
Benedict VI (973-974)
Benedict VII (974-983)
John XIV (983-984)
Boniface VII (984-985)
John XV (985-996)
Gregory V (996-999)
Sylvester II (999-1003)

ELEVENTH CENTURY
John XVII (1003)
John XVIII (1004-1009)
Sergius IV (1009-1012)
Benedict VIII (1012-1024)
Gregory VI (1012)
John XIX (1024-1032)
Benedict IX (1032-1044)
Sylvester III (1045)
Gregory VI (1045-1046)
  (John Gratian Pierleoni)
Clement II (1046-1047)
  (Suitgar, Count of
  Morsleben)
Damasus II (1048)
  (Count Poppo)
St. Leo IX (1049-1054)
  (Bruno, Count of Toul)
Victor II (1055-1057)
  (Gebhard, Count of
  Hirschberg)
Stephen IX (X) (1057-1058)
  (Frederick of Lorraine)
Nicholas II (1059-1061)
  (Gerhard of Burgundy)
Alexander II (1061-1073)
  (Anselmo da Baggio)
Honorius II (1061-1064)
St. Gregory VII (1073-1085)
  (Hildebrand of Soana)
Clement III (1080-1100)
Bl. Victor III (1086-1087)
  (Desiderius, Prince of
  Beneventum)
Bl. Urban II (1088-1099)
  (Odo of Chatillon)
Paschal II (1099-1118)
  (Ranieri da Bieda)
Theodoric (1100-1102)
Albert (1102)
Sylvester IV (1105)

TWELFTH CENTURY
Gelasius II (1118-1119)
  (John Coniolo)
Gregory VIII (1118-1121)

Italicized = Antipopes

THE POPES

Callistus II (1119-1124)
(Guido, Count of Burgundy)
Honorius II (1124-1130)
(Lamberto dei Fagnani)
Celestine II (1124)
Innocent II (1130-1143)
(Gregorio Papareschi)
Anacletus II (1130-1138)
(Cardinal Pierleone)
Victor IV (1138)
Celestine II (1143-1144)
(Guido di Castello)
Lucius II (1144-1145)
(Gherardo Caccianemici)
Bl. Eugene III (1145-1153)
(Bernardo Paganelli)
Anastasius IV (1153-1154)
(Corrado della Subarra)
Adrian IV (1154-1159)
(Nicholas Breakspear)
Alexander III (1159-1181)
(Orlando Bandinelli)
Victor IV (1159-1164)
Paschal III (1164-1168)
Calixtus III (1168-7118)
Innocent III (1179-1180)
(Lando da Sessa)
Lucius III (1181-1185)
(Ubaldo Allucingoli)
Urban III (1185-1187)
(Uberto Crivelli)
Gregory VIII (1187)
(Alberto del Morra)
Clement III (1187-1191)
(Paolo Scolari)
Celestine III (1191-1198)
(Giacinto Boboni-Orsini)
Innocent III (1198-1216)
(Lotario de Conti di Segni)

THIRTEENTH CENTURY
Honorius III (1216-1227)
(Cencio Savelli)
Gregory IX (1227-1241)
(Ugolino di Segni)
Celestine IV (1241)
(Goffredo Castiglione)
Innocent IV (1243-1254)
(Sinibaldo de Fieschi)
Alexander IV (1254-1261)
(Rinaldo di Segni)
Urban IV (1261-1264)
(Jacques Pantaléon)
Clement IV (1265-1268)
(Guy le Gros Foulques)
Bl. Gregory X (1271-1276)
(Tebaldo Visconti)
Bl. Innocent V (1276)
(Pierre de Champagni)
Adrian V (1276)
(Ottobono Fieschi)
John XXI (1276-1277)
(Pietro Rebuli-Giuliani)
Nicholas III (1277-1280)
(Giovanni Gaetano Orsini)

Martin IV (1281-1285)
(Simon Mompitie)
Honorius IV (1285-1287)
(Giacomo Savelli)
Nicholas IV (1288-1292)
(Girolamo Masci)
St. Celestine V (1294)
(Pietro Angelari da Murrone)
Boniface VIII (1294-1303)
(Benedetto Gaetani)

FOURTEENTH CENTURY
Bl. Benedict XI (1303-1304)
(Nicolò Boccasini)
Clement V (1305-1314)
(Raimond Bertrand de Got)
John XXII (1316-1334)
(Jacques Dueze)
Nicholas V (1328-1330)
(Pietro di Corbara)
Benedict XII (1334-1342)
(Jacques Fournier)
Clement VI (1342-1352)
(Pierre Roger de Beaufort)
Innocent VI (1352-1362)
(Étienne Aubert)
Bl. Urban V (1362-1370)
(Guillaume de Grimord)
Gregory XI (1370-1378)
(Pierre Roger de Beaufort, the Younger)
Urban VI (1378-1389)
(Bartolomeo Prignano)
Clement VII (1378-1394)
(Robert of Geneva)
Boniface IX (1389-1404)
(Pietro Tomacelli)
Benedict XIII (1394-1423)
(Pedro de Luna)

FIFTEENTH CENTURY
Innocent VII (1404-1406)
(Cosmato de Migliorati)
Gregory XII (1406-1415)
(Angelo Correr)
Alexander V (1409-1410)
(Petros Philargi)
John XXIII (1410-1415)
(Baldassare Cossa)
Martin V (1417-1431)
(Ottone Colonna)
Clement VIII (1423-1429)
Benedict XIV (1424)
Eugene IV (1431-1447)
(Gabriele Condulmer)
Felix V (1439-1449)
(Amadeus of Savoy)
Nicholas V (1447-1455)
(Tommaso Parentucelli)
Callistus III (1455-1458)
(Alonso Borgia)
Pius II (1458-1464)
(Aeneas Silvio de Piccolomini)
Paul II (1464-1471)
(Pietro Barbo)

Sixtus IV (1471-1484)
(Francesco della Rovere)
Innocent VIII (1484-1492)
(Giovanni Battista Cibo)
Alexander VI (1492-1503)
(Rodrigo Lanzol y Borgia)

SIXTEENTH CENTURY
Pius III (1503)
(Francesco Todoeschini-Piccolomini)
Julius II (1503-1513)
(Giuliano della Rovere)
Leo X (1513-1521)
(Giovanni de Medici)
Adrian VI (1522-1523)
(Adrian Florensz)
Clement VII (1523-1534)
(Giulio de Medici)
Paul III (1534-1549)
(Alessandro Farnese)
Julius III (1550-1555)
(Giovanni Maria Ciocchi del Monte)
Marcellus II (1555)
(Marcello Cervini)
Paul IV (1555-1559)
(Gian Pietro Caraffa)
Pius IV (1559-1565)
(Giovanni Angelo de Medici)
St. Pius V (1566-1572)
(Antonio Michele Ghislieri)
Gregory XIII (1572-1585)
(Ugo Buoncompagni)
Sixtus V (1585-1590)
(Felice Peretti)
Urban VII (1590)
(Giambattista Castagna)
Gregory XIV (1590-1591)
(Nicolò Sfondrati)
Innocent IX (1591)
(Gian Antonio Facchinetti)
Clement VIII (1592-1605)
(Ippolito Aldobrandini)

SEVENTEENTH CENTURY
Leo XI (1605)
(Alessandro de Medici-Ottaiano)
Paul V (1605-1621)
(Camillo Borghese)
Gregory XV (1621-1623)
(Alessandro Ludovisi)
Urban VIII (1623-1644)
(Maffeo Barberini)
Innocent X (1644-1655)
(Giambattista Pamfili)
Alexander VII (1655-1667)
(Fabio Chigi)
Clement IX (1667-1669)
(Giulio Rospigliosi)
Clement X (1670-1676)
(Emilio Altieri)
Bl. Innocent XI (1676-1689)
(Benedetto Odescalchi)

Alexander VIII (1689-1691)
(Pietro Ottoboni)
Innocent XII (1691-1700)
(Antonio Pignatelli)

EIGHTEENTH CENTURY
Clement XI (1700-1721)
(Gian Francesco Albani)
Innocent XIII (1721-1724)
(Michelangelo dei Conti)
Benedict XIII (1724-1730)
(Pietro Francesco Orsini)
Clement XII (1730-1740)
(Lorenzo Corsini)
Benedict XIV (1740-1758)
(Prospero Lambertini)
Clement XIII (1758-1769)
(Carlo Rezzonico)
Clement XIV (1769-1774)
(Lorenzo Ganganelli)
Pius VI (1775-1799)
(Gianangelo Braschi)

NINETEENTH CENTURY
Pius VII (1800-1823)
(Barnaba Chiaramonti)
Leo XII (1823-1829)
(Annibale della Genga)
Pius VIII (1829-1830)
(Francesco Saverio Gastiglioni)
Gregory XVI (1831-1846)
(Bartolomeo Alberto Cappellari)
Bl. Pius IX (1846-1878)
(Giovanni Mastai-Ferretti)
Leo XIII (1878-1903)
(Gioacchino Pecci)

TWENTIETH CENTURY
St. Pius X (1903-1914)
(Giuseppe Sarto)
Benedict XV (1914-1922)
(Giacomo della Chiesa)
Pius XI (1922-1939)
(Achille Ratti)
Ven. Pius XII (1939-1958)
(Eugenio Pacelli)
St. John XXIII (1958-1963)
(Angelo Roncalli)
St. Paul VI (1963-1978)
(Giovanni Battista Montini)
John Paul I (1978)
(Albino Luciani)
St. John Paul II (1978-2005)
(Karol Jozef Wojtyla)

TWENTY-FIRST CENTURY
Benedict XVI (2005-2013)
(Joseph Alois Ratzinger)
Francis (2013-   )
(Jorge Mario Bergoglio)

ART AND PHOTO CREDITS

Cover

Montage–*St. Peter's Basilica*, Rome; Pictorial Library of Bible Lands; Todd Bolen, photographer and St. Peter, Pierre Etienne Monnot, San Giovanni in Laterano, Rome

Introduction

Chapter 1

Chapter 2

ART AND PHOTO CREDITS

66 *Crucifixion*, Andrea del Castagno; National Gallery, London, England
67 *First Vatican Council*; Renaissance Museum, Rome, Italy; Archivo Oronoz
69 *St. Ambrose*, Luca de Robbia, Florence, Italy; Archivo Oronoz
71 *St. Jerome*, Student of Marinus van Reymerswaele; Prado Museum, Madrid, Spain; Archivo Oronoz
72 *St. John Chrysostom*; Vatican Museum, Vatican; Archivo Oronoz
73 *St. Cyril of Alexandria*, Osorio Meneses; Museum of Fine Arts, Seville, Spain; Archivo Oronoz
74 *St. Athanasius*, Master of St. Ildefon; Museum of Culture, Valladolid, Spain; Archivo Oronoz
75 Coin: *Emperor Constantius II*, Nicomedia mint, struck ca. AD 335-361; CoinArchives.com
77 *St. Basil* (detail), Alonso Sanchez Coello; Royal Monastery of St. Lawrence of Escorial, Madrid, Spain; Archivo Oronoz
79 *Emperor Theodosius Exiling Nestorius*, fresco; 16th Century Church, Cyprus
80 *St. Leo I*, mosaic; Patriarchal Basilica of Saint Paul Outside the Walls, Rome, Italy
83 *Ordination of St. Augustine*, Jaime Huguet; Catalonia Museum of Art, Barcelona, Spain; Archivo Oronoz
84 *Constantine*; Capitoline Museum, Rome, Italy; Pictorial Library of Bible Lands; Todd Bolen, photographer
85 *Roman Coin with Christogram*; AG Archives
86 *Emperor Theodosius I*, (detail) silver plate, fourth century; Royal Academy of History, Madrid, Spain
89 *St. Athanasius* (detail), Alonzo Sanchez Coello; Royal Monastery of St. Lawrence of Escorial, Madrid, Spain; Archivo Oronoz
90 *The Winged Victory of Samothrace*; Louvre, Paris, France
91 *St. Jerome*, Pedro Berruguete; Convent of St. Thomas, Avila, Spain; Archivo Oronoz
92 *The Triumph of St. Augustine*, Claudio Coello; Prado Museum, Madrid, Spain; Archivo Oronoz

Chapter 3

93 *St. Paul the Hermit and St. Anthony*, David Teniers the Younger; Prado Museum, Madrid, Spain; Archivo Oronoz
96 *The Baptism of Clovis*, Master of Saint Gilles; National Gallery of Art, Washington D.C.
97 *German Barbarian Chief*, Vermorcken; Private Collection, Paris, France; Archivo Oronoz
98 *The Meeting Between Leo the Great and Attila*, Raphael; Stanza di Eliodoro, Palazzi Pontifici, Vatican
99 *Attila and His Hordes Overrun Italy*, Delacroix; Bibliothèque, Palais Bourbon, Paris, France
100 Illustrated Manuscript, *Missal*; Archivo Oronoz
103 *St. Gregory the Great*, Francisco de Goya; Romantic Museum, Madrid, Spain; Archivo Oronoz
104 (left) *Dome of the Rock*, Jerusalem; Pictorial Library of Bible Lands; Todd Bolen, photographer
104 (right) *Three Worshipers Praying in a Corner of a Mosque*, Jean-Léon Gérôme; Private Collection
107 (top) *Clovis*, Private Collection, Paris, France; Archivo Oronoz
107 (bottom) *St. James Inspired with the Holy Spirit*, Pedro Bocanegra; Abadía del Sacromonte, Granada, Spain; Archivo Oronoz
108 *Council of Toledo*, Jose Marti Monso; Madrid Senate Museum, Madrid, Spain; Archivo Oronoz
109 *St. Patrick*, Holy Card (detail); AG Archives
110 *St. Columba*, Icon; AG Archives
111 *St. Augustine of Canterbury*, Icon; AG Archives
113 (left) *St. Bede*, Bartolome Roman; Prado Museum, Madrid, Spain; Archivo Oronoz
113 (right) *Ecclesiastical History of the English People* (front cover AD 731), St. Bede; Robert Cotton Library, British Museum, London, England
114 *Pagan god Thor*; AG Archives
115 *Sts. Cyril and Methodius*, Icon; AG Archives
116 *Glagolithic Alphabet*; AG Archives
117 *Otto III Enthroned*, from the Gospel Book of Otto III, folio 23v-24r; Bavarian State Library, Munich
120 *Fatih Sultan Mehmed Bridge* over the Bosporous Strait seen from over Rumelihisari; AG Archives
122 *Hagia Sophia*, Istanbul, Turkey; Pictorial Library of Bible Lands; Todd Bolen, photographer
124 *St. John of Damascus*, Greek Icon; from Skete of St. Anne, Hellenistic Ministry of Culture
125 *The Triumph of Orthodoxy*, Icon; British Museum, London, England
127 (top) *Charlemagne's Throne*; Palace Chapel, Aachen Cathedral, Aachen, Germany
127 (bottom) *Emperor Charlemagne*, Albrecht Dürer; German Natonal Museum, Nuremburg, Germany
128 (top) *Coronation of Charlemagne*; from the *Annals of Lorsch* (794-803), Richbod, Bishop of Tríves, National Library, Vienna, Austria
128 (bottom) *Charlemagne Receives Alcuin*, Victor Schnetz; Louvre, Paris, France
129 *Charlemagne's Crown*; Kunsthistorisches Museum, Vienna, Austria
130 *Hagia Sophia*, artist's concept of Justinian's Church; AG Archives
131 *Eastern Orthodox Liturgy* (3 images); AG Archives
133 *Hagia Sophia interior*, Istanbul, Turkey
134 *Pope Stephen X (IX)*, mosaic; Patriarchal Basilica of Saint Paul Outside the Walls, Rome, Italy
135 *Pope John Paul II* (2 images-2001); *Pope Paul VI and Patriarch Athenagoras* (1964); AG Archives
136 *Hagia Sophia* mosaic, Istanbul, Turkey
140 *Scene from the Life of St. Jerome*, Juan Espinal; Museum of Fine Arts, Seville, Spain; Archivo Oronoz, Istanbul, Turkey
142 *Battle of Nineveh*, Piero de Francesca; Church of San Francisco, Arezzo, Italy; Archivo Oronoz

Chapter 4

143 *Virgin of the Caves*, Francisco Zurbaran; Museum of Fine Arts, Seville, Spain; Archivo Oronoz
147 *Viking Navy*, Rafael Monleon; Naval Museum of Madrid, Spain; Archivo Oronoz
148 *St. Bruno and Pope Urban II*, Francisco Zurbaran; Museum of Fine Arts, Seville, Spain; Archivo Oronoz
149 (left) *Abbey of Cluny*; Cluny Museum, France
149 (right) *Bell Tower*, Cluny Abbey, France; Archivo Oronoz
151 *Otto I the Great*; Madrid National Library, Madrid, Spain; Archivo Oronoz
152 *William I the Conqueror*; Private Collection, Paris, France; Archivo Oronoz
154 *Pope Gregory VII*; Salerno Cathedral, Salerno, Italy; Archivo Oronoz
155 *Henry IV and Pope Gregory VII*, Pietro Aldi; Pitigliano Cathedral, Pitigliano, Italy; Archivo Oronoz
157 *Frederick I Enters Milan*, Villani; Vatican Library, Vatican; Archivo Oronoz

ART AND PHOTO CREDITS

ART AND PHOTO CREDITS

Chapter 6

ART AND PHOTO CREDITS

Chapter 7

309 *Science and Art,* Adriaen Van Stalbent; Prado Museum, Madrid, Spain; Archivo Oronoz
311 *Louis XIV,* Hyacinthe Rigaud; Louvre, Paris, France; Archivo Oronoz
312 *The Crossing of the Rhine by the Army of Louis XIV, 1672,* Joseph Parrocel; Louvre, Paris, France
313 (left) *Cornelius Jansen;* wikipedia.com, public domain
313 (right) *Ex Voto, Philippe de Champaigne;* Louvre, Paris, France
314 *Bust of Louis XIV,* Gian Lorenzo Bernini; Musée National de Versailles, Versailles, France
315 *Charles I, King of England,* Sir Anthony Van Dyck; National Gallery, London, England; Archivo Oronoz
316 *Oliver Cromwell,* Robert Walker; National Portrait Gallery, London, England; Archivo Oronoz
317 *King William III,* after Sir Peter Lely; National Portrait Gallery, London, England
318 *René Descartes,* Jan Baptist Weenix; Museo Central, Utrecht, Holland; Archivo Oronoz
319 *Heliocentric System of the Universe,* Nicolas Copernicus; Private Collection; Archivo Oronoz
320 (left) Diagram from *On The Revolutions of the Heavenly Bodies,* Nicolas Copernicus; High Altitude Observatory website
320 (right) Engraving from *Tycho's Astronomiae instaurata mechanica,* published in Wansbeck in 1598; High Altitude Observatory website
321 *The Trial of Galileo,* Cristiano Banti; High Altitude Observatory website
322 *Initiation of Mozart into the Lodge of Freemasons,* Freimaurer; Kunsthistorisches Museum, Vienna, Austria; Archivo Oronoz
323 (left) *Bust of Voltaire,* Marie-Anne Collot; Hermitage, St Petersburg, Russia
323 (right) *Elmens de la philosophie de Neuton,* Voltaire; A Amsterdam: Chez Etienne Ledet & Compagnie, 1738
324 *Jean-Jacques Rousseau,* Quintin Latour; Museum of Art, Geneva, Switzerland; Archivo Oronoz
325 *Empress Maria Theresa;* AG Archives
326 *King Charles III,* Anton Raphael Mengs; Prado Museum, Madrid, Spain
329 *Louis XVI,* Antonio Franc Callet; Prado Museum, Madrid, Spain; Archivo Oronoz
330 *Emmanuel Joseph Sieyès,* Jacques-Louis David; Fogg Art Museum, Harvard University, Cambridge, Massachusetts
331 *The Tennis Court Oath,* Jacques-Louis David; Musèe National du Chateau, Versailles, France
332 (top) *Prise de la Bastille* (Storming the Bastille), Jean-Pierre Louis Laurent Houel; National Library, Paris, France
332 (bottom) *The Declaration of the Rights of Man and Citizen;* Musèe Carnavalet, Paris, France; Archivo Oronoz
333 *Assault on Versailles,* Fery de Guyon; National Library, Paris France; Archivo Oronoz
335 (top) *Jean-Paul Marat;* Musèe Carnavalet, Paris, France; Archivo Oronoz
335 (bottom) *Decree Abolishing the Monarchy;* Private Collection, Paris, France; Archivo Oronoz
337 (top) *Feast of the Supreme Being,* De Machy; Musèe Carnavalet, Paris, France
337 (bottom) *Maximilien Robespierre;* Private Collection, Paris, France; Archivo Oronoz
338 *Procession of the Goddess of Reason;* National Library, Paris, France
339 *Pope Pius VII,* Jacques-Louis David; Louvre, Paris, France
340 *Napoleon Crossing the Great St. Bernard Pass,* Jacques-Louis David; Kunsthistorisches Museum, Vienna, Austria
341 *Charles Maurice de Talleyrand,* Francois Gerard; Palace Museum, Versailles, France; Archivo Oronoz
343 *The Meeting of Pope Paul VII and Napoleon;* Fontainebleau Palace Museum, Fontainebleau, France; Archivo Oronoz
345 *Napoleon I on His Imperial Throne,* Jean Auguste Dominque Ingres; Musèe de L'Armee, Paris, France
346 *Napoleon Crowning Himself Emperor Before the Pope,* Jacques-Louis David; Louvre, Paris, France; Archivo Oronoz
349 *Denis Diderot,* Louis-Michel van Loo; Louvre, Paris, France; Archivo Oronoz

Chapter 8

351 *The Strike,* Robert Koehler; Archivo Oronoz
354 (top) *Klemens Lothar Wenzel von Metternich* (Clement von Metternich), Thomas Lawrence; The Hermitage, St. Petersburg, Russia
354 (bottom) *James Monroe,* Gilbert Stuart; Metropolitan Museum of Art, New York
355 *Equestrian Portrait of Alexander I,* Franz Kruger; The Hermitage, St. Petersburg, Russia
356 *Francois-Rene de Chateaubriand,* Anne-Louis Girodet de Roussy-Trioson; Musée d'Histoire et du Pays Malouin, Saint-Malo, France
358 *Textile Factory-19th century;* Archivo Oronoz
359 *Child Laborer,* Newberry, South Carolina, 1908; wikipedia.com
360 *Revolution in the Streets of Paris-1848;* National Library, Paris, France; Archivo Oronoz
361 *Emperor Napoleon III,* Franz Xavier Winterhalter; Napoleon Museum, Rome, Italy
362 *Pope Pius IX,* Antonio Soubelt; Palace Real, Madrid, Spain; Archivo Oronoz
363 *John Henry Newman; The Oxford Illustrated History of Christianity,* John McManners, Editor, 1990
364 (bottom right) *The Immaculate Conception,* Bartolome Murillo; Prado Museum, Madrid, Spain; Archivo Oronoz
364 (inset) *St. Bernadette,* 19 years old, studio photograph at Tarbes, 1863; catholicpilgrims.com
365 *St. Bernadette at the Grotto in Lourdes-1862;* catholicpilgrims.com
366 *First Vatican Council;* Museo Renacimiento, Rome, Italy; Archivo Oronoz
367 Title page of *El Syllabus,* Bl. Pius IX; wikipedia.com
368 *Bl. Pius IX;* wikipedia.com
369 *Otto Bismarck;* Archivo Oronoz
371 (top) *Cartoon portraying British Imperialism;* wikipedia.com, public domain
371 (bottom) *David Livingstone;* David Livingstone Centre, Blantyre, Scotland
372 *Arriving at Manyema,* sketched by Henry Morton Stanley; *The Oxford Illustrated History of Christianity,* John McManners, Editor, 1990
374 *Pope Leo XIII,* Franz von Lenbach; Wallraf-Richartz Museum, Cologne, Germany

ART AND PHOTO CREDITS

375 (top) *Charles Darwin;* Private Collection, London, England; Archivo Oronoz
375 (bottom) *Karl Marx-1861;* public domain
377 *Pope Leo XIII;* Archivo Oronoz
378 *Pope Leo XIII;* wikipedia.com
380 *Pope Pius X;* Vatican Embassy, Madrid, Spain; Archivo Oronoz
381 *Pope Pius X;* wikipedia.com
382 (top) *Benedict XV;* wikipedia.com
382 (bottom) *First Meeting of League of Nations Assembly in Geneva-1920;* wikipedia.com
384 *St. Jacinta, St. Francisco, and Lucia Fatima;* public domain
385 *Pope Pius XI;* Vatican Embassy, Madrid, Spain; Archivo Oronoz
386 *St. Josemaría Escrivá,* Luis Mosquera; Opus Dei Prelature, Madrid, Spain; Archivo Oronoz
387 (left) *Eugenio Pacelli Leaving the Presidential Palace in Berlin-1929;* wikipedia.com
387 (right) *Cardinal Pacelli Signing the 1933 Concordat with Germany;* wikipedia.com
388 *Francisco Franco,* Genaro Lahuerta; Bank of Spain Art Collection, Madrid, Spain; Archivo Oronoz
389 *The Martyrdom of Blessed Miguel Pro, S.J.,* photograph; puffin.creighton.edu/jesuit/pro/index.html
390 (top) *Pope Pius XII;* Midwest Theological Forum Archives
390 (bottom) *Adolf Hitler at the Harvest Festival in Buckeberg,* Germany, 1938; Archivo Oronoz
391 (left) *St. Maximilian Kolbe,* Lorenzo Olaverri; Maximilian Kolbe Collection, Madrid, Spain; Archivo Oronoz
391 (right) *St. Teresa Benedicta (Edith Stein),* Lorenzo Olaverri; Maximilian Kolbe Collection, Madrid, Spain; Archivo Oronoz
392 (top) *Pope Pius XII;* Midwest Theological Forum Archives
392 (bottom) *Mao Tse-Tung Declares the Formation of The People's Republic of China-1949;* wikipedia.com
393 *Assumption of the Virgin,* Juan Martin Cabezalero; Prado Museum, Madrid, Spain
394 (left) *Pope John Paul II at the Wailing Wall;* from *Witness to Hope: The Life of Karol Wojtyla, Pope John Paul II* (2002); film by Judith Hallet, produced by Catherine Wyler
394 (right) *Prayer placed by Pope John Paul II at the Wailing Wall;* from *Witness to Hope: The Life of Karol Wojtyla, Pope John Paul II* (2002); film by Judith Hallet, produced by Catherine Wyler
395 *Arthur Wellesley, 1st Duke of Wellington with Sir Robert Peel,* Franz Xavier Winterhalter; Private Collection
396 *The Basilica at Lourdes,* France; Archivo Oronoz

Chapter 9

399 *Second Vatican Council;* St. Peter's Basilica, Vatican; Archivo Oronoz
401 *Pope John XXIII Signing Pacem in Terris;* wikipedia.com
402 *Pope John XXIII;* Venice, Italy; Archivo Oronoz
403 *Pope Paul VI Opening the Second Vatican Council;* St. Peter's Basilica, Vatican; Archivo Oronoz
405 *Pope Paul VI Celebrating Mass;* Archivo Oronoz
406 *Pope Paul VI and Patriarch Athenagoras I;* Archivo Oronoz
407 *Pope John Paul I;* from *Chronicle of the Popes,* published by Thames and Hudsen (197)
408 *Fr. Karol Wojtyla on a kayaking retreat in Poland;* from *Witness to Hope: The Life of Karol Wojtyla, Pope John Paul II* (2002); film by Judith Hallet, produced by Catherine Wyler
409 *Pope John Paul II;* Midwest Theological Forum Archives
410 *Pope Benedict XVI;* L'Osservatore Romano, Vatican City, wikipedia.com
411 *Pope John Paul II Visits with Mehmet Ali Agca in Prison-1983;* wikipedia.com
411a *Mother Marianne Cope-1883;* wikipedia.com
412 *Crucifixion,* Nicolas Tournier; Louvre, Paris, France
413 *St. Kateri Tekakwitha,* Fr. Claude Chauchetiere; Saint Francis Xavier Mission, Kahnawake, Quebec
414 *Commodore John Barry, USN,* Gilbert Stuart; White House, Washington D.C.
415 *Archbishop John Carroll,* Gilbert Stuart; Georgetown University, Washington, D.C.
416 (top left) *Bishop St. John Neumann;* wikipedia.com, public domain
416 (top right) *St. Elizabeth Seton Saying the Rosary;* Mother Seton School, Emmitsburg, Maryland website
416 (bottom) *Unveiling the Statue of Liberty,* Edward Moran; Public Collection
417 *A Family Visits the Lincoln Memorial in Washington, D.C.;* Archivo Oronoz
418 *Orestes Augustus Brownson,* George Peter Alexander Healy; National Portrait Gallery, Smithsonian Institution, Washington, D.C.
419 (left) *James Cardinal Gibbons and Teddy Roosevelt;* Maryland Historical Society, Baltimore, Maryland
419 (right) *James Cardinal Gibbons;* Antiquity Project, ironorchid.com
421 (top) *Al Smith, 1928;* wikipedia.com
421 (center) *Dorothy Day, 1933,* Vivian Cherry photographer
421 (bottom) *Bishop Fulton Sheen,* from his TV show *Life is Worth Living; How Sweet It Was,* published by Bonanza Books, New York (1966)
422 *President John F. Kennedy Meets with Pope Paul VI, 1963;* from *The Cultural Atlas of the World: Christian Church,* published by Stonehenge Press (1987)
424 *The Basilica of the National Shrine of the Assumption of the Blessed Virgin Mary* in Baltimore, Maryland; wikipedia.cpm
425 *Charles Carroll of Carrollton,* Chester Harding; National Portrait Gallery, Washington, D.C.
427 *Jacques Marquette and Louis Joliet Exploring the Mississippi River;* Library of Congress, Washington, D.C.
428 *Signing the Declaration of Independence,* John Trumbull; Yale University Art Gallery, New Haven, Connecticut

INDEX

INDEX

Baptism, 54-55, 118
    Baptism of Blood, 28
    definition of, 40
    effects of, 26-28
        communion with the Church, 307
        duties from Baptism, 307
        makes us members of Christ's Mystical Body, 141, 307
    Holy Spirit and, 8, 26
    in early Church, 26
    of adults, 26, 44
    of infants, 27-28, 41, 44
    religious consecration and, 142
    the Church and, 11
    Trinitarian formula, 28
Barbarians, 95-100
    conversion of, 106-107
Barnabas, St., Disciple, 14, 22
Bartholomew, St., Apostle, 14, 24
Basil I, 132
Basil II, 118-119
Basil the Great, St., 77, 100
Beatitudes, 6
Beauty
    art and, 142, 238
Bec, 153
Becket, St. Thomas à, 156-157
Bede the Venerable, St., 113
Beirut, 78
Belcastro, 193
Believer(s)
    the Church and, 307
    unity of believers in Christ, 141, 237
Believing
    gift of, 307
Benedict, St., 100-102
    Rule of St. Benedict, 102, 148, 159, 178
Benedict of Aniane, St., 149
Benedict VIII, 150
Benedict XV
    appeal to Our Lady for world peace (1917), 384
    Our Lady responds (Fatima, 1917), 384
Benedict XVI, 410-411b
    Resignation, 411b
Benevolence
    God's plan of loving goodness, 350
Bernadette, St., Soubirous, 365
Bernard of Clairvaux, St., 160-161, 169, 178, 364
Berno, St., Abbot of Cluny, 148
Bertha, 112
Bessette, St. Andre. See Andre Bessette
Bethlehem, 4, 70
Bible. See Sacred Scripture
Bishop(s). See Episcopacy
Black Sea, 119-120
Blood
    and water as symbols of Christ's Church, 43
    Baptism of Blood, 28
Bobbio, 110
Body of Christ, divisions between the members of, 237
Bohemia, 117, 160, 361
Boleslaus I, 117
Bologna, 187
    University of, 186-187
Boni viri (good men) and the Inquisition, 174-175, 178
Boniface, St., 114-115, 126, 137
Book of Kells, 7
Boris I, 133

Bosporus Straits, 119-120, 166
Bremen, 171
Britain, 55, 82, 108
Brother(s)
    in the Lord, 141, 307
Bruno, St., 160-161
Buddha, 65
Bulgaria, 132-133
Burgundians, 97
Burgundy, 107
Burial and catacombs, 30
Byzantine Christianity, 120-121
Byzantine Empire, 84, 118-122, 124-126, 128, 133, 166
Byzantium, 23, 33, 84, 118,
    See also Constantinople

C

Cabrini, St. Frances Xavier (Mother), 420
Cæcilian, 81
Caesarea, 17-18, 20
Caesaropapism, 87, 121, 130, 137
Caligula, Roman Emperor (AD 37-41), 47, 50
Call, God's
    and consecrated virgins and widows, 142
Callixtus, St., 30
Calvin, John, 249-251
    belief in the Bible as the only source of revelation, 249
    his belief in Predestination defined, 250
    his belief that human nature is totally corrupted, rotten and vicious, 249
    his influence on the French Huguenots, 251
    his influence on the Puritans in England, 251
    his teachings as a basis for John Knox's creation of the Presbyterian Church, 251
    his theocracy in Geneva, 250
    rejection of human freedom, 249
    rejection that man can merit through good works, 249
Canon law, 121, 127, 137, 154, 156, 184, 187-188, 244
Canon of Scripture
    and the Apocrypha, 72
    and the Didache, 37
    established by the Church, 7, 29, 34-35, 64
Canossa, 154-155
Canterbury, 111-112, 137, 153, 156, 158
Capitalism, 171
    the Church's judgment on some aspects of, 398
Carolingian dynasty, 126-130, 145, 147, 151-152, 178
Carthage, 82, 121
Carthusians, 159-161
Catacomb(s), 29-30
    in Rome, 30
Catechesis
    and Christian initiation, 44
Catechism of the Catholic Church, 11
Catechumenate, 26
    in early Church, 26
Catechumens, 26-27, 40
Catherine of Siena, St., 70, 210-212
    declared Doctor of the Church, 211, 270
    dedicated herself to the service of the poor and the sick, 211
    Dialogue, 211
    her body discovered incorruptible, 211
    mystical experiences and conversations with Christ, 210-211
    mystical marriage, 210

only the Blessed Sacrament for food, 211
    visions of hell, purgatory and heaven, 211
Catholic Church in the United States.
    See Church in the United States, Catholic
Catholic Reformation, 259, 290
Catholicity
    preaching the Gospel and, 141, 307
Celestine I, St., 79, 82, 109
Celestius, 82
Celts, 96, 111-112
    conversion of, 108-111
Chalons, Battle of, 97
Chaminade, Bl. William Joseph, 334
Charism
    of Consecrated Life, 142
    of infallibility, 43-44, 181
Charity, 18
    and martyrdom, 38
    charity as witness and service
        religious life and, 142
        the Church as the community of, 237, 307
        towards neighbor, 238, 308
Charlemagne, 127-130, 132-133, 144, 151, 153, 177
Charles Martel, 105, 126
Chartreuse, 160-161
Children's Crusade (1212), 166
China, 97, 168
Christ. See Jesus Christ
Christian Humanism, 218-219, 231
Christian(s)
    and society, 26
    early Christians, 26
        beliefs and practices of, 26-29, 32-35
        misunderstood by Romans, 49
Christianity
    foundational principles present at birth of Jesus, 4
Chrysostom, St. John. See John Chrysostom, St.
Church, 8, 11
    after fall of Rome, 94-95, 98, 100
    and Canon of Scripture, 7
    and state, 157, 159, 172
        caesaropapism, 87, 137
        lay investiture controversy. See Lay Investiture
    and the Holy Spirit, 2-4, 8, 11, 13, 62
    and the Niceno-Constantinopolitan Creed, 76
    Apostles as pillars of the Church, 14
    as Bride of Christ, 13
    as the Mystical Body of Christ, 11, 13, 18
    Attributes of the Church, 11, 13, 43
        Apostolic, 13
        Catholic, 13
            diversity in unity, 141, 307
            mission as a requirement of the Church's Catholicity, 141, 307
            relations with churches that are not, 307
        Holy, 13
        One, 13
            bonds of unity, 237
            seeking unity by the unity already given, 237
            wounds to unity, 141, 237
    Birth of the Church at Pentecost, 8-9
        definition of, 11, 40
        exists for Christ, 2
        founded by Christ, 2-3
        growth of, 2, 17-18, 22, 26
        make-up of the Church
            religious and consecrated life, 142
    "Catholic Church" first used, 51

INDEX

INDEX

INDEX

INDEX

INDEX

INDEX

INDEX

INDEX

INDEX

INDEX

State, political
    and personal freedom, 398
    and the early Church, 56, 85-86
    caesaropapism, 87
    in the Middle Ages, 172
    society of law, 308
Stein, Edith. See Teresa Benedicta of the Cross, St.
Stephen II, 126
Stephen X, 134
Stigmata, 197, 233
    definition of, 197, 233
Stoicism, 54
Submission, man's
    refusal to submit to the Supreme Pontiff (schism), 91, 237
Subsidiarity, 398
Substance (nature, essence)
    the Son, consubstantial with the Father, 91
Summa Theologiæ, 190
Superstition, 123
Supreme Pontiff, 13, 33, 67, 136
    [See individual name for specific Pope]
    infallibility of, 43, 81, 181
    offices, power, and authority of, 157
        Dictatus Papæ, 154
        historical evidence for, 33
    role of Supreme Pontiff in ecumenical councils, 67
    titles of
        bishop of Rome, 33
        Servus servorum Dei, 103, 138
        Vicar of Christ, 33, 41, 158, 179
        Vicar of St. Peter, 157
Switzerland, 97
    conversion of, 110
Syllabus of Errors, 366
    Bl. Pius IX's Encyclical, 366-367
    what it condemned, 366-367
Sylvester I, St., 75
Sylvester II, 151
Symbols of faith, 32
Synod of Rome (382), 34
Synod(s). See Councils, Local
Syria, 55, 196

T

Tacitus, Cornelius, 48, 219
Tancred, 163
Tartars, 171
Tekakwitha, St. Kateri. See Kateri Tekakwitha
Temple (in Jerusalem), 4
    and the Dome of the Rock, 104
Ten Commandments, 6
Teresa Benedicta of the Cross, St., (Edith Stein), 391
Teresa of Avila, St., 69
    The Way of Perfection, Foundations, 270
Tertullian, 27-28, 32, 35-37, 44, 65, 398
Teutonic Knights, 168, 171
Thagaste, 82-83
Thames River, 112
The Genius of Christianity (1802), 326
Theodelinda, 103
Theodora (empress wife of Justinian I), 122
Theodora (empress wife of Theophilus), 125
Theodore I, 81
Theodore Guerin, St., 411a
Theodoric, 95-96
Theodosius I (the Great), 70, 85-86, 119
Theodosius II, 78-79, 97, 119

Theology
    and St. Paul, 18
Theophilus, 125
Therese of Lisieux, St., 69
Thessalonica, 70, 115-116
Thirty Years War (1619-1648), 286-287
    final "War of Religion", 286
    Peace of Augsburg (1555), 287
Thomas Aquinas, St., 62, 82-83
Thomas, St., Apostle, 14, 25
Thuringia, 248
Titles and attributes of God. See God
Toulouse, 175
Tours
    Battle of (732), 105, 126
Tradition, 6, See Sacred Tradition
Traditor, meaning of, 81
Trajan, 50-52
    Trajan's Rescript (112), 50-51, 89
Translations of Scripture, 70-71
Trier, Germany, 70
Truth, 26
    as the way of salvation, 141
    neglect and rejection of the revealed, 91, 238
    seeking, 189-191, 308
    the Church's Magisterium in the service of, 43, 181
    truth, beauty, and sacred art, 142, 238
Turks, 164-167, 171

U

Ukraine, 23
    conversion of, 117-118
Umbria, 194
Uniate Catholic Church, 131
United States Conference of Catholic Bishops, 422
    created (1991), 422
Unity
    of the Church, 237-238
    union of Christians, 237-238
Universities, 184, 186, 189
    origin and rise of, 186-189
        academic coursework, 188
Urban II, Bl., 148, 150, 160, 162-163
    speech at Clermont (1095), 162

V

Valens, 78
Valentinian II, 70
Valentinian III, 80
Valerian, 57
Values
    hierarchy of values
    and economic activity, 398
    and social institutions, 430
    science, technology, and moral values, 236-238
Vandals, 94, 97, 121
Venerable
    meaning of title, 113
Veneration
    of icons, 124-125
    of relics, 215, 240, 251, 265
    of saints, 251, 265, 296
Verdun, Treaty of (843), 145, 179
Vespasian, Titus Flavius, 53
Vigilance in protecting the faith, 350
Vigilius, 122

Vikings, 118, 145, 152
    invasions of, 147-148
Virginity
    for the sake of the Kingdom of Heaven, 142
Visigoths, 95-96, 121
Vladimir, St., 117-118
Vocation
    of the laity, 307-308
Voltaire, 323
    considered Christianity foolish and absurd, 323
Vow
    definition of, 102, 138
Vulgate. See Sacred Scripture

W

War
    arms, 398
    duty to avoid, 308
    just, 182
Wars of Religion, 300
    Four Major Conflicts
        Revolt of the Low Countries (1559-1592), 272-274
        Huguenot Wars in France (1562-1593), 277
        Struggle for the British Isles (1561-1603), 281-282
        The Thirty Years War in Germany (1618-1648), 286-289
Wata. See Oak of Thor
Way(s)
    early Christians referred to the faith as "the Way", 46
    of God's plan, 11
Wessex, 114
Widow, 142
Wilfrid, St., 112
William I the Conqueror, 152-153, 163
William of Ockham, 205, 213-214
William (the Pious), Duke of Aquitaine (tenth century), 148
Willibrord, St., 114
Wisdom
    Hagia Sophia (Church of Holy Wisdom). See Hagia Sophia
Witness(es) to Christ
    martyrdom as the supreme, 38, 91-92
    of the Saints, 91
Word of God
    Christ as, 4
World
    and Christians, 26
    the Church "sent" into the whole, 308
Worms, 97
    Concordat of (1122), 156-157, 177
Worship
    of God (*latria*), 125
Wycliffe, John, 214, 234, 240, 244, 249

X

Xavier, St. Francis. See Francis Xavier, St.

Y

York, 112

Z

Zachary, St., 126
Zebedee, 14
    sons of, 23, 25